SIMS' SYMPTOMS IN THE MIND

Commissioning Editor: Alison Taylor
Development Editor: Clive Hewat
Project Manager: Jess Thompson
Design Direction: Erik Bigland
Illustration Manager: Merlyn Harvey
Illustrator: David Graham

SIMS' SYMPTOMS IN THE MIND

An Introduction to Descriptive Psychopathology

Femi Oyebode, MBBS MD PhD FRC Psych
Professor and Head of Department of Psychiatry,
University of Birmingham;
Consultant Psychiatrist,
Queen Elizabeth Psychiatric Hospital,
Birmingham, UK

FOURTH EDITION

SAUNDERS
ELSEVIER

EDINBURGH LONDON NEW YORK OXFORD PHILADELPHIA ST LOUIS SYDNEY
TORONTO 2008

SAUNDERS
ELSEVIER

Cover art
'Maison, Arbre et Personnage' – 1917/22
Anton Muller-Heinrich 1869–1930
With the kind permission of Kunstmuseum Bern, Switzerland.

First edition 1988
Second edition 1995
Third edition 2005
Fourth edition 2008

ISBN 978-0-7020-2885-4

British Library Cataloguing in Publication Data
A catalogue record for this book is available from the British Library

Library of Congress Cataloging in Publication Data
A catalog record for this book is available from the Library of Congress

Note
Neither the Publisher nor the Author assumes any responsibility for any loss or injury and/or damage to persons or property arising out of or related to any use of the material contained in this book. It is the responsibility of the treating practitioner, relying on independent expertise and knowledge of the patient, to determine the best treatment and method of application for the patient.

The Publisher

Printed in China

CONTENTS

This is dedicated to my late father, Dr Charles Sims, who, more than anyone else, taught me to be observant

Andrew Sims

For my father, Jonathan Akinyemi Oyebode (1918–1971)

Femi Oyebode

PREFACE TO THE FIRST EDITION

'If the word mind means anything, it means that which feels' (John Stuart Mill, 1811). That is the sense in which this book investigates the mind and its disturbances – emphasizing subjective experience and its description by the sufferer and the behaviour that results. The title *Symptoms or Signes in the Mind* is 'Partition 1, Section 3, Member 1, Subsection 2' of Robert Burton's *Anatomy of Melancholy* (1621). Burton claimed that one can dissect and display the essential elements of 'melancholy'. This is what I have attempted in this account of psychopathology in order to learn about them for subsequent research and treatment.

This book is aimed specifically at the recruit to psychiatry in his or her first year of training in the specialty. Such a person will have received some teaching in psychiatry as a medical undergraduate and some experience in dealing with those with emotional disturbance or personality difficulties in their medical practice since qualification, but is unlikely to have experience of the vast range of symptoms that patients present, nor is it likely he or she will have acquired a system for structuring abnormal subjective phenomena. I hope others, both in psychiatry and in related disciplines, will also find this book helpful; there has been a healthy revival of interest in descriptive psychopathology in the last few years, especially in British psychiatry. This has resulted in no small part from the enormous encouragement to high standards in the training of psychiatrists consequent upon the inception of the Royal College of Psychiatrists. Changes in the examination for membership of the College further emphasized the importance of clinical training in psychiatry and hence the need for a thorough grasp of descriptive psychopathology.

Psychopathology is a very complicated subject and the texts have not always been remarkable for their lucidity and conciseness. Writing about mental illness is a forlorn task, a matter of trying to describe the ultimately indescribable. Having had the temerity to attempt it, I have gone further and tried occasionally to represent the abstract visually and in tabular form. My apologies to all those who are offended by this, but I hope that by over-simplifying I may help some to start looking at mental illness in a more observant and comprehending way. This is not offered as a textbook of psychiatry; the classical syndromes are not usually dealt with in a simple section but scattered, according to the different elements of their psychopathology, in many chapters. This book took some fifteen years to write; the first few years were spent collecting information to fill it up and the latter few discarding it to slim it down.

For the sake of clarity some arbitrary lines have had to be drawn. The material of many chapters is not discrete but overlaps. There are still enormous areas of uncertainty in psychopathology; I hope these have not been spuriously simplified and that my own continuing quest for understanding is apparent. To this end I invite the reader to comment on any specific topics so that we (he, she, I) can continue to work together towards a more authoritative subsequent edition.

In the words of the Oxford English Dictionary the word *he* is used 'of things not sexually distinguished ... any man, any one, a person'. This convention has been used throughout; it reads more easily than interminable 'he or she' or genderless 'theys'.

There are very many people who have helped me in preparation and without whom this would never have appeared; they are not responsible for my errors. Dr Ruth Sims has helped throughout. I am very grateful for discussion with and useful suggestion from Professor Robert Bluglass; Mrs Marian Greenwood; Dr Peter McKenna; Professors Clive Mellor, Richard Mindham and Kenneth Rawnsley; Drs Keith Rix, Paula Salmons, Charles Sims and Philip Snaith; Professor Sir William Trethowan; and Dr Alfred White.

I acknowledge the help of successive groups of Leeds and Birmingham postgraduate and undergraduate students who have asked difficult questions and also perused my drafts with admirable astringency. Mrs Monika O'Connor, and at an earlier stage Mrs Barbara Rudge, have been endlessly patient in preparing repeated drafts. I am grateful to the Medical Illustration Department at St James's University Hospital, Leeds, for all their work over the years, some of which is included. The libraries of the Universities of Leeds and Birmingham and especially the staff at St James's Hospital library have been extremely helpful at all stages of preparation.

I suppose I should thank British Rail, who have been my hosts while much of this has been written, and who, by their relaxed attitude to punctuality, have given me much more time for work than I could have anticipated.

Many patients over the years have taken the trouble to explain to me exactly how they feel; they have taught me what I know, and also that I know little. I acknowledge my indebtedness to them and I hope that this work will partly repay my debt by improving understanding of their successors. Perhaps the chief difference between this book and others on this topic that have gone before is that it aims to put descriptive psychopathology in its social, psychological and biological contexts.

Andrew Sims

PREFACE TO THE FOURTH EDITION

Sims' Symptoms in the Mind has, since its first publication in 1988, become established as the leading introductory textbook on clinical psychopathology. In this new edition I have retained the original structure of the book but made some changes. There are shifts in emphasis and new material in a number of chapters. Easily recognizable modifications are evident in the chapters on disturbance of memory, disorder of time, pathology of perception, disorder of speech and language, affect and emotional disorders, and disorders of volition and execution. In the main these have been prompted by a desire to incorporate advances from neuropsychology and cognitive neuroscience. In some cases I have provided novel classifications of the abnormalities under consideration. Additional pathological phenomena are described in various chapters. Many of these phenomena are not new but rediscovered or imported from neurology. These phenomena include such experiences as palinopsia, palinaptia, teleopsia, pelopsia, akinetopsia, zëitraffer phenomenon, exosomesthesia and many others. One of the distinctive features of *Sims' Symptoms in the Mind* has been its use of figures, tables and illustrative case examples. I have kept to this and added boxes and additional case examples from the classical literature, autobiographical narratives and fiction.

I have been anxious not to do any harm to Professor Sims' work. I can only hope that the result of my interventions repays his trust in my judgement. I am indebted to many more people than I can list. Professor Tolani Asuni inspired my interest in psychiatry; Dr Frieda Schoenberg introduced me to psychopathology; and I have been influenced by Drs Ken Davison, Alan Kerr, Hamish McClelland, Kurt Schapira and Alan Stephens and by Professor Ian Brockington. The Birmingham Philosophy Group has been meeting monthly since 1992. Its members have contributed to my thinking about psychiatric phenomena. I am therefore grateful to Drs Man Cheung Chung, Lenia Constantine, Tom Harrison, Anupama Iyer, Simon O'Loughlin, Michael Radford and Sandy Robertson. Dr Jan Oyebode ensured that the contributions of psychologists and the many insights of neuropsychology and cognitive neuroscience were properly integrated into the potentially narrow view of a psychiatrist. Finally, without the patients who experience and endure these abnormal phenomena, and the students and psychiatric trainees who ask awkward questions and out of curiosity enquire into the nature of these phenomena, this book would definitely be the poorer.

Femi Oyebode
2008

PREFACE TO THE FOURTH EDITION

Section One

CONCEPTS AND METHOD

Fundamental Concepts of Descriptive Psychopathology

1

> “How the mind should be conceived for the purposes of psychopathology, what its faculties, functions or elements are (if there are any), how these can be distinguished, and how mental disorders can be comprehended by an application of these concepts are philosophical questions. *Manfred Spitzer (1990)*

Psychiatry is that branch of medicine which deals with morbid psychological experiences. By definition, in the medical conditions that are central to psychiatric practice psychological phenomena are important as causes, symptoms and observable clinical signs and also as therapeutic agents. The scope of psychiatry can be said to include minor emotional disturbances that are understandable reactions to environmental or psychosocial stress; profound psychological change that is unheralded by significant or meaningful stress; disturbances of personality that have a pervasive influence on behaviour such that the person or others suffer; psychological changes that are directly the consequences of demonstrable organic brain change; and psychological and behavioural consequences of the use of substances such as alcohol, cannabis, cocaine or heroin (Slater and Roth, 1977). In order to describe, delineate and differentiate these conditions, the morbid psychological phenomena that constitute the subjective experience of patients need to be carefully assessed, elicited and recorded. This is the territory of descriptive psychopathology.

It can be said that descriptive psychopathology is the fundamental professional skill of the psychiatrist; it is, possibly, the only diagnostic skill unique to the psychiatrist. It is considerably more than just carrying out a clinical interview of a patient, or even listening to the patient, although it necessarily involves both of these. Its accurate application involves the deployment of *empathy* and *understanding*. Of course, for the rational practice of psychiatry there is a need for knowledge of the basic neurosciences; appropriate factual knowledge of psychology, sociology and social anthropology is also required. With these, there is a need for a comprehensive working knowledge of general medicine, especially neurology and endocrinology. This could be considered to be the minimum knowledge base essential for practising psychiatry. However, it is descriptive psychopathology that provides the foundation of clinical psychiatric practice. The subjective phenomena that are revealed during the clinical assessment, coupled with observable behaviours, ultimately determine the clinical judgements that influence treatment and management decisions.

WHAT IS PSYCHOPATHOLOGY?

Psychopathology is the systematic study of abnormal experience, cognition and behaviour – the study of the products of a disordered mind. It includes the *explanatory psychopathologies*, in which there are assumed explanations according to theoretical constructs (for example on a cognitive, behavioural, psychodynamic or existential basis and so on), and *descriptive psychopathology*, which is the precise description and categorization of abnormal experiences as recounted by the patient and observed in his behaviour (Figure 1.1).

Berrios (1996) has described two formulations of descriptive psychopathology in the nineteenth century. Psychologists and brain scientists, predominantly, tended to regard morbid phenomena as quantitative variations on normal mental functions – the *continuity* view. Psychiatrists, working directly with the mentally ill (alienists), considered that some symptoms were too bizarre to have a counterpart in normal behaviour – the *discontinuity* view. Both formulations have contributed to the current state of descriptive psychopathology. Undoubtedly, the quality of empathy shown by the doctor contributes to an understanding of the patient, but there is a limit, for example with psychotic phenomena in which the patient's notions and behaviour may no longer be understandable using empathy and patient and doctor may be mutually alienated.

There are, therefore, two distinct parts to descriptive psychopathology: the *empathic assessment of subjective experience* and the *observation of behaviour*. *Empathy*, as a psychiatric term, means literally 'feeling oneself into'. It is sometimes used by those in the caring professions to describe a warm, soft feeling for other people's adversities. It is, of course, commendable to feel this way for our patients' difficulties, but that is not empathy but rather sympathy, that is, 'feeling with'. It is somewhat surprising to know that in modern Greek empathy means 'keeping your feelings inside', that is, bearing a grudge. This is not at all the way the term is used in psychiatry!

In descriptive psychopathology, the concept of empathy is like a clinical instrument that needs to be used with skill to measure another person's internal subjective state using the observer's own capacity for emotional and cognitive experience as a yardstick. Empathy is achieved by precise, insightful, persistent and knowledgeable questioning until the doctor is able to give an account of the patient's subjective experience that the patient recognizes as his own. If the doctor's account of the patient's internal experience is not recognized by the patient as his own, then the questioning must continue until the internal experience is recognizably described. Throughout the process, success depends on the capacity of the doctor as a human being to experience something like the internal

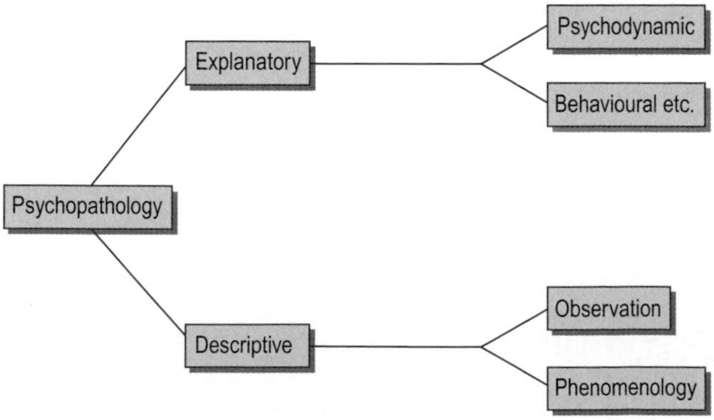

Figure 1.1 The psychopathologies.

experience of the other person, the patient; it is not an assessment that could be carried out by a microphone and computer. It depends absolutely on the shared capacity of both doctor and patient for human experience and feeling. It is empathy that allows the doctor to come to *understand* the patient's experiences. In this sense, it is empathy that makes it possible for us to know what it is like for another person, another subject of experience, to be in a particular mental state. When empathy fails to render a patient's subjective experience understandable, we can then talk about that experience as being *ununderstandable*. In other words, the farthest reaches of our intuitive comprehension of a phenomenon has been exceeded.

Accurate observation of behaviour is the other component of descriptive psychopathology. Subjective human experience becomes available to us for examination and exploration through verbal communication but also through meaningful gestures, bodily stance, behaviour and actions. Observation of the objective expression of subjective experience, that is, of behaviour, is extremely important and is a much more useful exercise than simply counting symptoms; the slavish use of a symptom checklist for their presence or absence is often an obstacle to genuine clinical observation. The objectivity that is facilitated by checklists is crucial, but there is a need also for the skilled observation of behaviour.

PHENOMENOLOGY AND PSYCHOPATHOLOGY

Psychopathology is concerned with abnormal experience, cognition and behaviour. *Descriptive psychopathology* avoids theoretical explanations for psychological events. It describes and categorizes the abnormal experience as recounted by the patient and observed in his behaviour. In its historical context, Berrios (1984) defines it as a cognitive system constituted by terms, assumptions and rules for its application, 'the identification of classes of abnormal mental acts'. *Phenomenology* is the study of events, either psychological or physical, without embellishing those events with explanation of cause or function. As used in psychiatry, phenomenology involves the observation and categorization of abnormal psychological events, the internal experiences of the patient and his consequent behaviour. An attempt is made to observe and understand the psychological event or phenomenon so that the observer can, as far as possible, know for himself what the patient's experience must feel like.

How can one use the word *observer* about someone else's internal experience? This is where the process of *empathy* becomes relevant. Descriptive psychopathology therefore includes subjective aspects (phenomenology) and objective aspects (description of behaviour). It is concerned with the variety of human experience, but it is deliberately limited in its scope to what is clinically relevant, for example it can say nothing about the religious validity of what James (1902) has called 'saintliness'.

How does this work in practice? Mrs Jenkins complains that she is unhappy. It is the business of *descriptive psychopathology* both to elicit her thoughts and actions without trying to explain them and to observe and describe her behaviour – the listless sagging of her shoulders, the tense gripping and wringing of her hands. *Phenomenology* demands a very precise description of exactly how she feels inside herself: 'that horrible feeling of not really existing' and 'not being able to feel any emotion'.

Some psychiatrists have held phenomenology in derision as archaic, hair-splitting or hare-chasing pedantry, but the diagnostic evaluation of symptoms is a task that the psychiatrist omits at his own and his patient's peril. Studying phenomenology whets diagnostic tools, sharpens clinical acumen and improves communication with the patient. The patient and his complaints deserve our scrupulous attention. If 'the proper study of mankind is man', the proper study of his mental illness starts with the description of how he thinks and feels inside – 'chaos of thought and passion, all confused' (Pope, 1688–1744).

A cavalier neglect of phenomenology can have serious repercussions for care of the patient. Eight people were sent separately to twelve admission units in American mental hospitals complaining of hearing these words said aloud: 'empty', 'hollow' and 'thud' (Rosenhan, 1973). In all cases save one, they were diagnosed as suffering from schizophrenia. They produced no further psychiatric symptoms after admission to hospital but acted as normally as they could, answering questions truthfully except to conceal their name and occupation. The ethics and good sense of the experiment can certainly be questioned, but what comes out clearly is not that psychiatrists should refrain from making a diagnosis but that their diagnosis should be made on a sound psychopathological basis. Neither Rosenhan, nor his colleagues, nor the admitting psychiatrists gave any information as to what symptoms could reasonably be required for making a diagnosis of schizophrenia; this requires a method based on psychopathology (Wing, 1978). With adequate use of phenomenological psychopathology, this failure of diagnosis would not have occurred.

Jaspers (1959) wrote, 'Phenomenology, though one of the foundation stones of psychopathology, is still very crude'. One of the great problems in using this method is the muddled nature of terminology. Almost identical ideas may be assigned different names by people from different theoretical backgrounds, for example the plethora of descriptions of how a person may conceptualize himself: self-image, cathexis, body awareness and so on.

There is considerable confusion over the meaning of the term *phenomenology*. Berrios (1992) has described four meanings in psychiatry.

> " P1 refers to its commonest clinical usage as a mere synonym for 'signs and symptoms' (as in 'phenomenological psychopathology'; this is a bastardized usage, and hence conceptually uninteresting. P2 refers to a pseudo-technical sense often used in dictionaries and which achieves spurious unity of meaning by simply cataloguing successive usages in chronological order; this approach is misleading in that it suggests false evolutionary lines and begs important questions relating to history of phenomenology. P3 refers to the idiosyncratic usage started by Karl Jaspers who dedicated his early clinical writings to the description of mental states in a manner which (according to him) was empathic and theoretically neutral. Finally, P4 refers to a complex philosophical system started by Edmund Husserl and continued by writers collectively named the 'Phenomenological Movement'. *(p. 304)*

Of these meanings, this chapter, and indeed this book, will concentrate entirely on the Jaspersian meaning of phenomenology, P3 of Berrios. Jaspers defines phenomenology perhaps 30 to 40 times in his writings in subtly different ways but always implying the *study of subjective experience*. Walker (1988, 1993a, b, 1994) has argued, very elegantly, that even though Jaspers himself thought that he had been influenced by Husserl and his system of phenomenology this was not in fact so, and his psychopathology owed more to Kantian concepts such as form and content. Walker (1995a, b) considers that Jaspers radically misconstrued Husserl's phenomenology. This view has been rebutted by others (Wiggins *et al.*, 1992). The implication for what follows in this chapter, and in the rest of the book, is that the concept of phenomenology used here comes directly from Jaspers and was probably influenced by both Kant and Husserl.

Phenomenology, the *empathic* method for the eliciting of symptoms, cannot be learned from a book. Patients are the best teachers, but it is necessary to know what one is looking for – the practical, clinical aspects in which the patient describes himself, his feelings and his world. The doctor tries to unravel the nature of the sufferer's experience, to understand it well enough and to feel it so poignantly that the account of his findings evokes recognition from the patient. The method of phenomenology in psychiatry is entirely subjugated to its single purpose of rendering the patient's experience *understandable* (this is a technical word in phenomenology and is described in more detail on p. 14–16; however, it incorporates the capacity for putting oneself in the patient's place) so that classification and rational therapy may proceed.

> “ The barrier to conspicuous advance in psychiatry has not been stinginess and prejudice on the part of those who decide whether a research project submitted to them should live or die; nor has it been lack of ability among those who are engaged in psychiatric research: it lies in the inherent toughness of the problems. *(Lewis, 1963: 1556)*

It is not the assimilation of abstruse facts or the accumulation of foreign eponyms that is most difficult in phenomenology, although either of these may be hard: it is the comprehension of a method of investigation and the ability to use new concepts. In an attempt to avoid the obscure and obvious, in the rest of this chapter some of these concepts are described in contrasted pairs.

NORMAL HEALTH

Some words are used very commonly but inconsistently, so, although we know what we mean by them, we are unable to assume that other people are using them in the same way. Two such words are *normal* and *healthy*. In a discussion of mental illness, they occur so frequently that they should be examined briefly before further excursion into psychopathology.

Health–illness

Psychopathology concerns itself with *illness of the mind*, but what is illness? This is a vast subject that has received discussion from philosophers, theologians, administrators and lawyers as well as from physicians. Doctors who spend most of their working time straddled between health and illness rarely ask this question and even less frequently attempt to answer it.

- The World Health Organization (1946) definition of health states, 'Health is a state of complete physical, mental and social well-being and not merely the absence of disease or infirmity'. If total well-being is required, perhaps virtually all of us are excluded.

- Illness may be thought of in physical terms as in Griesinger's (1845) dictum that mental diseases are diseases of the brain. Although this statement readily fits the 'organic' psychiatric states and can be broadened to encompass learning disability (mental retardation), there are problems in trying to include psychotic and neurotic disorders, the so-called functional disorders, within this compass, and personality disorders are particularly difficult to fit in.
- Similarly, diseases may be described in terms of *what doctors treat*. In defining this, Kräupl Taylor (1980) states, 'the diagnosis of patienthood has as its sufficient and necessary condition the experience of therapeutic concern by a person for himself and/or the arousal of therapeutic concern for him in his social environment'. *Mental illness* becomes, then, a term to describe the symptoms and condition of those people who are referred to a psychiatrist. This tautologous description of illness has some practical advantage, as it does not prevent therapeutic skills from being used over a wide spectrum of human problems. It does, however, have the disadvantage of allowing society to choose whom it will call mentally ill, and with a malignant social system the state may direct that those who are politically deviant should be deemed ill (Bloch and Reddaway, 1977).
- Illness may be considered as a statistical variation from the norm, carrying biological disadvantage. This concept was formulated by Scadding (1967) for physical illness and developed for psychiatric disease by Kendell (1975). Biological disadvantage implies reduced fecundity and/or a shortened life. This state of disadvantage becomes difficult to apply to modern man, as he has learned to control his environment and procreativity to such an extent that the very term *biological disadvantage* becomes arguable.
- Illness has legal implications. For instance, the circumstances that result in illness may merit compensation at law; if the behaviour arises from illness, this may mitigate punishment. Similarly, mental illness is a concept that can justify compulsory detention in hospital (Bluglass, 1983; Mental Health Act, 1983), and mentally ill offenders are dealt with by the law in a different way from other criminals (Bluglass and Bowden, 1990).

This distinction between normality and disease, health and illness, is by no means trivial.

> “A large part of medical ethics and much of the whole underpinning of current medical policy, private and public, are squarely based on the notion of disease and normality. Left to himself the physician (whether he realizes it or not) can do very well without a formal definition of disease... Unfortunately, the physician is not left alone to work his common sense. He is attacked from two angles: the predatory consumers and the pretentious advisors. *(Murphy, 1979)*

Normality–abnormality

The word *normal* is used correctly in at least four senses in the English language (Mowbray *et al.*, 1979). These are the *value* norm, the *statistical* norm, the *individual* norm and the *typological* norm. *Normal* is abused when it replaces unjustifiably the words *usual* or *usually*.

The *value* norm takes the ideal as its concept of normality. Thus the statement 'It is normal to have perfect teeth' is using normal in a value sense; in practice, most people have something wrong with their teeth.

The *statistical* norm is, of course, the preferred use the word retains in the scientific vocabulary; the abnormal is considered to be that which falls outside the average range. If a normal Englishman is 5 feet 8 inches tall, to be either 6 feet 2 inches or 5 feet 2 inches tall is equally abnormal statistically.

The *individual* norm is the consistent level of functioning that an individual maintains over time. Following brain damage, a person may experience a decline in intelligence that is certainly a deterioration from his previous individual level but may not represent any statistical abnormality from that of the general population (for example a decline in intelligence quotient from 125 to 105).

Typological abnormality is a necessary term to describe the situation in which a condition is regarded as normal in all the three meanings above and yet represents *abnormality*, perhaps even disease. The example given by Mowbray *et al.* is the infective condition of *pinta*. The mottling of the skin of this condition is highly prized by the South American Indians who 'suffer' from it, to the extent that 'non-sufferers' are excluded from the tribe. Thus, having the condition is normal in a value, statistical and individual sense, and yet it is pathological in the sense that it is the result of a spirochaetal skin infection. The pursuit of thinness by models and dancers in our society would be an everyday example.

Psychiatric sample–general population

While discussing health and normality, it is important to point out those dangerous generalizations that arise when the psychiatrist, often against her will, is thrust into the position of being the expert on the whole conduct of life. We cannot easily extrapolate from the abnormal to the normal or vice versa. Some normal psychological states, such as fear, may lie on a continuum with abnormal anxiety states, whereas the normal perception of the objective world by sight may be qualitatively different from abnormal visual experiences such as visual hallucinations. Because of her detailed knowledge of abnormal psychic processes and symptoms and their management, the psychiatrist is not necessarily also an expert on normal psychological processes or such diverse human tasks as bringing up children or providing a recipe for achieving a tranquil mind.

The sample of people seeing a psychiatrist is different in many respects from those consulting their family doctors with psychological symptoms, and this general practice population varies from the population at large (Goldberg and Huxley, 1980). While it is very necessary to concentrate on the individual and his symptoms, it is also useful to bear in mind the characteristics of the remainder of the population from which he comes. His behaviour and his understanding of the world have roots within his own individual psychopathology and also in the social milieu that is his usual context.

Having pointed out this difference, the similarities should be stressed. It is remarkable how constant is the psychopathological form in different parts of the world and in different cultures; this will become apparent with examples used from non-western societies in later chapters. It is also significant how constant is the form of symptoms over time. Beveridge (1997) gives a very clear account of schizophrenic abnormalities of language, delusions, hallucinations, disorders of mood and altered insight as evident in patients' letters from the Royal Edinburgh Asylum, 1873–1908. The fact that psychopathological form is relatively constant for different conditions over time and in different places is reassuring for its clinical use and validity.

Very often, one wants to argue from the particular to the general. On the basis of our experience with young patients with schizophrenia in a teaching hospital, we make assertions about *schizophrenia*. To be able to do this, we must know that the patients we have seen (our sample population) are representative of the target population (schizophrenia). We can make this claim only if our sample was randomly selected from all young persons suffering from schizophrenia, so that all such persons had a known, equal and greater than zero probability of getting into our sample. In practice, of course, this can never be so, and we must restrict our target population to a more limited group (the sample), and our claims for knowledge about them must be similarly restricted. The following axiom bears repeating: different populations have different characteristics.

The common–the esoteric

Descriptive psychopathology is sometimes in danger of indulging in the esoteric, with excessive interest in rare syndromes. To be of practical use, it needs to concentrate on the manifestations of abnormality that are shared by many patients.

- Observation of phenomena without preconceived theory is useful in reconciling different schools of psychopathology.
- The requirement of precise definition forms a basis for sound research. Rare syndromes have their value in learning psychopathological skills, but interest in them should not detract from the more important, if more mundane, application in day-to-day clinical practice.

UNDERSTANDING THE PATIENT'S SYMPTOMS

Understanding, in both an everyday and a phenomenological sense, cannot be complete unless the doctor has a detailed knowledge of the patient's background culture and specific information about his family and immediate environment. Neither can phenomenology concentrate solely on the individual isolated in a moment of time. It must be concerned with the person in a social setting; after all, a person's experience is largely determined by his interactions with others. It must also be concerned with the mental state and environment of the individual before the event of immediate interest and with what occurs afterwards.

The method of phenomenology facilitates communication: its use makes it easier for the doctor to understand his patient. The patient is also helped to have confidence in the doctor, because he realizes that his symptoms are understood and therefore accepted as 'real'. The precise description and evaluation of symptoms also helps communication between doctors.

Symptom–sign

Clinical medicine makes a clear distinction between signs and symptoms. The patient complains of *symptoms*: feeling agitated and uncomfortable in hot weather with hyperthyroidism. Physical *signs* are elicited on examination: soft goitre with audible bruit, loss of weight, rapid pulse and exophthalmos.

This distinction is not usually made with the phenomena of the mental state. The patient's description of an abnormal mental phenomenon is usually called a *symptom* whether he is complaining about something that distresses him or simply describing his mental experience, which appears pathological to an observer. In his account of his experiences, both these descriptions are therefore considered as symptoms. When these symptoms are aggregated, they may be regarded as the *signs* of whatever diagnosis is indicated.

Symptom, then, which is taken to include sign, may be either an item of complaint (for example a feeling of misery) or an item of phenomenological description that may represent no complaint from the patient (for example hearing quiet voices who discuss the patient with admiring awe). The feeling of misery may be a sign of depressive illness; the auditory hallucinations may be a sign of schizophrenia. There are also *behavioural* symptoms or signs, such as the patient who shouts at the ceiling; this may be regarded as a *sign* suggesting auditory hallucinosis. Schneider (1959) considers that a *symptom* in schizophrenia is a 'frequent and therefore a prominent characteristic of that state'. For a symptom to be used diagnostically, its occurrence must be typical of that condition and it must occur relatively frequently in this condition.

The method of empathy–the method of observation and experiment

The classical method in medicine of gaining information about the patient is from the history and by physical examination. The use of phenomenology in psychiatry is an extension of the *history* in that it amplifies the description of the present complaint to give more detailed information. It is also *examination* in that it reveals the mental state. It is not possible for me, the doctor, to observe my patient's hallucination or in any direct way to measure it. However, what I can do to comprehend him is to use those human characteristics I hold in common with him: my ability to perceive and to use language that I share with him. It is also important to be intellectually curious and genuinely interested in the inner life of another person. The inquiries that arise from this stance should aim to recreate for oneself or represent to oneself the subjective experiences of another person with the aim of understanding and making sense of them. The aim is thus to explore and test, through dialogue, the patient's subjective experience. I endeavour to create in my own mind what his experience must be like. I then test to see if I am correct in my reconstruction of his experience by asking him to affirm or deny my description. I also use my observation of his behaviour – the sad expression of his face or him thumping the desk with his fist – to reconstruct his experiences.

Listening and observing are crucial for understanding. Great care must be taken with asking questions. Doctors not infrequently identify symptoms incorrectly and come to the wrong diagnosis because they have asked leading questions with which the patient, through his submissiveness to the doctor's status and anxiety to cooperate, is only too willing to concur.

The method of empathy implies using the ability to feel oneself into the situation of the other person by proceeding through an organized series of questions, rephrasing and reiterating when necessary until one is quite sure of what is being described by the patient. The sequence might go as follows.

Question: 'You describe your thoughts changing; what happens to them?'
Answer: a description of how he has a recurring thought to kill people and this results from a pain in his stomach.

Question: (trying to isolate the elements of his experience) 'What is your thought of killing people like?' (obsession, delusion, fantasy, is likely to be acted on, etc.). 'Do you believe that your stomach affects your thinking?', 'Is this different from a person who knows that they become irritable when hungry?', 'In what way is it different from that?', What causes your pain in the stomach?'
Answer: he describes the details, which will include among irrelevant material the sort of information required for determining what symptoms are present.

Question: (the invitation for empathy) 'Am I right in thinking that you are describing an experience in which rays are causing pain in your stomach, and that your stomach in some way quite independent of yourself causes this thought, which frightens you, that you must kill somebody with a knife?' This is an account of the relevant symptoms that he has described in language he should be able to recognize as his own.
Answer: 'Yes' (we have then achieved our goal); 'No' (therefore I must try again to elicit the symptoms, experience them for myself and describe them back to him again).

To give examples of what this implies in practice: how do I, a clinician, decide whether an individual patient is depressed or not? This is not done by imitating a machine that might record units of vocal tone or of facial expression, adding up to a diagnosis of depression. For the clinical assessment, I go through the following process.

- I am capable of feeling unhappy, miserable and depressed and know what this feeling is like inside myself.
- If I were feeling as I observe the patient to be looking, speaking, acting and so on, I would be feeling miserable, depressed and unhappy.
- Therefore I assess the mood of the patient to be that of depression.

Of course, this mental process of diagnosis is not usually verbalized.

In another example, a patient says, 'the Martians are making me say swear words; it is not me doing it'. Empathic questioning reveals the false belief held by the patient that when swear words come from his mouth he believes that the cause is actually outside himself, 'Martians', rather than from inside himself. Questioning would include 'Do you actually *hear* the Martians? How do you know that it is Martians and no one else?' and so on.

A further, non-psychotic example would be a 20-year-old girl who has fainting attacks when she is criticized at work. The clinician has to place him or herself, even if a 55-year-old man from a different cultural background, into her position with a knowledge not only of her social history but also of the way that she, in the present, perceives that history; only then may the development of her symptoms become understandable. For instance, when it is known about her alcohol-abusing father, the rows he had with her epileptic mother, the very restricted cultural background that they experienced in an isolated fishing village and how her mother would have a fit when rows became intolerable, then one may begin to understand something of the development of the patient's own symptom. This is not achieved solely by explanation as an outside observer but by empathic understanding and the capacity for subjective experience by the doctor, who puts himself into, and therefore becomes, the 20-year-old girl for the process of the psychiatric interview.

It is the purpose of the phenomenological method therefore to (a) describe inner experiences, (b) order and classify them and (c) create a reliable terminology. Empathy is also invaluable therapeutically in establishing a relationship with the patient. Knowing that the doctor understands, and is even to some extent able to share his feelings, gives the patient confidence and a sense of relief. This empathy is also useful as a way of extending knowledge more generally in the field of psychiatry, as it allows a diagnostic terminology to be developed.

The undifferentiated whole–the significant part

Generally, classification of any sort requires detailed scanning of a large amount of material to identify the small, but significant, clue. This is true for phenomenology, when the significant part of psychological material for phenomenological evaluation may occur within a lengthy history and examination, in which most of the patient's conversation does not reveal any evidence of illness. One patient talked for several minutes and various things he said seemed rather strange, but I could not be sure that he was psychotic. However, when he said 'I shaved my eyebrows because they were ginger and when people saw ginger eyebrows they knew I was queer' (homosexual; in practice, he was not homosexual), it became obvious that he was probably harbouring abnormal beliefs, and this symptom was explored in more detail.

Using phenomenology diagnostically in the mental state may be compared with scanning the field of the microscope. One cannot expect to find the blood film meaningful by simply focusing and looking. One has to move the slide about and pick out a good example to demonstrate the point of interest from the undifferentiated mass. So the patient's conversation may have demonstrated many odd ideas and bizarre allusions, but perhaps only once can the interviewer obtain a description that is wholly satisfactory as being an example of a particular psychopathological symptom of diagnostic significance.

Random behaviour–meaning

A man cycling along a canal towpath met a large man walking in the opposite direction carrying a length of rubber pipe. The large man lifted his rubber pipe and thumped the cyclist on the shoulder, nearly knocking him into the canal. When he reached the next village, the cyclist reported the assault to the local policeman, who duly arrested his assailant. The police considered this behaviour senseless and therefore asked for a psychiatric opinion. When asked why he had assaulted the cyclist, the assailant said that he had had a pain in his stomach. He had heard a voice saying 'hit the man on the bicycle and the pain will go', and so he had done just that.

The casual layman commenting on 'mad' behaviour may say that it is meaningless, but because the meaning is not always apparent to an observer or even a victim, it does not negate its real, although psychotic, meaning to the patient. 'An action is on principle intentional' (Sartre, 1943).

It is important to try to reach the patient's subjective meaning and not just be satisfied that the response is abnormal. Phenomenological meaning is sometimes revealed in the type of response; for instance, when a schizophrenic patient was asked to explain the difference between a *wall* and a *fence* he answered 'you can see through a fence, but walls have ears' (Rawnsley, 1985, personal communication). In the same way that external events have causes that may be explained, so internal psychological events can be shown to emerge from each other meaningfully if the subject's internal state is understood empathically.

Understanding–explanation

Wilhelm Dilthey (1833–1911) argued that the natural sciences treat nature as objects and forces that can be explained through causal laws. In other words, the goal of such science is the formulation of general, universal laws, whereas the humanities, for example history and psychology, have the human subject as their focus and causal laws do not apply in these circumstances. For Dilthey, science 'explains' natural phenomenon by causal explanation. The humanities 'understand' human psychic phenomenon through the interpretation of the meaning structures revealed in texts or through dialogue with another person. This distinction between 'explanation' and 'understanding' continues to be influential in our thinking even today (Phillips, 2004). In science we come to know the object from outside, but in the humanities we are able to 'know' the subject from inside. We are able to represent to ourselves, if not 'know', the inner life of another person because we too have an inner life. We are able to understand the other person through the network of meanings associated with their behaviour. We start with the premise that behaviour means something; that is, it arises with internal consistency from psychological events. Wittgenstein (1953) has stated, 'We explain human behaviour by giving reasons not causes'.

Jaspers drew on Dilthey's formulation and contrasted understanding (*verstehen*) with explaining (*erklären*) and has shown how these terms may be used in both a 'static' and a 'genetic' sense. *Static* implies understanding or explaining the present situation from information that is available now; the *genetic* sense considers how the situation reached its present state by examining antecedents, the evolving process and emerging situation. This is represented in Table 1.1.

Understanding and explanation are both necessary parts of the psychiatric investigation. *Explanation* is concerned with accounting for events from a point of observation outside them, understanding from inside them. One understands another person's anger and its consequences; one explains the occurrence of snow in winter. Explanations also can be described as static or genetic. See Boxes 1.1 and 1.2.

Jaspers makes an important distinction between that which is *meaningful* and allows empathy and that which is ultimately *ununderstandable*, the essence of

Table 1.1 Diagram of understanding and explanation		
	Understanding	Explanation
Static	Phenomenological description	Observation through external sense perception
Genetic	Empathy established from what emerges	Cause and effect of scientific method

Box 1.1 Static and genetic understanding

Understanding is the perception of personal meaning of the patient's subjective experience.

- If we want to find meaning at a particular moment in time, the method of phenomenology is appropriate. The patient's subjective experience is dissected out, and a *static* picture is formed of what that thought or event meant to him at that particular time. No comment is made on how the event arose, and no prediction is made as to what will happen next. The meaning is simply extracted as a description of what the patient is experiencing and what this signifies to him now. A man feels angry: static understanding uses empathy to describe in detail exactly what it is like for him to feel angry. Have I, the examiner, experienced phenomena like these? Are they known to me through the experiences I have had in my lifetime?
- *Genetic* understanding, as opposed to static understanding, is concerned with a *process*. It is understood that when this man is insulted, he reacts with violence; when that woman hears voices commenting on her actions, she draws the curtains. For understanding the way that psychic events emerge one from another in the patient's experience, the therapist uses *empathy* as a method or a tool. He *feels himself into* the patient's situation. If that first event were to have occurred to him personally in the patient's total circumstances, the second event, which was the patient's reaction to it, might reasonably be expected to have followed. He understands the feelings he ascribed to the patient in terms of the action that results from these feelings. So if I were the patient with the same history, do I feel that I would have the same experiences and behave in the same way? An example would help to demonstrate the humanity of this approach and the universality of human experience: I must put myself into the shoes of another young woman, aged 19, also raised in an isolated fishing community, the eldest of eight siblings, who becomes stuporose during her second pregnancy. She is married to an alcoholic man aged 35, and her father is also alcoholic. I must understand how she dealt with her father's alcoholic behaviour as a child, what her pregnancy meant to her, how she regarded her mother's behaviour during her own pregnancies and so on.

> **Box 1.2** Static and genetic explanation
>
> - *Static* explanation is concerned with external sense perception, observing an event, for example 'I witnessed the 1999 eclipse in Plymouth'.
> - *Genetic* explanation consists of unravelling causal connections; it describes a chain of events and why they follow that sequence ('visual perception of the eclipse is the result of physiological changes in my retina, which in turn produce changes in my occipital cortex that ultimately cause me to see the eclipse').

the psychotic experience. There is, thus, a limit to understanding psychopathological phenomenon. Although one can empathize with the *content* of a patient's delusion and thereby understand how that content of the belief originated, the occurrence of the delusion itself is more recalcitrant to our empathy and understanding. It can be said that our understanding reaches its limit when it confronts the fact of the delusion itself. For that, we need to appeal to cognitive mechanisms or other natural science processes. We are in need of scientific explanation, not psychological understanding.

We can understand from a knowledge of the patient's background why, if her thinking is going to be disordered in form, the topic or content of that thinking should be concerned with persecution by the Nazis – perhaps because her parents escaped from Germany in 1937. But we can have no understanding of why she should believe something that is demonstrably false: that her persecutors are putting a tasteless fluid into her drinking water that makes her feel ill. The delusion itself, as psychopathological form, is *ununderstandable*. Meaningful connections, then, show the linkage between different psychological events by understanding how these events emerge one from another by a process of empathy.

Primary–secondary

Jaspers discusses the different meaning that can be given to the terms *primary* and *secondary* when applied to symptoms. The distinction may be in terms of understanding; what is primary is immediate and ultimate and therefore cannot be further reduced by understanding, for example hallucinations. What is secondary is what *emerges* from the primary in a way that can be understood, for example delusional elaboration arising from the healthy part of the psyche in response to hallucinations from the unhealthy part of the psyche. Again, the distinction between primary and secondary may be determined by the causal chain, in that what is primary is the proximate cause while what is secondary is the discernible distal effect: a cerebrovascular accident *causes* sensory aphasia and is therefore primary; the aphasia is the distal effect and is therefore secondary to the cerebrovascular accident.

These two distinct meanings of the term *primary* overlay the crucial distinction between meaningful connections and causal connections. For the avoidance of doubt in physics and chemistry, we make observations by experiment and then formulate causal connections and causal laws, whereas in psychopathology we experience another sort of connection wherein psychic events emerge out of one another in a way that can be understood – so-called *meaningful connections* (Robinson, 1984, personal communication).

THE ANALYSIS OF EXPERIENCE

What the patient considers important in giving his history of symptoms and causes of distress may not necessarily be identical to what the doctor or examiner regards as significant. The doctor may very well be trying to ascertain the psychopathological entities that are present, perhaps in order to make a diagnosis, while the patient is concerned to communicate the distress experienced, its intensity and the way it is perceived as a threat.

Form–content

Form and content are distinct in phenomenology. For Jaspers, 'form must be kept distinct from content which may change from time to time, e.g the fact of a hallucination is to be distinguished from its content, whether this is a man or a tree, threatening figures or peaceful landscapes. Perceptions, ideas, judgements, feelings, drives, self-awareness, are all forms of psychic phenomenon; they denote the particular mode of existence in which content is presented to us'. Thus, like warp and woof, form and content are essentially different but inextricably woven together. One way to think of *form* is to regard it as the sense modality in which a perception is presented to us or the cognitive domain in which a particular aspect of psychic life is experienced or enacted. The *form* of a psychic experience is the description of its structure in phenomenological terms, for example a delusion, or, as Berrios (1996) says, 'Form refers to those impersonal aspects of the mental symptoms that guarantee its stability in time and space; that is, its "constancy" elements'. Viewed in this way, *content* is the subjective colouring of the experience. The patient is concerned because he believes that people are stealing his money. His concern is that 'people are taking my money', not that 'I hold on unacceptable grounds a false belief that people are taking my money'. He is concerned about the content. Clearly, form and content are both important but in different contexts. The patient is concerned only with the content: 'that I am pursued by ten thousand hockey sticks'. The doctor is concerned with both form and content, but as a phenomenologist only with form, in this case a false belief of being pursued. As far as form is concerned, the hockey sticks are irrelevant. The patient finds the doctor's interest in form unintelligible and a distraction from what he regards as important, and he often demonstrates his irritation.

In Chapter 7, a patient is described who said, 'When I turn the tap on, I hear a voice whispering in the water pipe, "She's on her way to the moon. Let's hope she has a soft landing"'. The *form* of this experience is what demands the attention of the phenomenologist and is useful diagnostically. She is describing a *perception*; it is an auditory perception and a false or disordered auditory perception. It has the characteristics of a hallucination, and specifically of a *functional* hallucination. This is the form. While the psychiatrist is busy clarifying the form, the patient is getting very irritated because 'he is not taking any notice of what I am saying'. She is worried that she is being sent to the moon.

What will happen when she gets there? How will she get back? So the *content* is all important to her, and the doctor's absorption with form is incomprehensible and frustrating in the extreme.

The form is dependent on, and is therefore a diagnostic key to, the particular mental illness from which the patient suffers. For example, *delusional percepts* occur in schizophrenia, and when demonstrated as the form of the experience they indicate this condition. The finding of a visual hallucination suggests the likelihood of an organic psychosyndrome (Chapter 7). The nature of the content of these two examples is irrelevant in coming to a diagnosis. The content can be understood in terms of the patient's life situation with regard to culture, peer group, status, sophistication, age, sex, life events and geographical location. For example, another patient described himself as having been sent to the moon and back during the night within a fortnight of the first landing by man on the moon. Describing one's thoughts as being controlled by television is necessarily confined to those people who have seen that invention. A colleague has informed me that in the fortnight following Elvis Presley's death, three self-confessed reincarnations of the famous singer attended his emergency room.

Hypochondriacal content can occur in more than one form. It could take the form of an auditory hallucination in which the patient hears a voice saying 'you have cancer'. It could be a delusion, in that he believes falsely and with delusional evidence that he has cancer. It could be an overvalued idea, in that he spends a major part of every day checking on his health believing himself to be ill. It could be an abnormality of affect that manifests itself in extreme hypochondriacal anxiety or in depressive hypochondriacal despondency.

The significance of culture and individual variation in ascertaining the detailed complaint of the patient should be stressed. Because the psychiatrist needs to assess whether this notion of the patient demonstrates the specific psychopathological form of delusion, it does not diminish the parallel need to understand the patient's philosophical, religious, political and social beliefs, and know how they fit, or fail to fit, into the patient's larger, national and more intimate, subcultural social contexts (Fabrega, 2000).

Alongside the need of the psychiatrist to acquire skills in psychopathology and the elucidating of mental symptoms is the parallel requirement for cultural education and sensitivity. Both aspects are necessary for every patient–doctor interaction. If anything, the painstaking and detailed study of phenomenology increases the awareness of the cultural context and how it influences cognition and behaviour.

Subjective–objective

Objectivity in science has come to be revered as the ideal, so that only what is external to the mind is considered to be real, measurable and valuable. This is a mistake, because objective assessments are necessarily subjectively value-laden in what the observer chooses to measure, and this subjective aspect can be made more precise and reliable. There are always value judgements associated with both subjective and objective assessments. The process of making a scientific evaluation consists of various stages: receiving a sensory stimulus, perceiving, observing (making the percepts meaningful), noting, coding and formulating hypotheses. This is a progressive process of throwing away information, and it is the subjective judgement of what is valuable that determines the small amount of each stage that is retained for transmission to the next part of the process. 'There is no such thing as an unprejudiced observation' (Popper, 1974).

Objective assessments in psychiatry have covered many aspects of life. A few examples are, in addition to many physiological measures, the measurement of body movements, facial expression, patients' writings, learning capacity, responses to an operant conditioning programme, memory span, work efficiency and evaluation of logical content of the patients' statements. All these can be quantified and analysed objectively. Subjective analysis can be made, for example, from facial expression or from the patient's description of himself, of his own writing or of his inner events. When a doctor says about a patient 'she looks sad', he is not measuring the patient's facial expression in 'units of sadness' by some objective yardstick. He is going through this process: 'I associate her facial expression with the affect that I recognize in myself as feeling sad; seeing her expression makes me feel sad'. *Rapport* is this quality that the patient establishes with the doctor during the clinical interview. In order for it to happen, the doctor has to be receptive to this communication. He has to be able to establish rapport himself, to have a capacity for human understanding. This is necessarily a subjective experience for the doctor, but that is not to say that it is unreal or even that it cannot be measured. The method of phenomenology tries to increase our knowledge of subjective events so that they can be classified and ultimately quantified.

Aggernaes (1972) has defined subjectivity and objectivity for immediate everyday experiences.

> “When an experienced something has a quality of 'sensation', it is also said to have a quality of 'objectivity' if the experiencer feels that under favourable circumstances, he would be able to experience the same something with another modality of sensation than the one giving the quality of sensation. When an experienced something has a quality of 'ideation', i.e. is not being directly sensed at the moment, it is also said to have a quality of 'objectivity' if the experiencer feels that under favourable circumstances, he would nevertheless be able to experience the same something with at least two modalities of sensation.

> “An experienced something has a quality of 'subjectivity' if the experiencer feels that under no circumstances would he be able to experience this something with two or more modalities of sensation.

Thus I can look at the table in front of me as a visual perception or I can turn my head and still fantasize it as a visual image. As I 'see' it, in either way, the fact that I can imagine both hearing a sound if I were to hit it with a spoon and bruising my knuckles if I were to punch it confirms its quality of objectivity. If I use my imagination to create in my mind a visual image of a Chippendale chair that I have never actually seen but is a composite of objects and pictures I have seen, I know that I will never be able to feel or hear this actual chair; it is a subjective image without external, objective reality.

Process–development

In the same way that understanding or explaining depends on the perspective of the interviewer – empathically from inside or observing from the outside – so process or development depends on whether the person experiences an event as within their usual pattern of life or outside it. Development implies that an experience is understandable in terms of the person's constitution and history; personality aberrations would be seen as disorders of development. Process is seen as the imposition of an event from outside; epilepsy would be experienced as an occurrence of disease quite separate from normal development – the disease process has interrupted the normal course of life. Similarly, the onset of a schizophrenic illness often produces a definite 'break' in the life history of a late adolescent.

THEORETICAL STANCES OF PSYCHOPATHOLOGY

There are myriad psychopathologies. Any explanation for abnormal behaviour has the germ of a theory of psychopathology. *Descriptive psychopathology* as distinct from other forms of psychopathology eschews explanation of the phenomena that it describes. It simply describes, thereby avoiding arguments about aetiology. Explanatory psychopathologies often assume that mental phenomena are meaningful. There are other radically different models of psychology that regard mental experience, including thoughts, moods and drives, as *epiphenomena*, that is, as no more than froth on top of the beer. In these models (radical materialism or eliminative materialism), mental life is illusory; it is only the material, organic processes that are real. The significance the thinker attaches to subjective experience is regarded as purely illusory. Such a position poses difficulties for psychological enquiry and treatment.

Descriptive–dynamic psychopathology

Psychopathology is the study of abnormal psychic processes. Descriptive psychopathology is concerned with describing the subjective experiences and also the resultant behaviour during mental illness. It does not venture explanations accounting for these experiences or behaviour, nor does it comment on the aetiology or the process of development. The aim is to do full justice to what the patient is actually experiencing, to describe this fully and exclusively, without postulating causes, motives or other origins of the patient's experiences, unless these are actual mental experiences of the patient's (Wiggins *et al.*, 1992). Hence descriptive psychopathology guards against and avoids theory, presupposition or prejudice. This constraint of descriptive psychopathology acts to secure the conceptual framework of the subject on phenomenology, that is, the actual experience of the patient.

This approach to abnormal psychic phenomena contrasts quite sharply with other theoretical frameworks of psychopathology, for example the psychoanalytic. In psychoanalysis, at least one of several basic mechanisms are assumed to be taking place and the mental state becomes understandable within this framework. Explanations of what occurs in thought or behaviour are based on these underlying theoretical processes, such as *transference* or *ego defence mechanisms*. For example, with a delusion descriptive psychopathology tries to describe what it is that the person is believing, how he describes his experience of believing, what evidence he gives for its veracity and what is the significance of this belief or notion to his life situation. An attempt is made to assess whether this belief has the exact characteristics of a delusion and, if so, of what type of delusion. Having made this phenomenological evaluation, the information gained can be used diagnostically, prognostically and hence therapeutically. Some of the contrasts between descriptive and psychoanalytic psychopathology are summarized in Table 1.2.

Analytic or dynamic psychopathology, however, would be more likely to attempt to explain the delusion in terms of early conflicts repressed into the unconscious and now able to gain expression only in psychotic form, perhaps on a basis of projection. The content of the delusion would be considered an important key to the nature of the underlying conflict, which has its roots in early development. Descriptive psychopathology makes no attempt to say why a delusion is present; it solely observes, describes and classifies. Dynamic psychopathology aims to describe how the delusion occurred and why it should be that particular delusion, on the evidence of that person's experience in early life. This is related to genetic understanding, as described above, and has been called *prescient understanding* by Mellor (1985, personal communication), indicating presumed foreknowledge of how the events of mental life must unfold because they will necessarily conform with theoretical postulates for development.

Conscious–unconscious

Phenomenology cannot be concerned with the unconscious because the patient cannot describe it, and so the doctor cannot empathize. Descriptive psychopathology has no theory of the unconscious, nor does it deny its existence.

Table 1.2 Psychopathology: descriptive versus psychoanalytic

	Descriptive	Psychoanalytic
Summary	Empathic evaluation of patient's subjective experience	Study of the roots of current behaviour and conscious experience through unconscious conflicts
Terminology	Description of phenomena	Theoretical processes demonstrated
Methods	Understanding the patient's subjective state through empathic interview	Free association, dreams, transference
Differences in practical application	Makes distinction between understanding and explanation: understanding through observation and empathy	Understanding in terms of notional theoretical processes
	Form and content clearly separated: form of importance for diagnosis	No distinction made; concerned with content
	Process and development distinguished: process interferes with development basis	No distinction made; symptoms seen as having unconscious psychological basis

Unconscious mind is simply outside its terms of reference, and psychic events are described without recourse to explanations involving the unconscious. Dreams, the contents of hypnotic trance and slips of the tongue are described according to how the patient experienced them, that is, according to how they manifest in consciousness.

Organic–symptomatic

Psychopathology is essentially a non-biological approach to abnormal mental processes, so that, even when the organic causes of a condition are known, psychopathology is involved in ordering the symptoms and the experience of the patient rather than with its organic pathology. There are now many links known between different psychiatric illnesses and identifiable organic pathology. However, it is not with these links that psychopathology is concerned, and its usefulness is not dependent on ultimately finding the localization in the brain of a delusion or any other psychic event. Early, organically oriented psychiatrists, such as Griesinger and Wernicke, were not concerned with the psychopathological in psychiatry but much more with charting the diseased brain. This paid a rich dividend, for example in elucidating the nature and treatment of cerebral syphilis. Similarly, some modern behaviourists have been uninterested in phenomenology. Phenomenology is not ultimately concerned with organic pathology or with behaviour per se but with the patient's subjective experience of his world.

For a long time, symptomatic psychiatry, descriptive psychopathology, seemed to have lost contact with organic psychiatry, in which evidence of mental illness is sought in disease of the brain. There has now developed what Mundt (2000) describes as a 'fresh wind from the experimental field of psychopathology, neuropsychology and biological neurosciences'. This linkage is still at an early stage, but it has potential for the future study of symptoms and of brain pathology.

Organic has not been contrasted with the conventional *functional*, because functional is a most misleading term. It causes conceptual fog rather than enlightenment. A logical person who is innocent of medical jargon would be baffled to know why disturbance of human function by psychological mishap should be called functional while similar disturbance of function from organic disease is not. It is the *symptomatic* elements of disease that phenomenology can explore: the nature of the symptoms and with what they are associated.

Brain–mind

René Descartes (1596–1650) examined, formulated and restated views on the separation of body and soul. He described *l'âme raisonable*, 'the soul that reasons', lodged in the machine and having its principal seat in the brain. He described the soul as the engineer who altered the movements of the machine, the body (Descartes, 1649). Descartes was a man of his time, reflecting as well as developing then current dichotomous views. An example of this Cartesian dualism occurring before Descartes is the following obituary inscription to Lady Doderidge, who died in 1614.

"As when a ruinous clocke is out of frame
a workman takes in peeces small the same
and mendinge what amisse is to be found
the same rejoynes and makes itt treppe and gow
so god this ladie into two partes tooke
too soone her soule her mortall corse forsooke
But by his might att length her bodie sound shall rise
rejoynd unto her soule now crownd
Till then they rest in earth and heaven sundred
at which conjoined all such as live we then wondred

This clear affirmation of an absolute separateness between body and soul occurs on her tomb, which is to be found in Exeter Cathedral.

From this dualism comes our tendency to think in terms of body and mind – mental and physical illness. The whole discipline of psychiatry tacitly accepts a dualistic background for its very existence, although it resents this and tries hard to teach medicine of the whole person. Our language continually brings us back to dualistic words and expressions, and we are constantly in danger of either a 'mindless' or a 'brainless' psychiatry (Eisenberg, 1986, 2000).

The method of phenomenology has in this regard the advantage of being a bridge across this otherwise irreconcilable chasm. As it is concerned with subjective experience, it is involved with mind not body, but the mind can perceive only the stimuli that the body has received and there can be no perception without the state of consciousness of the mind. 'The body is not just a *caused mechanism*, but essentially an *intentional* entity always goal-directed. The *lived-body* is that experience of our body which cannot be objectified' (Gold, 1985, Gold's italics). The term *mind* is not intended to represent some psychological homunculus resident, perhaps upside down, in the cerebral cortex; it is purely an abstraction referring to one aspect of our humanity. Like any other aspect or view, what is held in focus is fairly clear, but the edges of the field are blurred and so we cannot say what precisely lies within the confines of *mind*. Neither can we discriminate absolutely between body and mind, nor would we say that mankind is wholly explicable in terms of body and mind (Sims, 1994).

The philosophy of mind is a thriving area of research. The current focus is on elucidating the nature of consciousness. The structure of the arguments parallels the debates about mind–brain duality. Since Popper and Eccles (1977) developed Cartesian dualism further and elaborated a trichotomous concept – mind, body and self – further body–mind theories have been elaborated. Their relationships to psychiatry have been well summarized by Granville-Grossman (1983) and more recently by Cutting (1997), who follows Schoppenhauer and Bergson and develops a framework of duality: two aspects of the external world, two minds and, of course, two hemispheres. The debate is still ongoing, but its resolution is not essential for the more pragmatic nature of descriptive psychopathology. *Mind* is used hereafter as an abstraction, a way of looking at part of the phenomena of man. These issues have necessarily been dealt with summarily in this opening chapter, in which the purpose has been to look at illness and not to dissect the mind; 'the study of the distinctive characteristics which manifest themselves' (Pinel, 1801).

REFERENCES

Aggernaes A (1972) The experienced reality of hallucinations and other psychological phenomena. *Acta Psychiatrica Scandinavica 48*, 220–38.

Berrios GE (1984) Descriptive psychopathology: conceptual and historical aspects. *Psychological Medicine 14*, 303–13.

Berrios GE (1992) Phenomenology, psychopathology and Jaspers: a conceptual history. *History of Psychiatry iii*, 303–27.

Berrios GE (1996) *The History of Mental Symptoms: Descriptive Psychopathology Since the Nineteenth Century*. Cambridge: Cambridge University Press.

Beveridge A (1997) Voices of the mad: patients' letters from the Royal Edinburgh Asylum 1873–1908. *Psychological Medicine 27*, 899–908.

Bloch S and Reddaway P (1977) *Russia's Political Hospitals*. London: Victor Gollancz.

Bluglass R (1983) *A Guide to the Mental Health Act*. Edinburgh: Churchill Livingstone.

Bluglass RS and Bowden P (1990) *Principles and Practice of Forensic Psychiatry*. Edinburgh: Churchill Livingstone.

Cutting J (1997) *Principles of Psychopathology: Two Worlds – Two Minds – Two Hemispheres*. Oxford: Oxford University Press.

Descartes R (1649) Les Passions de l'Âme. In *Descartes' Philosophical Writings* (transl. Kemp Smith N, 1952). London: Macmillan.

Eisenberg L (1986) Mindlessness and brainlessness in psychiatry. *British Journal of Psychiatry 148*, 497–508.

Eisenberg L (2000) Is psychiatry more mindful or brainier than it was a decade ago? *British Journal of Psychiatry 176*, 1–5.

Fabrega H (2000) Culture, spirituality and psychiatry. *Current Opinion in Psychiatry 13*, 525–30.

Gold J (1985) Cartesian dualism and the current crisis in medicine – a plea for a philosophical approach: discussion paper. *Journal of the Royal Society of Medicine 78*, 663–6.

Goldberg D and Huxley P (1980) *Mental Illness in the Community: a Pathway to Psychiatric Care*. London: Tavistock.

Granville-Grossman K (1983) Mind and the body. In Lader MH (ed.) *Mental Disorders and Somatic Illness: Handbook of Psychiatry 2*, pp. 5–13. Cambridge: Cambridge University Press.

James W (1902) *The Varieties of Religious Experience*. London: Penguin.

Jaspers K (1959) *General Psychopathology*, 7th edn (transl. Hoenig J and Hamilton MW, 1963). Manchester: Manchester University Press.

Kendell RE (1975) The concept of disease and its implications for psychiatry. *British Journal of Psychiatry 127*, 305–15.

Lewis AJ (1963) Medicine and the affections of the mind. *British Medical Journal ii*, 1549–57.

Mental Health Act (1983) London: HMSO.

Mowbray RM, Ferguson Rodger T and Mellor CS (1979) *Psychology in Relation to Medicine*, 5th edn. Edinburgh: Churchill Livingstone.

Mundt C (2000) Editorial. *Psychopathology 33*, 2–4.

Murphy EA (1979) The epistemology of normality. *Psychological Medicine 9*, 409–15.

Phillips J (2004) Understanding/explanation. In Radden J (ed.) *The Philosophy of Psychiatry: a Companion*. Oxford: Oxford University Press.

Pinel P (1801) *Traite Médico-philosophique sur la Manie*, 2nd edn (transl. Zilboorg G and Henry GW, 1941). New York: Norton

Pope A (1688–1744) *An Essay on Man*. New York: WW Norton.

Popper K (1974) *Unended Quest*. Harmondsworth: Penguin.

Popper KR and Eccles JC (1977) *The Self and its Brain*. Berlin: Springer-Verlag.

Rosenhan DL (1973) On being sane in insane places. *Science 179*, 250–8.

Sartre JP (1943) *Being and Nothingness* (transl. Barnes HE, 1958). London: Methuen.

Scadding JG (1967) Diagnosis: the clinician and the computer. *Lancet ii*, 877–82.

Schneider K (1959) *Clinical Psychopathology*, 5th edn (transl. Hamilton MW). New York: Grune & Stratton.

Sims ACP (1994) 'Psyche': spiritual as well as mental? *British Journal of Psychiatry 165*, 441–6.

Slater E and Roth M (1977) *Clinical Psychiatry*. London: Baillière Tindall.

Spitzer M (1990) Why philosophy? In Spitzer M and Maher BA (eds) *Philosophy and Psychopathology*. New York: Springer-Verlag.

Taylor FK (1980) The concepts of disease. *Psychological Medicine 10*, 419–24.

Walker C (1988) Philosophical concepts and practice: the legacy of Karl Jasper's psychopathology. *Current Opinion in Psychiatry 1*, 624–9.

Walker C (1993a) Karl Jaspers as a Kantian psychopathologist. I The philosophical origins of the concept of form and context. *History of Psychiatry 4*, 209–38.
Walker C (1993b) Karl Jaspers as a Kantian psychopathologist. II The concept of form and context in Jaspers' psychopathology. *History of Psychiatry 4*, 321–48.
Walker C (1994) Karl Jaspers and Edmund Husserl: 1: the perceived convergence. *Philosophy, Psychiatry and Psychology 1*, 117–34.
Walker C (1995a) Karl Jaspers and Edmund Husserl: II: the divergence. *Philosophy, Psychiatry and Psychology 2*, 245–65.
Walker C (1995b) Karl Jaspers and Edmund Husserl: III: Jaspers as a Kantian phenomenologist. *Philosophy, Psychiatry and Psychology 2*, 65–82.
Wiggins OP, Schwartz MA and Spitzer M (1992) Phenomenological/descriptive psychiatry: the methods of Edmund Husserl and Karl Jaspers. In Spitzer M, Uehlein F, Schwartz MA and Mundt C (eds) *Phenomenology, Language and Schizophrenia*. New York: Springer-Verlag.
Wing JK (1978) Clinical concepts of schizophrenia. In Wing JK (ed.) *Schizophrenia: Towards a New Synthesis*. London: Academic Press.
Wittgenstein L (1953) *Philosophical Investigation* (transl. Anscombe GEM). Oxford: Blackwell.
World Health Organization (1946) Constitution of the World Health Organization. *Official Record of the World Health Questionnaire 2*, 100.

Eliciting the Symptoms of Mental Illness

2

"Human beings are like parts of a body,
Created from the same essence.
When one part is hurt and in pain,
The others cannot remain in peace and be quiet.
If the misery of others leaves you indifferent
And with no feelings of sorrow,
You cannot be called a human being. *Sa'adi (thirteenth century), Persian*

Eliciting the symptoms involves listening to a narrative account of the person's complaints and his internal state and observing the whole repertoire of behaviour and then reducing these to a few summarizing phrases. It is a difficult task, requiring an ability to actively listen and communicate, a sensitivity to the needs and feelings of a person who is bewildered and distressed, a knowledge of the possible conditions of complaint. A genuine interest in the human condition and its manifold expressions, as well as a curiosity about intrapsychic experiences, is essential. This cannot be learned from a book alone, but a structure for case taking that suggests likely areas for exploration is invaluable. There are many comprehensive schemes, and they can often be traced to earlier textbooks with only slight modification. A summary of the scheme on which this chapter is based is shown in Box 2.1. A practical guide to history taking and evaluation of the mental state, diagnosis, formulation and management is found in the *Handbook for Trainee Psychiatrists* (Rix, 1987). A useful approach to making the patient information available for diagnosis and planning treatment is *Making Sense of Psychiatric Cases* (Greenberg *et al.*, 1986). A further account of the areas to be considered and the modifications of the history and examination required in particular circumstances is to be found in Sims and Curran (2001).

There is a significant conflict of interest between the patient and the interviewer. The patient describes untoward and distressing experiences. He wants to be rid of these experiences. One patient may, for example, say that he is depressed and miserable, or another may complain that his thoughts are being sucked out of his head by the Martians. In both instances, the patient wants the symptom to be relieved and he feels that describing it to the doctor in the way that it is affecting him is the first stage in achieving this. The doctor needs to learn a lot of things from the patient that the latter would consider irrelevant. She needs to have a precise description of the symptoms and of the patient's state of mind. She needs to know about the context of the patient's symptoms, including the patient's developmental history, and about his adjustment to his social environment in general and to his symptoms in particular. To return to

Box 2.1 Outline for psychiatric examination

Patient's name: ______________ Age: ___ Occupation: _______ Marital status: ____
Address: ______________________ Source of referral: __________________

- Reason for referral
- Present illness: symptoms and their chronology
- Previous medical history
  - i Physical
  - ii Psychiatric
- Family history: father, mother, siblings, other relations, atmosphere at home
- Personal history
  - i Pregnancy
  - ii Infancy
  - iii Childhood and adolescence
  - iv Education at school
  - v Further education
  - vi Occupation (and military service)
  - vii Sexual history: puberty, menstruation
  - viii Marital history
  - ix Children
- Social data
  - i Life situation: currently working, housing situation, financial problems, relationships
  - ii Crime, delinquency
  - iii Alcohol, drugs, tobacco
  - iv Social and religious affiliations and beliefs
- Premorbid personality
- Mental state
  - i Appearance and behaviour
  - ii Talk and thought
  - iii Mood: subjective, objective, rapport
  - iv Thoughts and beliefs: phobias, obsessions, compulsions, suicidal thoughts, delusions, misinterpretations
  - v Experience and perception:
    - a of the environment (hallucinations, illusions, derealization)
    - b of the body (hypochondriasis, somatic hallucinations)
    - c of the self (depersonalization, thought passivity)
  - vi Cognitive state: orientation, attention, concentration and memory
  - vii Insight
- Diagnosis and assessment
  - i Diagnosis and differential diagnosis
  - ii Evidence for diagnosis
  - iii Aetiological factors
  - iv Management
  - v Prognosis

our examples, the doctor needs to know not only that the patient feels depressed; she must enquire about the precise nature of the 'depression', what the word implies to the patient, how the affect disturbs the routine of his life and whether there are any other associated symptoms.

The person suffering at the hands of the Martians will be only too ready to talk about Martians. However, they are largely irrelevant to the interviewer, who is interested in exactly what the experience of 'thoughts being extracted' entails. What is the patient's evidence that this happens? What other abnormal mental phenomena are experienced? The reader can perhaps understand the patient's irritation if he can imagine that, after he had paid his gas bill, a final demand notice with an intimation that his gas supply was to be cut off came through the letterbox. On explaining to the authorities that his bill was already paid, they did not apologize or say that they would correct their computer, but they started interrogating the harassed consumer as to why he should be so upset about it, and what was his evidence that he had been especially picked on by the authorities. Understandably, there is a real conflict of interest between the patient's wish for relief of symptoms and the doctor's need to start by making a diagnosis. A compromise is necessary.

The patient will quite quickly tire of the effort required to answer phenomenological questions. Several short interviews are preferable to a marathon session: 'never ask today what you can ask tomorrow'. This method should encourage the examiner to bracket out all preconceptions, and the patient to reflect on his experiences under guidance from the examiner, who should not be digging for phenomena like a dog at a rabbit hole. It is important for the examiner to distinguish quite clearly between observations and inferences.

DIAGNOSIS AND LABELLING

Why make a diagnosis? Medical classification of diseases allows a cluster of symptoms to be brought under a single term that embodies the essence of a given condition. The diagnostic term carries information in an efficient manner. But there are disadvantages, including the unreliability of diagnostic terms as well as the risk of undue labelling and the associated stigma of psychiatric diagnosis. It is central to the work of a professional that her first task is to carefully collect information so that she knows exactly what clinical problem confronts her within her professional competence, and therefore what action would be appropriate; this is what diagnosis implies.

In psychiatry, a multifactorial approach to the understanding of disorder is the rule rather than the exception. This is the basis of the biopsychosocial approach to psychiatric disorders. This means that a narrow diagnosis, in purely organic or purely behavioural terms, is inadequate. The diagnosis needs to be made in the context of an understanding of the biological, psychological and social antecedents, which in turn determine the biological, psychological and social management of the condition.

THE PSYCHIATRIC HISTORY

This account is chiefly interested in the way *taking the history* sheds light on the *mental state*. The nature and type of *referral* is noted and recorded, for example from a general practitioner as an urgent problem, from a solicitor for a court report and so on. After recording the reason for referral, the history will usually begin with the patient's *verbatim* description of his *present symptoms*, including the duration of each symptom and an account of the development of the illness. Using the patient's own words is valuable in giving insight into his state of mind and how he himself views his symptoms. It is helpful after receiving a catalogue of complaints to ask 'Which is the very worst of all these symptoms?' This reveals how the patient conceptualizes his problem and also suggests a preliminary target for treatment.

Often, the patient's history of his present complaint is literally his story; there is nothing wrong in recording this in narrative style provided this is accurate. A chronological account of the present illness reveals how the patient regards the development of his symptoms as well as giving information on the actual history. In the history, one wants to know about the sequence of symptoms and the effects these symptoms had on the patient's lifestyle, about changes in behaviour and about alterations in physical function. It is appropriate at this point to note psychiatric symptoms of which the patient has been aware in the past but for which he has never consulted a doctor or received treatment. They may have relevance in the total picture of how the illness developed, and it is known that the majority of people with psychiatric conditions of clinical severity do not seek medical consultation, let alone come to the attention of a psychiatrist (Andrews *et al.*, 2001).

The patient feels it to be innately reasonable to describe chronologically and meticulously his previous *illnesses*, operations and accidents. He also will appreciate the logic of giving details of hospital and general practice treatment for mental illness and will usually give accurate information with regard to dates, duration, nature of treatment, in what hospital and whether he was an in-patient or outpatient. Treatment received from the family doctor is recalled less well; the dates are less reliable, and often the patient does not know what was the nature of treatment or what it was for.

The *family history* is concerned with genetic and environmental, pathoplastic features. History of mental illness, suicide, nature of treatment and so on is relevant for the first-degree relatives (those sharing 50 per cent of the genetic material with the patient: parents, siblings, children) and more distant relatives. It is important to know about the quality of relationships, emotional bonding and interpersonal conflicts, both for the family in which the patient was a child and for the family in which the patient may be a parent. Relationships between individual members of the family are described, and also the general emotional atmosphere and social and financial problems. The occupations of different family members give information about the social context; a record of health may be relevant, as may a description of their personalities. Of course, the family is seen through the patient's eyes; this means that it is not just a factual description but rather an account of the emotional impact the patient feels his family has made on him. If the history from the patient is supplemented by an account from another *informant*, this bias of the patient's will itself give information that may be useful in subsequent treatment.

The *personal history* traces the stages of the patient's development, health and forming of relationships from conception, birth and infancy through childhood, school experiences, adolescence and further education to an occupational, marital and sexual history. The factual details of these stages need to be recorded, and also the way they have influenced the personality and attitudes of the patient, how he feels about them, how he has related to other people (for example teachers and workmates) and how all these details are connected with the psychiatric condition. There are at least two processes at play in taking a history. There is the simple business of taking a factually accurate account of a patient's history of complaints as well as the family, personal and social history. In addition to this approach, there is the requirement to grasp the meaning of the patient's history, that is, his story, in order to understand how he sees himself in relation to the world and how his development and circumstances have been influential in provoking, exacerbating or ameliorating his present illness. The factual history is the foundation of the clinical diagnosis. Human beings live in a world of meanings, and the symbolic and social dimension of the history are the basis of an adequate and humane response to the patient's illness and distress.

PREMORBID, PREVIOUS OR USUAL PERSONALITY

Assessment of personality is the most complex and problematic task that a psychiatrist faces. In clinical interviews, the doctor assesses the patient's personality using three areas of information. First, the examiner asks the patient to describe in detail his relationships with other people, interests and activities. Second, the examiner studies the way in which the patient reacts to the examiner in the interview situation. Third, the examiner tries to help the patient to describe and demonstrate what he, the patient, is like as a person; how he feels inside himself in different situations; and his interests, goals and standards.

Personality assessment is not the exclusive preserve of psychiatrists or psychologists but an important learned skill of many professionals who deal with people, for example schoolteachers, lawyers and even bank managers, although their terminology is different. Personality is that part of a person, excepting his physical characteristics, that makes him individual, that is, different from other people. Personality is revealed by a person's characteristic behaviour; if one can predict how he will react, what his behaviour will be in particular circumstances, then the basis of that prediction is the evaluation of his personality. Subjectively, personality is shown in the totality of a person's aims and goals, formed of everything that he values and to which he aspires. Personality is not a *thing* but an abstraction, one way of looking at human beings. Furthermore, it is multidimensional and is best defined in action. Verbal description is unlikely to exhaust the essence of any individual.

Categorization into normal and abnormal personality requires a further level of abstraction. *Normal*, an ordinary word in everyday use, needs to be used more rigorously in this context (see Chapter 1). In medicine, the term *normal* is often used to denote a statistical norm, that is, what occurs in the majority of people. Equally, the term is also used to mean 'ideal', in the sense of a description that conforms to an 'ideal' type. In relation to personality, classification and definitions of personality disorders depend on deviance from the norm but the definitions depend on 'ideal' descriptions of personality types.

A normal personality conforms therefore in its characteristics and the extent to which they are developed with the majority of mankind. Abnormal personality has some characteristics developed or underdeveloped to such an extent as to be quantitatively different from the mass of people. In other words, abnormalities of personality are differences of degree; the deviant traits are shared in common with others but exaggerated in expression.

In the clinical interview, there are various areas of dialogue with the patient that are likely to lead to useful information for depicting the detail and colouring of his personality – the *personality type*. Painting the picture and defining the type are both necessary clinical exercises. Social relations are investigated. How does he relate to his family? Is he detached or overdependent? What sort of friendships does he form, with what sort of people, and are they close knit or superficial, with an exclusive few or an unlimited crowd? How do his interests and leisure activities involve him with others? Social or solitary, structured or informal? How does he relate to bosses, workmates and employees at work? Is he a leader or a follower, an organizer or an isolant? Is he pliant or truculent, cooperative, sympathetic or clubbable? His sexual preferences and relationships should be noted.

The nature of his *interests* and activities is informative. What does he like doing in his spare time? If he is interested in sport, it is useful to know if he can feel partisan and involved and also whether he is a participant or an observer. Enquiry is made of his preference and interests in films and literature: how he observes, criticizes and enjoys the material. To what social organizations does he belong? Religion requires more than a single word designating religious affiliation in the case notes. The phenomenological method is equally relevant for this area of life. What is the individual's self experience of his religious beliefs and how do these interact with psychiatric symptomatology (Sims, 1994)?

An account of his predominant *mood* is requested, and whether his mood is fluctuating or stable, responsive to precipitants or endogenous. Character traits imply a detailed adjectival list, for example irritable, reserved, fussy and so on. It will, of course, be helpful to corroborate his description with an account from another person. Enquiry is made about his attitudes and values; his views about himself and his body; how he regards others close to him; his more general social values in religion, morality, politics and economics; how he feels events occur and can be made to occur. Drive and energy and the way these are expressed in ambition, lethargy, effectiveness and persistence are an important aspect of personality.

Study of his *fantasy* life is made: the frequency and duration of daydreams and their content; whether these are goal-directed and realistic or dissociated from any expectation of fulfilment. Dreams and other supposed signs of unconscious psychic activity are useful, especially when the subject attempts to interpret them. We may comment on his habits of ingestion, inhalation and excretion; whether they are regular and to what extent he depends on this regularity; if there is an indication that there should be a more detailed history and exploration of current habits of eating, smoking, drinking alcohol and taking other drugs. As the patient unfolds the facets of his personality, so the overall emphases that he puts in areas of description become illuminating in understanding him as a whole person.

DIFFERENTIATION OF PERSONALITY DISORDER

Allocating the patient to a personality type without taking into account the infinite variability of individuals is quite inadequate. However, certain characteristics tend to occur together and are of clinical significance. Allocation to a particular category of personality disorder is made on the relative predominance of these different character traits. Having decided that a certain definite trait or traits are present in this individual to an abnormal extent, does the abnormality of personality cause the person himself or other people to suffer? That is, is personality disorder present?

If personality disorder is considered to be present, it is recommended that one of the classification systems described in Chapter 21 be used (American Psychiatric Association, 1994; Tyrer and Alexander, 1979; World Health Organization, 1992). None of these classifications is perfect, but conforming to an established scheme will facilitate communication. With greater consistency and the use of clearly laid-down operational definitions, it is hoped that research in this area will advance and this will have considerable clinical application.

More than one abnormal type of personality may be present in any individual; they are not mutually exclusive. In formulating the psychiatric history and evaluation of mental state, comment on premorbid personality should always be made, even if it is only to state that due to the ravages of the mental illness it is impossible to assess premorbid state. The predominant traits should be described, preferably with verbatim comments of the patient to illustrate them. The interviewer should decide whether these traits are there to a statistically abnormal extent and, if so, whether this amounts to personality disorder. The type of disorder should be differentiated.

THE MENTAL STATE EXAMINATION

The mental state examination is the special area of expertise of psychiatrists. It is the psychiatrist's equivalent of the neurological examination. The mental state examination is guided by the same principles and communication skills as for any other clinical interview (Box 2.2). It is dependent on facility with language, because that is the tool with which psychiatric practice is conducted. The clinician uses 'open' questions at the beginning of clinical inquiries and utilizes 'closed' questions to clarify specific points. There are specific techniques for signalling active listening. These include the use of 'summary statements' to summarize what the clinician has made of what the patient is saying and provide the opportunity for the patient to correct any misapprehension on the part of the clinician. Furthermore, 'normalizing statements' can be used to introduce difficult subjects, for example the clinician could introduce the issue of suicidal thoughts by saying, 'It is not uncommon for people who are depressed to find that they feel hopeless and that life is not worth living; have you felt like that?' Statements that comment on the emotional aspects of the patient's communication or behaviour, such as 'I can see that it must be very difficult for you to talk about these experiences', may help to deepen the rapport between clinician and patient. Further practical advice on conducting the psychiatric examination is found in Leff and Isaacs (1990).

Box 2.2 Communication skills techniques

- Introductory statements and setting the context: 'My name is Dr Smith. I have a letter from your GP informing me that you have been feeling low for the past 6 weeks.' etc.
- Open questions: 'Can I start off by asking how you have been feeling lately?'
- Closed questions: 'I understand that you have been hearing voices for several weeks now. Are these voices there all the time?'
- Summary statements: 'From what you have been saying, I understand that you have been feeling low for the past 6 weeks, and that this has been steadily getting worse to the degree that you are now tearful all the time and for no good reason, and that your sleep has also been badly affected.'
- Normalizing statements: 'It is not uncommon for people in your kind of situation to feel so low that life no longer seems worth living. Have you felt like that?'
- Reflective and empathic statements: 'As I understand it, when your husband lost his job you had a lot of money worries. That must have been quite difficult for you, especially with the new baby too.'
- Concluding statements: 'I now have a good grasp of how things have been for you in the past year. Are there things that you wanted to tell me that you have not yet had the opportunity to bring up?'

As the interviewer asks each question, she should be thinking what the possible answers to that question could be from a *reasonable* person in *this* context. In everyday conversations, one is conditioned to avoid asking embarrassing questions and so, when someone makes an odd remark, the tendency is to fill in the meaning of the response in order to make it ordinary, sensible and avoid asking further questions in this area. This is exactly the opposite to phenomenological investigation, in which the interviewer is looking for ways into the patient's private way of thinking. When the patient says something unreasonable, odd or unexpected, the interviewer must note it and, without embarrassing or disturbing the patient's equanimity, clarify the inner experience partly revealed. This will entail the use of the empathic method described in Chapter 1. One of the difficulties for the aspiring phenomenologist is to know when to pursue what the patient reveals in more detail – when to make the incision for the psychopathological operation.

Words limit as well as liberate. The clinical interviewer needs to be very careful not to restrain her patient's answers by imposing the shackles of psychiatric technical jargon. Careful attention must be paid to the patient's use of language and, as far as possible, the clinician should be using language that mirrors the patient's language. It is important to be certain that both clinician and patient are using words in the same sense. The question 'Do you hear voices?' is a good example of this. The patient may truthfully answer 'No' and yet be suffering from almost continuous auditory hallucinations. This particular perceptual experience is most often described by patients and their doctors as 'voices'. However, phonemes may be thought of by the patient in quite other terms. He may make no distinction at all between these auditory perceptions, 'voices' he hears for which an outside observer realizes there is an appropriate stimulus, and auditory hallucinations. He may be largely oblivious of the form of the communication as *auditory* and *hallucinatory* because he is totally absorbed with its *content* (an order telling him to go to Strasbourg and preach). Obviously, another patient may answer the question 'Do you hear voices?' truthfully in the affirmative and yet have a quite different form of phenomenological experience from auditory hallucination (see Chapter 7).

Almost every *technical term* in general medicine has diagnostic implications. This is also true in psychiatry. A symptom may not be pathognomonic of a certain condition but nevertheless predominantly found with that illness. If the doctor uses the term *perseveration* in describing her patient's mental state to a colleague, she is by inference suggesting a diagnosis of an organic psychiatric state. If this is not the diagnosis, she has some hard explaining to do to justify the use of that word. Is it really perseveration or just the repetitious use of words and phrases in a person who is retarded and shows poverty of expression? To avoid misunderstanding, it is best to use longer descriptions until the interviewer is sure that the symptom is truly present.

Observation of the *appearance* and *behaviour* of the patient is an invaluable supplement to his self-description. The observations of others, and at times other than the interview, need to be taken into account. As the interview proceeds, the interviewer more definitely pursues her real intention of finding out the meaning behind the words the patient uses. What is the patient feeling and experiencing? His own account may be a blind to prevent other people, or even himself, seeing how bad he really feels. The *empathic method* is invaluable in working out what he is implying. So also is acute, insightful and trained observation. *Observation* may reveal white lines across the knuckles of an anxious person talking about what upsets him most and that renders him impotently angry. Empathy allows the observer to employ his own capacity for emotion as a diagnostic and therapeutic tool. Training and experience are essential for knowing in which areas delving will be rewarded with useful information: how to ask questions that are comprehensible to patients of different verbal abilities and cultural backgrounds, and which will result in appropriate answers; how to avoid damaging the patient still further with well-directed but brutal questions. Observation and empathy must always be used together in eliciting the mental state. Note also the double meaning of the word *observant*: not only noticing what is going on around but also conforming with the cultural mores of the immediate society. A good phenomenologist will be observant in both senses of the word.

SYSTEMATIC ENQUIRY

The *appearance* and *behaviour* of the patient are observed for the clinical medical information they carry. Does the patient look ill? Is he alert, oriented, fully conscious, fluctuating in his mental state? Are there any behavioural or neurological abnormalities? Observation is also useful for assessing non-verbal communication (Argyle, 1975). From his posture, gestures, facial expression and so on he betrays his state of emotion, information about his personality and his attitude to the observer and to others despite his silence or contradictory verbal communication. Obviously, observation of behaviour also indicates psychiatric symptomatology such as tics, catatonic movements, possible hallucinatory perception, feeding and excreting disorders. Posture can be revealing to the acute observer, for instance the *pharaonic posture*, and the slow deliberate movements of head and neck of the patient with schizophrenia. If the patient is mute, observed behaviour is the only source of clinical information, but the importance of observation needs to be stressed also for those patients who do speak. Observation may be valuable to corroborate the patient's complaints, to make clear the degree of emotional involvement he has in his symptoms, or sometimes to contradict his statement, for example the person who manifests physically extreme anxiety yet denies any worries on enquiry.

Talk reveals *thought*. Listening to and studying the patient's utterances is usually the most important part of assessing his mental state. Thought disorder and the interpretation of abnormalities in the use of words, syntax and association of ideas are discussed in more detail in Chapter 9. The flow of talk merits notice. Does he talk volubly and easily or in taciturn monosyllables? Does he just answer questions or speak spontaneously? Is his conversation appropriate to the social context, and is it coherent? Is the train of thought readily distracted? Throughout the interview, as much as possible of the patient's speech should be recorded verbatim. This provides a clearer flavour of this individual person's inner milieu, and also the data of self-experience will allow another person to evaluate the diagnosis. It is useful, in investigating thought processes, to give the patient proverbs to interpret. Using proverbs that he will not have come across before, for example 'the image maker does not worship the gods', is preferable, as they will prevent an automatic response (Rawnsley, 1985). Tests of *similarity* are also useful. How is an aeroplane like a car? In what way are ice and water similar? Unexpected answers may reveal psychopathology of thought processes.

As the interviewer enquires about and forms her own assessment of *mood*, she has three areas for exploration: *subjective* and *objective* description of mood and evaluation of *rapport*. There is much more to mood than just depression or elation; the finer nuances of this person's *subjective* emotional experience must be carefully dug out like truffles, using a sensitive nose and delicate extraction. A person anticipating an event may be acutely apprehensive, exquisitely excited but rather anxious, hopelessly resigned and so on; 'afraid of the future' is not an adequate description. Mood can be studied for its direction (depression or elation), its consistency (stable or labile), its appropriateness, its amplitude and the degree of discrepancy between subjective description and objective observation.

Of course, there is really no such thing as wholly objective assessment of mood. The doctor comments on the mood state of her patient from her observation of the patient's demeanour and the general tone of his conversation during the interview. She makes the comment, 'He appears depressed; he is agitated and tense'. In fact, this comment on her patient's emotion abbreviates the empathic process through which she goes to make this judgement. The doctor observes the patient and picks up available cues for mood, relating these to her experience with other patients and other people through her life, and ultimately to her knowledge of her *own* affective state. Her assessment runs 'If I felt how my patient looks, speaks and acts, I would feel profoundly depressed and agitated; he is, on observation, depressed and agitated.'

Rapport is a useful measure of the patient's ability to communicate his feelings to another person. The interviewer needs to make herself into a yardstick, a *constant rapport maker*, against which the patient's ability to make rapport can be measured. To do this, the doctor requires clinical experience and an objectivity in which she knows how she reacts to, and communicates with, many different sorts of people. She knows herself and her own competence well enough to exclude this from the assessment of rapport so that, as far as possible, it is only the patient's capacity for emotional communication that is being tested.

The *ideas* and *beliefs* the patient holds and *abnormalities of perception* he experiences are ascertained and explored during the interview. In ordinary conversation, there is a great deal of filling in or editing to eliminate the deficiencies of communication. A person talks and comes to a halt halfway through a sentence for loss of a word. The other person provides the word and thus continues the conversation to both parties' satisfaction. There is a tendency for those coming new to dialogue with the mentally ill to bring into their conversation these social niceties that are used to save embarrassment. The doctor tends to note what she thinks the patient meant to say, as if the latter's thinking processes were similar to her own, rather than concentrating on what he actually said. A lot of significant psychopathology is thus missed. Delusions and hallucinations are not volunteered by the patient as symptoms for the obvious reason that they are not experienced as different from the rest of the person's thinking or perceiving. To the patient, subjectively, a delusion is indistinguishable from any other idea, a hallucination is indistinguishable from any other normal perception. Skill in interviewing therefore comes very much in knowing when to look for a delusion and how to make a clear distinction between what the person describes as experience and what it reveals phenomenologically.

Passivity or delusions of control, *obsessions*, *compulsions* and *depersonalization* may be obvious or only made plain with some difficulty. It is important to try to categorize the type of experience as early in the course of exposure to professional enquiry as possible, because patients' explanations tend to become contaminated on repeated questioning. When passivity, for example, is suspected, it is generally best to follow up the clues right away and decide once and for all whether the symptom is present.

Assessment of the *cognitive state* includes, at least briefly, testing for orientation, attention, concentration and memory. The Mini-Mental State Examination (Folstein *et al.*, 1975) is a widely used standardized bedside test of cognitive function that is useful to administer in the clinical setting.

The doctor, from specific questions and from the interview in general, needs to form an idea of her patient's attitude to his illness, difficulties and prospects. To what extent does he have *insight* into his condition? Any illness of some severity will alter the patient's world and view of the world. Insight assesses the awareness of this change by the patient and the accurate labelling of this change as originating from a mental illness that requires treatment. Insight is therefore highly complex as a function. It is the ability of the individual to be self-aware and to be sensitive to inner subjective change. The capacity to correctly attribute the subjective psychological change to pathological causes is evidence of intact self-awareness despite evidence of mental illness. It is potentially an extremely valuable part of the mental state examination, as it is associated with compliance with treatment and also with the likelihood of treatment under compulsion. In summary, insight has three components: recognition of subjective psychological change, labelling of this change as pathological in nature and recognition of need for treatment as well as compliance with treatment (David, 1990; see Chapter 12).

Many textbooks and numerous psychiatric institutions have their own scheme for psychiatric interviewing. This account is a general commentary rather than yet another scheme. Box 2.1 contains a memorandum of key areas to be covered in the history and examination of a psychiatric patient.

REFERENCES

American Psychiatric Association (1994) *Diagnostic and Statistical Manual of Mental Disorders*, 4th edn. Washington: American Psychiatric Association.

Andrews G, Issakidis C and Carter G (2001) The shortfall in mental health service utilisation. *British Journal of Psychiatry 179*, 417–25.

Argyle M (1975) *Bodily Communication*. London: Methuen.

David AS (1990) Insight and psychosis. *British Journal of Psychiatry 156*, 789–808.

Folstein MF, Folstein SE and McHugh PR (1975) 'Mini-mental state'. A practical method of grading the cognitive state of patients for the clinician. *Journal of Psychiatric Research 12*, 189–98.

Greenberg M, Szmuckler G and Tantam D (1986) *Making Sense of Psychiatric Cases*. Oxford: Oxford University Press.

Leff JP and Isaacs AD (1990) *Psychiatric Examination in Clinical Practice*, 3rd edn. Oxford: Blackwell Scientific.

Rawnsley K (1985) *Workshop on the Teaching of Descriptive Psychopathology to Postgraduates in Psychiatry*. Leeds: Association of University Teachers of Psychiatry.

Rix KJB (1987) *Handbook for Trainee Psychiatrists*. London: Baillière Tindall.

Sims A (1994) 'Psyche' – spirit as well as mind? *British Journal of Psychiatry 165*, 441–6.

Sims A and Curran S (2001) Examination of the psychiatric patient. In Henn F, Sartorius N, Helmchen H and Lauter H (eds) *Contemporary Psychiatry*. Berlin: Springer.

Tyrer P and Alexander J (1979) Classification of personality disorder. *British Journal of Psychiatry 135*, 163–7.

World Health Organization (1992) *The ICD-10 Classification of Mental and Behavioural Disorders: Clinical Description and Diagnostic Guidelines*. Geneva: World Health Organization.

Section Two

CONSCIOUSNESS AND COGNITION

Consciousness and Disturbed Consciousness

3

> "Psychiatry and neuropathology are not merely two closely related fields, they are but one field in which only one language is spoken and the same laws rule. *Wilhelm Griesinger (1868)*
>
> I have always been intrigued by the specific moment when, as we sit awaiting in the auditorium, the door to the stage opens and a performer steps into the light, or, to take the other perspective, the moment when a performer who waits in semidarkness sees the same door open, revealing the lights, the stage, and the audience. . . . as I reflect on what I have written, I sense that stepping into the light is also a powerful metaphor for consciousness, for the birth of the knowing mind, for the simple and momentous coming of the self into the world of the mental. *Antonio Damasio (1999)*

To be able to experience, one must be conscious. So the logical starting place for the study of symptoms, from a subjective standpoint, is that which allows subjectivity to exist (consciousness). Until quite recently, studies of consciousness were looked on with suspicion by neuroscientists, thereby leaving clinicians, both neurologists and psychiatrists, in intellectual darkness. This has been rectified in the past decade through combining and sharing the perspectives of different disciplines: philosophy, psychology, medicine and neurosciences (Bock and Marsh, 1993).

Although it is essential for our clinical work concerning disturbances in consciousness that we use the principles of descriptive psychopathology and applied phenomenology, we need to be aware of the limitations (Dennett, 1991). Dennett has pointed out that from Descartes via Locke, Berkeley and Hume phenomenology has tended to describe consciousness from the first person plural: 'according to longstanding philosophical tradition we all agree on what we find when we "look inside" at our own phenomenology'. We may not all be the same inside, and even if we are, we m[...] when we try to describe our inner experiences. He also questi[...] person perspective of behavioural psychology and adv[...] Heterophenomenology'. This depends, for its authenti[...] precision of the questions asked, the objectivity of r[...] (three stenographers preparing separate documents fr[...] ing the 'intentional stance' (assuming that the sub[...] intending to make a statement about something) a[...] When this process has been followed, the text 'is tak[...] expression and to be a *single, unified subject* of tha[...] opinions'. It becomes clear that this process is sir[...]

structured for research purposes, to the separate steps in the *method of empathy*, as described in Chapter 1.

Terminology in this area is appallingly confused. This and subsequent chapters have attempted to clarify the words used, sometimes at the expense of sacrificing altogether terms with a long history, and sometimes lumping as a single concept words between which there are only minute differences of meaning. One major problem is that different disciplines use different terms to cover partly overlapping meanings.

CONSCIOUS AND UNCONSCIOUS EXPERIENCES

Consciousness

The words *consciousness, conscious mind* and *awareness* are used very freely in psychiatry but often without a precise meaning. *Consciousness* 'is a state of awareness of the self and the environment' (Fish, 1967); also, consciousness 'is to be conscious, to know about oneself and the world' (Scharfetter, 1980); and, 'by consciousness, I simply mean those subjective states of sentience or awareness that end when one goes to sleep at night or falls into a coma, or dies, or otherwise becomes as one would say, unconscious' (Searle, 1994). Consciousness is characterized by its subjective nature and privacy. Furthermore, consciousness appears to have a unique quality, termed *qualia*, that is recalcitrant to any external physical description. This is the particular character of any object of our conscious experience, for example the redness of the colour red as we perceive it. Consciousness is also intentional, by which we mean that it is directed towards objects; that is to say that consciousness has content – it is always about something. Finally, our conscious experience is unified into a whole and not given to us in fragments or unintegrated parts.

The term, as used by clinicians, refers first to the inner *awareness* of experience as opposed to the categorizing of events as they occur. Second, it refers to the subject reacting to objects *intentionally*. Third, it denotes a knowledge of a conscious *self*.

Unconsciousness

Unconscious, according to Jaspers (1959), 'means something that is not an inner existence and does not occur as an experience; secondly, something that is not thought of as an object and has gone unregarded; thirdly, it is something which has not reached any knowledge of itself'.

In clinical practice, the term *unconscious* is used in three quite different ways that have in common only the phenomenological element in that there is *no* subjective experience (Figure 3.1).

- A person suffering from serious brain disease may be unconscious; consciousness in this instance is seen as being on a continuum, with a normal state of consciousness at one end and death at the other.
- Someone who is asleep is unconscious; again, there is a continuum from full wakefulness to deep sleep.
- ...n alert and healthy person is aware of only certain parts of his ...onment both externally and internally; of the rest, he is unconscious. ...also a continuum here from full vigilance directed towards the ...bject of awareness to total unawareness.

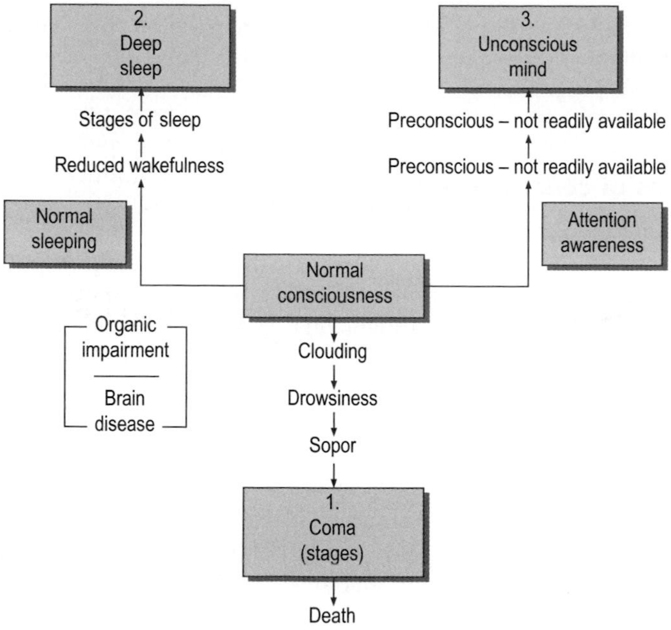

Figure 3.1 Three dimensions of unconsciousness.

The organic state of the brain as, for instance, demonstrated by the electroencephalogram is utterly different in these three situations.

The third meaning of unconsciousness implies that certain mental processes cannot be observed by introspection alone, even when the brain is normal and healthy. Among such processes, for which there is good evidence of their existence, frequency and complexity, there are some that have been, or may yet become, conscious. This is what Freud called the *preconscious* (Frith, 1979). Whereas there is a strict limit to the number of items available in the conscious state and that are therefore capable of being memorized (approximately seven, for example a number with seven digits), there is very much more information stored at the preconscious level. If a stimulus is ambiguous, only one interpretation is possible in consciousness at any one time; however, multiple meanings are available preconsciously. It is very difficult to carry out more than one task at a time consciously, but undertaking parallel tasks is usual at a preconscious level. Preconscious processes are automatic, whereas conscious ones are flexible and strategic. This function of the preconscious was well known long before Freud, for example Brodie (1854):

> “ But it seems to me that on some occasions a still more remarkable process takes place in the mind, which is even more independent of volition than that of which we are speaking; as if there were in the mind a principle of order which operates without our being at the time conscious of it. It has often happened to me to have been occupied by a particular subject of inquiry; to have accumulated a store of facts connected with it; but to have been able to proceed no further. Then, after an interval of time, without any addition to my stock of knowledge, I have found the obscurity and confusion, in which the subject was originally enveloped, to have cleared away; the facts have all seemed to have settled

> themselves in their right places, and their mutual relations to have become apparent, although I have not been sensible of having made any distinct effort for that purpose.

Dimensions of consciousness

Consciousness, then, is the awareness of experience. There may be awareness of objects or self-reflection. Awareness of objects includes the capacity to be aware of oneself as an object (see Chapter 14); self-reflection refers to the subjective experiencing of self. The three dimensions of consciousness (contrasted with unconsciousness, as in Figure 3.1) are vigilance, lucidity and self-consciousness.

Vigilance (wakefulness)–drowsiness (sleep)

Vigilance is taken to mean the faculty of deliberately remaining alert when otherwise one might be drowsy or asleep. This is not a uniform or unvarying state, but it fluctuates. Factors inside the individual that promote vigilance are interest, anxiety, extreme fear or enjoyment, whereas boredom encourages drowsiness. The situation in the environment and the way the individual perceives that situation also affect the vigilance–drowsiness axis. Some abnormal states of health increase vigilance, while many diminish it.

As well as the contrast between vigilance and drowsiness, there are qualitative differences in the nature of wakefulness. The vigilant state of mind of a person scanning a radar screen for a possible enemy interceptor is very different from the rapt attention of a music lover listening to a symphony. These aspects of attention and their abnormalities are discussed in Chapter 4.

Lucidity–clouding

Consciousness is inseparable from the object of conscious attention: lucidity can be demonstrated only in clarity of thought on a particular topic. The *sensorium*, the total awareness of all internal and external sensations presenting themselves to the organism at this particular moment, may be clear or clouded. Obviously, lucidity is not unrelated to vigilance: unless the person is fully awake, he cannot be clear in consciousness.

Clouding of consciousness denotes the lesser stages of impairment of consciousness on a continuum from full alertness and awareness to coma (Lishman, 1997). The patient may be drowsy or agitated and is likely to show memory disturbance and disorientation. In clouding, most intellectual functions are impaired, including attention and concentration, comprehension and recognition, understanding, forming associations, logical judgement, communication by speech and purposeful action.

Consciousness of self

Alongside full wakefulness and clear awareness is an ability to experience self, and an awareness of self, that is both immediate and complex. This is considered in more detail in Chapter 13.

PATHOLOGY OF CONSCIOUSNESS

It has proved complicated to describe exactly what is disordered in pathological states, hence this rather convoluted definition of a disturbed state of consciousness (DSC) by Aggernaes (1975):

> “a state in a person in which he has no experiences at all, or in which all of his experiences are deviant, concerning other or more qualities than tempo and mood coloring, from those he would have under similar stimulus conditions in his habitual waking state. The state is a DSC only if the individual cannot return to, and remain in, his habitual state by deciding to do so himself, and if others bring about a lasting return to his habitual state by the application of a simple social procedure.

Most abnormal states of consciousness show a lowering or diminution of consciousness. However, *heightened* consciousness occurs in which there is a subjective sense of richer perception: colours seem brighter and so on; there are changes in mood, usually exhilaration, perhaps amounting to ecstasy; there is *subjective* experience of increased alertness and a greater capacity for intellectual activity, memory and understanding. There may also be *synaesthesiae* (a sensory stimulus in one modality resulting in sensory experience in another, for example hearing a fingernail drawn down a blackboard results in a cold feeling down the spine). Such states, both heightening of consciousness and synaesthesiae, may occur in normal, healthy people, especially in adolescence or at times of emotional, social or religious crisis: when falling in love, on winning a large sum of money, at sudden religious conversion and so on.

Heightened awareness is not uncommon with certain drugs, notably with the hallucinogens, for example lysergic acid diethylamide, and central nervous system stimulants, for example amphetamine. A similar state of awareness may occur occasionally in early psychotic illness, especially mania, or less often in schizophrenia.

Consciousness is clearly associated with the arousal systems of the organism. A conjectural representation of this relationship is shown in Figure 3.2.

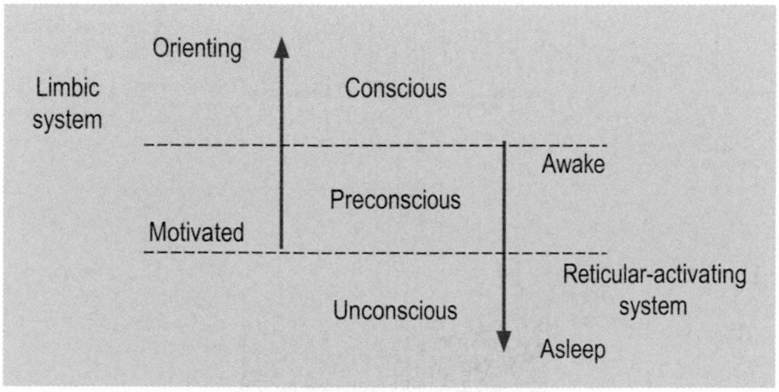

Figure 3.2 Arousal systems of consciousness.

Quantitative lowering of consciousness

As mentioned above, consciousness may be considered as a continuum from full alertness and awareness to coma. In that sense, consciousness may be regarded as quantitative (Figure 3.3). Impairment of consciousness is the primary change in acute organic reactions and holds a fundamentally important place in the detection of acute disturbance of brain function and in assessment of severity (Lishman, 1997).

Some conditions may produce a variable level of diminution of consciousness; that occurring with migraine, for example, may range from blunted awareness through lethargy and drowsiness to loss of consciousness (Lishman, 1997).

Clouding of consciousness

This represents the lesser stages of impairment of consciousness, with deterioration in thinking, attention, perception and memory and, usually, drowsiness and reduced awareness of the environment. There are important differences between the reduced wakefulness before falling asleep and clouding in an organic state (Lipowski, 1967). Although the patient's awareness is *clouded*, he may be agitated and excitable rather than drowsy. Clouding may be seen in a wide variety of acute organic conditions, including drug and alcohol intoxication, head injury, meningeal irritation caused by infection and so on. *Drowsiness* as a descriptive term simply means diminished alertness and attention that is not under the patient's control.

The term *clouding* should be used for the psychopathological state: impairment of consciousness, slight drowsiness with or without agitation and difficulty with attention and concentration. This will usually occur with organic impairment of function, for instance with cerebral tumour, after head injury or with raised intracranial pressure. If it occurs in schizophrenia, it is as a part of the cognitive deficit that has been shown sometimes to occur in schizophrenia (Frith, 1979). It is suggested that in this condition there is an awareness of automatic processes that normally occur below the level of consciousness. These processes are concerned with the selection of appropriate interpretation of stimuli and of response.

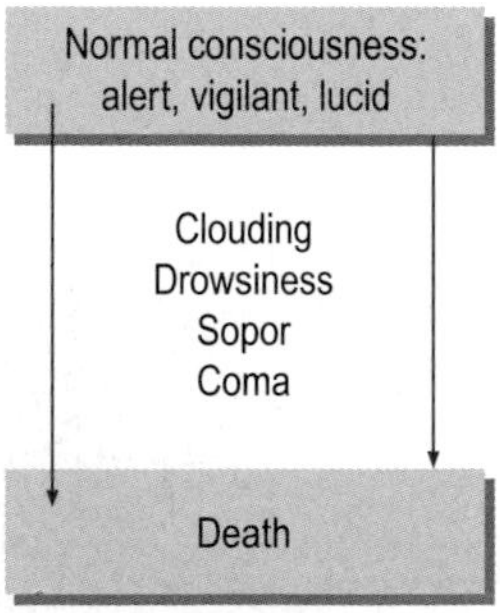

Figure 3.3 Levels or stages of diminished consciousness.

Drowsiness

As a persistent state, this is the next level of progressive impairment. The patient is 'awake' but will drift into 'sleep' if left without sensory stimulation. He is slow in actions, slurred in speech, sluggish in intention and sleepy on subjective description. There is an attempt at avoidance of painful stimuli. Reflexes, including coughing and swallowing, are present but reduced; muscle tone is also diminished.

In psychiatric practice, this is commonly seen following overdosage with drugs that have a central nervous system depressant effect (for example tricyclic antidepressants). From the psychiatrist's point of view, it means, of course, that interviewing the patient is impossible. These levels of diminished consciousness are quite non-specific and occur whatever the nature of the cause: head injury, tumour, epilepsy, infection, cerebrovascular disorder, metabolic disorder or toxic state.

Coma

Whereas the drowsy patient is conscious but lapsing at times into unconsciousness, in coma the patient is unconscious. In lighter states, with strong stimuli, he may be momentarily rousable. There are no verbal responses or responses to painful stimuli. The righting response of posture has been lost; reflexes and muscle tone are present but greatly reduced; breathing is slow, deep and rhythmic; the face and skin may be flushed.

In later stages, the patient is no longer rousable; he is deeply unconscious. Distinct stages of coma have identifiable physical signs ultimately culminating in brain death, but these are not discussed further in this book – they are *beyond* psychiatry (Conference of Medical Royal Colleges and their Faculties, 1976). Practical assessment of the depth and duration of impaired consciousness and coma has been quantified in the scale devised by Teasdale and Jennett (1974).

These stages are all those that occur progressively and quantitatively with lowering of consciousness. *Qualitative* variations are now discussed further.

Qualitative changes of consciousness

Various other organic disturbances in brain function are recognized. These are virtually always associated with some degree of quantitative impairment. The use of terminology in this whole area of discourse is, unfortunately, very muddled, with the same term sometimes having different meanings and similar phenomena being described by different words.

Delirium

Lipowski (1990) defines delirium as 'a transient organic mental syndrome of acute onset, characterized by global impairment of cognitive functions, a reduced level of consciousness, attentional abnormalities, increased or decreased psychomotor activity, and a disordered sleep–wake cycle'. The recognition that the term *delirium* should refer to a syndrome involving global disturbance was incorporated in the *Diagnostic and Statistical Manual of Mental Disorders*, fourth edition (DSM-IV; American Psychiatric Association, 1994). In DSM-IV, the term describes a disturbance of consciousness that is accompanied by a change in cognition that cannot be better accounted for by a pre-existing or evolving dementia. There is a reduction in the clarity of awareness of the environment. Similarly, the *ICD-10 Classification of Mental and Behavioural Disorders* (World Health Organization, 1992) uses the term *delirium* in a generic and global sense:

> “An etiologically nonspecific syndrome characterized by concurrent disturbances of consciousness and attention, perception, thinking, memory, psychomotor behaviour, emotion, and the sleep–wake cycle. *(p. 57)*

Fluctuation of consciousness

Fluctuation in conscious level is seen in various conditions. It occurs in health, in sleep and in fatigue. In patients with epilepsy, there is fluctuation in relation to fits and it may occur before, during or after the seizures. Alterations of conscious level are described with third-ventricle tumours associated with variations in intracranial pressure (Sim, 1974). In delirious states, there may be considerable diurnal fluctuation of consciousness. Characteristically, the patient becomes more disoriented, disturbed in mood and distracted perceptually with illusions and hallucinations in the late evening and shows greatest lucidity mid-morning. Such variation of conscious level is also described and observed with drugs, for instance mescaline, in which there may also be fluctuations of time sense.

Confusion

The concept of *confusion* was originally developed in France (confusion mentale) and later in Germany (Verwirrtheit) in the nineteenth century (Berrios, 1981). It is a term, imprecisely defined, referring to subjective symptoms and objective signs indicating loss of capacity for clear and coherent thought. It is purely a descriptive word and does not only apply to clouding of consciousness. When physicians, psychiatrists and nurses were asked what *confusion* meant, marked discordance was found. The term should be used only if clearly defined (Simpson, 1984). It occurs with impairment of consciousness in acute organic states and with disruption of thought processes due to brain damage in chronic organic states, but it is also seen in non-organic disturbance. Thus, confusion of thinking may occur as part of the picture in functional psychoses and also in association with powerful emotion in neurotic disorders. It should therefore be used simply to describe these disturbances of thought and not as a term pathognomonic of organic psychosyndromes.

To simplify, therefore, *confusion* of thinking can be described as occurring either when the individual describes his own thinking as being confused or when the external observer considers that the thought processes are disturbed and confused. Phenomenologically, therefore, it is simply a description of the patient's self-experience or the doctor's observation.

Other terms

Twilight state

Twilight state is a well-defined interruption of the continuity of consciousness (Sims *et al.*, 2000). It is usually an organic condition and occurs in the context of epilepsy, alcoholism (*mania à potu*), brain trauma and general paresis; it may also occur with dissociative states. It is characterized by (a) abrupt onset and end; (b) variable duration, from a few hours to several weeks; and (c) the occurrence of unexpected violent acts or emotional outbursts during otherwise normal, quiet behaviour (Lishman, 1997). If the term is reserved for these three features in combination, as a psychopathological entity, then it should be used whenever they concur, irrespective of cause.

The forensic implications of this condition are therefore important, and it has been used as a legal defence for violent behaviour for which the person had subsequent amnesia.

Consciousness may be markedly impaired or relatively normal between episodes. There may be associated dream-like states, delusions or hallucinations. It is sometimes associated with the temporal lobe seizures of epilepsy; it may occur with other organic states without epilepsy; similar behaviour may occur in apparent hysterical dissociation; and it is also described as an acute reaction to massive catastrophe. In the forensic context, it is important to demonstrate (a) the occurrence of similar episodes with inexplicable behaviour before the key happening and (b) other, objective evidence of physical or mental illness. The *Ganser state* (described with memory disorders in Chapter 5) is, in practice, a sort of twilight state in which the organic element is often dubious.

Mania à potu (pathological intoxication)

This is one type of twilight state specifically associated with alcoholism. It is important to distinguish this syndrome of acute pathological intoxication with alcohol from delirium tremens, which is a symptom of *withdrawal*. Keller (1977) has defined *mania à potu* as:

> “ an extraordinarily severe response to alcohol, especially to small amounts, marked by apparently senseless violent behaviour, usually followed by exhaustion, sleep and amnesia for the episode. Intoxication is apparently not always involved and for this reason *pathological reaction to alcohol* is the preferred term. The reaction is thought to be associated with exhaustion, great strain or hypoglycaemia, and to occur especially in people poorly defended against their own violent impulses.

Coid (1979) describes four components:

- the condition follows the consumption of a variable quantity of alcohol
- senseless, violent behaviour then ensues
- there is then prolonged sleep
- total or partial amnesia for the disturbed behaviour occurs.

Because there is often doubt as to whether intoxication really followed the consumption of an inappropriately small amount of alcohol, and because several of the other causal factors are diagnostic categories in their own right (hypoglycaemia, epilepsy), Coid would do away with the diagnostic category of *pathological* intoxication in the definition above, leaving only either acute drunkenness or another condition associated with alcohol intake.

Automatism

Automatism implies action taking place in the absence of consciousness. It has been defined by Fenwick (1990) as follows:

> "An automatism is an involuntary piece of behaviour over which an individual has no control. The behaviour itself is usually inappropriate to the circumstances, and may be out of character for the individual. It can be complex, co-ordinated, and apparently purposeful and directed, though lacking in judgement. Afterwards, the individual may have no recollection, or only partial and confused memory, for his actions.

Epileptic automatism may be defined as a state of clouding of consciousness that occurs during, or immediately after, a seizure and during which the individual retains control of posture and muscle tone and performs simple or complex movements and actions without being aware of what is happening (Fenton, 1975). It occurs as part of the clinical presentation of psychomotor epilepsy, most often arising from discharge in the temporal lobes. It was particularly common in those patients with chronic epilepsy who were resident in an epilepsy colony or a mental hospital.

An *aura* may be the first sign of an epileptic attack with temporal lobe automatism and may be manifested as abdominal sensations; feelings of confusion with thinking; sensations elsewhere in the body, especially the head; hallucinations or illusions (especially olfactory or gustatory); and motor abnormalities such as tonic contracture, masticatory movement, salivation or swallowing.

Behaviour during automatism is usually purposeful and often appropriate, for instance continuing to dry the dishes. Awareness of the environment is impaired; the patient appears to be only partly aware of being spoken to and does not reply appropriately. Initially, activity is diminished, with staring eyes and slumped posture; it then becomes stereotyped, with repetitive movements, lip smacking, fumbling and other actions. Finally, more complex purposeful behaviour occurs, such as walking about, making irrelevant utterances, removing clothing and so on. Sometimes, the patient may continue, during automatism, with whatever he was doing before, for example driving his car, although there is subsequent amnesia and the behaviour or speech at the time never appears entirely normal.

Violence is rare during automatism, and when it occurs it usually amounts to resisting restraint. However, automatism is, rarely, cited as an explanation for a person's violent and criminal action of which he is unaware afterwards. The legal definition then becomes 'The state of a person who though capable of action, is not conscious of what he is doing. . . . it means unconscious, involuntary action and it is a defence because the mind does not go with what is being done' (Kilmuir, 1963). Clearly, when such violent behaviour occurs automatism fulfils the criteria for the definition of *twilight state* as defined above (see p. 49).

Speech automatism occurs when there is utterance of identifiable words or phrases at some stage during the epileptic attack, for which the patient has no memory later. Phenomenologically, then, automatism is action without any knowledge of acting, and it is the latter claim that requires careful investigation.

Dream-like (oneiroid) state

This is an unsatisfactory term not clearly differentiated from twilight state or delirium. The patient is disoriented, confused and experiences elaborate hallucinations, usually visual. There is impairment of consciousness and marked emotional change, which may be terror or enjoyment of the hallucinatory experiences; there may also be auditory or tactile hallucinations. The patient may appear to be living in a dream world, and so-called *occupational delirium* could be mentioned in this context, for instance the ship's petty officer, admitted after a head injury at sea (associated with excess alcohol intake), who kept shouting 'Man the boats'.

It is important to look for other symptoms or organic states to make the important distinction between physical illness and a dissociative non-organic condition.

Stupor

'Stupor names a symptom complex whose central feature is a reduction in, or absence of, *relational* functions: that is, action and speech' (Berrios, 1996). It is distinct from coma and does not lie on a continuum from wakefulness to coma. This term should be reserved for the syndrome in which mutism and akinesis occur; that is, the inability to initiate speech or action in a patient who appears awake and even alert. It usually occurs with some degree of clouding of consciousness but does not refer solely to a diminished level. The patient may look ahead or his eyes may wander, but he appears to take nothing in.

This syndrome is characteristic of lesions in the area of the diencephalon and upper brainstem, and also the frontal lobe and basal ganglia, and the term *akinetic mutism* has sometimes been reserved by neurologists to describe a much more narrowly defined organic syndrome. A rare but specific condition involving the motor pathways in the ventral pons is called the *locked-in syndrome*, in which there is full alertness and feeling but aphonia and total muscle paralysis, apart from blinking, and jaw and eye movements (Plum and Posner, 1972). It is important to realize, however, that the symptoms of akinesis and mutism in a conscious patient also occur with schizophrenia, with affective psychoses (both depressive and manic) and in dissociative states.

The difference between psychogenic (so-called functional) and neurological (organic) causes of stupor can be clinically extremely perplexing. Psychiatric definitions have demanded that the condition occurs when there is 'a complete absence, in clear consciousness, of any voluntary movements' (Wing *et al.*, 1974). Of course, it is not possible at the time of observation to know whether consciousness is quite clear or not; and even for functional stupors, subsequent amnesia is common. A phenomenological definition of stupor must, therefore, exclude the state of consciousness of a mute patient, and diagnosis of stupor must then be followed by investigation of the differential diagnosis which includes both organic and non-organic conditions.

Sleep disorders

These are discussed in Chapter 4.

REFERENCES

Aggernaes A (1975) The concepts: disturbed state of consciousness and psychosis. *Acta Psychiatrica Scandinavica 51*, 119–33.

American Psychiatric Association (1994) *Diagnostic and Statistical Manual of Mental Disorders*, 4th edn. Washington: American Psychiatric Association.

Berrios GE (1981) Delirium and confusion in the 19th century: a conceptual history. *British Journal of Psychiatry 139*, 439–49.

Berrios GE (1996) *The History of Mental Symptoms: Descriptive Psychopathology Since the Nineteenth Century*. Cambridge: Cambridge University Press.

Bock GR and Marsh J (1993) *Experimental and Theoretical Studies of Consciousness*. Chichester: John Wiley.

Brodie BC (1854) *Psychological Inquiries: in a Series of Essays*. London: Longman, Brown, Green & Longman.

Coid J (1979) Mania à potu: a critical review of pathological intoxication. *Psychological Medicine 9*, 709–19.

Conference of Medical Royal Colleges and their Faculties (1976) Diagnosis of brain death. *British Medical Journal ii*, 1187–8.

Damasio A (1999) *The Feeling of What Happens: Body and Emotion in the Making of Consciousness*. London: William Heinemann.

Dennett D (1991) *Consciousness Explained*. London: Allen Lane.

Fenton GW (1975) Epilepsy and automatism. In Silverstone T and Barraclough B (eds) *Contemporary Psychiatry*, pp. 429–39. Ashford: Headley Brothers.

Fenwick P (1990) Automatism. In Bluglass R and Bowden P (eds) *Principles and Practice of Forensic Psychiatry*. Edinburgh: Churchill Livingstone.

Fish F (1967) *Clinical Psychopathology*. Bristol: John Wright.

Frith CD (1979) Consciousness, information processing and schizophrenia. *British Journal of Psychiatry 134*, 225–35.

Griesinger W (1868) In Zilboorg G and Henry GW (eds) (1941) *A History of Medical Psychology*. New York: WW Norton.

Jaspers K (1959) *General Psychopathology* (transl. Hoenig J and Hamilton MW, 1963). Manchester: Manchester University Press.

Keller M (1977) A lexicon of disablements related to alcohol consumption. In *Alcohol Related Disabilities*. Geneva: World Health Organization.

Kilmuir, Viscount (1963) Bratty V Attorney General for Northern Ireland AC 386; (1961) 3WLR965; (1961) 3 All ER 523.

Lipowski ZJ (1990) *Delirium: Acute Confusional States*. Oxford: Oxford University Press.

Lipowski ZS (1967) Delirium, clouding of consciousness and confusion. *Journal of Nervous Mental Diseases 145*, 227–55.

Lishman WA (1997) *Organic Psychiatry: the Psychological Consequences of Cerebral Disorder*, 3rd edn. Oxford: Blackwell Scientific.

Plum F and Posner JB (1972) *Diagnosis of Stupor and Coma*, 2nd edn. Philadelphia: Davis.

Scharfetter C (1980) *General Psychopathology: an Introduction*. Cambridge: Cambridge University Press.

Searle JR (1994) The problem of consciousness. In Revonsuo A and Kamppinen M (eds) *Consciousness in Philosophy and Cognitive Neuroscience*. Hillsdale: Lawrence Erlbaum Associates.

Sim M (1974) *Guide to Psychiatry*. Edinburgh: Churchill Livingstone.

Simpson CJ (1984) Doctors and nurses use of the word 'confused'. *British Journal of Psychiatry 145*, 441–3.

Sims A, Mundt C, Berner P and Barocka A (2000) Descriptive phenomenology. In Gelder MG, López-Ibor JJ and Andreasen N (eds) *New Oxford Textbook of Psychiatry*. Oxford: Oxford University Press.

Teasdale G and Jennett B (1974) Assessment of coma and impaired consciousness: a practical scale. *Lancet ii*, 81–4.

Wing JK, Cooper JE and Sartorius N (1974) *The Measurement and Classification of Psychiatric Symptoms*. Cambridge: Cambridge University Press.

World Health Organization (1992) *The ICD-10 Classification of Mental and Behavioural Disorders: Clinical Description and Diagnostic Guidelines*. Geneva: World Health Organization.

Attention, Concentration, Orientation and Sleep

4

"Come, Sleep! O Sleep, the certain knot of peace
The baiting – place of wit, the balm of woe,
The poor man's wealth, the prisoner's release,
Th' indifferent judge between the high and low.
Sir Philip Sidney (1554–1586), Astrophel and Stella, sonnet 39

The terms attention, concentration and orientation have often been used very loosely. It is suggested that their use is restricted to the following. *Attention* is the active or passive focusing of consciousness on an experience such as sensory inputs, motor programmes, memories or internal representations. The concept overlaps with the terms *alertness, awareness* and *responsiveness*. *Voluntary* attention occurs when the subject focuses his attention on an internal or external event; *involuntary* when the event attracts the subject's attention without his conscious effort. *Concentration* is only one aspect of attention. It involves focused or selective attention. Other aspects of attention include sustained attention or *vigilance*, divided attention and alternating attention. *Orientation* is an awareness of one's setting in time and place and of the realities of one's person and situation. It is not a discrete function but closely bound up with memory and the clarity or coherence of thought.

This chapter is concerned with cognitive function, but it is not limited to the functions that are disturbed by organic lesions and covers a wider field than just consciousness and its disorders.

ATTENTION, AWARENESS AND CONCENTRATION

Attention is a different function from consciousness, but it is dependent on it. Thus, variable degrees of attention are possible with full consciousness, but complete attention and concentration are impossible with diminished consciousness. A central feature of attention is its limited *capacity*. This refers to the fact that only so much cognitive processing activity can be carried out at any one time. Attentional capacity is usually tested by the digit span, and although it is a relatively stable feature of attention it is prone to influence by, for example, fatigue, depression and brain injury.

There are four other aspects of attention. *Focused* or *selective attention* refers to the capacity to highlight the one or two important stimuli or ideas being dealt with while suppressing awareness of competing distractions. This aspect of attention is usually referred to as *concentration*. Serial sevens is usually employed to assess this aspect of attention, and it requires focused attention as well as other cognitive processes. *Sustained attention* or *vigilance* involves the ability to maintain attentional activity over a period of time. It is usually measured by vigilance tests. *Divided attention* involves the ability to respond to more than one task at a time or to multiple elements within a task. *Alternating attention* allows for shifts in focus of attention and tasks (Lezak *et al.*, 2004; Table 4.1).

Automatic cognitive processes, that is, those that occur without intention, that are involuntary and that do not interfere with other ongoing activities, exist in parallel to those that require attentive processes (Kolb and Whishaw, 1996). These automatic processes allow for the effortless extraction of features of a perception in bottom-up fashion, whereas attentive processes allow for the top-down processing of information (Figure 4.1).

Alteration of the degree of attention

Attention is decreased in normal people in sleep, dreams, hypnotic states, fatigue and boredom. It may be pathologically decreased in organic states, usually with lowering of consciousness, for instance with head injury, acute toxic confusional states such as drug- and alcohol-induced conditions, epilepsy, raised intracranial pressure and brainstem lesions. In psychogenic states, attention may be altered, for example diminished in hysterical dissociation. Narrowing of attention is also prominent in depressive illness, in which the morbid mood state results in attention being limited to a restricted number of themes – mostly unhappy.

A severe deficit of attention is a prominent feature in the hyperkinetic disorders in childhood (World Health Organization, 1992) but also occur in adult life (see Chapter 3). Observation of the child's behaviour by adults such as parents or teachers concentrates on three aspects: inattention, impulsiveness and hyperactivity. Inattention is shown in that the child, most often a boy and usually aged between 3 and 10, fails to finish activities he starts, appears not to listen, is easily distracted, has difficulty in concentrating on any task requiring sustained attention and has difficulty sticking to a play activity.

Lack of attention and concentration denotes an inability to focus on an object in a purposeful way, implying weakening of the *determining tendency*. This is a feature of mania and hypomania and also occurs in organic states. These

Table 4.1 Aspects of attention

Aspect of attention	Definition
Focused attention	This is the capacity to highlight important stimuli while suppressing awareness of competing distractions
Sustained attention or vigilance	This refers to the capacity to maintain attentional activity over a prolonged period
Divided attention	This involves the ability to respond to more than one task at a time, including taking account of the multiple elements within a complex task
Alternating attention	This is the ability to shift attentional focus from task to task
Attentional capacity	This is the extent of the processing ability inherent in the attentional system; it is often considered to be a form of working memory

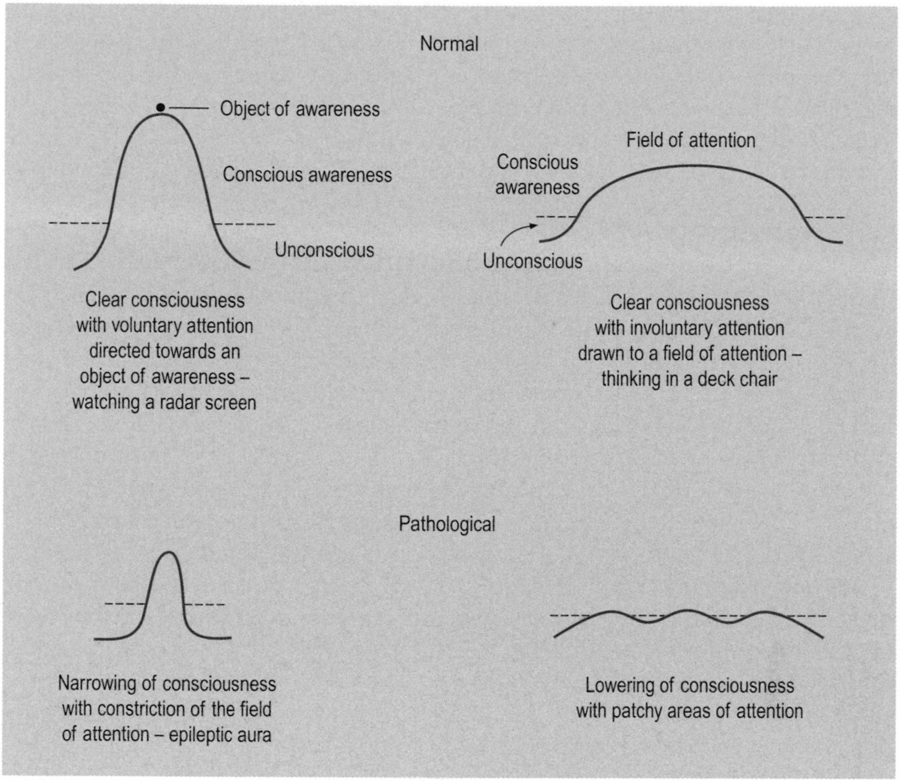

Figure 4.1 Variations in level of awareness.

features combine to show the symptoms of *distractibility*, which is prominent in mania and some organic states.

Narrowing of attention entails the ability of the subject to focus on a small part of the field of awareness and occurs in conditions in which involuntary attention is directed elsewhere – by hallucinations, by delusions or by strong emotion. After an unprofitable conversation with a patient with schizophrenia in which she repeatedly ignored questions, she said, 'I wish you would not interrupt when I am being given my instructions'.

Psychosis and attention

Alteration of external perception is associated with change of attention. For instance, as the auditory hallucinations gradually disappear with successful treatment in schizophrenia, the patient sometimes describes having to concentrate fully to hear the voices anymore, 'and even then they seem faint and unimportant'. In other situations, psychotic experiences occur only with lowered attention. Thus *functional hallucinations* (Chapter 7) tend to occur associated with a normal perception that is in the background and not the focus of attention: 'I only hear the voices when the water pipes are noisy'. A *visual pseudohallucination* (Chapter 7) may be removed by directly looking at it. However, *pareidolic illusions* become more clear-cut with a greater degree of attention.

Depressed mood is often associated with preoccupation with gloomy thoughts to such an extent that concentration and attention are impaired. In such a situation, misinterpretations of perception influenced by the mood state frequently arise. Every hearse is believed to be there to carry the patient to the graveyard, and a passing black car is noticed just sufficiently to be considered as strengthening this belief. Similarly, acute anxiety often results in diminished attention.

ORIENTATION

Orientation is the capacity of a person to gauge accurately time, space and person in his current setting. This enables him to make sense of, and be at home in, his environment. This is virtually the same faculty as intellectual grasp, in that various perceptual cues are used, and with correct sense of time and place the person is able to come to appropriate conclusions from his context. A man suffering from an advanced dementia was being interviewed by a doctor in the presence of a dozen student nurses, who were taking notes with pen and notebook. When asked where he was, he looked around the rather dingy hospital classroom and said, 'Well, we're waiting to see the doctor'. He had picked up certain clues that reminded him of a general practitioner's waiting room; he had totally missed the fact that all the nurses were in uniform, that they were taking notes and that he was being asked formal questions. He was disoriented in place and in person.

Orientation in *time* is labile and quite readily disturbed by rapt concentration, strong emotion or organic brain factors (for example alcoholic intoxication). Milder degrees of disorientation are shown by inaccuracy of more than half an hour for the time of day or duration of interview. More advanced states are demonstrated with incorrect day of the week, year or period of day. Yet further disturbance is shown when the season of the year is not known correctly.

Orientation in *space* is disturbed later in the disease process than time. A patient may be unable to find his way, especially in an area that is relatively new to him. It may take him an inordinate length of time to learn his way to the dining table in the ward after admission. Disorientation in time and place are, when clearly established, evidence of an organic mental state; they may be the earliest signs in a dementing process.

In disorientation for *person*, the patient fails to remember his own name. Loss of knowledge of the patient's own name and identity occurs at a very late stage of organic deterioration. Loss of intellectual grasp (apprehension) occurs in organic states as a form of disorientation, usually combined with other evidence of deterioration. Such a person cannot understand the context of his present situation and connects outside objects and events with himself. Disorientation may occur with a disturbance of consciousness, attention, perception or intelligence. In severe intellectual defect and severe disturbances of memory, orientation is impaired even when consciousness is clear (Scharfetter, 1980).

Disorientation

Orientation may fluctuate in some organic conditions, for example a patient with an acute toxic state associated with congestive cardiac failure was disoriented in time every evening but quite clear mentally in the morning.

Disorientation in time and loss of intellectual grasp (situational disorientation) usually occur first in a progressive illness; disorientation in place usually occurs later and, in person, last of all. Disorientation for one's own identity occurs at a later stage than for that of other people. An elderly woman who knew who she was and her previous status as a professor's wife, kept on referring to her daughter as 'that minx who comes in every time the doctor visits'.

Delusions that mimic disorientation

It is, of course, important to understand the phenomenological distinction between disorientation and a delusion that results in misinterpretation of place, of situation or of person. Disorientation is usually associated with other organic features, such as lowering of consciousness or disturbance of memory. Delusions of misorientation have the features of a delusion (Chapter 8): a person on the ward may believe himself to be in prison, and a visiting relative may be considered to be an interrogator from the Gestapo.

Dissociation and disorientation

Definite, undisputed disorientation is indicative of either an acute organic brain syndrome, if coupled with lowering of consciousness, or chronic organic deterioration. Hysterical dissociation may mimic this, however, with apparent disorientation. Careful examination of the mental state is likely to reveal suggestive discrepancies, for example disorientation for person may be much more marked than for time or may be bizarre to an excessive extent. A patient is described in the next chapter who lived in Birmingham, United Kingdom, but who found himself after a hysterical fugue in Montreal. Although apparently disoriented, he actually showed an abnormality of memory as part of a dissociative state.

SLEEP DISORDERS

Sleep, deep, satisfying and undisturbed, is conventionally associated with well-being and good health, as exemplified by the quotation with which this chapter begins; its absence or poor quality, equally, is held to account for disorder of mood and misery. There is a relationship between disturbed sleep and psychiatric disorder; mental illness may cause and manifest as sleep disturbance, disturbed sleep may precipitate psychiatric symptoms or the two may occur together but independently.

Frequently, we are dealing with normal phenomena about which some people complain, rather than definite pathology, although there are explicit sleep disorders. The loss of consciousness that occurs in sleep is quite different from that occurring in organic states, for example following head injury. The alerting and arousal mechanisms are suspended but can readily be brought into action, and the essential, psychological self remains in touch with meaningful stimuli. Many doctors have experienced the extraordinarily selective mechanism of waking instantly to the sound of the telephone when they are on duty, but excluding entirely other extraneous noises and the sound of a telephone in a neighbouring room when they are not on call. The sense of time is also preserved in sleep and can be demonstrated by the accuracy with which a person may wake at a predetermined hour.

The objective assessment of sleep is usually carried out electrophysiologically. Five stages of sleep can be identified (Rechtschaffen and Kales, 1968); see Table 4.2. Using an electroencephalogram and electromyogram of the external ocular muscles, the durations of the different stages are recorded. It has been shown that rapid eye movement (REM) sleep is associated with dreaming. With current neuroimaging techniques, it is possible, by showing changes in regional cerebral blood flow, to localize and represent visually altered activity, especially in the medial thalamus, associated with different stages of sleep from relaxed wakefulness to the slow-wave sleep of stage 4. There are also changes in the visual and auditory cortex, possibly associated with dreaming (Hofle *et al.*, 1997). When considering the quality and duration of sleep and its stages and whether this amounts to a symptom, it is important to take into account the age of the patient, any medication he may be taking and whether he has slept during the day. The subjective experience, as described by the patient, may be very different from the objective findings of observation and measurement. The psychiatrist should investigate the meaning of this discrepancy phenomenologically and conclude what are the consequences for diagnosis and treatment.

Insomnia

Insomnia implies subjective dissatisfaction with the duration or quality of sleep (Oswald, 1981); however, in many psychiatric conditions there is also objective disturbance of sleep. The individual may complain that the duration of sleep is too short; or that sleep feels broken, less refreshing or insufficiently deep; or that the pattern of sleep has changed for the worse. Insomnia is more common in women and in older people and is more often associated with a feeling of excessive mental arousal than bodily disorder. Causes of dissatisfaction include unrealistic expectations from the elderly that they will sleep for as long as when they were younger and from the sedentary that they will sleep as deeply as after exhausting physical activity. Complaints of sleeping poorly are extremely common, occurring in many psychiatric disorders, including depression,

Table 4.2 The five stages of sleep identified with an electroencephalogram

Stage	Characteristics
1	Low voltage, mixed frequency without REM
2	12 to 14 cycles per second with sleep spindles and K complexes on a background of low voltage and mixed frequency
3	Moderate amounts of high-amplitude, slow-wave activity
4	Large amounts of high-amplitude, slow-wave activity
REM sleep	Relatively low voltage, mixed frequency, with episodic REMs and low-amplitude electromyogram

REM, rapid eye movement.

generalized anxiety, panic and phobia, and hypochondriasis, and with personality disorders. They are among the most frequent symptoms in neurotic and affective disorders. Comparing those people with neuroses with a normal population, Jovanovic (1978) found that neurotic patients complained of more wakefulness in the first third of the night; they spent more time lying awake in bed, they awoke during the night more frequently, they spent a relatively shorter period in deep sleep and their sleep was more likely to be impaired by unfamiliar surroundings. Those with major depressive disorder suffer from disturbed sleep, in which they take longer to fall asleep and spend less time asleep because of periods of wakefulness during the night and early morning wakening.

Early insomnia, or difficulty in getting off to sleep, occurs in normal people who are aroused through anxiety or excitement. Their thoughts tend to dwell on the affect-laden experiences of the immediate past and also to rehearse ways of dealing with problems. Fatigue is experienced, but there is also a high level of arousal that prevents the necessary relaxation and withdrawal from perception that is required for sleeping. *Late insomnia* is particularly characteristic of the depressive phase of affective disorders. The patient may wake frequently in the night after getting off to sleep satisfactorily and thenceforward sleep only fitfully and lightly. Alternatively, he may wake early in the morning and be unable to get to sleep again. The important characteristic of depression is that there is a marked change in sleep rhythm from the normal pattern for that person. In depression, the early morning wakening is often associated with marked diurnality of mood, with the most severe feelings of despondency and retardation occurring in the early morning. There is also often a marked reduction of sleep requirement in mania.

The mean sleep requirement diminishes with increasing age. It is usually about 7 to 8 hours through the middle adult years but is markedly reduced from about 50 years onwards. With insomnia, intermediate stages of light, restless sleep occur. These are often associated with abnormal experience in the sleepy state, such as *hypnagogic* and *hypnopompic* hallucinations (Chapter 7). Pseudohallucinations also occur and vivid imagery that is difficult to distinguish from hallucination. Normally, passage into sleep is rapid and occurs passively rather than with active intention to sleep. Waking is also normally rapid, and the slowing of this process of becoming awake may be described as a symptom: a complaint of feeling drowsy and being incompetent and incoordinated for an excessive time on wakening – in other words, *sleep drunkenness*.

Hypersomnia

Hypersomnia may occur either as sleeping for significantly longer periods at night or episodes of somnolence during the day. These cases are more often seen by a neurologist than a psychiatrist and are reported only briefly here.

In the *Kleine–Levin syndrome*, attacks of somnolence occur, usually in young men. The condition is rare, and usually the attack ends spontaneously. The patient sleeps excessively by day and night but is rousable as from normal sleep. When awake, the patient eats voraciously (megaphagia) and may show marked irritability (Critchley, 1962).

Hypersomnia with sleep drunkenness is more common: the patient has difficulty in achieving complete wakefulness and exhibits confusion, disorientation, a readiness to return to sleep and motor incoordination (Lishman, 1997). Such patients may sleep for 17 hours or more and always require vigorous stimulation to wake them. The condition may persist throughout life.

In the *Pickwickian syndrome*, named after the fat boy of *The Pickwick Papers* (Dickens, 1837), profound daytime somnolence is associated with gross obesity and cyanosis due to hypoventilation. Breathing is periodic during sleep and somnolence, with apnoeic phases that may last for up to a minute.

Sustained drowsiness may occur with organic lesions of the midbrain or hypothalamus of various causes. Hunger, weight gain, excessive thirst and polyuria may also occur.

Hypersomnia may also occur as a psychogenic symptom. There may be a state amounting to hysterical stupor, and other conversion symptoms may be present. Other patients with neurotic disorders complain persistently of daytime somnolence and an inability to concentrate.

Somnambulism

Sleepwalking is more characteristic of children than adults and males more than females. Activity is usually confined to aimless wandering and purposeless repetitive behaviour for a few minutes. The sleepwalker may reply monosyllabically to questions, and there is little awareness of the environment, but injury is unusual. Frequently there is a family history, and enuresis is often associated. As sleepwalking occurs in deep sleep (stages 3 and 4), usually during the first third of the night, it is unlikely to be the acting out of dreams. It is not the same phenomenon as epileptic automatism, which may also result in a person, who is apparently asleep, getting up and walking around. It is important to establish the diagnosis in each case.

Night terrors also occur in deep sleep early in the night and often in the same individual who sleepwalks. Intense anxiety is manifested, the subject may shout and there is rapid pulse and respiration. Usually, there is complete amnesia for the experience on waking. It is not the same experience as a nightmare, because the latter is a type of dream, occurring in lighter states of sleep, and is remembered vividly if the person awakes immediately after the experience. Most children grow out of night terrors and sleepwalking.

Claims have been made that automatic, violent behaviour has taken place during a night terror. A person who commits a criminal act while asleep is not conscious of his actions and cannot be held legally responsible for them; the law calls this *sane automatism* (Fenwick, 1986). If the act, for instance homicide, is remembered by its perpetrator as following a chain of psychic events ('being chased by Japanese soldiers'), these images are most likely to have occurred in the context of a nightmare and the act therefore took place on waking from the dream and would be regarded as motivated. During the nightmare itself, sleep paralysis will prevent violent emotions being acted on. For the act to be convincingly ascribed to night terror, neither the act nor its antecedent storyline should be remembered and all the evidence should point to the individual being asleep at the time. Previous evidence of night terror and sleep activity is important for corroboration.

Narcolepsy

Narcoleptic attacks are short episodes of sleep (10 to 15 minutes) that occur irresistibly during the day; they usually begin during adolescence and persist throughout life. Narcolepsy is often associated with *cataplexy*, during which the subject falls down because of sudden loss of muscle tone provoked by strong emotion. *Hypnagogic hallucinations* and *sleep paralysis* may also occur, but less commonly, in this syndrome. There is usually no structural brain disease present. Hypnagogic hallucinations are usually auditory but may be visual or tactile. They occur between wakefulness and sleep, less commonly between sleep and wakening (hypopompic hallucination). Sleep paralysis is the inability to move during the period between wakefulness and sleep (in either direction).

DREAMS

How does phenomenology view dreams, their significance and their interpretation? First, phenomenology can be concerned only with what is conscious; it cannot comment on that which is unconscious, although it may infer the existence of unconscious mind. Second, the meaning belongs to the dreamer and not to an interpreter or theorist. This has implications for the way in which the phenomenological approach will be used in therapy.

Phenomenology can make a contribution to the understanding of dreaming. Both by introspecting and by taking accounts from patients while actually dreaming, we know that memory is accurate and detailed, sometimes very detailed. Also, the process of reasoning is faultless, both for when bizarre elements are intruded and also for when they are not. These bizarre elements, therefore, demonstrate neither deficient memory nor incapacity for rational thinking. They appear to be *premises* – the Euclidean 'let'. In dreaming, fantasy is permitted so that we say, or dream, let Bill Snooks (who lives in Heckmondwike and has never met the President of the United States of America) travel on a barge down the Amazon; what, then, would happen next? This phenomenological theory of dreams could be explored experimentally; if attitudes can be changed in consciousness by cognitive reprocessing, then the constructs that are used in dreams should also be capable of change.

Orthodox sleep (stages 1 to 4) and *paradoxical* sleep (REM sleep) have been distinguished from each other using sleep electroencephalographic tracings in human subjects (Oswald, 1980). Normal reflex activity occurs in the stages of orthodox sleep, but localized activity is seen in paradoxical sleep while other muscle actions are paralysed. REMs in paradoxical sleep are to some extent associated with dreaming. Nightmares are unpleasant dreams; often, the particular horror of a nightmare is that there is nothing the sufferer can do about the terrifying experience. Dreaming occurs in REM (paradoxical) sleep, and the transfixed sensation of the nightmare is an accurate representation of the sleep paralysis that occurs in that phase.

Dreams have been used to establish elaborate psychiatric theories concerning the origins of conflict; it is outside the scope of this book to enter into any discussion of this area. It is, of course, a topic that was extensively written about by Sigmund Freud (1976). More recently, the meaning of dreams has been explored empirically by Kramer *et al.* (1976). Dreams are remembered and described as a psychic event: nightmares (unpleasant dreams) are often complained of and may be a prominent symptom, for instance in depression. Dreams are highly complex experiences and, so far, have defied adequate analysis and explanation. However, certain characteristics can be described.

There is a loss of some of the structures of waking consciousness, thus there is a loss of self-awareness and awareness of the confines of one's own body. The margin between self and not-self becomes indefinite. The dreamer may dream of himself merging or transforming into someone else without contradiction. Time sense is also lost: there is no sense of progression of events but only immediate awareness of the present. Events occurring in the dream include those in which the dreamer himself is instrumental. There is often a loss of the sense of his having circumstances within his control, and there is also a loss of the physical and mental associations between the different parts of a whole experience. There are, therefore, gaps unaccounted for in space as well as in time and causation.

As well as the loss of temporal and spatial connections, there is a loss of the psychological associations between events. There is no progressive sequence of serial ideas or pictures. The dream is often like a group of short excerpts from very different films.

In addition to the loss of structure that is typical of the dreaming state, there are also elements that do not occur in the normal waking state. These are best called dream images, as they are not accurately delusions, hallucinations, false memories or other abnormalities of perception or ideation characteristic of being awake. These images are more vivid than fantasy and have a characteristic of immediacy and importance, so it is not surprising that from the beginnings of time people have acted on their dreams as if they were instructions.

To regard dreaming as a symptom rather than merely a remembered experience, it has to become invested with unpleasant affect. A patient may describe pleasant dreams if requested, but he does not usually complain of these as symptoms or ask for their removal. However, if the dream is associated with anxiety, terror, gloom or foreboding, and especially if the content or the theme is recurrent, it will be complained of and will indicate a prevailing affect; possibly, the areas of conflict that have precipitated the distress will be revealed in the content of the dream. Unpleasant dreams in which a part of the traumatic event is re-experienced are a diagnostic feature of post-traumatic stress disorder following major disaster or catastrophe.

HYPNOSIS

It has been suggested by Marcuse (1959) that we 'define hypnosis by what it does rather than by what it is'. At one extreme, hypnosis is considered to be a very different state of awareness from normal waking consciousness. At the other extreme, Merskey (1979) considers that 'the phenomena of hypnosis are identical with those of hysteria: they involve self-deception and the production of alternative symptoms or behaviour to solve a problem, even if not a conflict'. Merskey further goes on to propose as definition:

“Hypnosis is a manoeuvre in which the subject and hypnotist have an implicit agreement that certain events (e.g. paralysis, hallucinations, amnesias) will occur, either during a special procedure or later, in accordance with the hypnotist's instructions. Both try hard to put this agreement into effect and adopt appropriate behavioural rules and the subject uses mechanisms of denial to report on the events in accordance with the implicit agreement. This situation is used to implement various motives whether therapeutic or otherwise, on the part of both participants. There is no trance state, no detectable cerebral physiological change, and only such peripheral physiological responses as may be produced equally by non-hypnotic suggestions or other emotional changes.

Superficially, hypnosis appears to resemble sleep, but there are no electroencephalographic findings to distinguish hypnosis from other states of relaxed wakefulness. The trance in hypnosis is produced, therefore, in a waking state by one person on another using suggestion with compliance (Marcuse, 1959). It has been claimed to occur in non-human species, but this state cannot necessarily be considered identical with hypnosis. Hypnosis has been used for the control of pain, in the treatment of hyperemesis gravidarum, for various sexual difficulties and especially in the control of anxiety (Waxman, 1984).

The induction of hypnosis requires the implicit contract Merskey implies. The subject must be willing and cooperative; he or she relaxes and exercises imagination. The field of consciousness is narrowed to include only the instructions of the hypnotist. The subject relinquishes some degree of control to the hypnotist and accepts reality distortion. Following the successful induction of hypnosis, autohypnosis can become established. Marcuse considers the following to be the characteristics of a hypnotic state:

- the subject ceases to make his own plans
- attention is selectively directed, for example towards the voice of the hypnotist
- reality testing is diminished and distortions are accepted
- suggestibility is increased
- the hypnotized subject readily enacts unusual roles
- post-hypnotic amnesia is often present.

Suggestion, for the hypnotic subject, is straightforward and obvious; it does not imply gullibility or loss of will-power. It describes the emotion of trust occurring within the implicit relationship in which the subject accepts the hypnotist's statements, acts on his commands and denies evidence from his own senses that would contradict those statements.

A capacity for fantasy is necessary for hypnosis to take place. The relaxation that accompanies hypnosis may progress to normal sleeping, even during a hypnotic session. The alteration in conscious awareness occurring in hypnosis is similar to that in dissociative states but different from the fluctuations of conscious level occurring in organic psychosyndromes.

Suggestion has been used to produce many physical sequelae, for example blisters, alterations in pulse and blood pressure, levitation of an arm, opisthotonus, absence of pain sensation and so on. The psychological effects are equally variable and include alterations to perception, cognition, ideation, memory and affect. The subject enters a dramatically altered state in which he temporarily surrenders responsibility for his actions to the hypnotist. In his turn, the hypnotist retains the confidence of the subject only as long as he keeps within the limits of behaviour that the subject finds acceptable; beyond this, the subject will relinquish his dependent relationship and come out of the hypnotic state.

REFERENCES

Critchley M (1962) Periodic hypersomnia and megaphagia in adolescent males. *Brain 85*, 627–56.

Dickens C (1837) *The Posthumous Papers of the Pickwick Club*. London: Penguin.

Fenwick P (1986) Murdering while asleep. *British Medical Journal 293*, 574.

Freud S (1976) *The Interpretation of Dreams* (transl. Strachey J). Harmondsworth: Penguin.

Hofle N, Paus T, Reutens D, *et al*. (1997) Regional cerebral blood flow changes as a function of delta and spindle activity during slow wave sleep in humans. *Journal of Neurosciences 17*, 4800–8.

Jovanovic UJ (1978) Sleep profile and ultradian sleep periodicity in neurotic patients compared with the corresponding parameters in healthy human subjects. *Waking and Sleeping 2*, 47–55.

Kolb B and Whishaw IQ (1996) *Fundamentals of Human Neuropsychology*, 4th edn. Basingstoke: WH Freeman.

Kramer M, Hlasny R, Jacobs G and Roth T (1976) Do dreams have meaning? An empirical enquiry. *American Journal of Psychiatry 133*, 778–81.

Lezak MD, Howieson DB and Loring DW (2004) *Neuropsychological Assessment*, 4th edn. Oxford: Oxford University Press.

Lishman WA (1997) *Organic Psychiatry: the Psychological Consequences of Cerebral Disorder*, 3rd edn. Oxford: Blackwell Scientific.

Marcuse FL (1959) *Hypnosis: Fact and Fiction*. Harmondsworth: Penguin.

Merskey H (1979) *The Analysis of Hysteria*. London: Baillière Tindall.

Oswald I (1980) *Sleep*, 4th edn. Harmondsworth: Penguin.

Oswald I (1981) Assessment of insomnia. *British Medical Journal 283*, 874–5.

Rechtschaffen A and Kales A (1968) *A Manual of Standardized Terminology, Techniques and Scoring System for Sleep Stages of Human Subjects*. Bethesda: US Department of Health, Education, and Welfare.

Scharfetter C (1980) *General Psychopathology: an Introduction*. Cambridge: Cambridge University Press.

Waxman D (1984) *Psychological Influences and Illness: Hypnosis and Medicine*. London: Macmillan.

World Health Organization (1992) *The ICD-10 Classification of Mental and Behavioural Disorders: Clinical Description and Diagnostic Guidelines*. Geneva: World Health Organization.

Disturbance of Memory

5

> "Cans't thou not minister to a mind diseas'd;
> Pluck from the memory a rooted sorrow;
> Raze out the written troubles of the brain;
> And with some sweet oblivious antidote
> Cleanse the stuff'd bosom of that perilous stuff
> Which weighs upon the heart? *William Shakespeare (1606)*

Disturbance of memory is always of significance for the sufferer; sometimes, however, forgetting is equally important and is an active process, as in the quotation above. That memory disturbance was a specific feature following head injury and other conditions was recognized in neuropsychiatric writings in the mid-nineteenth century; Hughlings Jackson (1887) considered it to be an integral part of deterioration in organic mental functioning. The earliest detailed study of disordered memory from a psychological standpoint was by Ribot (1882). Korsakov (1890) subsequently described his eponymous condition, pointing out that gross disorder of memory may occur in patients in whom other intellectual functions and judgement are preserved.

MECHANISMS OF MEMORY

One of the major justifications for using psychopathology in the description of memory disturbance is that there exists no good analogue of memory in animals. Conventionally, disturbance of memory is described in terms of the length of time information has been retained. If one concentrates on the phenomenological aspects, the analysis of experience, it is in fact quite arbitrary to make a distinction between memory and perception as they are both stages in information processing (Weinman, 1981). Memory *storage* is organized in three ways.

SENSORY MEMORY

Sensory memory is the initial and early phase of memory. It holds large amounts of incoming information briefly. It is a selecting and recording system via which perceptions enter the memory system (Lezak *et al.*, 2004). Fleeting visual image, *iconic* memory, lasts up to 200 milliseconds, whereas auditory, *echoic* memory, lasts up to 2000 milliseconds. The information selected and recorded at this level needs to be further processed as short-term memory or it quickly decays and is lost.

SHORT-TERM MEMORY

Short-term memory is conceptualized as a limited capacity system that operates as a set of subsystems. While it is theoretically distinguishable from attention, in practice it is profitably equated with a simple span of attention limited to six or seven items and lasting 15 to 30 seconds unless the items are rehearsed. Baddeley and Hitch (1974) hypothesized a model of working memory comprising of a *central executive*, a *visuospatial scratch pad* and a *phonological loop*. In this system, the *central executive* is the attentional controller assisted by the *visuospatial scratch pad* that allows for the temporary storage and manipulation of visual and spatial information. The *phonological loop* holds memory traces of verbal information for a couple of seconds combined with subvocal rehearsal (Baddeley, 1986; Baddeley *et al.*, 2002).

LONG-TERM MEMORY

Long-term memory can be conceptualized into two long-term and retrieval systems: a *declarative* system, or *explicit* memory, that deals with facts and events and is available to consciousness for declaration, and a non-declarative or implicit system (Lezak *et al.*, 2004). The declarative system can be further divided into *semantic* (fact memory) and *episodic* (memory for specific autobiographical incidents) memory. In other words, *semantic memory* is the storage of information in pure form without specification of time or place ('*General Psychopathology* was written by Karl Jaspers'), whereas *episodic memory* refers to personally experienced events ('I had a kipper for breakfast today' (Baddeley, 1990). Long-term memory can hold information for between a few minutes to many decades, and the capacity is very large. Forgetting may be by loss of information or failure of retrieval. Normal forgetting rates are determined by such variables as personal meaningfulness of the material, conceptual style and age. Storage in, and also retrieval from, the long-term memory is impaired in the *dysmnestic syndromes*. Information is stored in reorganized and sometimes distorted form.

Description of the requirements for memory is chiefly referable to long-term memory and can be subdivided *phenomenologically* into the following five functions.

- *Registration* or *encoding* is the capacity to add new information to the memory store.
- *Retention* or *storage* is the ability to maintain knowledge that can subsequently be returned to consciousness.
- *Retrieval* is the capacity to access stored information from memory by recognition, recall or implicitly by demonstrating that a relevant task is performed more efficiently as a result of prior experience.
- *Recall* is the effortful retrieval of stored information into consciousness at a chosen moment. It requires an active, complex search process. It is influenced by *primacy* (first item) and *recency* (last item) effects. The question 'What is the capital of France?' requires the recall function.
- *Recognition* is the retrieval of stored information that depends on the identification of items previously learned and is based on either

remembering (effortful recollection) or *knowing* (familiarity-based recollection). In this process, a stimulus triggers awareness; remembering or knowing then takes place. The question 'Which of the following is the capital of France: Paris, Lille or Lyon?' tests the recognition function.

Abnormality of memory may occur in any of these areas. In other words, there can be impairment of encoding, impairment of storage or impairment of retrieval.

ORGANIC IMPAIRMENT OF MEMORY

Memory disturbances can be separated into those that are psychogenic, sometimes occurring in healthy people, and those that are organic, associated with disease of the brain. The latter are referred to as *organic* or *true* amnesia and can be described in terms of the different functions of memory.

Impairment of registration

In *anterograde amnesia*, the impairment is usually demonstrated in the failure of retrieval of information encountered after the onset of a clinical disorder. This impairment of retrieval may, of course, be due to problems at the registration (encoding) stage, particularly in patients with Korsakov's syndrome. There is evidence that these patients may have difficulty in spontaneously encoding the semantic features of information to a sufficient level at input, and this failure results in poor memory (Mayes, 2002). It is therefore problems in the initial analysis and representation of information and inability to select the salient semantic features of information that underlie impairment of registration. In a list-learning test situation, for example, the semantic features of the words, such as the fact that the words are derived from a list of the names of flowers, fails to assist the subject to encode the new information.

Impairment of retention

Retrograde amnesia is the loss of memory for events preceding the onset of brain injury. As with anterograde amnesia, the deficit is demonstrated in the impairment of retrieval, but it is thought to be due to impairment of retention (storage), particularly in cases of cerebral trauma. Usually, it is of short duration of less than 30 minutes. Typically, it follows a temporal gradient in which newer memories are more vulnerable to loss than older ones. There is a dissociation between anterograde and retrograde amnesia that suggests that the anatomical structures involved in new learning and retrieval of old memories are distinct.

Impairment of retrieval or recall

Retrieval is the capacity to access information from memory stores. Impairment of retrieval can be due to deficit in either *direct retrieval*, in which a cue elicits a memory automatically, or *strategic (indirect) retrieval*, in which a cue provokes a strategic search process that produces a result. In *direct retrieval*, the question 'Have you ever been in Lagos?' acts as a cue that elicits a memory automatically. In *strategic retrieval*, the question 'Who won the World Cup before the current champions?' instigates a strategic process that frames the memory problem, initiates the search and constrains it, guiding it towards local, proximal cues that then activate associative memory processes. The memory output is then monitored for accuracy and placed in a proper temporal–spatial context in relation to other memories (Gilboa and Moscovitch, 2002). *Direct retrieval* is thought to be dependent on medial temporal lobes and related structures, whereas *strategic retrieval* is dependent on the ventromedial prefrontal cortex. Confabulation is a good example of a condition that is a result of impairment of retrieval. It results from a faulty memory system creating faulty cue–memory associations, faulty search strategies and defective monitoring of faulty memories (Gilboa and Moscovitch, 2002).

Impairment of recognition

Recognition is the retrieval of stored information that depends on the identification of items previously learned. In episodic memory, that is, memory for events that includes the context, time, place and emotions associated with the event, recognition can take the form of either conscious recollection (*remembering*) or *knowing* based simply on a sense of familiarity. This is the so-called remember–know paradigm, and it proposes a dual-process memory system, one relying on conscious recollection and the other based on familiarity. In other words, the phenomenal experience that accompanies the recognition of a previously presented stimulus seems to take at least two forms. Recognition can occur when the stimulus evokes some specific experience in which the stimulus was previously involved, or alternatively the stimulus gives rise only to a feeling of familiarity without any recollective experience. A 'remember' response indicates that recognizing the stimulus brings back to mind some conscious recollection of its prior occurrence, whereas a 'know' response indicates that recognizing the stimulus is not accompanied by any conscious recollection of its prior occurrence (Dalla Barba, 1997; Tulving, 2000). Impairment of recognition has been described in Alzheimer's disease (Dalla Barba, 1997) and in schizophrenia (Drakeford *et al.*, 2006).

VARIOUS DISTURBANCES OF MEMORY

Déjà vu and related phenomena (identifying paramnesia)

Déjà vu is not primarily a memory disorder but a disturbance in which the associated feeling of familiarity that normally occurs with previously experienced events occurs with a novel event, that is, when the event is experienced for the first time. In *jamais vu*, an experience that the patient knows he has experienced before is not associated with the appropriate feeling of familiarity. The patient may also have the feeling that some important memory is about to be recalled, although it does not actually arrive.

Déjà vu and *jamais vu* are common, normal experiences but may also be significant symptoms of temporal lobe epilepsy or with cerebrovascular disorder (Lishman, 1998). An epileptic patient said, 'I feel that I've done something terribly wrong'. However, these experiences on their own, or associated only with vague feelings of depersonalization, should not be accepted as evidence of temporal lobe epilepsy, as these symptoms are also frequently experienced both in neurotic patients and in normal individuals.

Confabulation

This is a falsification of memory occurring in clear consciousness in association with an organically derived amnesia (Berlyne, 1972). It is probably best to conceive of confabulation as a loose term that covers a wide range of qualitatively different memory phenomena. The term is used to describe mild distortions of an actual memory, such as intrusions, embellishments, elaborations, paraphrasing or high false alarm rates on tests of anterograde amnesia. It can also refer to highly implausible bizarre descriptions of false realities such as claiming to be a space traveller temporarily resident on earth (Gilboa and Moscovitch, 2002; Box 5.1).

Bonhoeffer (1901) observed that confabulation in Korsakov's syndrome could take two forms.

- Confabulation of *embarrassment* was a direct result of the memory loss and depended for its presence on a certain attentiveness and activity. This form of confabulation is *momentary* in nature. The patient tries to cover an exposed memory gap by an *ad hoc* confabulated excuse relating to his recent behaviour. It does, therefore, reveal social awareness and some realization of the requirements of the situation in terms of social behaviour.
- In other cases, confabulation exceeded the needs of the memory impairment; the patient describes spontaneously adventurous experiences of a *fantastic* nature. The spontaneity is a key characteristic of this form of confabulation. Such memory disturbance may occur with organic deterioration following alcohol abuse and also in the 'organic amnesic syndrome, not induced by alcohol and other psychoactive substances' (ICD-10; World Health Organization, 1992), in which there is severe memory impairment, especially for recent memory; evidence for disorder of the brain; and absence of a defect in immediate recall, a disturbance of attention and consciousness, and global intellectual impairment.

Box 5.1 Characteristics of confabulation

- It is a falsely retrieved memory, often containing false details within its own context.
- The patient is unaware that he or she is confabulating and often unaware of the existence of memory deficit. In other words, confabulations are not intentionally produced.
- Patients may act on their confabulation, confirming their belief in the false memory.
- Confabulation is most apparent in autobiographical memory.

(From Gilboa and Moscovitch, 2002, with permission of John Wiley.)

Suggestibility is a prominent feature of the confabulating patient and was considered by Pick (1921) to be dependent on clouding of consciousness, weakened judgement and the interplay of fantasy; it may, in fact, closely resemble daydreams. The confabulating patient may produce mutually contradictory statements consecutively and not make any attempt to correct them. The material of confabulations has been likened to dreams (Scheid, 1934). It has also been explained, in terms of memory disturbance, that confabulations are actual experiences taken out of their chronological order (Van der Horst, 1932) and that the individual's wishes and interests guide confabulation in the same way as in dreams and fantasy.

It seems probable that confabulation is related to the normal mechanisms of recollection. All the owners of a certain model of car were asked by the police, as part of a large-scale murder hunt, what they were doing on a particular Monday about 9 months previously. To answer this question, an individual would have no recollection for that particular Monday, so he would recreate a typical programme with regular movements and times of appointments for a Monday from about that period. It would seem that the mechanism of *social confabulation* is of that order. To the question 'What did you do yesterday?', the confabulating patient mentioned above said, 'I pushed my baby in the pram down to the office to see my old workmates there'. This could indeed have happened 12 years previously when she had resigned her job in that office during her pregnancy. The *fantastic* type of confabulation is also directly associated with memory. Normally, one has a clear memory of which sensations and events were experienced and which were fantasized, yet with confabulation it is probable that distant fantasies are remembered, but it is not remembered that they were fantasy rather than reality. Such confabulations, like the *momentary* type, are autobiographical. The momentary or embarrassment confabulation is very much more common than the fantastic type and is a true memory displaced in its time context (Berlyne, 1972).

Fantastic confabulation with persecutory content has been described by Roth and Myers (1969). This is a falsification of memory occurring in clear consciousness. Typically, the patient believes others are stealing his money or trying to defraud him. Memory falsifications of various types occur in schizophrenia, depressive illness, dissocial personality disorder and obsessional states. The more definite, fantastic and gap-filling features of organic confabulations are always associated with memory defect.

Confabulation has been described in schizophrenia (Nathaniel-James and Frith, 1996). When subjects were presented with narratives and asked to recall them, confabulation was defined as recall of information not present in the narrative. Schizophrenic patients spontaneously rearranged the original narratives to produce new ideas. The amount of confabulation was found to be related to difficulties in suppressing inappropriate responses and formal thought disorder but unrelated to understanding of the gist or moral of the narratives. The examples given would suggest that the content of these confabulations is germane to the predominant thinking of the schizophrenic patient.

Perseveration

Perseveration usually occurs in association with disturbance of memory and is a sign of organic brain disease, perhaps the only pathognomonic sign in psychiatry. It occurs with clouding of consciousness and is particularly useful in distinguishing this from dissociative abnormalities (Allison, 1962). Perseveration is defined as a response that was appropriate to a first stimulus being given inappropriately to a second, different stimulus. This may be demonstrated verbally or in motor activity. The interviewer, while conducting the mental state examination, asks 'What is the capital of Italy?' – 'Rome', and then subsequently 'What is the object that you wear that tells you the time?' – 'Rome'. Alternatively, the examiner asks the patient to put his right hand on his left shoulder, which he does correctly, and then, on asking him to put his left hand on his left knee, he again puts his right hand on his left shoulder.

Memory disturbance and electroconvulsive therapy

There is always some memory disturbance immediately after electroconvulsive therapy (ECT). This includes impaired learning ability, defective retrieval and apparent loss of memory stores. Memories of events immediately preceding the treatments (retrograde amnesia) are most likely to be permanently lost, and more recent personal (autobiographical) memories are more vulnerable to loss than older ones (Cahill and Frith, 1995; Stern and Sackeim, 2002). There is also some anterograde amnesia, with difficulty in retention for some hours after treatment. Defect of memory for current events at about the time of the treatment may persist for a few weeks after completing a course of treatment. This memory disturbance is similar to other organic amnesic states.

The retention defect is related to the strength and duration of electrical stimulation and to the duration of the seizure. Confusion and memory disturbance have been claimed to be less after unilateral, non-dominant ECT. There is no evidence for loss of the ability to acquire new patterns of behaviour or execute established ones, even after a long course of ECT.

Using a very wide-ranging battery of tests to examine all areas of cognitive function, Weeks *et al.* (1981) state that ECT does not produce lasting impairment when used in everyday clinical circumstances. Memory functions tested included recall, releasing rate and recognition in the auditory–verbal and visuospatial modalities. Similarly, Fraser (1982) considers that the memory loss that follows ECT is minimal and can be detected for only a few hours after treatment. Unilateral placement of electrodes accelerates postictal recovery and shortens the duration of amnesia (Fraser, 1982). In summary, it seems now that ECT does not cause more than a temporary disturbance in memory (Williams *et al.*, 1990).

Memory impairment in schizophrenia

Earlier writers tended to play down the significance of intellectual impairment in schizophrenia (Bleuler, 1911; Kraepelin, 1913). However, decline in intellectual performance (Rogers, 1986), impairment with neuropsychological test batteries (Taylor and Abrams, 1984), sometimes a dementia-like syndrome (Liddle and Crow, 1984) and substantial memory deficit (Cutting, 1985; McKenna *et al.*, 1990) have been demonstrated. Memory deficit has been shown not to be restricted to patients with chronic schizophrenia.

Tamlyn *et al.* (1992) studied 60 schizophrenic patients encompassing all grades of severity and chronicity using detailed assessment of memory, including the Rivermead Behavioural Memory Test, and more general evaluation of intellectual and cognitive impairment. Memory deficit in schizophrenia was found to be prevalent throughout the range of severity and chronicity, often substantial in extent and impairing function and also disproportionate to global intellectual performance, which was sometimes only minimally impaired. This memory impairment could not readily be accounted for by lack of cooperation of the patient, poor attention or motivation, neuroleptic or anticholinergic medication or a physical procedure such as ECT. Memory deficit was significantly and positively associated with severity and chronicity of illness, with the presence of negative schizophrenic symptoms and with formal thought disorder (Chapter 9).

There are deficits in long-term memory, including evidence of impaired retrieval in both recall and recognition. There is also evidence of impaired short-term memory, demonstrated by deficit of forward digit span. Furthermore, there is evidence of impairment of working memory and semantic memory, but procedural or implicit memory is intact (McKenna *et al.*, 2002).

Temporal lobe disorder

It is useful to summarize at this stage the psychopathological phenomena of temporal lobe dysfunction: disturbance of memory, perception and affect. Disorder of memory includes the hippocampal defects of diminished storage and accelerated forgetting; *déjà vu* and *jamais vu* also occur, as described above (see p. 68). There may be altered states of consciousness such as a fugue, with impaired registration. *Panoramic recall*, in which the patient may feel that he is rapidly re-enacting long periods of his life, is also described.

Perceptual disturbances of temporal lobe dysfunction occur with all the major abnormalities described in Chapter 7 but especially visual, olfactory, gustatory, visceral and auditory hallucinations. Disturbance of speech and behaviour, as described in Chapter 3, may occur. Abnormal affect, associated with the attack but not accounted for by external circumstances, include rage, terror or marked suspiciousness.

AFFECTIVE DISORDER OF MEMORY

Memory is not only disturbed by organic damage to the brain itself; it is also affected by emotion. This is certainly true of normal, healthy people, in whom the affective state strongly influences the processes of remembering and forgetting. It is also true of those with affective and schizophrenic psychoses, and of neuroses and personality disorders. Depression is linked to self-reported memory problems. There is also substantial evidence of an association between depression and generic memory impairment. It is thought that mood disorder, such as depression, reduces the amount of cognitive processing resources available for a given task, and in the memory domain this is manifest as deficits in the elaboration, organization, encoding and retrieval of material into and out of memory (Dalgleish and Cox, 2002). There is also evidence of memory bias for affectively toned material, such that information that has an emotional valence is more likely to be retrieved if it is congruent with the individual's mood during retrieval. This *mood-congruent memory* effect is similar but distinct from *state-dependent memory*, which refers to the memory bias for material that is learned in a particular mood and is more easily retrieved if the individual is in that same mood during retrieval.

Selective forgetting

In normal forgetting, there is loss of or diminished access to recently acquired and stored information. Rates of forgetting are influenced by the personal meaningfulness of the information, the conceptual style of the individual, the degree of processing and elaboration of the information and age. It is likely that normal forgetting is determined by disuse or interference by more recently learned or more vivid material and underpinned by physiological or metabolic processes (Lezak *et al.*, 2004). The process of *selective forgetting*, however, suggests that forgetting is not simply down to errors in the filing and retrieval mechanism. Forgetting is subject to the influence of affect: which sensations are registered, what is retained and for how long and what information is available for recall. *Falsification* always occurs to some extent because of this interplay of memory with affect. This was commented on by Nietzsche (1889): 'Memory declares that I did this; I could not have done this, says my pride; and memory loses the day'. Certain *catastrophic events*, which lowered self-esteem, are remembered remarkably vividly, with the attendant feelings of embarrassment and humiliation. These, especially in those with anankastic or paranoid personality types, are prone to become affect-laden complexes associated with the development of emotional symptoms.

Usually, however, there is a tendency for painful and embarrassing events to be obliterated and distorted by memory in time. The event itself may be accurately remembered, but the craven attitude of the subject may be distorted so that he remembers his part in the drama to be one of unadulterated heroism. The selective nature of forgetting is produced as evidence of the existence of the *unconscious*. It is important evidence for the psychodynamic concept of *ego defence mechanisms*. Descriptive psychopathology neither explains phenomena in terms of defence mechanisms nor denies their existence. As the theoretical supposition is that they are unconscious functions of the self, description can be made only when they are manifested in conscious experience or behaviour. We remember pleasant experiences better than unpleasant ones and unpleasant better than emotionally neutral experiences.

Falsification of memory

In *pseudologia fantastica* – fluent plausible lying – the untruthful statements are often grandiose and extreme. Questions are answered with fluency, and the story appears to be believed implicitly by the pseudologic himself. This usually occurs with an associated personality disorder of histrionic or dissocial type, and often when the individual is experiencing a major life crisis such as facing criminal proceedings. Often, the picture is of a very isolated person, without family or friends, drifting into the accident and emergency department of a large hospital in a strange city late at night, with stories of his own exploits and importance and the unfortunate vicissitudes he has experienced. There is overlap with the so-called Münchausen's syndrome (Chapter 15).

With personality disorders and also with affective disorders, especially at times of heightened emotion, memory is falsified and distorted and events and circumstances are misrepresented. The advice of doctors may be grossly misconstrued. An ophthalmic surgeon examined a depressed patient's eyes and informed her that her visual acuity was satisfactory and no treatment was required. She reported this to her psychiatrist; her 'eyesight would be bad for evermore and the surgeon has told me that nothing can be done about it'.

Memory impairment is a regular feature of organic states. When there is a defect of reasoning and judgement, falsification occurs. So the grandiose delusions and memory disturbance of *general paresis* may result in falsification and distortion of events remembered. Similarly, confabulation as in the Korsakov state is associated with falsification.

In schizophrenia, remembered circumstances often take on a new meaning: 'I remember last week three red cars following me at the traffic lights in Stafford. . . .I realized that I have become involved in politics'. This was stated by a patient who had quite suddenly come to believe that all her actions were being observed and, subsequently, her behaviour controlled. Memory is accurate, but its significance is distorted. A distinction should be made between delusional memories, in which the primary delusional experience is described as a memory, and delusional retrospective falsification. This is a backdating of delusion to a time before the patient was ill, based on an admixture of remembered true events and delusional interpretations of the meaning of those events. A person who believed that she was 'much more of a genius than Albert Einstein' considered that her powers to heal people had started as a child, because her hands had sometimes been shiny.

Inaccuracy of recall is sometimes called *paramnesia*. As well as occurring in the normal state and in personality disorders, it is a prominent feature of affective disturbances. A woman with depressive illness falsified the events of her life: 'I am not married. My children are illegitimate. We do not own this house. We are bankrupt' (see Chapter 18). All these statements were untrue, and the falsification of her memory occurred in response to her severe depressive mood. Memory itself was accurate, but on remonstrating on any particular point of fact, further depressive explanations of events would be given. For instance, the marriage licence was described as a forgery, and complicated legal explanations were given as to why the house did not belong to her and her husband. In mania, unacceptable events or opinions may be brushed aside as not having occurred and unrealistic goals pursued as though there were nothing to prevent their attainment.

While a clear-cut, organic disturbance of retention occurs in dementia, more subtle, and not necessarily pathological, disturbances of memory are found as part of the normal ageing process. Ribot's law of memory regression (1882) formulates the finding that memory for recent events is lost before memory for more remote events. Earlier periods of life are remembered best, and one reason for the predilection for reminiscence of an old person is the sense of security this engenders in talking about facts that are well remembered rather than discussing areas in which he is afraid that his defective memory will let him down so that he makes a fool of himself. As dementia progresses, a multilingual person will forget the later-attained foreign languages to a much greater extent than his original mother tongue. More recently acquired words are lost first, so that a word such as 'wireless' might be used rather than 'radio'.

Psychogenic disturbance of memory

Cryptamnesia is the experience of not remembering that one is remembering! A person makes a witty remark, or writes a haunting melody, without realizing that he is quoting (plagiarizing) rather than producing something original. The process is seen when words or phrases come into popular usage for a few months or years by some process of mass spread, in which people using the expression believe they are introducing a new idea.

Generally, unpleasant and uncomfortable experiences are not remembered accurately or completely – 'forgetting of the disagreeable'. This is a defect of recall that can be seen as a successful *defence mechanism*; it helps to maintain the integrity of the person. However, in the *affect of hopelessness*, reactivation of memories of previous failures is a frequent reason for perpetuating neurotic thinking and behaviour (Engel, 1968; Chapter 22). Psychogenic amnesia may appear without any organic disease present, but the presentation of organic brain disease is always modified by psychogenic factors (Pratt, 1977).

Misnaming objects and momentary loss of memory for words in healthy subjects may result from faulty retrieval from short- and long-term memory stores rather than from the psychoanalytic explanation of repression. Such errors may be categorized as *acoustic* or *semantic*, acoustic tending to occur in short-term stores up to 30 seconds and semantic in long-term stores after more than 5 minutes (Shallice and McGill, 1977).

Dissociative (hysterical) fugue

The symptoms pertaining to dissociative (conversion) disorders (hysteria) in the *International Classification of Diseases* (World Health Organization, 1992) are of two types: conversion and dissociation. In dissociation, there is a narrowing of the field of consciousness, with subsequent amnesia for the episode. In many ways, dissociative symptoms represent a layman's impression of 'madness'. In dissociative (hysterical) fugue states, there is narrowing of consciousness, wandering away from normal surroundings and subsequent amnesia. The person appears to be in good contact with his environment and usually behaves appropriately, maintaining basic self-care, although he sometimes displays disinhibition. There is quite often loss of identity or assumption of another, false identity. The duration of the episode can be very variable, from a few hours to several weeks, and the subject may travel considerable distances. A citizen of Birmingham, United Kingdom, described a state in which he 'came to' in a city he did not recognize and where people were speaking French. As he walked about the streets, he found he was near an airport terminal and, to his surprise, he discovered that he was in Montreal. Germane to his adventure was the history of a catastrophic row and the breakdown of his marriage just before he took off. Thus the features of dissociative fugue are dissociative amnesia, purposeful travel beyond the usual everyday range and maintenance of basic self-care (World Health Organization, 1992).

Ganser state

The original paper by Ganser (1898) has been much misunderstood. In it, he described four criminals who showed the following symptoms.

- *Vorbeigehen* ('to pass by') or *approximate answers*, described by Ganser thus: 'In the choice of answers the patient appears to pass over deliberately the indicated correct answer and to select a false one, which any child could recognize as such'.
- Clouding of consciousness with disorientation.
- 'Hysterical' stigmata.
- Recent history of head injury, typhus or severe emotional stress.
- 'Hallucinations', auditory and visual (from his description, they are more like pseudohallucinations).
- Amnesia for the period during which the above symptoms were manifest.

The Ganser state is very rarely seen in English prisons but, when it does occur, it is more likely in those awaiting trial than those already sentenced (Enoch, 1990).

There has been considerable argument as to whether this condition is primarily hysterical or an organic psychosis, with different authors supporting each contention (Latcham *et al.*, 1978). A case that illustrated both the hysterical (dissociative) and organic elements was that of a female university student, aged 20 years, who experienced head injury with concussion when in Italy. Her premorbid personality was markedly histrionic and theatrical and, at the age of 13 years, she had developed a hysterical inability to walk for a few weeks. After transfer from the Italian hospital to Britain, she demonstrated approximate answers thus:

Question: 'What is the capital of Italy?'
Answer: 'Naples.'
Question: 'How many legs has a centipede?'
Answer: 'Seven.'

This was accompanied by interference in the treatment of other patients, flirtatious behaviour towards male staff, lability of mood and a facetious manner. On serial testing of intellectual function on the Wechsler Adult Intelligence Scale, initial testing 12 days after head injury had to be abandoned; after 1 month, there was marked impairment, worse for *performance* than for *verbal* items. Intellectual function had eventually returned to her premorbid, superior level by 9 months. Whitlock (1967) considers the distinction between the Ganser state and pseudodementia to lie in disturbed consciousness, present in the former and not the latter. However, sometimes clouding of consciousness in an organic state cannot be distinguished from the altered mental state of dissociative disorder in the absence of other organic signs.

Enoch and Trethowan (1979) have regarded the four main features of Ganser's syndrome as:

- approximate answers
- clouding of consciousness
- somatic conversion features
- pseudohallucinations (not always present).

It should be noted that approximate answers are not the random inaccuracies of the quick guess but responses that appear deliberately just to have missed the correct answer. These authors regard the syndrome as a hysterical dissociative reaction and have pointed out the similarity of features with those exhibited by normal people asked to simulate mental disorder, the difference being that the Ganser subjects were subsequently amnesic for their abnormal behaviour. Ungvari and Mullen (1997) have classified Ganser's syndrome with the controversial group of reactive psychoses so that a stressful life event is the usual predisposing factor.

Multiple personality

This is described in more detail in Chapter 13. There is considerable doubt about the authenticity of multiple personality disorder (F44.81, ICD-10; World Health Organization, 1992), often being considered iatrogenic, created by the medical interest shown in the case, or simulated, used by the patient during criminal proceedings. There is a lack of information on the reliability of diagnosis, the prevalence or the role of selection bias (Fahy, 1988). However, in supposed *bona fide* cases, there is often complete amnesia subsequently for one or more of the personalities: one personality may claim not to know of the existence of another personality (with a different name) within the same person.

Recovered memory and false memory syndrome

This is currently one of the most hotly debated issues in psychiatry and clinical psychology. Those working with survivors of traumatic experiences noted in their patients the recovery of additional memories during clinical sessions after apparent psychogenic amnesia for a long time, sometimes decades. Recovered memory has been particularly associated with the return of memory for childhood sexual abuse. Brewin (1996) reviews the evidence for such events being 'forgotten' and then recalled after many years and the mechanisms that may account for this amnesia. He concludes that memories may be recovered from total amnesia and they may sometimes be essentially accurate. Equally, such 'memories' may sometimes be inaccurate in whole or in part.

The term *false memory syndrome* came into use in 1992, when the False Memory Syndrome Foundation was set up to represent the interests of parents who had been accused of abusing their children sexually. In the opinion of Merskey (1998), sufferers from false memory syndrome are typically female and are usually participating in some type of psychotherapy. They report sexual abuse in childhood, which it is claimed has been forgotten and recovered only in adult life, having been repressed from 8 to 40 years. It is considered that these 'memories' have been implanted during therapy by a process of suggestion similar to that thought to occur in multiple personality disorder. Another situation in which false memories have been thought to develop has been in nursery daycare, when caregivers have been subjected to grave and bizarre accusations.

These two opposing viewpoints are held with great fervour by their protagonists. It is probable that childhood trauma is sometimes only recovered in adult life, although this is not likely to be frequent. It is also probable that on occasions adults may 'remember' as trauma events that may not have happened to them.

REFERENCES

Allison RS (1962) *The Senile Brain*. London: Edward Arnold.

Baddeley AD (1986) *Working Memory*. Oxford: Clarendon.

Baddeley AD (1990) *Human Memory: Theory and Practice*. Hove: Erlbaum.

Baddeley AD (2002) The psychology of memory. In Baddeley AD, Kopelman MD and Wilson BA (eds) *The Handbook of Memory Disorders*, pp. 3–15. Chichester: John Wiley.

Baddeley AD and Hitch G (1974) Working memory. In Bower GA (ed.) *Recent Advances in Learning and Motivation*, vol. 8, pp. 47–89. New York: Academic Press.

Berlyne N (1972) Confabulation. *British Journal of Psychiatry 120*, 31–9.

Bleuler E (1911) *Dementia Praecox or the Group of Schizophrenias* (transl. Zinkin J, 1950). New York: International Universities Press.

Bonhoeffer K (1901) *Die akuten Geisteskrankheiten der Gewohnheitstrinker*. Jena: Gustav Fischer. Cited by Berlyne N (1972).

Brewin CR (1996) Scientific status of recovered memories. *British Journal of Psychiatry 169*, 131–4.

Cahill C and Frith C (1995) Memory following electroconvulsive therapy. In Baddeley AD, Wilson BA and Watts FN (eds) *The Handbook of Memory Disorders*. Chichester: John Wiley.

Cutting JC (1985) *The Psychology of Schizophrenia*. Edinburgh: Churchill Livingstone.

Dalgleish T and Cox SG (2002) Memory and emotional disorder. In Baddeley AD, Kopelman MD and Wilson BA (eds) *The Handbook of Memory Disorders*, 2nd edn. Chichester: John Wiley.

Dalla Barba G (1997) Recognition memory and recollective experience in Alzheimer's disease. *Memory 5*, 657–72.

Drakeford JL, Edelstyn NM, Oyebode F, *et al.* (2006) Auditory recognition memory, conscious recollection, and executive function in patients with schizophrenia. *Psychopathology 39*, 199–208.

Engel GL (1968) A life setting conducive to illness: the giving up-given up complex. *Annals of Internal Medicine 69*, 293–300.

Enoch MD (1990) Hysteria, malingering, pseudologia fantastica, Ganser syndrome, prison psychosis and Münchausen's syndrome. In Bluglass R and Bowden P (eds) *Principles and Practice of Forensic Psychiatry*. Edinburgh: Churchill Livingstone.

Enoch MD and Trethowan WH (1979) *Uncommon Psychiatric Syndromes*. Bristol: John Wright.

Fahy TA (1988) The diagnosis of multiple personality disorder: a critical review. *British Journal of Psychiatry 153*, 597–606.

Fraser M (1982) *ECT: a Clinical Guide*. Chichester: John Wiley.

Ganser SJM (1898) A peculiar hysterical state. *Archiv fuer Psychiatrie und Nervenkrankheiten 30*, 633 (transl. Schorer CE, 1965, *British Journal of Criminology 5*, 120–6).

Gilboa A and Moscovitch M (2002) Cognitive neuroscience of confabulation. In Baddeley AD, Kopelman MD and Wilson BA (eds) *The Handbook of Memory Disorders*, 2nd edn. Chichester: John Wiley.

Jackson JH (1887) Remarks on evolution and dissolution of the nervous system. In Taylor J (ed.) (1931) *Selected Writings of John Hughlings Jackson*, vol. 2. London: Hodder & Stoughton.

Korsakov SS (1890) Eine psych. Storung combiniert mit multipler Neuritis. *Allgemeine Zeitschrift fuer Psychiatrie 46*.

Kraepelin E (1913) *Dementia Praecox and Paraphrenia* (transl. Barclay RM, 1919). Edinburgh: Livingstone.

Latcham RW, White AC and Sims ACP (1978) Ganser syndrome: the aetiological argument. *Journal of Neurology, Neurosurgery and Psychiatry 41*, 851–4.

Lezak MD, Howieson DB and Loring DW (2004) *Neuropsychological Assessment*, 4th edn. Oxford: Oxford University Press.

Liddle PF and Crow TS (1984) Age disorientation in schizophrenia is associated with global intellectual impairment. *British Journal of Psychiatry 144*, 193–9.

Lishman WA (1998) *Organic Psychiatry: the Psychological Consequences of Cerebral Disorder*, 3rd edn. Oxford: Blackwell Scientific.

Mayes AR (2002) Anterograde amnesia. In Baddeley AD, Kopelman MD and Wilson BA (eds) *The Handbook of Memory Disorders*, 2nd edn. Chichester: John Wiley.

McKenna PJ, Tamlyn D, Lund CE, Mortimer AM, Hammond S and Baddeley AD (1990) Amnesic syndrome in schizophrenia. *Psychological Medicine 20*, 967–72.

McKenna PJ, Ornstein T and Baddeley AD (2002) Schizophrenia. In Baddeley AD, Kopelman MD and Wilson BA (eds) *The Handbook of Memory Disorders*, 2nd edn. Chichester: John Wiley.

Merskey H (1998) Prevention and management of false memory syndrome. *Advances in Psychiatric Treatment 4*, 253–62.

Nathaniel-James DA and Frith CD (1996) Confabulation in schizophrenia: evidence of a new form? *Psychological Medicine 26*, 391–9.

Nietzsche F (1889) *Twilight of the Idols* (transl. Hollingdale RS, 1968). Harmondsworth: Penguin.

Pick A (1921) Neues Zur Psychologie der Konfabulation Msschr. *Psychiatria et Neurologia 49*, 314–21. Cited by Berlyne N (1972).

Pratt RTC (1977) Psychogenic loss of memory. In Whitty CWM and Zangwill OL (eds) *Amnesia: Clinical, Psychological and Medicolegal Aspects*. London: Butterworth.

Ribot E (1882) *Diseases of Memory: an Essay in the Positive Psychology*. London: Kegal Paul, Trench.

Rogers D (1986) Cognitive disturbances: real or apparent? *Psychiatry in Practice 5*, 6–8.

Roth M and Myers DH (1969) The diagnosis of dementia. *British Journal of Hospital Medicine 2*, 705–17.

Scheid W (1934) Zur Pathopsychologie des Korsakow Syndroms. *Zeitschrift fuer Neurologie und Psychiatrie 151*, 346–69. Cited by Berlyne N (1972).

Shakespeare W (1606) Macbeth V, iii, 41–6.

Shallice T and McGill J (1977) Attention and purpose. In Requin J and Bertelson P (eds) *The Origins of Mixed Errors*. New York: Academic Press.

Stern Y and Sackeim HA (2002) Neuropsychiatric aspects of memory and amnesia. In Yudofsky SC and Hales RE (eds) *American Psychiatric Publishing Textbook of Neuropsychiatry and Clinical Neurosciences*, 4th edn. Washington: American Psychiatric Publishing.

Tamlyn D, McKenna PJ, Mortimer AM, Lund CE, Hammond S and Baddeley AD (1992) Memory impairment in schizophrenia: its extent, affiliations and neuropsychological character. *Psychological Medicine 22*, 101–15.

Taylor MA and Abrams R (1984) Cognitive impairment in schizophrenia. *American Journal of Psychiatry 141*, 196–201.

Tulving E (2000) Concepts of memory. In Tulving E and Craik FIM (eds) *Oxford Handbook of Memory*. Oxford: Oxford University Press.

Ungvari GS and Mullen PE (1997) Reactive psychoses. In Bhugra D and Munro A (eds) *Troublesome Disguises: Underdiagnosed Psychiatric Syndromes*. Oxford: Blackwell Science.

Van der Horst L (1932) Ueber die Psychologie des Korsakowsyndroms. *Monatsschrift fuer Psychiatrie und Neurologie 83*, 65–84.

Weeks D, Freeman CPL and Kendell RE (1981) Does ECT produce enduring cognitive deficits? In Palmer RL (ed.) *Electroconvulsive Therapy. An Appraisal*. Oxford: Oxford University Press.

Weinman J (1981) *An Outline of Psychology as Applied to Medicine*. Bristol: John Wright.

Whitlock FA (1967) The Ganser syndrome. *British Journal of Psychiatry 113*, 19–29.

Williams KM, Iacono WI, Remick RA and Greenwood P (1990) Dichotic perception and memory following electroconvulsive treatment for depression. *British Journal of Psychiatry 157*, 366–72.

World Health Organization (1992) *The ICD-10 Classification of Mental and Behavioural Disorders: Clinical Description and Diagnostic Guidelines*. Geneva: World Health Organization.

Section Three

AWARENESS OF REALITY: TIME, PERCEPTION AND JUDGEMENT

Disorder of Time

6

“There are men I know who can wake themselves at any time to the minute. They say to themselves literally, as they lay their heads upon the pillow, ‘Four-thirty’, ‘Four-forty-five’, or ‘Five-fifteen,’ as the case may be; and as the clock strikes they open their eyes. It is very wonderful this; the more one dwells upon it, the greater the mystery grows. Some Ego within us, acting quite independently of our conscious self, must be capable of counting the hours while we sleep. Unaided by clock or sun, or any other medium known to our five senses, it keeps watch through the darkness. At the exact moment it whispers ‘time!’ and we awake. The work of an old riverside fellow I once talked with called him to be out of bed each morning half an hour before high tide. He told me that never once had he overslept himself by a minute. Latterly, he never even troubled to work out the tide for himself. He would lie down tired, and sleep a dreamless sleep, and each morning at a different hour this ghostly watchman, true as the tide itself would silently call him. *Jerome K. Jerome (1900)*

“Space and time are always present in sensory processes. They are not primary objects themselves but they invest all objectivity. Kant calls them ‘forms of intuition’. They are universal. No sensation, no sensible object, no image is exempt from them. Everything in the world that is presented to us comes to us in space and time and we experience it only in these terms. *Jaspers (1959)*

This is how Jaspers, the philosopher, looks at human subjective experience. He continues, ‘If we want to bring these primary things home to ourselves in some neat phraseology we may say that they both represent the sundered existence of Being, separated from itself. Space is extended being (the side-by-side) and time is sequential being (the one-after-the-other)’. Sense of time is clearly very central to the concept of self and its relationship with the outside world. Disturbance of sense of time or time-related disorder, although not always of great importance to the functioning of the organism, is a sensitive indicator that something is going wrong in the mechanisms of the individual. Sense of time and time-related disorders of biological rhythm will be considered separately in this chapter. There is no widely agreed classification of disorders of time. However, it is possible to divide the disorders of time into two broad categories: disorder of objective time and disorder of subjective time (Box 6.1).

Objective (Clock) time and subjective (Personal) time

An important distinction is that between *objective (clock) time* and *subjective (personal) time*. Objective time – chronological, physical or historical time – is

Box 6.1 Classification of disorders of time

Disorder of objective time
- Disorder of knowledge of time:
  disorientation in time
  age disorientation
- Disorder of duration of time
- Disorder of chronology (temporal order)

Disorder of subjective time
- Disorder of flow of time
- Disorder of direction of time
- Disorder of uniqueness of time
- Disorder of quality of time

quantitative and independent of the self. It depends on accurate measurement and is objective to the degree that it is shared with others and verifiable. Subjective time is the inner, subjective experience of time. Aspects of both kinds of time may be affected by psychiatric illnesses. Objective time may be altered so that the knowledge of time, that is, the orientation to time including age disorientation and appreciation of time duration and of chronology may be adversely affected. Subjective time may be altered so that the experience of time duration, flow of time, meaning of time, uniqueness of time and succession of time may be affected.

Biological rhythms and time

Although our units of time are to some extent arbitrary, natural and biological time operates within definite periods. The four periods that have the most relevance to mental illness are circadian rhythms (about 24 hours – night and day), monthly cycles, seasonal variations and life epochs (from birth to death). All these rhythms are important for the mental state in times of health and form the basis for such conditions as early morning wakening in depression, premenstrual tension, seasonal affective disorder and involutional melancholia. Many of these biological rhythms with variation of mood are biochemically mediated through the endocrine system.

Personal time (and also, to a lesser extent, clock time) is often described in relation to these biological rhythms. Our whole notion of the progression of time is closely related to processes of physical function: birth, growth and decay.

DISORDER OF OBJECTIVE TIME

An ability to separate events into past, present and future, even if limited; the capacity to estimate duration; and the ability to put events in the correct sequence are necessary for intellectual processes to be carried out satisfactorily. Disorder of knowledge of time is closely associated with disturbance of consciousness, attention and memory.

Disorientation in time

Disorientation for time is demonstrated by the inability to correctly tell the time without recourse to a clock, to indicate the date, day and season. This impairment is closely associated with impairment of attention, concentration, consciousness and memory. It is a feature of delirium and dementia. It is also a good clinical criterion for distinguishing between organic and function disorders (Cutting, 1997). The second abnormality is impairment of the ability to assess the *duration of time*, and this is also disturbed in organic states.

Age disorientation

The term *age disorientation* was first used by Zangwill (1953) in relation to Korsakov's syndrome to describe a 'fixed, stable disorientation for age, which was impervious to logical correction'. *Age disorientation*, now defined as a 5-year discrepancy between the patient's actual age and what the patient states to be his own age, has been considered to correlate clinically with intellectual impairment in chronic schizophrenia (Crowe and Stevens, 1978). Such patients were much less able than chronic schizophrenic patients without age disorientation to answer questions about date and the duration of time. They systematically underestimated the present year and the duration of their stay in hospital, and sometimes their own age.

This gives quantitative support to the observation that for some chronic patients 'time stands still'; they remain in the cultural set of the time when they developed their illness. Such patients tend to use the idiomatic language, sing the popular songs, wear the modish clothes and tell the characteristic jokes of the time before their illness became established. It is a mistake to believe that they are indulging in nostalgia; their cultural life is still firmly fixed within that particular period. Not only in the back ward of an old-fashioned mental hospital, but also in a hostel in the community, these patients live in their own time capsule with invisible, but impregnable, walls.

Disorder of time duration

Estimation of time duration has been studied using various methods, but the results have been inconsistent. Objective measures of estimation of the passage of time, for example, show that patients with depressive illness tend to underestimate the passage of 30 seconds, on average, by 6 seconds. This compared with overestimation of the passage of time by normal controls by on average 10 seconds (Kuhs *et al.*, 1991). That is to say that depressed patients on average estimated 30 seconds' duration as 24 seconds and the normal controls estimated 30 seconds' duration as 40 seconds. In other words, time appeared to flow more slowly for patients with depression than it did for normal controls. It is important to emphasize that this refers to estimation of the passage of momentary time. Other investigations have demonstrated an overestimation of time duration in depression (Kitamura and Kumar, 1984; Munzel *et al.*, 1988). There is more consensus on the subjective experience of time in depression (see below).

Disorder of chronology (temporal order)

Memory for the temporal order of events is an aspect of time sense that is often ignored. There is evidence that patients with diencephalic lesions compared with those with medial temporal lobe lesions have distinct deficits in temporal order memory tasks. These patients are unable to correctly indicate the temporal order of learned words on a list or the sequence of presentation of particular stimuli. This has led to the suggestion that diencephalic structures may have a function in the encoding of temporal information (O'Connor and Verfaellie, 2002). Frontal lobe lesions are also associated with impairment of function on temporal order tasks. In addition to this, an aspect of temporal order coding, namely frequency estimation, which involves estimating how often an event has happened, is known to be impaired by left frontal but not temporal lesions (Baldoa and Shimamura, 2002).

Clinically significant disorders of temporal order for past and current events have been reported. These take the form of intact memory for autobiographical events but impaired appreciation of the duration and timing of these events. These impairments are associated with organic lesions in the cingulate gyrus, the parietal lobes and the left anterior frontal areas (Cutting, 1997).

DISORDER OF SUBJECTIVE (PERSONAL) TIME

Disorder of subjective time is characterized by abnormalities in how time is experienced. This can involve the experience of (a) flow of time, (b) direction of time, (c) uniqueness of time and (d) quality of time. These disorders go to the heart of how the world is experienced. Any alteration in how time is experienced will by definition influence the experience of the objective world and may come to imbue perceptions of the objective world with an alien hue.

Disorder of flow of time

The flow (passage) of time may slow down or speed up. In some instances, it may become arrested and stand still. Tolstoy's (1895) short story *Master and Man* is true to life – or death. Lost at night in a Russian snowdrift, his character, Vasilii Andreich,

> “got up and lay down a couple of dozen times. The night seemed it would never end. It must be getting on for morning now, he thought once as he raised himself and looked around. Let's have a look at my watch. ... He could not believe his eyes. ... It was only ten past twelve. The whole night still lay ahead.

Time, as a modality of personal experience, is disturbed in mood disorders. It has been observed both clinically and experimentally that those with depressive illness feel that time passes slowly (Wyrick and Wyrick, 1977). Lewis (1967) quotes a patient who was depressed with *affective functional psychosis*:

> “Everything seems very much longer. I should have said it was afternoon, though they say it is midday. They always tell me it is earlier than I think ... and it looks as if I'm wrong and I can't help feeling I'm right ... I cannot see any end to anything, only end to the world.

The flow of time can also be arrested such that time appears to stand still. The patient feels that time is standing still, that in some way everything temporal has come to an end. This is described not uncommonly with psychotic depression. A patient says, ‘I have stopped being, I have just stopped, everything else has just stopped as well'. The incessant sequential march of events no longer impresses the person with its inevitability.

This feeling of time standing still may also be experienced in ecstasy states, in which the person may feel that he is existing in the past, the present and the future all at the same time. Such states may occur with mania, with some neurotic conditions or in normal people undergoing an exceptional psychological experience.

When the disturbance in the sense of the passage of time occurs in the setting of depression, the depressed mood is also apparent. Another of Lewis' (1967) patients said, 'I never know any moment what is going to happen. It's the most terrible outlook I've ever had to look to. It's all perpetual. I've got to suffer perpetually'. This last sentence is perhaps the key to the abnormal psychopathology. It is the abnormal mood associated with time sense that is significant, so depressive in-patients were significantly more likely to feel that time was passing more slowly than healthy 'control' subjects (Kitamura and Kumar, 1982).

In mania, time passes rapidly, but the picture is uncertain in schizophrenia (Orme, 1966). The flow of time is also known to be affected in organic brain conditions. Patients with Korsakov's syndrome underestimate the passage of time, and subjects who have had thalamotomy experience the flow of time as speeded up (Cutting, 1997).

A distinct but related disturbance of the flow of time is the *Zeitratter* phenomenon. *Zeitratter* phenomenon is literally time-lapse phenomenon. This phenomenon was first described in the German literature in the 1930s, and Cutting (1997) has now brought it to the attention of the English-speaking world. The characteristic features are (a) the speeding up or slowing down of events; (b) its association with increased speed, pitch and volume of auditory perceptions; and (c) alterations in the fluency of observed movements. There may also be visual hallucinations, anomalous experience of space such as distortions of horizontal and vertical lines. Invariably, this phenomenon occurs in the setting of acute organic brain disease such as cerebrovascular accident.

The original case was described by Hoff and Potzl (1934, quoted in Cutting, 1997):

> “Doctors and nurses were first of all moving with a measured step, conspicuously, as if on a film. Then the tempo of things became very erratic, sometimes coming at a furious pace, 'like moving pictures speeded up' as if the people involved were 'running a race'... Music, whose source was to his left, sounded very loud and very fast, as if 'several radios were all blaring away together ... as if all the instruments wanted to show how much noise they could make'. Sometimes, other people's speech seemed excessively fast and incomprehensible 'as if the doctors and nurses were practising for a world record'. However, if he were addressed directly, the rate appeared quite normal and he could understand it quite well. It was when someone was speaking away to the left that it sounded most peculiar – shriller, louder and faster than when to away to the right.

Disorder of direction of time

It seems such a fundamental aspect of our experience of time that the arrow of time travels from the past through the present to the future. It is incomprehensible that anyone could experience time as if events were being played in 'rewind mode' backwards. This phenomenon is reported by one of Lewis' patients (1967): 'Whenever anyone said anything to me, it referred back to some part of my life... One mind was living back and my mind forward'. One of Fischer's (quoted in Cutting, 1997) patients said, 'There is no present anymore, only a sense of the past. Is there a future? There used to be, but now it is shrinking. The past is so obtrusive... I'll give you an example of what it's like. I'm like a machine, which stands in one place only, working away, yes, but one which tears everything to shreds... Or else I'm like a flaming arrow which can only go backwards'.

Disorder of uniqueness of time

Part of our experience of time is the sense of uniqueness of the time, momentary or otherwise, that we live through. This uniqueness of time experience is instantiated in the unique events that populate time. This means that every moment is given its singular identity by the context, by the events played out in a given place, by particular personalities and by association with specific emotions. These coordinates of time stamp each moment with its specific unique feeling.

The *déjà vu* experience can be conceptualized as an alteration of the feeling of uniqueness that time and events are invested with. When this is disrupted, novel events and the time and place in which they occur seem familiar. In this conceptualization, *déjà vu* is the experience of this feeling of familiarity for events and times that have not been previously encountered. *Jamais vu* is the absence of this feeling of familiarity for events that have been previously encountered. In other words, even previously encountered situations are experienced as novel, that is, as unique. Although it is possible to conceptualize these experiences as disorders of time, it is probably more appropriate to regard them as aspects of memory disturbance (Chapter 5).

Déjà vu occurs in the normal state and in pathological conditions. The composer Ralph Vaughan Williams, in describing his first hearing of the tune used in *Dives and Lazarus*, explained, 'I had that sense of recognition – here's something which I have known all my life, only I didn't know it' (Kennedy, 1964). Most people can recall similar *déjà vu* experiences. It is also commonly associated with temporal lobe epilepsy. A patient described his aura before a fit experienced in hospital: 'I went into the kitchen. The window looked as if I'd seen it before. I felt very peculiar'. *Déjà vu* and *jamais vu* are quite often described in schizophrenia.

Déjà vu has been produced with brain stimulation. Penfield and Kristiensen (1951) were able to reproduce a sensation of familiarity with stimulation of a brain electrode in epileptic patients. This stimulation clearly produced an abnormality of the feeling of familiarity, not an abnormality of memory. It was a disturbance of the feeling of recognition that accompanies recall in the process of memory. Janet considered *déjà vu* to be a form of loss of reality or negation of the present (Taylor, 1947), while Freud (1901) regarded it as being associated with the recall of unconscious fantasies.

In a more extreme form, the disorder of the uniqueness of time presents as *reduplication of time*. The term was first used by Weinstein *et al.* (1952). Petho

(1985) described a case in which the patient's central symptom was the belief that she had lived through this life once before. The patient experienced a reduplication of every event, and in relation to attending the 1976 Olympic Games said, 'It could happen that I will go; I have a memory of it. But I also have a memory that I won't go to those Games so that that memory wont come back to me'.

Disorder of the quality of time

In these conditions, the normal experience of the quality of time is either lost or distorted in some way. What is central to these experiences is that the 'taken for granted' aspect of time is replaced by a degree of alienation from time such that time becomes salient, obtrusive and even unreal.

In depersonalization and derealization, there can be a loss of the feeling of reality for time experience; there may also be alteration in the sense of duration or in the perspective of time (Freeman and Melges, 1977). The person can assess time span quite accurately, and there is no loss of memory. However, he has no feeling that things are happening or time is passing; the abnormality is always one of experience. Time itself takes on a feeling of unreality, and he feels unable to initiate action.

This phenomenon can also occur in schizophrenia. One of Cutting's (1997) patients said, 'Time is somewhat changed. Time isn't supposed to be the way it is. I don't know in what way'. Fischer described a number of cases (quoted in Cutting, 1997), of which one said, 'Time stood still. Then it became different. Then it disappeared entirely... Then a new time emerged. This new time was endless, more manifold than the previous one, hardly deserving the name 'time' as we know it. Suddenly it came to me that this time did not only lie in front of and behind me, but spread out in all directions'.

BIOLOGICAL RHYTHMS AND THEIR RELATION TO PSYCHIATRY

Daily, there are profound changes in the body and brain associated with the external rhythm of the world. During the waking day we are active, and at night we rest, recuperate and repair our body parts. This biological rhythm is driven by an internal clock. The primary internal body clock is located in the suprachiasmatic nuclei, a cluster of approximately 100 000 neurons located on either side of the midline above the optic chiasma, about 3 centimetres above the eyes (Hastings, 1998). There is strong evidence that the clock is an autonomous property of the suprachiasmatic nuclei, and individual cells, *in vitro*, continue to fire rhythmically for several weeks with only the slightest deviation from 24 hours. It is known that this clock can be desynchronized by jet lag, shift work and depression (Arendt, 1995). However, there is still a great deal of ignorance about the connections with different mental illnesses. In this section, brief reference is made to daily, monthly and annual rhythms, and also to the association with the stage of life. Among psychiatric disorders, most information is available on affective disorder and its associations with daily and annual rhythms (Thompson, 1988).

Circadian rhythms

Comparing internal time with clock time, repeated estimates of fixed time spans show a gradual increase in time of the estimate, suggesting that there is a slowing of the internal clock. Subjects were asked repeatedly to guess a fixed duration of time; their estimate started by being slightly longer than actual time and became progressively longer. The intrinsic period of the circadian rhythm in humans is approximately 25 hours, but this is usually modified by external cues such as daylight (Wher and Goodwin, 1983). This has been likened to the finding in vigilance experiments, in which there is a gradual decrease of efficiency. There was also found to be a greater overestimation of fixed intervals in the morning, as compared with in the afternoon, and this was found to be correlated with body temperature. The internal clock accelerates when the body temperature is raised.

There is considerable circumstantial, but little direct, evidence that circadian rhythms are causally associated with affective disorders (Thompson, 1984). Early morning wakening and diurnal variation in mood, with the mood most depressed in the early morning, are considered as biological symptoms of depression and have been postulated as *phase advance* of the sleep–wake cycle; that is, each point of the rhythm occurs earlier than usual relative to the light–dark cycle. There is a change in depression in that rapid eye movement sleep occurs earlier, rather than later, in the night, and this also may point to phase advance of the circadian rhythm. Sleep deprivation has been used with variable success in the treatment of depression; there has been research into the genetic and familial aspects of sleep disturbance, into sleep disorders in depression and other neuropsychiatric conditions and into the relationship of sleep disturbance in depression and other neuroendocrine changes (Linkowski and Mendlewicz, 1993; Vogel *et al.*, 1980).

Although diurnality of mood usually manifests itself by the subject feeling worse in the early morning, sometimes this is reversed. Styron (1991) describes this for his own severe depressive illness: 'there was now something that resembled bifurcation of mood: lucidity of sorts in the early hours of the day, gathering murk in the afternoon and evening'.

In depression, changes of body temperature and cortisol levels over the 24 hours have also been interpreted as phase advance of the circadian rhythm, but results are equivocal. The action of antidepressant drugs has been investigated in terms of their effect on the rhythm by lengthening the intrinsic cycles of rest, temperature and sleep, but again the evidence is not clear. Corroboration studies of air travellers crossing time zones have suggested that travel from east to west is more likely to be associated with depression and from west to east with hypomania (Jauhar and Weller, 1982). However, physiological studies of jet lag would not support such an association (Arendt and Marks, 1982).

It has been suggested that there may be a shortened rhythm, of less than 24 hours, in patients with long-term schizophrenia. Abnormalities of circadian rhythm have also been described, but not fully substantiated, in anorexia nervosa and in people with abnormal personalities.

Monthly cycles

Clearly, the most obvious human biological rhythm to recur monthly is the menstrual cycle, and this has been linked with changes in the mental state, but premenstrual syndrome remains controversial in terms of its definition, management and politicosocial implications (Bancroft, 1993). Similar psychological mood swings with a monthly cycle have been sought in the male but not convincingly found. Estimates for the frequency of *premenstrual syndrome* have varied in the general population between 30 per cent and 80 per cent of women of reproductive age (Clare, 1982). Psychological symptoms include lethargy, anxiety, irritability and depression, but many symptoms are both psychological and physical (headache, feeling bloated, loss of energy). It is the timing rather than the nature of the symptoms that indicates the diagnosis, and there are clearly differing constellations of complaint within the syndrome (Sampson, 1989).

Much numerical data have been provided by Dalton (1984) to support the contention that there is increased psychopathology of various types during the 8 days of the premenstruum and the menstrual period itself relative to the rest of the cycle. She stated that 46 per cent of emergency psychiatric admissions, 53 per cent of attempted suicides, 47 per cent of admissions for depression and 47 per cent of admissions for schizophrenia of women of reproductive age occur during these stages. However, these figures have not yet been substantiated. Premenstrual syndrome is the recurrence of symptoms in the premenstruum with absence in the postmenstruum. Disabling tension has been described, as have mood swings of severe proportion and sudden onset, varying from genial equanimity to murderous irritability, suicidal depression and incapacitating lethargy. At a more general level, four psychiatric syndromes have been identified as related to reproductive function in women: postpartum depression, premenstrual syndrome, post-hysterectomy depression and involutional melancholia (Gitlin and Pasnau, 1989). The relationship between these conditions and other psychiatric disorders, and between their psychosocial and endocrinological aetiology, is not yet clear.

Seasonal variation

Season of the year has been invoked for the onset of episodes of many psychiatric illnesses. Understandably, this is more pronounced at increasingly higher latitudes in the northern hemisphere. Similar associations of illness with summer or winter have been observed in the southern hemisphere.

In schizophrenia, patients show an excess of birth dates in the winter months in northern and southern hemispheres (Hare, 1988); this is most strikingly found for those without a family history of the illness (O'Callaghan *et al.*, 1991). There is a higher rate for admission to psychiatric hospital during the summer months.

For every decade since 1921, suicide rates in England and Wales have been highest in the quarter containing April, May and June (Morgan, 1979). There appears to be no association between season of birth and affective illness; however, the onset of depressive illness and the administration of electroconvulsive therapy both become more common in spring and autumn (Rawnsley, 1982). Symonds and Williams (1976) found a peak for the admission of female manic patients in August and September.

Seasonal affective disorder (recurrent depressive disorder, F33 in ICD-10; World Health Organization, 1992) is characterized by repeated episodes of depression, which may vary in severity from mild to severe and recur with an onset at the same time of year, most often late winter or spring. It is more common in women than in men and tends to start later in life, often about the fifth decade. There are often a large number of episodes of depression in seasonal affective disorder (10 to 17 per patient), each episode lasting from 17 to 23 weeks; anxiety, irritability, hypersomnia and gain in appetite and weight were prominent symptoms (Thompson and Isaacs, 1988). The distinctive symptoms of this condition have been measured using the Seasonal Pattern Assessment Questionnaire (Thompson *et al.*, 1988). It occurs more frequently in higher latitudes in the northern hemisphere. In a study conducted in Finland (Saarijärvi *et al.*, 1999), in which prominent symptoms included lack of energy, hypersomnia, excessive eating, weight gain and a craving for carbohydrates in addition to other depressive symptoms, there was lower prevalence among Lapps, who were ethnically and genetically different from Finns living at the same latitude.

Life epochs

Virtually the whole of psychopathology is mediated through, and influenced by, changes in situation and life epoch. It is important to take into account the relative preponderance of different factors: biological change, pressure of social context and individual perception of life situation. It is outside the scope of this book to chart these associations in detail, but an impressionistic sketch is offered in Figure 6.1. The psychological effects of important life changes have

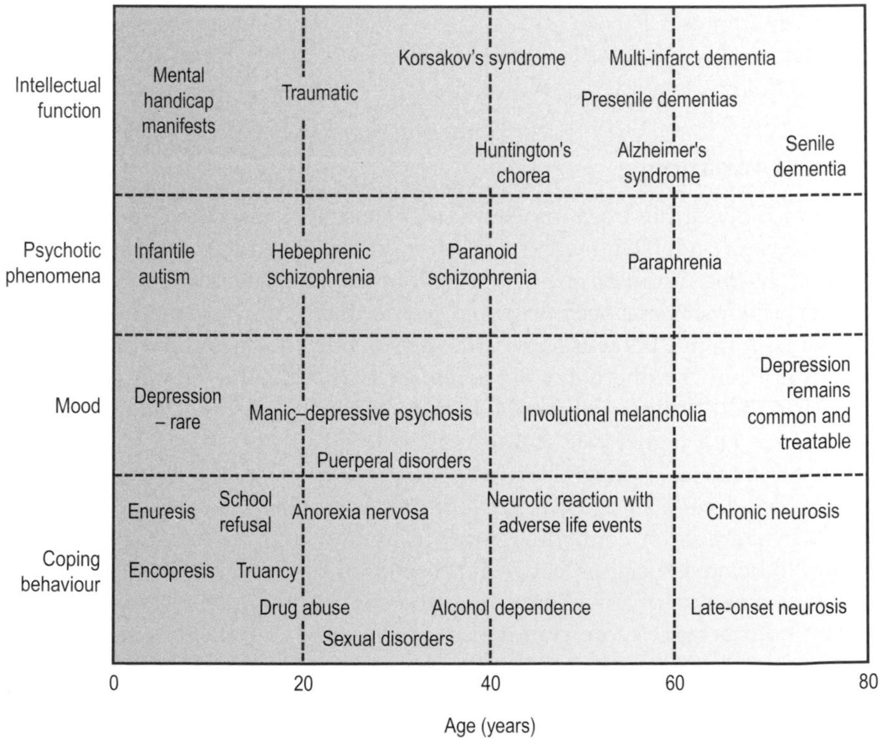

Figure 6.1 Psychiatric disturbance and life epoch.

been studied in primary care situations: birth of the first child (Jewell, 1984), starting school (Pitt and Browne, 1984), puberty (Howe and Page, 1984) and leaving school (Brown, 1984).

Some of the abnormal mental states associated with life changes of female gender could equally well be discussed with life epoch. These are discussed further in Chapter 16.

REFERENCES

Arendt J (1995) *Melatonin and the Mammalian Pineal Gland*. London: Chapman & Hall.

Arendt J and Marks V (1982) Physiological changes underlying jet lag. *British Medical Journal 284*, 144–6.

Baldoa JV and Shimamura AP (2002) In Baddeley AD, Kopelman MD and Wilson BA (eds) *The Handbook of Memory Disorders*, 2nd edn. Chichester: John Wiley.

Bancroft J (1993) The premenstrual syndrome – a reappraisal of the concept and the evidence. *Psychological Medicine Monograph Supplement* 24.

Brown A (1984) Leaving school. *British Medical Journal 288*, 1884–6.

Clare AW (1982) Psychiatric aspects of premenstrual complaint. *Journal of Psychosomatic Obstetrics and Gynaecology 1*, 22–31.

Crowe TJ and Stevens M (1978) Age disorientation in chronic schizophrenics: the nature of the cognitive deficit. *British Journal of Psychiatry 133*, 137–42.

Cutting J (1997) *Principles of Psychopathology: Two Worlds – Two Minds – Two Hemispheres*. Oxford: Oxford University Press.

Dalton K (1984) *The Premenstrual Syndrome and Progesterone Therapy*, 2nd edn. London: Heinemann.

Freeman AM and Melges FT (1977) Depersonalization and temporal disintegration in acute mental illness. *American Journal of Psychiatry 134*, 679–81.

Freud S (1901) The psychopathology of everyday life. In *Standard Edition of the Complete Works of Sigmund Freud*, vol. VI, p. 151 (transl. Stanley J, 1960). London: Hogarth Press.

Gitlin MJ and Pasnau RO (1989) Psychiatric syndromes linked to reproductive function in women: a review of current knowledge. *American Journal of Psychiatry 146*, 1413–22.

Hare E (1988) Temporal factors and trends, including birth seasonality and the viral hypothesis. In Nasrallah HA (ed.) *Handbook of Schizophrenia*, vol. 3. Amsterdam: Elsevier.

Hastings M (1998) The brain, circadian rhythms, and clock genes. *British Medical Journal 317*, 1704–7.

Howe C and Page C (1984) Puberty. *British Medical Journal 288*, 1809–11.

Jaspers K (1959) *General Psychopathology* (transl. Hoenig J and Hamilton MW, 1963). Manchester: Manchester University Press.

Jauhar P and Weller MPI (1982) Psychiatric morbidity and time zone changes: a study of patients from Heathrow Airport. *British Journal of Psychiatry 140*, 231–53.

Jerome JK (1900) *Three Men on the Bummel*. Gloucester: Alan Sutton.

Jewell MD (1984) Birth of the first child. *British Medical Journal 288*, 1584–6.

Kennedy M (1964) *The Works of Ralph Vaughan Williams*. London: Oxford University Press.

Kitamura T and Kumar R (1982) Time passes slowly for patients with depressive state. *Acta Psychiatrica Scandinavica 65*, 415–20.

Kitamura T and Kumar R (1984) Controlled study on time reproduction of depressive patients. *Psychopathology 17*, 24–7.

Kuhs H, Hermann W, Kammer W and Tolle R (1991) Time estimation and the experience of time in endogenous depression (melancholia): an experimental investigation. *Psychopathology 24*, 7–11.

Lewis A (1967) The experience of time in mental disorder. In *Inquiries in Psychiatry*, pp. 3–15. London: Routledge & Kegan Paul.

Linkowski P and Mendlewicz J (1993) Sleep encephalogram and rhythm disturbances in mood disorders. *Current Opinion in Psychiatry 6*, 35–7.

Morgan HG (1979) *Death Wishes? The Understanding and Management of Deliberate Self-Harm*. Chichester: John Wiley.

Munzel K, Gendner G, Steinberg R and Raith L (1988) Time estimation of depressive patients: the influence of interval content. *European Archives of Psychiatry and Neurological Science 237*, 171–8.

O'Callaghan E, Gibson T, Colohan HA, *et al* (1991) Season of birth in schizophrenia. Evidence for confinement of an excess of winter births to patients without a family history of mental disorder. *British Journal of Psychiatry 158*, 764–9.

O'Connor M and Verfaellie M (2002). The amnesic syndrome. In Baddeley AD, Kopelman MD and Wilson BA (eds) *The Handbook of Memory Disorders*, 2nd edn. Chichester: John Wiley.

Orme JE (1966) Time estimation and the nosology of schizophrenia. *British Journal of Psychiatry 112*, 37–9.

Penfield W and Kristiensen K (1951) *Epileptic Seizure Patients*. Springfield: Thomas.

Petho B (1985) Chronophrenia – a new syndrome in functional psychosis. *Psychopathology 18*, 174–80.

Pitt G and Browne MJ (1984) Starting school. *British Medical Journal 288*, 1655–7.

Rawnsley K (1982) Epidemiology of affective psychoses. In Wing JK and Wing L (eds) *Handbook of Psychiatry 3: Psychoses of Uncertain Aetiology*, pp. 129–33. Cambridge: Cambridge University Press.

Saarijärvi S, Lauerma H, Helenius H and Saarilehto S (1999) Seasonal affective disorders among rural Finns and Lapps. *Acta Psychiatrica Scandinavica 99*, 95–101.

Sampson GA (1989) Premenstrual syndrome. *Baillières Clinical Obstetrics and Gynaecology 3*, 687–704.

Styron W (1991) *Darkness Visible: a Memoir of Madness*. London: Jonathan Cape.

Symonds RL and Williams P (1976) Seasonal variations in the incidence of mania. *British Journal of Psychiatry 129*, 45–8.

Taylor WS (1947) Pierre Janet 1859–1947. *American Journal of Psychology 60*, 637–45.

Thompson C (1984) Circadian rhythms and psychiatry. *British Journal of Psychiatry 145*, 204–6.

Thompson C (1988) Biological rhythms and mental illness. *Current Opinion in Psychiatry 1*, 66–71.

Thompson C and Isaacs G (1988) Seasonal affective disorder – a British sample: symptomatology in relation to mode of referral and diagnostic subtype. *Journal of Affective Disorders 14*, 1–11.

Thompson C, Stinson D, Fernandez M, Fine J and Isaacs G (1988) A comparison of normal, bipolar and seasonal affective disorder subjects using the Seasonal Pattern Assessment Questionnaire. *Journal of Affective Disorders 14*, 257–64.

Tolstoy L (1895) *Master and Man* (transl. Foote P, 1977). London: Penguin.

Vogel DW, Vogel F, McAbee RS and Thurmond AJ (1980) Improvement depression by REM sleep deprivation. *Archives of General Psychiatry 37*, 247–53.

Weinstein EA, Kahn RL and Sugarman LA (1952) Phenomenon of reduplication. *Archives of Neurology and Psychiatry 67*, 808–14.

Wher TA and Goodwin FK (1983) *Circadian Rhythm in Psychiatry*. Pacific Grove: Boxwood Press.

World Health Organization (1992) *The ICD-10 Classification of Mental and Behavioural Disorders: Clinical Description and Diagnostic Guidelines*. Geneva: World Health Organization.

Wyrick RA and Wyrick LC (1977) Time experience during depression. *Archives of General Psychiatry 14*, 1441–3.

Zangwill OL (1953) Disorientation for age. *Journal of Mental Science 99*, 698–701.

Pathology of Perception

7

“ I flew her body back to the Bar to be buried, because I felt that was where she belonged. I couldn't complain about our marriage anymore then. She'd gone and left me behind after forty-two years. We'd lived through thick and thin, good times and bad. We'd had a rough life and been forced to eat tucker we didn't like, but we'd raised six kids and survived. . .

I was lying on my bed with my arm over my head when my cattle dog gave one sharp yelp. The kids were all asleep and I didn't look up at first because I thought it was probably my son Johnny coming in, as I was expecting him. When I did look up who did I see sitting on the end of my bed but Susie. I was so stunned I rolled back and hid my face, when I looked again she was still there. She sat there for a while and then just disappeared.

The next day I went and saw some of our people and told them what had happened. They said, 'Yes, that's right, we seen her too'.

Later some of the children and grandchildren saw her. She continued to appear to different ones on and off in Port Hedland and Marble Bar for twelve months, and then she was gone. I think it takes them that long to say goodbye to their family. *Sally Morgan (1989)*

For almost 7 years – except during sleep – *I have never had a single moment in which I did not hear voices*. They accompany me to every place and at all times; they continue to sound even when I am in conversation with other people, they persist undeterred even when I concentrate on other things. *Daniel Schreber (1842–1911)*

Disorders of perception, particularly auditory hallucinations or 'hearing voices', have a central place in psychopathology. Along with delusions (Chapter 8), they are thought of as synonymous with mental illness. This apparent association with mental illness has come to imply that 'hearing voices' is a sign of serious mental illness and that hallucinations portend madness. In this chapter, the nature of sensation, perception and imagery is discussed as a prelude to examining the nature of disorders of perception.

Sensation and perception

Sensation is only the first stage in receiving information from outside the self. The sensory system includes the visual, auditory, tactile, olfactory, gustatory, kinaesthetic and proprioceptive pathways. These pathways deal with the receipt, transformation and transmission of raw and disparate sensory data from peripheral receptors to the central nervous system. The transformation of raw sensory stimuli into sensory information that is decoded into meaningful perception at the cortical level involves active processes that are influenced by attention, affect, cultural expectations, context, prior experiences and memory and, most importantly, prior concepts. It is therefore the case that perception is not a passive process but an active process that involves the construction of an external world that depends on internal templates.

Much of what we know about sensation and perception derives from our understanding of the visual system. In the visual system, light sensation is received by the retina and transformed into a neural code that is transmitted from the retinal ganglion cells to the primary visual cortex via the lateral geniculate nucleus of the thalamus. Perception occurs when a stimulus has undergone processing according to its form, colour, motion and meaning.

The distinction between sensation and perception is well illustrated by the dissociation between intact sensation and impaired perception in the agnosias. In visual object agnosia, the subject is able to recognize that an object is in his field of vision (that is, sensation is intact), but he is unable to recognize what the object or its function is (impaired perception). This visual model of perception is likely to have counterparts within the other sensory systems.

Oliver Sachs (1995) recounts the story of Virgil, a 51-year-old man who had been blind since infancy. He had a cataract extraction, but the return of visual sensation was unaccompanied by uncomplicated perception. Virgil was able to 'pick up details incessantly – but would not be able to synthesize them, to form a complex perception at a glance. This was one reason the cat, visually was so puzzling; he would see a paw, the nose, the tail, an ear, but could not see all of them together, see the cat as a whole'. This case is reminiscent of Gregory's patient (2004), S.B., who when he was first shown a lathe 'was quite unable to say anything about it, except he thought the nearest part was a handle.... He complained that he could not see the cutting edge, or the metal being worked, or anything else about it, and appeared rather agitated. ... S.B. was allowed to touch the lathe. The result was startling.... He ran his hands eagerly over the lathe, with his eyes shut. Then he stood back a little and opened his eyes and said: "Now that I've felt it I can see." These two cases underline the distinction between sensation and perception and confirm that 'we are not given the world: we make our world through incessant experience, categorisation, memory, reconnection' (Sachs, 1995).

There are various competing models of how recognition is achieved by the visual system. Detailed description of these models is outside the scope of this chapter (see Smith and Kosslyn, 2007). Bottom-up processing consists of the primary processes that transform sensation into the perception of objects that have form, colour, motion and location in space. On the other hand, top-down processes involve the influence of learned experience of perceiving objects to narrow the competition between the possible interpretation of the sensory information. The alternative models of the top-down processes that attempt to explain object recognition, that is, perception, are the template-matching model, the feature-matching model, the recognition-by-components model and the configural models.

The template-matching model requires an internal template in memory to which an object can be matched against. The weakness of this model is that the template must accommodate object size and orientation, for example, and must still be rapid and reliable. The feature-matching model requires only that a distinct and discriminating feature of an object on its own should specify what the object is. Trees need only be specified by the fact that they have a trunk and branches. The exact location of the branches and size of the trunk do not matter. The recognition-by-components model requires a knowledge of the correct arrangement of parts in three-dimensional space. Thus, irrespective of the perspective, a bicycle is still recognized as a bicycle. Finally, the configural model is a refinement of the recognition-by-components model. It deals with the mechanism whereby individual examples of a class are recognized. This is the distinction between different makes of cars, the variation that determines that one car is a Mercedes and another is a Volvo.

Imagery

Imagery is the internal mental representation of the world and is actively drawn from memory. Imagery underlies our capacity for many crucial cognitive activities, such as mental arithmetic, map reading, visualizing and imagining places previously visited and recollecting spoken speech. In day-to-day life, it is common to refer to 'seeing in the mind's eyes' or 'hearing in the mind's ears'. These terms refer to imagery. Jaspers (1962) described the formal characteristics of images as follows: (a) images are figurative and have a character of subjectivity; (b) they appear in inner subjective space; (c) they are not clearly delineated and come before us incomplete; (d) although sensory elements are individually the equal of those in perception, mostly they are insufficient; (e) images dissipate and always have to be recreated; and (f) images are actively created and are dependent on our will (Table 7.1).

Functional imaging studies have demonstrated that the same cortical areas are implicated in visual imagery and visual perception (Kosslyn and Thompson, 2003), and transmagnetic resonance studies have also shown that transmagnetic resonance applied repeatedly to visual areas reduces the capacity for visual imagery (Kosslyn *et al.*, 1999). Furthermore, behavioural experiments have shown that participants are able to construct mental images that have perceptual qualities such as colour, size, shape and orientation. These images are uneven, with the level of detail depending on the degree of visual attention (Smith and Kosslyn, 2007).

Table 7.1 Formal characteristics of normal perception and imagery

Normal perception	Imagery
Perceptions are of concrete reality	Images are figurative and have a character of subjectivity
Perceptions occur in external objective space	Images appear in inner subjective space
Perceptions are clearly delineated	Images are incomplete and poorly delineated
The sensory elements are full and fresh	The sensory elements are relatively insufficient
Perceptions are constant and remain unaltered	Images dissipate and have to be recreated
Perceptions are independent of our will	Images are dependent on our will

(After Jaspers, 1962, with permission of Manchester University Press.)

The study of imagery remains a controversial area within cognitive neuroscience. Theories of visual imagery have borrowed from the language and model of the camera; this is referred to as the *pictorial* or *depiction* theory of mental imagery. The foremost proponent of this approach is Kosslyn. A detailed account of the theory and its difficulties is outside the scope of this book (see Kosslyn, 2004; Pylyshyn, 2004). Kosslyn argues that a mental image is figuratively accurate, as each point of the image corresponds to each point on the represented object. This means that there is a point-to-point representation such that performing particular operations on the image takes as much time as it would take performing the same operation on the object. In other words, the time to scan a mental image is the same as the time to scan the object. Pylyshyn, on the other hand, argues that there are decisive differences between retinal or cortical images and mental images.

Imagery is important for psychopathology because an understanding of the formal characteristics or nature of imagery is required for examining the nature of perceptions, hallucinations and pseudohallucinations. Functional imaging studies and case reports have shown that the mechanisms responsible for visual perception of objects and those responsible for imagery may be similar. In other words, the neural substrates of perception and imagery at the very least overlap (Martin, 2006). Ultimately, these investigations may shed light on the mechanisms uniting imagery and abnormal perceptions.

ABNORMAL PERCEPTION

We will now divide abnormal perception into *sensory distortions*, in which a real perceptual object is perceived distorted, and *false perceptions*, in which a new perception occurs that may or may not be in response to an external stimulus. *Illusions*, *hallucinations* and *pseudohallucinations* will be included under false perceptions. The possibility of a neurological deficit affecting perception also needs to be considered.

Subjectively, *hallucination* is similar to sense perception: it is experienced as a *normal* perception and it can be distinguished from the fantasy elements that invest it. In *vivid imagery*, the whole experience is imaginary. *Pseudohallucination* has a close affinity to imagery but also has some aspects that are characteristic of sense perception or hallucination: vividness, definition, constancy and apparent independence from volition.

Sensory distortions

Disturbance of the mental state, with or without organic brain pathology, may cause sensory distortion. This distortion may involve any of the components or elementary aspects of perception, such as uniqueness, size, shape, colour, location, motion or general quality. What is significant is that the perceived object is correctly recognized and identified yet there is a deviation from its customary appearance without prejudicing the knowledge of the kind of thing that it is (Cutting, 1997).

Elementary aspects of visual perception

In visual perception, the recurrence or prolongation of a visual phenomenon beyond the customary limits of the appearance of the real event in the world is termed *palinopsia* (Cutting, 1997). Critchley (1951) gave a number of examples: a cat noticed in the street one day kept appearing at various times and various situations over the next few days, and the words 'Pullman Springs' noticed on the back of a van kept appearing on other vehicles over the next few months.

The size of the perception can be either larger (*macropsia*) or smaller (*micropsia*) than expected. In some cases, there can be apparent reduction in one hemifield of vision (*hemimicropsia*). These anomalies are common in temporal lobe epilepsy. Alteration in the customary shape of the perceived object is termed *metamorphopsia*. Usually, this may involve the appearance of things taking on a different aspect: 'One woman saw people upside down, on their heads' (Bleuler, 1950). This is an example of inversion. When metamorphopsia affects faces, it is referred to as *paraprosopia*. Typically, these perceptual distortions of faces are rapidly fluctuant and dynamic. Schreber (1955) describes his experience as follows: 'At the same time I repeatedly witnessed that [some patients] changed heads during their stay in the common room; that is to say without leaving the room and while I was observing them, they suddenly ran about with a different head'. Bleuler (1950) also describes 'wardmates change their faces the very moment that one looks at them'. One of Cutting's patients (1997) said, 'Man behind a lorry was pulling hideous faces'.

Different aspects of colour perception can be affected. The intensity of the colour (*visual hyperaesthesia*), the actual hue and the quality of the colour can all be affected. Cutting (1997) gives several examples: (a) 'colours are brighter', 'colours more vivid – red, yellow, orange stood out'; (b) 'black looked brown sometimes', 'brown looked different; trouble with pink as it comes across as green'; and (c) 'this colour looks like an old blue – something horrible'. Bleuler (1950) describes 'one patient sees everything as coloured red; another sees everything as white', and Jaspers 'I only see black; even when the sun is shining, it is still all black'. These perceptual distortions of colour occur in schizophrenia. In organic conditions, *achromatopsia*, which is the complete absence of colour, has been described following unilateral or bilateral occipital lesions, usually of the lingual and fusiform gyri. *Dyschromatopsia* refers to the perversion of colour perception and occurs following unilateral posterior lesions.

The spatial location of a perceived object may be distorted. *Teleopsia* involves the object appearing far away, and *pelopsia* the object appearing nearer than it should. *Alloaesthesia* is the term for when the perceived object is in a different position from what is expected so that the patient, for example, experiences the transposition of objects from left to right.

Akinetopsia is the impairment of visual perception of motion in which the individual is unable to perceive the motion of objects. It is very rare and is said to follow bilateral posterior cortical damage. Zeki (1993) quotes Zihl's case: 'She had difficulty, for example, in pouring tea or coffee into a cup because the fluid appeared to be frozen, like a glacier. In addition, she could not stop pouring at the right time since she was unable to perceive the movement in the cup (or a pot) when the fluid rose'.

The general quality of perception can be affected. This usually involves an indefinable alteration in the visual appearance of the perceived world so that everything seems different from what it used to be: 'People [look] like toys – almost dead and lifeless, carrying out automatic movements with special meaning' (Cutting, 1997); 'people look dead, pale, cold' (Cutting, 1997);

'A factory-worker sees a grass-hopper and becomes very disturbed and excited at the sight of this *very strange* [my emphasis] and unknown animal' (Bleuler, 1950). These experiences are examples of derealization. Normally, perception is accompanied by affect, which may be a feeling of familiarity, of enjoyment, of dislike, of involvement, of proximity and so on. This is usually appropriate and so ignored. However, changes in these feelings may present as symptoms, for example, 'everything looks clear but it all looks miles away', 'I feel in seclusion. It is like looking through the wrong end of a telescope'. These, and many other feelings, are described under *derealization* (Chapter 14). There is a feeling of unreality in the perceptual field, an alteration in the feelings associated with the objects of perception.

A patient who exemplified both the loss of intensity of sensation and the change in feelings associated with perception in the context of a depressive illness was a 23-year-old Sri Lankan Buddhist priest. Following a session of meditation, he became very frightened one night after assaulting another young priest, apparently in his sleep. In the next few days, he felt that he had lost all sensation. Things he saw and heard he could not understand properly. He could see only the things that were nearby. He could not get any sensations from his skin. He said that he could not read nor understand, nor feel sadness or happiness. He said that he could not feel anything: 'all is numbed, body and mind'. He admitted to feeling low, that life was not worth living and that he had thought of ending his life. There was no neurological or other physical abnormality.

Elementary aspects of auditory perception

The elementary elements of auditory perception that can be disturbed include the uniqueness of the experience, the intensity and the spatial position (Cutting, 1997). In *palinacousis*, the uniqueness of a perceptual experience is disturbed and there is persistence of sounds that are heard. A subject returned to answer the door several times during a 30-minute period after the doorbell had actually rung (Jacobs *et al.*, 1973). The *intensity* of auditory perception may be altered so that it is either heightened or diminished. For example, heightening in the auditory modality is called *hyperacusis*, a symptom in which the patient complains of everything sounding abnormally loud, saying 'I can't bear the noise'. Ordinary conversation may sound intolerably noisy, and even whispering at a distance may be found uncomfortable. There is, of course, no true improvement of auditory perception but simply a lowering of the threshold at which noise becomes unpleasant. The symptom occurs in depression, migraine and some toxic states, for example the *hangover* following acute alcohol excess. The spatial position of a sound may be disturbed so that the sound appears as if it was nearer, further or displaced in position.

Splitting of perception

This rather rare phenomenon is described sometimes with organic states and also with schizophrenia: the patient is unable to form the usual, assumed links between two or more perceptions. A patient watching television experienced a feeling of competition between the visual and auditory perceptions. She felt that the two were not coming from the same source but were competing for her attention and conveying opposite messages. *Splitting of perception* occurs when the links between different sensory modalities fail to be made, and so the sensations themselves, although in fact associated, appear to be quite separate and even in conflict.

False perception

Now we turn from the altered perception of real objects to consider the perception of objects that are not there; these are *new perceptions* that include illusion, hallucination and pseudohallucination. Illusions were separated phenomenonologically from hallucinations by Esquirol (1817) and later also by Hagen, who introduced the term *pseudohallucination* (Berrios, 1996). He described them as transformations of perceptions, coming about by a mixing of the reproduced perceptions of the subject's fantasy with natural perceptions.

Illusion

Three types of illusion are normally described: *completion illusion*, *affect illusion* and *pareidolic illusion*. Completion illusions depend on inattention for their occurrence. The faded lettering of an advertisement outside a garage is represented in Figure 7.1. Being more interested in music than cars, the author regularly misread this as 'Vivaldi'. We commonly miss the misprints in a newspaper because we read the words as if they were written correctly. As soon as our attention is drawn to the mistake, our perception alters. An incomplete perception that is meaningless of itself is filled in by a process of extrapolation from previous experience to produce significance.

Completion illusion demonstrates the principle of *closure* in gestalt psychology (see Chapter 10): there is a human tendency to complete a familiar but not quite finished pattern (Beveridge, 1985). It is necessary for us to make sense of our environment; when the sensory cues are nonsensical, we alter them slightly with remembered or fantasy material so that the whole perceptual experience becomes meaningful.

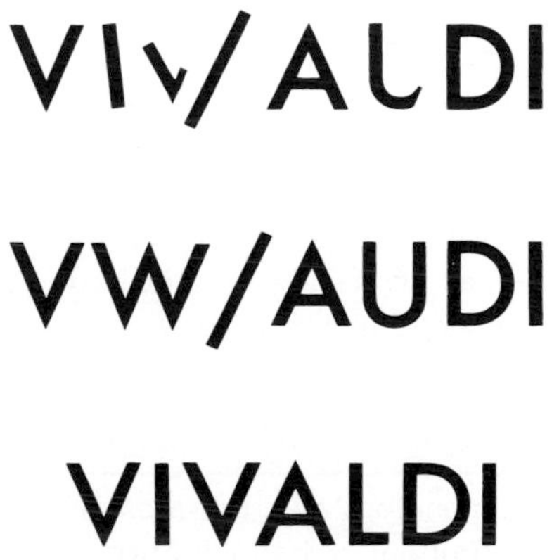

Figure 7.1 Illusion.

When *illusion* arises through *affect*, perception of everyday objects is changed. The illusion can be understood only in the context of the prevailing mood state. A child who is frightened of the dark wakes up in the half light and mistakes a towel hanging by the wall for a person moving. The experience lasts only a short time and disappears when the intense fear goes: the illusion is banished by attention. Of course, there is no absolute distinction between these different types of illusion. The degree of completion, or of affect involved, is variable. For example, a man looking through advertisements for a post found a job that he liked and misread the written word '*suitable*' for the illusional word '*superior* ... applicant is required'. Clearly, this was both an affective and a completion illusion. Similarly, in the stage of *searching* that occurs following bereavement, momentary recognition of the dead person may occur for someone in a crowd. Close observation of the individual immediately dispels the feeling of familiarity.

Pareidolia occurs in a considerable proportion of normal people. It may also be provoked by psychomimetic drugs. Typically, images are seen from shapes in pareidolic illusion. For example, the author used to see the head of a spaniel in a chip on the first paving stone of the path leading to the house where he lived as a child; the image was not just a dog but definitely a spaniel.

Pareidolic illusions are created out of sensory percepts by an admixture with imagination. The percept takes on a full and detailed appearance: 'a Victorian lady with a crinoline and frilled bloomers'. The person experiencing it, like someone seeing a photograph, knows that it is not truly there as an object but that it is pictorial. However, he cannot dismiss what he sees. Completion and affect illusions occur during inattention; they are banished by attention, which will, if anything, increase the intensity of pareidolic illusions as they become more intricate and detailed.

Pareidolic illusion occurs in children more than in adults. It should be distinguished from the following conditions.

- *Perceptual misinterpretation*, that is, simply making a mistake as to the nature of perception without that perception being particularly influenced by emotion mixed with fantasy.
- *Functional hallucination*, which occurs when a certain percept is necessary for the production of a hallucination, but the hallucination is not a transformation of that perception. For example, the patient hears voices when the tap is turned on; he hears voices in the running water, but the voices and the noise of water are quite distinct and can be heard separately and synchronously like any other voice that is heard against a background noise. The perception of hearing running water is necessary to produce the hallucination, but the hallucination is not a transformation of that perception.
- *Fantastic interpretations* or elaborate *daydreaming* can be very similar to pareidolic illusions and, as we have already discussed, there is a large admixture of fantasy in such illusions.

HALLUCINATION

Hallucinations are, phenomenologically, the most significant type of false perceptions. Here are five definitions of hallucination.

- A perception without an object (Esquirol, 1817).
- Hallucinations proper are false perceptions that are not in any way distortions of real perceptions but spring up on their own as something quite new and occur simultaneously with and alongside real perception (Jaspers, 1962).
- A hallucination is an exteroceptive or interoceptive percept that does not correspond to an actual object (Smythies, 1956).
- According to Slade (1976a), three criteria are essential for an operational definition: (a) percept-like experience in the absence of an external stimulus; (b) percept-like experience that has the full force and impact of a real perception; and (c) percept-like experience that is unwilled, occurs spontaneously and cannot be readily controlled by the percipient. This definition is derived from Jasper's formal characteristics of a normal perception (see Table 7.1).
- A hallucination is a *perception without an object* (within a realistic philosophical framework) or the *appearance of an individual thing in the world without any corresponding material event* (within a Kantian framework), according to Cutting (1997).

One of the simplest facts about hallucinations is often one of the most difficult to comprehend. That is, to the patient what the doctor calls a hallucination is a *normal sensory experience*. Although the standard definitions of hallucination imply that, subjectively, a hallucination is indistinguishable from a normal percept, some authors argue that hallucinatory percepts may be distinct from normal percepts (see below). One of the clues that the sufferer uses to grasp the fact that he might be hallucinated is that there is no corroborative evidence for the percept in other modalities. A woman hears voices giving a commentary on her activity: 'She is going to the sink. She is putting the coffee on'. She sees no one else in the room but recognizes the voices of her neighbours. She cannot understand how she can be hearing them, but she is so convinced by the reality of the voices that she draws the curtains and takes the mirrors off the walls. There is some conflict in her mind: she hears voices but can see no person to account for them. However, she resolves this conflict in what is a rational way, assuming that she believes implicitly in the genuineness of the perception: 'someone must have fixed a device or altered my sense of hearing'. What is notable is that she does not doubt the reality of the percept.

Horowitz (1975) has investigated hallucinations using a cognitive approach, looking at each of the following four constructs in terms of coding, appraising and transforming information.

> "Hallucinations are mental images that (1) occur in the form of images, (2) are derived from internal sources of information, (3) are appraised incorrectly as if from external sources of information, and (4) usually occur intrusively. Each of these four constructs refers to a separate set of psychological processes, although together they comprise a holistic experience.

This provides a conceptual framework for investigating the phenomena of hallucination.

This idea has been developed further by Bentall (1990), who considers that hallucinations represent faulty judgements about the origin of their perceptions, tending to attribute them to an external source. The content of hallucination was thought to be explained, at least in part, by the need to defend the individual's own self-esteem. Hallucinations may result from a failure of the metacognitive skills involved in discriminating between self-generated and external sources of information. This explanation was given further support by the finding that hallucinators more often misattributed auditorily presented answers to difficult clues to an experimenter than either a deluded but not hallucinated group of patients or normal control subjects (Bentall *et al.*, 1991).

Attempts to explain hallucinations in terms of underlying neurochemistry and neuropathology have so far not made much progress. An attempt has been made to incorporate concepts of biological vulnerability and psychological influences in the aetiology and clinical presentation of hallucinations, but research has produced no single mechanism to account for them (Asaad and Shapiro, 1986).

Hallucinations can take place at the same time as normal sensory stimuli are received. In this way, they are unlike dreams, which in fact have more of the characteristics of illusions. Hallucinations are like normal percepts, of which several can be perceived simultaneously or in rapid succession. Thus, the patient can hear hallucinatory voices at the same time as he is seeing his interviewer and listening to him speak. Hallucination is like *after-image*, *pareidolia* or the observation of a normal sensory object, in that attention will not remove it.

The sense of reality experienced by patients when they hallucinate has been studied by Aggernaes (1972), developing the concepts of Rasmussen. He pointed out six qualities of which normal people can be aware when they experience a sensation, which also occurred in over 90 per cent of a series of hallucinations.

- With normal sensation, we are able to distinguish *perceiving* with our sense organs from *imagining* the same objects; hallucinations similarly are experienced as *sensation* and not as *thought* or *fantasy*.
- When a subject experiences something, he realizes its possible *relevance* for his own emotions, needs or actions; hallucinations also have this quality of behavioural relevance.
- Normal sensation has a quality of *objectivity*, in that the experiencer feels that under favourable circumstances he would be able to experience the same something with another modality of sensation; this is also the experience of the hallucinator.
- An object is considered to *exist* if the observer feels certain that it still exists even though nobody else is experiencing it at that time; perceived objects and hallucinations share this quality.
- Experience of object perception and hallucination is *involuntary*, in that the experiencer feels that it is impossible or extremely difficult to alter or dismiss the experience simply by wishing to do so.
- Normally, the experiencer is aware, or through simple questioning becomes aware, that his experience is not simply the result of being in an unusual mental state; this quality of *independence* is present with normal perception and with hallucination.

One further quality of normal object perception was found to be absent more often than not with hallucination. This is the quality of *publicness*, in which the experiencer would be aware that anybody else with normal sensory faculties would be able to perceive this something. Often, the hallucinator does not believe that others could share his experience (delusional explanation may be given for this).

Clearly, cultural factors influence the manner in which subjects describe their abnormal perceptions. It has been claimed by Andrade (1988) that because patients in India were more prepared to accept paranormal explanations for phenomena, false perceptions or 'true hallucinations' are more likely to be ascribed with objectivity and veridicality. Even if this is so, and it is not proven, the qualities described by Aggenaes would still be useful in recognizing hallucination from other abnormalities of perception.

Cutting (1997) has argued that hallucinatory experiences are hardly plausible everyday occurrences, and that therefore it is not that hallucinatory percepts are indistinguishable from normal percepts but rather that they are taken for reality despite the fact that they are distinct from everyday reality. He makes the point that, for example, Lilliputian hallucinations in delirium and complex hallucinations involving comic characters are obviously not plausible perceptions in the real world yet they are taken as real! However, Cutting ignores the fact that it is precisely because hallucinatory phenomena have the quality of a normal experience that they are taken for reality despite being, as he points out, implausible. Other authors, such as Spitzer (1994), argue that hallucinations are not like normal perceptions, in that patients can distinguish between real perceptual experiences and their hallucinatory experiences. This is one reason why patients are able to understand the reference to *'hearing voices'* in interactions with clinicians; both parties know what this way of speaking stands for. Indeed, Wernicke (1906) had already drawn attention to this fact when he pointed out that the notion of 'hearing voices' was not invented by psychiatrists but rather was used by patients to indicate that somehow their experience was akin to hearing other people talk but also different from this as well. Junginger and Frame (1985) showed that a substantial proportion of patients (40 per cent) rated their voices as more akin to inner speech than to external spoken or heard speech, thus emphasizing that hallucinations may not always have the hallmark of normal perception.

Auditory hallucination

Hallucinations can occur in any of the areas of the five special senses and also with somatic sensation. We will start by discussing *auditory hallucinations*, as they are most often of supreme diagnostic significance. In acute organic states, the auditory hallucinations are usually unstructured sounds – *elementary hallucinations*, for example the patient hears whirring noises or rattles, whistling, machinery or music. Often, the noise is experienced as very unpleasant and frightening. Of interest are musical hallucinations, which tend to occur in older women with deafness or brain disease and no history of psychiatric illness (Berrios, 1990). There are, therefore, similarities with Charles Bonnet's syndrome, described below in the section on visual hallucinations.

Hearing voices is, of course, characteristic of schizophrenia, but it also occurs in other conditions, for example *chronic alcoholic hallucinosis* or *affective psychoses* occasionally. These voices are sometimes called *phonemes* (confusion exists, unfortunately, because the word is used with a totally different meaning in linguistics, in which phonemes are the units of speech-sound from which words are made). Usually in *organic states* the phonemes are simple words or short sentences, often spoken to the patient in the second person as either peremptory orders or abusive remarks. These abusive or imperative phonemes also occur in schizophrenia, but other more complicated speech is also heard; the voices may be single or multiple, male or female or both, people known and recognized by the patient or not known. They are experienced as coming from outside his head or his self. The voice is clear, objective and definite and is assumed by the patient to be a normal percept that at the same time may be baffling and incomprehensible in its import. Particularly characteristic of schizophrenia are voices that say the patient's *own thoughts out loud*, which give a *running commentary* on the patient's actions or voices, which *argue* or *discuss* vigorously *with each other*. They refer to the patient in the third person (Schneider, 1959).

In a series of 100 current patients experiencing auditory hallucinations, all of which were described as 'hearing voices', 61 suffered from schizophrenia and 78 from schizophrenia-related conditions (Nayani and David, 1996). Fifty-two per cent of the patients had an experience of sadness, and 45 per cent experienced churning or butterfly sensations in the stomach at or before onset. Most voices spoke in conversational tones, but a few whispered and a few shouted; half of the sample heard their voices through their ears as external stimuli. Most voices were male, often a middle-aged man, usually speaking in a different accent from the patient, for example 'an upper-class voice'. Subjects heard a mean of 3.2 different voices and usually knew the identity of at least one; in half of the subjects, the voices signified forces of Good or Evil. Half of the subjects were able to exert some control over their voices, and two-thirds had developed coping mechanisms to deal with them; high levels of distress were found among those with little control and few means of coping. The majority of subjects ascribed reality characteristics to their voices. A long history of auditory hallucinations tended to be associated with more hallucinated words, more voices, a greater range of emotional expression and grammatical style and greater likelihood of interpreting the voices delusionally.

Auditory hallucinations in schizophrenia are generally private events, but several early writers observed vocalizations that corresponded with the content of the voices taking place at the same time as the hallucinations. Normal people occasionally vocalize their own thoughts *sotto voce*; in the psychotic equivalent of this, it seems that sometimes those with schizophrenia are vocalizing their hallucinations at the same time as they experience them. Green and Preston (1981) increased the audibility of the whispers of such a patient to an intelligible level using auditory feedback.

Sometimes, patients with schizophrenia describe abnormal perceptions in both the visual and the auditory modalities. The examiner should be careful not to assume that there are both auditory and visual hallucinations present; there may be a different *form*, particularly for the visual experience. A man aged 45 described his experience as follows: 'I hear my nephews talking [about me]. "He is a poofter [homosexual] and a pervert"... I see them as well. The curtains move and I know that it is them moving them'. This is a description of a persecutory auditory hallucination, but the visual experience is a delusional interpretation of a normal perception, not a visual hallucination.

Patients' descriptions of their phonemes vary greatly. Sometimes, patients talk openly and quite blandly about their 'voices'. Not uncommonly, a patient may deny voices but assert that he hears 'spoken messages' or 'transmissions' or some other spoken sound, and it may be difficult to decide whether this is a real perception or an auditory hallucination. The phonemes may be so insistent, compelling and interesting that ordinary conversation with the doctor is found boring, and even unreal, in comparison. The voices may form an insistent background to life, so ensuring that a large part of the patient's speech and behaviour is occupied in answering and obeying the voices. Psychiatric nursing staff often observe that the auditory hallucinations described by patients are as real to them as any other remembered conversations, and both hallucinatory and real auditory perceptions form the memories on which patients base their life and behaviour in the present.

Auditory hallucinations occur when there is a combination of vivid mental imagery and poor reality testing in the auditory modality (Slade, 1976b). This has been investigated using a battery of tests including the *verbal transformation effect*. The word 'tress' was repeated on a tape recorder to the subjects for 10 minutes. After a time, subjects began to hear other words and syllables. Normal subjects and schizophrenics who were not auditorily hallucinated usually heard words that were phonetically linked to the original monosyllable, but psychotic patients who were auditorily hallucinated heard words that were quite different phonetically as often as those that were linked.

It appears that auditory hallucinations are dependent on the meaningfulness of sensory input. When various types of auditory input were presented to schizophrenic patients with hallucinations, it was found that it was not the degree of external stimulation that was required to diminish hallucinations but the nature of the stimulus and the degree of attention it received. When active monitoring of material was required by the subject reading aloud a prose passage and deciding the content afterwards, this produced a greater decrease of hallucinatory experience than any of the conditions in which sounds were played to the subject through earphones (Margo *et al.*, 1981). Morley (1987) reported the psychological treatment of a 30-year-old man with auditory hallucinations. Distraction by means of music presented by a portable cassette produced a transient reduction in the frequency and clarity of hallucinations. Subsequently, these hallucinations were totally abolished by the unilateral placement of a wax earplug: attention was considered more effective than distraction. The patient located the hallucination 'about a foot away from my right ear', and the plug was only effective in the right ear.

Schizophrenic patients experiencing auditory hallucinations were found to be impaired in cognitive processing in the aspects of tolerance of ambiguity and availability of alternative meanings. *Tolerance of ambiguity* was tested by asking the patient to recognize a spoken word, which was obscured by a masking noise of people reading. The masking noise was gradually reduced in volume until recognition occurred. *Alternative meanings* tests the subject's knowledge of less familiar meanings of words. These two processes reduced the quality of perception (resulting in hallucination) by introducing errors of premature judgement without the safeguard of subsequently considered alternatives (Heilbrun and Blum, 1984).

Some auditory hallucinations are considered to be 'first rank symptoms of schizophrenia' (Schneider, 1959); these are *audible thoughts*, *voices* heard *arguing* with each other and *voices commenting* on the patient's behaviour. These three perceptual disturbances, as other first-rank symptoms, each represent a massive interference with the boundaries of self-image, the discrimination of what is 'I' from what is 'not I' (Sims, 1991).

The mechanisms used by chronic schizophrenic patients to cope with persistent auditory hallucinations were discussed by Falloon and Talbot (1981). The strategies used to cope with intrusive voices could be classified as changes in behaviour, in sensory or affective state and in cognition. Changes in behaviour included alteration of posture, such as lying down, or seeking out the company of others. Physiological arousal was altered to cope with hallucinations through relaxation or physical exercise such as jogging. Cognitive methods included control of attention or active suppression of hallucinations. These authors believe that the common-sense application of strategies used by patients can be beneficial in the control of these distressing symptoms.

Visual hallucination

Visual hallucinations characteristically occur in *organic states* rather than in the functional psychoses. A 69-year-old married man was referred to the duty psychiatrist in a casualty department for assessment. He said that his life was at an end and he deserved to die, as he had been caught masturbating by his daughter-in-law and grandchildren that afternoon. His wife said that this was not true; he had become very agitated and distressed over 12 hours and no one had visited the house that day. During interview, he was intensely agitated and put his hands in front of his face. He claimed that he could see clearly a sheet of glass half a metre in front of him, which he attempted to move. Later, he described seeing dust falling down everywhere and was trying to catch it. He manifested clouding of consciousness. A diagnosis of viral encephalitis was made on the basis of the history of persistent headache, the neurological signs and the finding of lymphocytosis in the cerebrospinal fluid.

It is often difficult to decide whether the full criteria for the presence of a hallucination have been fulfilled in the visual modality. Distortion of visual percepts, based on either sensation of external stimuli or internal interference with the visual pathway, may produce disturbances that are similar to those occurring with entirely new perceptions. Sometimes, the account of his experience given by the patient sounds like a sensory transformation rather than a hallucination, but the bizarre and complex nature of the experience renders phenomenonological description difficult.

Visual hallucinations occur with *occipital lobe tumours* involving the visual cortex, for example tuberculous granuloma in the left occipital lobe caused a 'starburst' effect in the right visual field (Werring and Marsden, 1999). Hallucinations and other visual disturbances may occur with other physical lesions, such as *loss of colour vision*, *homonymous hemianopia* (loss of half of the field of vision, the same half in both eyes; Komel, 1985), *dyslexia* (inability to read at a level appropriate to the individual's age and intelligence) and *alexia* in a dominant hemisphere lesion, and *cortical blindness* (blindness due to a lesion of the cortical visual centre). They may, as in delirium tremens, be associated with an affect of terror or with an affect of hilarious absurdity. Similar visual hallucinations, illusions and changes in mood occur in other forms of delirium. Visual hallucinations also occur in the *post-concussional state*, in *epileptic twilight states* and in metabolic disturbances, for example *hepatic failure*. Visual hallucinations have also been described in association with various dementing processes, including Alzheimer's disease (Burns *et al.*, 1990), senile dementia (Haddad and Benbow, 1992), multi-infarct dementia (Cummings *et al.*, 1987), Pick's disease (Ey, 1973) and Huntington's chorea (Lishman, 1989). Among referrals to a psychogeriatric service, visual perceptual disturbance occurred in 30 per cent of patients; there was a strong correlation between the presence of visual hallucination and eye pathology (Berrios and Brook, 1984). In fact, visual hallucinations are common in elderly patients with a wide variety of medical conditions and often no psychiatric history (Barodawala and Mulley, 1997).

Hallucinations have also been described by individuals after sniffing glue and petrol. The drugs mescaline and lysergic acid diethylamide are potent causes of visual perceptual change. Visual hallucinations are infinitely variable in their content. They range from quite crudely formed flashes of light or colour (elementary hallucinations), through more organized patterns and shapes, to complex, full, visual perceptions of people and scenes. Visual and auditory hallucinations may occur synchronously in organic states, for example in *temporal lobe epilepsy* a visual hallucination of a human figure was also heard to speak.

With psychomimetic drugs, there are alterations in spatial perception, in the perception of movement and in the appreciation of colour, and visual illusions and hallucinations may occur. *Synaesthesiae* also occur with lysergic acid diethylamide and similar drugs, although only rarely (Anderson and Rawnsley, 1954), that is, a sensory stimulus in one modality is perceived as a sensation in another modality. One mescaline subject 'felt, saw, tasted and smelt the noise of the trumpet'.

Visual hallucinations are very uncommon in schizophrenia (although some of the earlier writers used the term *hallucination* for other visual abnormalities that occurred). Persaud and Cutting (1991) cautiously refer to 'anomalous perceptual experiences in the visual modality' in schizophrenic patients as, for example, the patient who although still recognizing a face considers it to be distorted. These authors report four such cases of perceptual disturbance in one visual field, always the left field. Visual hallucinations are not reckoned to occur in uncomplicated affective psychoses. It is common in schizophrenia for the patient to describe auditory hallucinations associated with visual *pseudo-hallucinations*. Although the phonemes are complete and appear to have all the characteristics, subjectively, of a normal percept, the visual experiences are often inferred on the basis of the auditory hallucinations and of contemporaneous delusions. It is possible to see, in most instances, how psychotically disordered fantasy accounts for the content of the visual experiences. Vivid elaborate scenic hallucinations have been described in *oneiroid* states of schizophrenia. In these states, there is also an altered state of consciousness.

Sometimes, visual hallucinations do not appear to be associated with any other psychiatric abnormality. Charles Bonnet's syndrome (phantom visual images) is a condition in which individuals experience complex visual hallucinations in association with impaired vision without demonstrable psychopathology or disturbance of normal consciousness (Schultz and Melzack, 1991). Although more common in the elderly, it can occur at any age and is usually associated with central or peripheral reduction in vision. Episodes may last from days to years, with images of people, animals, buildings and scenery being most frequently reported, the images being static, moving in the visual field or animated. Clearly, this condition is of importance in the differential diagnosis.

In most cases of Charles Bonnet's syndrome, and in musical hallucinosis in the deaf, to which it has been likened, there is no demonstrable brain pathology (Fuchs and Lauter, 1992). The features of this syndrome have been considered by Podoll *et al.* (1990) to be as follows.

- Elderly persons with normal consciousness experience visual hallucinations.
- None of the following are present: delirium, dementia, organic affective or delusional syndromes, psychosis, intoxication or neurological disorder with lesions of the central visual cortex.
- There is reduced vision, resulting from eye disease in most cases.

Hallucinations in this condition are always located in external space, are usually coloured and are much more vivid and distinct than the patient's impaired vision would otherwise permit. The content is *elementary* in about one-third of cases, such as photisms or geometric patterns. Complex objects are most often human figures, less often animals, plants and inanimate objects; these objects may be fragmented and may change over time – figures gliding through the room. The percepts may be modifiable by voluntary control, for example closing the eyelids, and there is usually insight concerning their 'unreality'. This is sometimes associated with fear of mental illness and would suggest that these phenomena may be pseudohallucinations rather than 'true' hallucinations in some cases.

Delirium tremens

The alcoholic withdrawal syndrome of *delirium tremens* is a specific form of acute organic syndrome and is characterized by gross changes in perception, mood and conscious state (see Chapter 3). Pareidolic or affective illusions are often prodromal in delirium tremens, and these are followed by visual and haptic *Lilliputian* hallucinations, which are often of little animals or diminutive men. There is a bizarre intermingling of affect so that the patient experiences stark terror and, at the same time, a sort of crazy comicalness especially common with these disorders.

The hallucinations in delirium tremens may change so rapidly that the patient has difficulty in describing them. A patient experiencing such visual phenomena tried to portray this in Figure 7.2. Illusions are frequently associated with hallucinations, especially affective illusions, in which, through the predominant mood state of terror, cracks in the wall of the ward, or curtains moving in the breeze, may be misinterpreted in a frightening way. At the same time, such patients are highly suggestible and can form abnormal visual experiences as a result of suggestion.

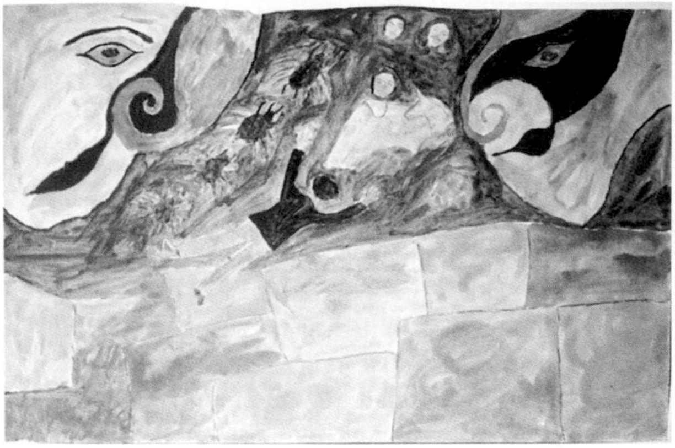

Figure 7.2 The experience of delirium tremens.

Autoscopic hallucination

Like so many topics of considerable phenomenological interest, the term *autoscopy* has been used with different meanings and definitions since its first use by Féré in 1891. The experience concerns how the individual regards the boundaries of self and is discussed further with other disorders of self-image. It is best to reserve autoscopy for abnormalities of visual perception involving *seeing oneself*; 'visual experiences where subjects see an image of themselves in external space viewed from within their own physical body' (Dening and Berrios, 1994).

Although this topic has been of considerable literary interest over the years, clinical cases with definite perceptual abnormality are not common. Dening and Berrios have reviewed 56 cases, 53 from the literature and 3 of their own. Males predominated, with a ratio of 2:1, and the mean age of subjects was 40 years. Both neurological and psychiatric disorder occurred in about 60 per cent of cases (different subjects), with epilepsy in approximately one-third. Decreased consciousness occurred in 45 per cent and delirium in 18 per cent, and 9 per cent of subjects were dead within 1 year. Visual imagery or narcissism was present in one-third of subjects, and depersonalization in 18 per cent. The commonest psychiatric diagnosis was depression. Usually, autoscopic episodes lasted for less than 30 minutes. Almost always, the subject saw his own face; quite often, he was lying in bed at the time. The experience often provoked distress, fear, anxiety and depression. This subjective experience was complex, with different components and causes rather than unitary.

Hallucination of bodily sensation

It has been convincingly argued by Berrios (1982) that diverse 'perceptions without object' were brought together by Esquirol (1817) within the term *hallucination*, which was relevant for 'distance senses' such as vision, hearing and, to a lesser extent, smell and taste, but not really applicable to touch. So-called *tactile hallucinations* appear to be different phenomenologically and only superficially resemble hallucinations of the distance senses. It would seem for tactile hallucinations that the most important corroborating diagnostic factor is the concurrence of a delusional component. Berrios concludes that the concepts of hallucination and delusion may be closer to each other than has often been considered, especially in British psychiatry.

Hallucinations of bodily sensation may be *superficial*, *kinaesthetic* or *visceral*. Superficial hallucinations affecting skin sensation may be *thermic*, an abnormal perception of heat and cold ('my feet on fire'); *haptic*, of touch ('a dead hand touched me'); or *hygric*, a perception of fluid ('all my blood has dropped into my legs and I can feel a water level in my chest'). *Paraesthesiae* is the term describing the sensation of tingling or 'pins and needles'. These may be delusionally ascribed, although of course they are often neurologically mediated, for example ulnar nerve compression causing pins and needles in the forearm.

Kinaesthetic hallucinations are those of muscle or joint sense. The patient feels that his limbs are being bent or twisted or his muscles squeezed. Such hallucinations in schizophrenia are often linked with bizarre somatic delusions. A man suffering from schizophrenia described the experience thus: 'I thought my life was outside my feet and made them vibrate' – he experienced kinaesthetic hallucinations of vibration. Kinaesthetic hallucinations may occur in organic states: 'a feeling of being rocked about'. Abnormal kinaesthetic perceptions have also been described in the withdrawal state from benzodiazepine drugs (Schopf, 1983) or from alcohol intoxication. A man, after recovery, described his episode of delirium tremens, saying, 'I felt as if I was floating in the air about fifty feet above the ground'. He illustrated this feeling with the picture in Figure 7.2.

Visceral hallucinations are false perceptions of the inner organs. There is only a limited range of possible visceral sensation, for example pain, heaviness, stretching or distension, palpitation and various combinations of these, such as throbbing. However, the possible range of bizarre schizophrenic false perceptions and interpretations is limitless. One man believed that he could feel semen travelling up his vertebral column into his brain, where it became laid out in sheets.

Hallucinations of bodily sensation are quite common in schizophrenia and are almost always delusionally elaborated, often *delusions of control* (Chapters 8 and 9). Haptic hallucinations may be experienced as touch ('like a hand stroking me') or painful ('knives stabbing my neck'). A patient believed that the smoke sensor in the ward was an infrared camera, 'because I feel it warm on my neck'. Another patient described a haptic hallucination in which she experienced genital stimulation that she ascribed to having sexual intercourse simultaneously with 'both Kennedy brothers all the time'. It is important to realize that there is both a hallucinatory and a delusional component in such experiences. One particularly unpleasant form of haptic hallucination is called *formication* (Latin: *formica*, 'ant'), the sensation of little animals or insects crawling over the body or just under the skin. This is especially associated with some drug states and withdrawal symptoms, for example cocaine addiction and alcohol withdrawal. It is often associated with *delusions of infestation*, but the latter may occur without hallucination.

Olfactory and gustatory hallucination

Hallucinations of smell and of taste frequently occur together, and it may be difficult or impossible to distinguish them from each other. This is not surprising, as a lot of what a layperson ascribes to taste is actually smell: 'the eucalyptus fragrance of this wine from the Barossa Valley'.

Olfactory hallucinations

Olfactory sensation or memory is often associated with powerful emotional resonances; it is not surprising therefore that hallucinations are also invested with a strong affective component. Olfactory hallucinations occur in schizophrenia, in epilepsy and in some other *organic* states. The patient has a hallucination of smell. The smell may or may not be unpleasant, but it usually has a special and personal significance (Aggernaes' quality of *relevance*), for example it may be associated with the belief that people are pumping a poisonous or an anaesthetic gas into the house, which the patient alone can smell. Sometimes, patients have an olfactory hallucination relating to themselves: 'I smell repulsive, unbearable – like a corpse, like faeces'. This particular patient killed himself. He felt that he created such a stench that he was intolerable in any reasonable society. Sometimes, patients misinterpret and *overvalue* normal body odours. A delusion in which a patient believes himself to smell malodorously without an accompanying olfactory hallucination is quite common in schizophrenia and related paranoid states.

Olfactory hallucinations occur in epilepsy, especially in association with a temporal lobe focus, and commonly form the aura (or earliest phase) of such fits. A patient described a smell of burning rubber regularly just before he became unconscious. Visual, auditory, gustatory and visceral hallucinations also occur in temporal lobe epilepsy.

Gustatory hallucinations

Gustatory hallucinations occur in various conditions. In schizophrenia, they sometimes occur with delusions of being poisoned. There may be a persistent taste, for example 'onions', 'a metallic taste' or some more bizarre type of taste. In depression and in schizophrenia, the flavour of food may disappear altogether or become unpleasant. Changes in gustatory perception may occur with some organic states, such as temporal lobe epilepsy, and also with some psychotropic drugs, for example lithium carbonate or disulfiram. It is often difficult to describe how this disturbance of taste is mediated and, therefore, whether it is hallucinatory or not.

Differentiation of hallucinations

Before deciding that a patient is hallucinated, the possibility of other perceptual experiences must be considered. These are not necessarily of pathological significance. The differential diagnosis of hallucination includes illusion, pseudohallucination, hypnagogic and hypnopompic images and, of course, vivid imagery and normal perception.

PSEUDOHALLUCINATIONS

Pseudohallucination is one of the least understood phenomena in psychopathology. As Berrios (1996) remarks, 'it has been used to refer to real perceptions perceived as "unreal", isolated hallucinations which do not fit into favoured diagnoses, side effects of drugs, withdrawal hallucinations, diabetic hallucinations, etc'. Berrios goes on to say, 'unrestrained, usage has strayed even wider, pseudohallucinations being sometimes applied to (i) phenomena which meet criteria for hallucinations or illusions, (ii) hallucinations in people without mental illnesses (e.g. the bereaved), (iii) the false perceptions of people recovering from psychotic illnesses, (iv) factitious hallucinations in malingerers, and (v) occasionally, normal but unusual perceptions which initially seem to be hallucinations (e.g. radio reception in dental amalgam or intracranial shrapnel fragments)'. Furthermore, part of the confusion over the meaning of the term *pseudohallucination* has arisen because it is often used in two different and mutually contradictory ways, according to Kräupl Taylor (1981). On one hand, it refers to hallucinations with insight (Hare, 1973), and on the other hand to vivid internal images. Hallucinations with insight would be those hallucinatory experiences in which the subject is aware that the hallucinatory percepts do not correspond to external reality despite the perceptions being veridical and in external objective space. Vivid internal images are those phenomena that have all the clarity and vividness of a normal percept except that they occur in inner subjective space.

Jaspers (1962) identified pseudohallucination as similar to normal perception except that it occurs in inner subjective space. This characteristic, pseudohallucination, shares with imagery. In other words, for Jaspers, pseudohallucination is a perceptual experience that is figurative and occurs in inner subjective space, not in external objective space. But it has all the vividness and clarity of a normal perception and can be retained unaltered. It occurs independent of the subject's will and therefore cannot be deliberately evoked. Jaspers derived this description of pseudohallucination from Kandinsky.

Kandinsky (1849–1889) based his description of pseudohallucination on his own personal experiences. He committed suicide at the age of 40 years while a patient at St Nicholas Hospital, St Petersburg, where he had once been medical superintendent (Lerner *et al.*, 2001). In 1885, he described *pseudohallucination* as a separate form of perception from true hallucination and wrote, 'subjective perceptions which in vividness and character are real hallucinations except that they do not have objective reality' (quoted in Berrios, 1996). Pseudohallucinations can be identified in the visual, auditory or tactile modalities.

Hare (1973) has given as an example of pseudohallucination the voice heard by an obsessional or depressed person. It is described by the patient as a voice but is actually recognized as his own thoughts. Pseudohallucinations are not pathognomonic of any particular mental illness. A patient with histrionic personality disorder saw a robed figure at the foot of her bed lifting his index finger to his mouth to caution her to silence. The image was sharp and vivid but was recognized as being seen with the inner eye. The patient knew that the figure was not at the foot of the bed and that other people in the room could not see him. When she tried to relate the figure in space to the background of her field of vision, in this case the walls and curtains of the room, she realized that she could not do so; it had no definite location in outer space, that is outside herself.

To summarize, the significance of hallucination is that it almost always denotes morbid mental state. The significance of pseudohallucination is in its differential diagnosis from hallucination, as pseudohallucination is not necessarily psychopathological.

OTHER ABNORMALITIES OF PERCEPTION

Autoscopy

Autoscopy is the experience of *seeing* oneself and knowing that it is oneself (see also visual hallucination, p. 111). It is sometimes called the *phantom mirror image*. It is one of the abnormalities of unity of self described in Chapter 13, but in *autoscopy* the experience is necessarily visual. Autoscopy may take the form of a pseudohallucination, for instance a person sees himself distinctly and vividly, the image lasts for some time and did not seem to be conjured up voluntarily and the phenomenon is considered to be in the subject's 'mind's eye' rather than in precisely located external space. Schizophrenic patients may have such pseudohallucinations, but they also occur in organic states such as temporal lobe epilepsy and parietal lobe lesions. On occasions, autoscopy may take the form of true visual hallucination; this is likely to be associated with an organic state.

Various abnormalities of body image of a perceptual nature occur in organic states in which the person may see himself or part of himself replicated. Autoscopy is quite different from *Capgras' syndrome*, which is not an abnormality of perception at all but a delusional misidentification of a person or people close to the patient. *Negative autoscopy* has also been described, in which, for instance, the patient looks in the mirror and sees no image at all.

Extracampine hallucination (concrete awareness)

'I know that there is someone behind me on the right all the time; he moves when I move', 'I keep on hearing them talking about my disease down in the post office' (half a mile away) – these hallucinations are experienced outside the limits of the sensory field, outside the visual field or beyond the range of audibility. They are not of diagnostic importance, as they occur in schizophrenia, epilepsy and other organic states and also as *hypnagogic hallucinations* in healthy people. The phenomenon is quite definitely experienced as a perception by the patient and not just as a belief or an idea.

Hypnagogic and hypnopompic hallucination

These are perceptions that occur while going to sleep (*hypnagogic*) and on waking (*hypnopompic*). According to Zilboorg and Henry (1941), hypnagogic hallucinations were first mentioned by Aristotle. It is known that the conscious level fluctuates considerably in different stages of sleep, and both types of abnormal perception probably occur in a phase of increasing drowsiness: the structure of thought, feelings, perceptions and fantasies and, ultimately, self-awareness becomes blurred and merged into oblivion. These experiences occur in many people in good health. They are also described with *narcolepsy*, *cataplexy* and *sleep paralysis* to form a characteristic tetrad of symptoms (see p. 61 for descriptions). *Toxic states* such as glue sniffing, acute fevers (especially in children), postinfective *depressive states* and phobic anxiety neuroses are other conditions that may be associated.

The perception may be visual, auditory or tactile. It is sudden in occurrence, and the subject believes that it woke him up, for example a loud voice in the street below saying 'world war!', a feeling of someone pushing him over the bed or seeing a man coming across the bedroom. The importance of these phenomena in psychopathology is to recognize their nature and realize that they are not necessarily abnormal, even though they may be truly hallucinatory.

Functional hallucination

This is the strange phenomenon in which an external stimulus is necessary to provoke hallucination, but the normal perception of the stimulus and the hallucination in the same modality are experienced simultaneously. A schizophrenic patient heard hallucinatory voices only when water was running through the pipes of his ward. He heard no phonemes for most of the time, but when he heard water rushing through the pipes along the wall he became very distressed by voices that told him to damage himself. He was terrified of the content of these voices because he was afraid he might act on them. He could readily separate the noise of water from the voices, and the latter never occurred apart from the former, but both perceptions were recognized as distinct and *real*. Another patient heard voices when the radio or television was switched on, alongside the broadcast voices; he had persecutory delusions that these activities were carried out deliberately to upset him and he became very distressed, and at times violent, as a result.

Reflex hallucination

As a doctor was writing in his case notes during his interview of a female patient, she said, 'I can feel you writing in my stomach'. The patient saw and heard the act of writing and was quite sure that it accounted for the tactile sensation in her abdomen. A stimulus in one sensory modality producing a hallucination in another is called a *reflex hallucination*. This is, in fact, a hallucinatory form of *synaesthesia*, mentioned earlier as the experience of a stimulus image in one sense modality producing an image in another, for example the feeling of discomfort caused by seeing and hearing somebody scratch a blackboard with their fingernails. Another reflex hallucination occurred in a woman who experienced pain whenever certain words were mentioned. Functional and reflex hallucinations are not themselves of great diagnostic or theoretical significance, but they require mentioning for completeness and recognition in order to identify other more important symptoms with confidence.

Abnormal imagery

Mental imagery tasks are designed to assess a subject's capacity for mental representation of the perceived world. In cases of hemineglect, there has been interest in whether the observed deficits in imagery are due to inattention or to impairment of mental imagery. Bisiach and Luzzatti (1978) described abnormalities in individuals with hemineglect. Their patients were asked to describe the Piazza del Duomo in Milan from two standpoints: facing the cathedral and with their backs to the cathedral. From both standpoints, the subjects were unable to describe the right side of the scene despite having correctly described it from the previous standpoint. In other words, even in imagination the mental representation of the piazza was unilaterally deficient for the right side. In these cases, inattention influenced the capacity for imagery. Guariglia *et al.* (1993) report a patient without hemineglect in whom impairment of imagery for objects in the left visual field was demonstrated. For the first time, this showed that without hemineglect, that is, visual inattention for space, failure of imagery was still possible.

Sensory deprivation

Continuing perception is necessary for consciousness. The field of sensation varies all the time as individual sensations in different modalities from the outside world and from inside oneself compete for attention. *Consciousness* consists of the integration of this changing field to form a composite awareness of oneself in one's environment. The essential nature of sensation has been explored by studying its absence, as revealed by research on the effects of sensory deprivation (Zubek, 1969). This topic is only given brief mention, as it is somewhat peripheral to psychiatry.

Sensory deprivation was studied using Canadian college students as volunteers (Bexton *et al.*, 1954). The subjects, wearing translucent goggles and gloves with cardboard cuffs, lay on a bed in a light but partially soundproof room; there was a continual background noise. This experience was found to be extremely unpleasant and, despite being paid, subjects were not prepared to remain in this state for more than 3 days.

This technique has been refined subsequently to blot out external sensations more completely. Various perceptual abnormalities are experienced. Visual hallucinations of varying complexity were described, but further study of these perceptual changes resulted in their being considered, more cautiously, to be 'reported visual sensations' and 'reported auditory sensations' (Zuckermann, 1969). These were classified into 'meaningless sensations' and 'meaningful integrated sensations'. Some of the latter are more like hallucinatory experiences. Depending on the completeness of deprivation of other sensations, abnormal perception occurs in modalities other than vision. Subjects show an altered affective state: they become panicky, restless, irritable or, alternatively, bored and apathetic.

Despite considerable neuropsychological research with valuable findings for investigating the sensory environment in growth and development, developing brain interconnections, neurochemistry and neurophysiology, the study of sensory deprivation has not so far made as big an impact on descriptive psychopathology as was initially expected. There are various difficulties to be accounted for. What part of the effects of deprivation is due to failure of development and what to loss of behaviours already established? How can one use animal work to explore subjective symptoms? How can one extrapolate from the experience of normal individuals in a highly abnormal environment to those who are psychiatrically ill? Many studies in sensory deprivation are described by Riesen (1975), who links the experimental data to neurological function and development.

The distinction has been made between *sensory deprivation* and *perceptual deprivation*. The latter is achieved by rendering the sensations patternless and meaningless, rather than by preventing sensations, by using such devices as translucent goggles and continuous 'white' noise. The deleterious effects of sensory deprivation have been considered by Slade (1984) as:

- inability to tolerate the situation
- perceptual changes
- intellectual and cognitive impairments
- psychomotor effects
- physiological changes in terms of the electroencephalograph and galvanic skin response measures.

Fantasy is often used as a means of reducing the unpleasant affective component of sensory deprivation. The subject may become disoriented and show increasing difficulty with problem solving and concentration. For perception and maintenance of the normal state of consciousness, it is necessary to have a variety of sensory stimuli available and for these stimuli to be changeable. If the objects of perception do not themselves change, the observer will move his point of observation in order to create change.

REFERENCES

Aggernaes A (1972) The experienced reality of hallucinations and other psychological phenomena. *Acta Psychiatrica Scandinavica 48*, 220–38.

Anderson EW and Rawnsley K (1954) Clinical studies of lysergic acid diethylamide. *Monatsschrift fuer Psychiatrie und Neurologie 28*, 38–55.

Andrade C (1988) Free hallucinations as culturally sanctioned experience. *British Journal of Psychiatry 152*, 838–9.

Asaad G and Shapiro B (1986) Hallucinations: theoretical and clinical overview. *American Journal of Psychiatry 143*, 1088–97.

Barodawala S and Mulley GP (1997) Visual hallucinations. *Journal of the Royal College of Physicians of London 31*, 42–8.

Bentall RP (1990) The illusion of reality: a review and integration of psychological research on hallucinations. *Psychological Bulletin 107*, 82–95.

Bentall RP, Baker GA and Havers S (1991) Reality monitoring and psychotic hallucinations. *British Journal of Clinical Psychology 30*, 213–22.

Berrios GE (1982) Tactile hallucinations: conceptual and historical aspects. *Journal of Neurology, Neurosurgery and Psychiatry 45*, 285–93.

Berrios GE (1990) Musical hallucinations: a historical and clinical study. *British Journal of Psychiatry 156*, 188–94.

Berrios GE (1996) *The History of Mental Symptoms: Descriptive Psychopathology Since the Nineteenth Century*. Cambridge: Cambridge University Press.

Berrios GE and Brook P (1984) Visual hallucinations and sensory delusions in the elderly. *British Journal of Psychiatry 144*, 662–4.

Beveridge A (1985) *Language disorder in schizophrenia*. M.Phil. thesis, University of Edinburgh.

Bexton WH, Heron W and Scott TH (1954) Effects of decreased variation in the sensory environment. *Canadian Journal of Psychology 8*, 70–6.

Bisiach E and Luzzatti C (1978) Unilateral neglect of representational space. *Cortex 14*, 129–33.

Bleuler E (1950) *Dementia Praecox or the Group of Schizophrenias* (transl. Zinkin J). New York: International University Press.

Burns A, Jacoby R and Levy R (1990) Psychiatric phenomena in Alzheimer's disease 2. Disorders of perception. *British Journal of Psychiatry 157*, 76–81.

Critchley M (1951) Types of visual perseveration: 'palinopsia' and 'illusory visual spread'. *Brain 74*, 267–99.

Cummings JL, Miller B, Hill MA, *et al.* (1987) Neuropsychiatric aspects of multi-infarct dementia of the Alzheimer type. *Archives of Neurology 44*, 389–93.

Cutting J (1997) *Principles of Psychopathology: Two Worlds – Two Minds – Two Hemispheres*. Oxford: Oxford University Press.

Dening TR and Berrios GE (1994) Autoscopic hallucinations: a clinical analysis of 56 cases. *British Journal of Psychiatry 165*, 808–17.

Esquirol JED (1817) *Hallucinations (reprinted in Des Maladies Mentales, 1938)*. Paris: Baillière.

Ey H (1973) *Traité Des Hallucinations*. Paris: Masson.

Falloon IRH and Talbot RE (1981) Persistent auditory hallucinations: coping mechanisms and implications for management. *Psychological Medicine 11*, 329–40.

Féré C (1891) Note sur les hallucinations autoscopiques ou spéculaires et sur les hallucinations altruistes. *Comptes Rendus Hebdomadaires des Séances et Memoires de la Société de Biologie 3*, 451–3.

Fuchs T and Lauter H (1992) Charles Bonnet syndrome and musical hallucinations in the elderly. In Katona C and Levy R (eds) *Delusions and Hallucinations in Old Age.* London: Gaskell.

Green P and Preston M (1981) Reinforcement of vocal correlates of auditory hallucinations by auditory feedback: a case study. *British Journal of Psychiatry 139*, 204–8.

Gregory RL (2004) Recovery from blindness. In Gregory RL (ed.) *The Oxford Companion to the Mind*, 2nd edn. Oxford: Oxford University Press.

Guariglia C, Padovani A, Pantano P and Pizzamiglio L (1993) Unilateral neglect restricted to visual imagery. *Nature 364*, 235–7.

Haddad PM and Benbow SM (1992) Visual hallucinations as the presenting symptom of senile dementia. *British Journal of Psychiatry 161*, 263–5.

Hare EH (1973) A short note on pseudohallucinations. *British Journal of Psychiatry 122*, 469–76.

Heilbrun AB and Blum NA (1984) Cognitive vulnerability to auditory hallucinations: impaired perception of memory. *British Journal of Psychiatry 144*, 508–12.

Horowitz MJ (1975) A cognitive model of hallucinations. *American Journal of Psychiatry 132*, 789–95.

Jacobs L, Feldman M, Diamond SP and Bender MB (1973) Palinacousis: persistent or recurring auditory sensations. *Cortex 9*, 211–6.

Jaspers K (1962) *General Psychopathology* (transl. Hoenig J and Hamilton MW). Manchester: Manchester University Press.

Junginger J and Frame CL (1985) Self-report of the frequency and phenomenology of verbal hallucinations. *Journal of Nervous and Mental Diseases 173*, 149–55.

Kandinsky V (1885) *Kritische und klinische.* Betrachtungen im Gebiete der Sinnestanschangen.

Komel HW (1985) Complex visual hallucinations in the hemianopic field. *Journal of Neurology, Neurosurgery and Psychiatry 48*, 29–38.

Kosslyn SM (2004) Mental imagery: depictive accounts. In Gregory RL (ed.) *The Oxford Companion to the Mind*, 2nd edn. Oxford: Oxford University Press.

Kosslyn SM and Thompson WL (2003) When is early visual cortex activated during visual mental imagery? *Psychological Bulletin 129*, 723–46.

Kosslyn SM, Pascual-Leone A, Felician O, *et al.* (1999) The role of area 17 in visual imagery: convergent evidence from PET and rTMS. *Science 284*, 167–70.

Kräupl Taylor F (1981) On pseudohallucinations. *Psychological Medicine 11*, 265–72.

Lerner V, Kapstan A and Witztum E (2001) The misidentification of Clerambault's and Kandinsky–Clerambault's syndromes. *Canadian Journal of Psychiatry 46*, 441–3.

Lishman WA (1989) *Organic Psychiatry: the Psychological Consequences of Cerebral Disorder*, 2nd edn. Oxford: Blackwell Scientific.

Margo A, Hemsley DR and Slade PD (1981) The effects of varying auditory input on schizophrenic hallucinations. *British Journal of Psychiatry 139*, 122–7.

Martin GN (2006) Human neuropsychology. Harlow: Pearson Education.

Morgan S (1989) *Wanamurraganya: the Story of Jack McPhee*. Fremantle: Arts Centre Press.

Morley S (1987) Psychological modification of auditory hallucinations: distraction versus attention. *Behavioural Psychotherapy 15*, 240–51.

Nayani TH and David AS (1996) The auditory hallucination: a phenomenological survey. *Psychological Medicine 26*, 177–89.

Persaud R and Cutting J (1991) Lateralized anomalous perceptual experiences in schizophrenia. *Psychopathology 24*, 365–8.

Podoll K, Schwartz M and Noth J (1990) Charles Bonnet-Syndrom bei einem Parkinson-Patientem mit beidseitigen Visusverlust. *Nervenarzt 61*, 52–6.

Pylyshyn ZW (2004) Mental imagery. In Gregory RL (ed.) *The Oxford Companion to the Mind*, 2nd edn. Oxford: Oxford University Press.

Riesen AH (1975) *The Developmental Neuropsychology of Sensory Deprivation.* New York: Academic Press.

Sachs O (1995) *An Anthropologist on Mars.* London: Picador.

Schneider K (1959) *Clinical Psychopathology*, 5th edn (transl. Hamilton MW). New York: Grune & Stratton.

Schopf F (1983) Withdrawal phenomena after long-term administration of benzodiazepines: a review of recent investigations. *Pharmacopsychiatry 16*, 1–8.

Schreber D (1955) *Memoirs of My Nervous Illness* (transl. Macalpine I and Hunter RA). London: Dawson.

Schultz G and Melzack R (1991) The Charles Bonnet syndrome: 'phantom visual images'. *Perception 20*, 809–25.

Sims ACP (1991) An overview of the psychopathology of perception: first rank symptoms as a localizing sign in schizophrenia. *Psychopathology 24*, 369–74.

Slade PD (1976a) Hallucinations. *Psychological Medicine 6*, 7–13.

Slade PD (1976b) An investigation of psychological factors involved in the predisposition to auditory hallucinations. *Psychological Medicine 6*, 123–32.

Slade PD (1984) Sensory deprivation and clinical psychiatry. *British Journal of Hospital Medicine 32*, 256–60.

Smith EE and Kosslyn SM (2007) *Cognitive Psychology: Mind and Brain*. Upper Saddle River: Prentice Hall.

Smythies JR (1956) A logical and cultural analysis of hallucinatory sense-experience. *Journal of Mental Science 102*, 336.

Spitzer M (1994) The basis of psychiatric diagnosis. In Sadler JZ, Wiggins OP and Schwartz MA (eds) *Philosophical Perspectives on Psychiatric Diagnostic Classification*. Baltimore: Johns Hopkins University Press.

Wernicke C (1906) *Grundri der psychiatrie in klinischen vorlesun gen*. Leipzig: Thieme.

Werring DJ and Marsden CD (1999) Visual hallucinations and palinopsia due to an occipital lobe tuberculoma. *Journal of Neurology, Neurosurgery and Psychiatry 66*, 684.

Zeki S (1993) *A Vision of the Brain*. Oxford: Blackwell.

Zilboorg G and Henry GW (1941) *A History of Medical Psychology*. New York: Norton.

Zubek JP (1969) *Sensory Deprivation: Fifteen Years of Research*. New York: Appleton-Century-Crofts.

Zuckermann M (1969) In Zubek JP (ed.) *Sensory Deprivation: Fifteen Years of Research*, pp. 47–84. New York: Appleton-Century-Crofts.

Delusions and Other Erroneous Ideas

8

> I cannot pretend to agree with him, when I know that his mind is working altogether under a delusion. *Trollope (1869)*

Anthony Trollope, in his novel *He Knew He Was Right*, describes not only the totally destructive effect of delusional jealousy on the individual himself but also the extraordinary dilemma this poses for other people who come into contact with him: whether to humour the individual and risk reinforcement or to confront him and risk violence. Fundamental to clinical practice in psychiatry, using the phenomenological or empathic method, is obtaining a clear account of the ideas or notions that the subject, the patient, actually holds. Although delusions are often referred to as beliefs, there is a growing literature questioning whether they are beliefs at all. *False beliefs* include primary and secondary delusions, overvalued ideas and *sensitive ideas* of reference. As already discussed, the association between delusion and hallucination is close although they are phenomenologically distinct.

IDEAS, BELIEFS AND DELUSIONS

Very rarely does anyone claim to be deluded, and usually what such a patient thought was a delusion does not prove to be so. A delusion is a false, unshakeable idea or belief that is out of keeping with the patient's educational, cultural and social background; it is held with extraordinary conviction and subjective certainty. Subjectively, or phenomenologically, it is indistinguishable from a true belief. A man who is a Bachelor of Medicine of the University of London holds a delusion that he is being used as 'an envoy from Mars'. He believes that he is both a doctor and an envoy, and neither thought seems to him to be delusional or imaginary. He likes to imagine himself a rich man with an estate in Gloucestershire. He has not the slightest difficulty in identifying this latter idea as fantasy. To the man himself, a delusion is much closer to a true belief than imagination, and the reasons enlisted to support its veracity are produced in the same way that a person would prove any other notion on which he was challenged. Normally, fantasy is easily distinguished from reality, although the subject may show great reluctance in accepting his aspirations as 'mere fantasy'. Similarly, there is usually very little difficulty for the external observer in deciding whether a false belief is a misinterpretation of the facts based on false reasoning, or a delusion.

Meaning of delusion

The delusions of the mad are not well received by the sane. At best, they have been treated as harmless and humorous, but often they have been regarded as deliberate attempts to deceive or as evidence of demonism. The English word *delude* comes, of course, from Latin and implies playing or mocking, defrauding or cheating. The German equivalent *Wahn* is a whim, false opinion or fancy, and makes no more comment than the English on the subjective experience. The French equivalent, *délire*, is more empathic; it implies the ploughshare jumping out of the furrow (*lira*), perhaps a similar metaphor to the ironical 'unhinged'.

Delusions and insanity in law

Delusion has been considered in law to be the fundamental feature of *insanity*. 'Delusions therefore, when there is no frenzy or raving madness, is the true character of insanity', stated Lord Erskine defending Hadfield, who, when clearly mentally ill, fired at King George III in 1800 (West and Walk, 1977).

The special verdict of *not guilty by reason of insanity* can be brought in English law only when the degree of insanity satisfies the *Rules Laid Down by Judges*, generally called the *McNaughton Rules*. These rules were drawn up in the mid-nineteenth century by judges in the House of Lords as definitive guidance following the attempted assassination of the Prime Minister by McNaughton. They state, 'To establish a defence on the ground of insanity it must be clearly proved that, at the time of committing the act, the party accused was labouring under such a defect of reason from disease of the mind, as not to know the nature and quality of the act he was doing was wrong'. The rules would be fulfilled by a man who bisects his victim with a meat cleaver believing the latter to be a carcass of beef, or by someone who shoots another person believing them to be an enemy assassin and himself to be the Queen's personal bodyguard. These McNaughton Rules are restrictive and exclude many defendants who are undoubtedly psychotic; more detailed consideration will be found in Wasik (1990). They are now rarely employed, the plea of *diminished responsibility* being more frequently used in defence for homicide, but the McNaughton Rules remain the basis for the legal concept of insanity.

Definition of delusion

There continues to be much debate and controversy about the definition of delusions. The standard approach is to follow Jaspers' (1959) claim that delusions are manifest in judgements and arise in the process of thinking and judging. For Jaspers, the characteristics of delusions are that (a) they are false judgements, (b) they are held with extraordinary conviction and incomparable subjective certainty, (c) they are impervious to other experiences and to compelling counterargument and (d) their content is impossible. Each of these criteria have been subjected to criticism. Delusions may not be false insofar as the content is concerned. This is best exemplified in delusional jealousy, whereby the belief may correspond to objective truth and is therefore not false. Delusions may not be held with extraordinary conviction but, equally, normal beliefs may be held with extraordinary conviction. Delusional beliefs may also be amenable to counterargument, although it is rare that this by itself will alter the belief. Finally, delusional content need not be impossible.

There is a growing body of opinion that delusions are not beliefs at all. Spitzer (1994), for example, argues this case. He makes the distinction between 'to know that' and 'to believe that'. In Spitzer's view, delusions make knowledge claims rather than belief claims. In other words, patients are asserting that they 'know such and such' rather than they 'believe such and such', which is why delusional statements are expressed with conviction and certainty and not subject to discussion and inquiry. Berrios (1996) comes to the same conclusions. He states that 'delusions are empty speech acts which assert themselves as beliefs'. Furthermore, he makes the point that the content of delusions is incidental to the fact of the phenomenon being a delusion. In Berrios' view, the content of delusions is randomly chosen; the content merely reflects whatever is in the environment at the time the delusion is formed. The content is lacking in informational quality and is not 'symbolic expression of anything'. These critiques of the current definitions and understanding of delusions underline the complexity of the conceptual status of delusions and show that there is still fruitful theoretical work to be done in psychopathology. For the purpose of this book, it is best to conceive of delusions as false beliefs.

The decision to call a belief or judgement *delusional* is not made by the person holding the belief but by an external observer. There can be no phenomenological definition of delusion, because the patient is likely to hold this belief with the same conviction and intensity as he holds other non-delusional beliefs about himself, or as anyone else holds intensely personal non-delusional beliefs. In this respect, delusions are to ideation what hallucinations are to perception. Subjectively, a delusion is simply a belief, a notion or an idea. Stoddart's definition of a delusion (1908), 'a judgement which cannot be accepted by people of the same class, education, race and period of life as the person who experiences it', has some advantages. However, it could include as delusional falling in love with a person others regard as unsuitable, having a minority religious belief or holding any unusual idea without acknowledging reasonable argument to the contrary.

Hamilton (1978) defined delusion as 'A false unshakeable belief which arises from internal morbid processes. It is easily recognisable when it is out of keeping with the person's educational and cultural background'.

Rather than suggest a unitary definition for delusion, Kendler *et al.* (1983) have proposed several poorly correlated dimensions or vectors of delusional severity.

- Conviction: the degree to which the patient is convinced of the reality of the delusional beliefs.
- Extension: the degree to which the delusional belief involves areas of the patient's life.
- Bizarreness: the degree to which the delusional beliefs depart from culturally determined consensual reality.
- Disorganization: the degree to which the delusional beliefs are internally consistent, logical and systematized.
- Pressure: the degree to which the patient is preoccupied and concerned with the expressed delusional beliefs.

Two other dimensions that might also be considered are as follows.

- Affective response: the degree to which the patient's emotions are involved with such beliefs.
- Deviant behaviour resulting from delusions: patients sometimes, but not always, act on their delusions.

The term *delusion* is used frequently in ICD-10 but is not defined there. It is referred to in all the major categories of organic mental disorders, substance misuse, schizophrenia and affective disorders, and its presence excluded from the category of neurotic disorders (see Chapter 23; Sims, 1991).

Delusions are entirely different from thought disorder, which is considered in Chapter 9: delusions are ideas that the patient believes to be true but an observer considers false; *formal thought disorder* is the alteration from normal that the patient himself describes subjectively in his thinking processes.

PRIMARY AND SECONDARY DELUSIONS

The confusing subject of primary and secondary delusions requires some explanation. It is probably most meaningful to use the term *primary* to imply that delusion is not occurring *in response* to another psychopathological form such as mood disorder. *Secondary* delusion is used in the sense that the false belief is *understandable* in present circumstances – because of the pervasive mood state or because of the cultural content.

Gruhle (1915) considered that a primary delusion was a disturbance of symbolic meaning, not an alteration in sensory perception, apperception or intelligence. Primary delusions occur in schizophrenia and not in other conditions; they include both delusional perception and delusional intuition (Cutting, 1985). However, delusional intuition, notion or idea is not pathognomonic of schizophrenia, because in any individual case there is too much scope for arguing whether this delusion is indeed *primary*, that is, ultimately ununderstandable, or *secondary* in nature. Secondary delusions occur in many conditions other than schizophrenia and can sometimes be understood in terms of the person's background culture or emotional state.

Wernicke (1906) formulated the concept of an *autochthonous idea*, an idea that is 'native to the soil', aboriginal, arising without external cause. The trouble with finding supposed autochthonous or primary delusions is that it can be disputed whether they are truly autochthonous. For this reason, they are not considered of *first rank* in Schneider's (1957) classification of symptoms. It is too difficult to decide in many cases whether a delusion is autochthonous. Several writers have claimed that all delusions are understandable if one knows enough about the patient.

The ultimately ununderstandable

Jaspers' detailed exposition of delusion has been carefully reviewed by Walker (1991). Jaspers' concepts of the *ununderstandable*, and of *meaningful connections*, are relevant here. If we ask an offender to describe the psychic world in which he lives – his attitudes, his feelings and how these developed through his childhood until now – we may be able to understand his sexual cruelty, which at first seemed quite incomprehensible: the behaviour becomes *meaningful* in the context of abuse by his stepfather and surviving as an adolescent in a harsh urban subculture with violence, humiliation and frustration. However, when we consider the middle-aged schizophrenic spinster who believes that men unlock the door of her flat, anaesthetize her and interfere with her sexually, we find an experience that is ultimately not understandable. We can understand, on obtaining more details of the history, how her disturbance centres on sexual experience, why she should be distrustful of men, her doubts about her femininity and her feelings of social isolation. However, the *delusion*, her absolute conviction that these things really are happening to her, that they are true, is not understandable. The best we can do is to try to understand externally, without really being able to feel ourselves into her position (*genetic empathy*, Chapter 1), what she is thinking and how she experiences it. We cannot understand how such a notion could have developed.

This is the core of the primary or autochthonous delusion: it is *ultimately ununderstandable*. The patient described above also believed the police were using rays to observe her. One does not have to try to find which delusion came first, the anaesthesia or the observation by rays, to decide which is primary; *primary* is not dependent on temporal relationships. In that both delusions are not ultimately understandable, they are both primary delusions. A delusion can still be primary in this, Jaspers' sense, although it arises on the basis of a memory, an atmosphere or a perception. The protagonist in Gogol's (1809–1852) *Diary of a Madman* (Gogol, 1972) says, 'There is a King of Spain. He has been found at last. That king is me. I only discovered this today'. This sudden and inexplicable belief arose autonomously and unpremeditated. Thereafter, it dictated the protagonist's every behaviour and influenced his view of the world.

How ideas and delusions are initiated

A delusion is a belief, an idea, a thought, a notion or an intuition, and it arises in the same type of setting as any other idea – in the context of a perception, a memory or an atmosphere – or it may be autochthonous, appearing to occur spontaneously.

Ideas are initiated in the following ways.

- An example of an idea occurring on the basis of a *percept*: I smell food cooking and then form the idea that I will go and eat.
- Ideas may follow *memory*: I remember listening to a string quartet and form the idea of playing a compact disc.
- Ideas may arise out of an *atmosphere* or a mood state: I already feel irritable, and when I collect my car from the garage and it makes an unexplained noise I become unreasonably angry and blame the mechanic for not repairing it satisfactorily.
- An idea may be *autochthonous*. I visit a ward of the hospital on an afternoon when I never normally go there. Although I accept that all behaviour has an explanation for its occurrence, I do not know why on this particular occasion I did this. Theoretical explanations may be given as to where such ideas come from, for example the *unconscious*, but subjectively they seem to have occurred *de novo*. Delusions occur in similar settings on the basis of percept, memory, atmosphere or *de novo* – 'out of the blue'.

In our discussion of primary delusions, we will see how the same four situations also account for the onset of delusions: percept, memory, mood or autochthonous. In this sense, delusion *is* an idea.

Secondary delusions

Primary delusions differ from secondary delusions in that the former are ultimately not understandable. Secondary delusions are understandable when a detailed psychiatric history and examination are available. That is, they are understandable in terms of the patient's mood state and/or life history. A manic patient claimed to be Mary, Queen of Scots. She accepted that the queen in question lived and died centuries ago but claimed descent from her and felt fully entitled to say that she *was* she. The belief could be understood in terms of her elated and expansive mood and disappeared as her affective state subsided. A depressed patient believed that he had committed the 'unforgivable sin'. Discussion and persuasion, even with a person whose religious views he respected, was of no avail in giving him relief. The belief could be seen as an integral part of his depressed mood. Depressive delusions may remain after treatment has resulted in improvement from retardation, and they account for suicide occasionally occurring in the recovery phase of depression. A secondary delusion may become understandable when the patient's social background is known and the doctor knows the beliefs of the subculture from which he comes. It has been suggested that there may be a decline in the prevalence of delusion occurring with depressive illness, but Eagles (1983), studying admissions to hospital in Edinburgh from 1892 to 1982, considered there to be no genuine reduction.

Secondary delusions (*delusion-like ideas*) can be traced for their origins to the circumstances of that person's life, to his current mood state, to the beliefs of his peer group and to his personality. They are understandable and often transient. There is no *subjective* distinction between a secondary delusion and an overvalued idea, for the distinction between the two can reliably be made only on the evidence given for holding them. A delusion, whether primary or secondary in nature, is based on delusional *evidence*: the reason the patient gives for holding his belief is like the belief itself – false, unacceptable and incorrigible.

TYPES OF PRIMARY DELUSION

Kurt Schneider (1957) discusses the dilemma of primary symptoms in schizophrenia extremely lucidly by giving six different possible meanings for the term *primary*, but he still leaves us in doubt as to whether the belief is primary or not. He makes it clear, however, that primary symptoms are not the same as *first-rank symptoms* of schizophrenia. Primary symptoms are those that arise without understandable cause in the context of the psychotic illness. They are therefore the necessary manifestations of the underlying psychopathology, in the same way that swelling and redness are a necessary consequence of physical trauma. First-rank symptoms, on the other hand, are, according to Schneider, simply a useful empirical list of symptoms that are found commonly in schizophrenia and not in other conditions. Describing their presence makes no claim as to how they arose.

True delusions, or *delusions proper*, are distinguished by Jaspers from *delusion-like ideas*. *True delusions* become, therefore, synonymous with primary delusions, and delusion-like ideas with secondary delusions. Delusion-like ideas can be seen to *emerge* understandably from the patient's internal and external environment, especially from his mood state. True delusions cannot be so explained; they are psychologically irreducible. They have, according to

Jaspers, the following types: (a) autochthonous delusion (delusional intuition), (b) delusional percept, (c) delusional atmosphere and (d) delusional memory.

Autochthonous delusion (delusional intuition)

These are delusions that appear to arise suddenly 'out of the blue'; they are phenomenologically indistinguishable from the sudden arrival of a normal idea. The patient gropes for explanations for the occurrence of his delusion in answering the interviewer's question, in the same way that a healthy person would find it difficult to account for the arrival of any idea if he were asked to explain it. The difference lies in the ability of the observer to empathize with, to understand, a non-delusional idea even though it may be bizarre and destructive, but he cannot understand how a person can have come to *believe* his delusion.

Schneider regarded the term *delusional idea* as based on outmoded psychology, and he felt it should therefore be abandoned. It is often confused with *delusion-like idea*, even in some textbooks, and this is another good reason for abandoning it. *Delusional intuition* is perhaps the most satisfactory translation of the German *Wahneinfall*. Delusional intuition occurs as a single stage, unlike *delusional perception*, which occurs in two stages: perception and then false interpretation. Like delusional perceptions, delusional intuitions are self-referent and usually of momentous import to the patient.

Delusional percept

This is present when the patient receives a normal perception that is then interpreted with delusional meaning and has immense personal significance. It is a *first-rank symptom of schizophrenia*. Jaspers delineated the concept of delusional percept, and Gruhle (1915) used this description to cover almost all delusions – he minimized the importance of delusional intuition. Schneider (1949) considered the essence of delusional perception to be the abnormal significance attached to a real percept without any cause that is understandable in rational or emotional terms; it is self-referent, momentous, urgent, of overwhelming personal significance and, of course, false.

It is often difficult to decide whether a delusion is truly a delusional percept or is being used to explain the significance of certain objects of perception within a delusional system. A woman said, 'every night blood is being injected out of my arms [*sic*]'. When asked for her evidence, she explained that she had little brown spots on her arms and therefore knew that she was being injected. The interviewer looked at the spots on her arms, rolled up his sleeve and showed her spots identical in appearance on his own arm. He said that they had been on his arm as long as he could remember and were called 'freckles'. She agreed that both sets of spots looked similar and accepted his explanation of his own spots, but she still insisted that her freckles proved that she was being injected in her sleep. This was a delusional percept.

Another example of what was probably a delusional percept caused considerable problems in surgical management, ultimately resulting in the death of the patient (Porter and Williams, 1997). A 65-year-old woman had flooded her house by leaving all the taps on.

“On admission she was unkempt, with unwashed hair, wearing a dirty dress and vest. She was bringing up bile stained vomit and was reluctant to be interviewed. She expressed delusional beliefs that her stomach had been blown up with ether over several weeks and that it was liable to burst as a result of a citizens band radio which was located in her stomach. She believed that the IRA had been after her for years and experienced auditory hallucinations of voices which she identified as coming from the CB receiver. One 'voice' told her not to let anyone examine her. There was no evidence of an acute confusional state and the diagnosis was consistent with a long-term paranoid psychosis.

“On physical examination her abdomen was soft but distended with a hard, craggy, immobile, central mass. The liver and spleen were of normal size and the kidneys were not palpable. Bowel sounds were loud. A diagnosis of possible intra abdominal malignancy was made.

She refused any investigation or treatment. She developed acute renal failure and ultimately died; ascitic fluid revealed adenocarcinomatous cells probably of ovarian origin.

Another patient, who had other delusional symptoms, believed that many of the patients in the hospital were well-known citizens cunningly disguised with wigs, make-up and false beards. She recognized that they did not look like the people whom she presumed them to be but considered this to be part of a gigantic hoax, in which she was herself involved, to 'help people spiritually'. Although her percepts were normal and her interpretations delusional, this was not considered to be a delusional percept but a misinterpretation. All the circumstances in her life were explained in terms of an immensely complicated delusional system, and these perceptions had no immediate personal significance beyond the significance that she found in all the objects and events around her.

In a delusional percept, there is a direct experience of meaning for this particular normal percept; it is not simply an interpretation of this percept to fit in with other established delusional beliefs. Delusional perception is, therefore, a direct experience of meaning that the patient did not have previously. Objects or persons take on new personal significance that is delusional in nature, even though the perception itself remains unchanged. This is different from a delusional misinterpretation, in which the delusional system affects all aspects of the patient's life, and so every event or perception is interpreted as being involved with that delusion. A patient sees that a doorknob is missing; this is not the precipitant of immediate *new* personal significance of a delusional nature, rather, it further confirms the belief he already held that people are trying to trap him and subject him to vivisection.

Perception, when considering delusional percept, can be understood in quite a wide sense. There is no difference, in subjective experience, between perceiving an object by means of a sense organ and perceiving or understanding the sense of written or spoken messages, although the perceptual routes are different. Thus delusional perception includes delusional significance attached to words and sentences as well as to purely sensory objects. For example, an in-patient at Rubery Hill Hospital walked to an entrance of the hospital and saw a dilapidated notice: 'R U B E ... ILL'. She suddenly realized that this was a concealed message just for her – 'Are you be(ing) ill?', that people were concerned to help her and that she would get better. The delusional interpretation was attached to the meaning of the letters of the notice.

There are two distinct stages in delusional perception:

- the object becomes meaningful within a field of sensations and is perceived; this is usually visual perception (Mellor, 1991)
- that object becomes invested with delusional significance.

These two stages need not be simultaneous for the experience to be a delusional percept. On occasions, they have been separated by an interval of years. A patient believed that his mind was being jammed by an electronic device. He claimed that this had started when, 5 years before, he had lifted the telephone receiver and heard an unusual clicking noise. The delusional belief he had held for only a few months.

Delusional atmosphere

For the patient experiencing delusional atmosphere, his world has been subtly altered: 'Something funny is going on', 'I have been offered a whole world of new meanings'. He experiences everything around him as sinister, portentous, uncanny, peculiar in an indefinable way. He knows that he personally is involved but cannot tell how. He has a feeling of anticipation, sometimes even of excitement, that soon all the separate parts of his experience will fit together to reveal something immensely significant. This is, in fact, what usually happens, as delusional atmosphere is part of the underlying process and, often, the first symptom of schizophrenia and the context in which a fully formed delusional percept or intuition arises. The mood of the atmosphere is very important, and this experience is often referred to as *delusional mood*. The patient feels profoundly uncomfortable, often extremely perplexed and apprehensive. When the delusion becomes fully formed, he often appears to accept it with a feeling of relief from the previous unbearable tension of the *atmosphere*.

A middle-aged man presented initially as a psychiatric outpatient with apparent obsessional symptoms. He kept checking that his neighbours could not hear what he was saying in his home. He had resigned from several jobs because he believed that his employers would not accept his religious beliefs. He felt that people around him were hostile and implacably opposed to him, although he could not define quite how – he just 'felt it'. He kept moving house, but the feeling stayed with him. This continued for several years, and he then arrived at a casualty department claiming that his neighbours were talking about his actions and controlling his thoughts. The atmosphere had developed insidiously over years, and eventually he manifested *auditory hallucinations* and *passivity of thought* (see Chapter 9).

German psychopathologists never used the term *delusional atmosphere* but always referred to *delusional mood*, according to Berner (1991), but he considers that atmosphere is to be preferred, as it allows the distinction to be made between a cognitive, perceptual disturbance provoking an emotional response and a modification of mood causing a changed perception of the outside world. It is considered that delusional atmosphere is a common end state resulting from different pathways: vulnerability to cognitive disturbance, as in 'Bleulerian' schizophrenia; dynamic derailment, as in affective disorders such as puerperal depression or psychogenic vulnerability; without either of the other two, with stressful life events. Berner considers that this state is not restricted to sufferers from schizophrenia.

The prodromal phases of schizophrenic illnesses are very variable in nature, and often another diagnosis has been given before the definitive symptomatology becomes established. In an instructive review of the literature on the simulation of psychosis, and study of six patients who were thought to be feigning a schizophrenic psychosis, Hay (1983) commented on the nature of *feigned psychosis*. In his opinion, simulation of schizophrenia is generally a prodromal phase of a schizophrenic psychosis occurring in people with extremely deviant premorbid personalities. All but one of his patients were found to be suffering from schizophrenia at the time of follow-up.

Delusional memory

In much the same way that delusional percept is a delusional interpretation of a normal percept, delusional memory is the delusional interpretation of a normal memory. These are sometimes called *retrospective delusions*. An event that occurred in the past is explained in a delusional way. A man aged 50 whose mental illness had lasted for about 2 years claimed that his health had been permanently affected since the age of 16, when he had had 'an operation to remove his appendix'. He now believed that the operation had been an excuse to 'implant a golden convolvulus' in his bowels.

If delusional meaning is attached to a normal percept that is remembered, this then becomes a *delusional percept*. It has the two components that were described as being necessary for delusional percept: the image of the remembered percept and the attachment to this percept of delusional significance. A married woman remembered years previously seeing a man standing in a pub 'with a sad look on his face'. She 'realized', at the start of her schizophrenic illness 2 weeks before admission to hospital, that he had been in love with her then, and she tried to locate his name in the telephone directory and make contact again, feeling that they were involved in a special relationship.

Of course, it is a mistake to expect phenomenological symptoms to reveal themselves tidily from the patient's conversation. There is no absolute demarcation between delusional memory and delusional percept or intuition. The patient describes a delusion. Did this occur 1 hour, 1 week or 10 years ago? At what point will this be delusional memory, not delusional intuition? Similarly, there is no absolute distinction between a normal event, perception or idea that occurred in the past and is remembered with a delusional interpretation, and a delusional event, perception or idea that occurred in the past and is also remembered with a delusional interpretation. In other words, there are two senses to the term *delusional memory*. There is the sense in which a normal memory is misinterpreted in the present, and another sense in which the actual memory is itself a false memory that is imbued with delusional interpretation. Both these are delusional memories, and it is not always possible to know how much of the event was factual and how much delusional. A woman with schizophrenia, aged 34, described 12 years ago picking up a telephone to ring a man she liked very much: 'God moved my arm and made me put the telephone back'. It was not possible to decide exactly what part of this experience was factual and what delusional, and at what time the delusion occurred.

Fine distinctions are sometimes imposed on the classification of primary delusions but are more collector's items than features of useful clinical significance. *Delusional awareness* is an experience that is not sensory in nature, in which ideas or events take on an extreme vividness as if they had additional reality. *Delusional significance* is the second stage of the occurrence of delusional perception. Objects and persons are perceived normally but take on a special significance that cannot be rationally explained by the patient.

THE ORIGINS OF DELUSION

What is the origin of delusions? This question drives at how far delusions are by definition different from normal beliefs and, if they are different from normal beliefs, what the mechanisms are that are involved in their development and manifestation. Jaspers' (1959) own view was that delusion was a primary phenomenon and that it implies a transformation in the total awareness of reality. This means that a delusional belief involves and implicates practical activity, behaviour, the meanings that are immanent in objects, and radically transforms the basic experience of the world. A person who is deluded that he is loved by a celebrity approaches the world with this certainty and knowledge and acts accordingly, by writing to, telephoning or attempting to visit the celebrity. This erroneous belief invests the patient's world with new meanings. In these terms, *reality* lies in the interpretation of, or the significance attached to, events that occur interpreted in the light of the primary erroneous belief.

An understanding of how delusions radically alter the patient's world as described does not help us to explain how delusions form in the first place. The factors involved in delusion formation have been summarized by Brockington (1991); see Box 8.1.

Fish (1967) has made a useful précis of the earlier German theories of the origins of delusion. Conrad proposed five stages in the development of delusional psychosis.

- *Trema*: delusional mood representing a total change in perception of the world.
- *Apophany*: a search for, and the finding of, new meaning for psychological events.
- *Anastrophy*: heightening of the psychosis.
- *Consolidation*: forming of a new world or psychological set based on new meanings.
- *Residuum*: eventual autistic state.

Gruhle (1915) considered *delusional perception* to be the most significant form of delusion, a normal percept taking on a new meaning. This results in a disturbed relationship of the understanding of events. Matussek considered that with delusional perception there is a change either in the significance of the words used or in the actual nature of the perception itself. These writers, and also Schneider, regard *delusional perception* as the key to understanding the nature of delusional experience.

Box 8.1 Factors involved in the germination of delusions

- Disorder of brain functioning
- Background influences of temperament and personality
- Maintenance of self-esteem
- The role of affect
- As a response to perceptual disturbance
- As a response to depersonalization
- Associated with cognitive overload

Hagen regarded *delusional atmosphere* as primary, arising for reasons unknown and resulting in a rearrangement of meanings in the world around the patient, who gropes for an answer to this problem of understanding and finds it in creating a delusion. It is easier to bear the certainty of a delusion than the uncertain foreboding of the atmosphere. Jaspers considered that there is a subtle change of personality due to the illness itself, and this creates the condition for the development of the delusional atmosphere in which the delusional intuition arises.

All these theories assume that the delusion is *primary* and *ultimately not understandable* in the same sense that Jaspers considers the experience of reality to be primary. Experience holds a symbolic implication beyond the fact of the event itself, for example the doctor writing a prescription for his patient in the consulting room means much more to the latter than if the doctor were doodling on his prescription block. (A patient in North Africa in the nineteenth century ate the prescription his doctor gave him, so great was his confidence in, and veneration for, the doctor; Sims, 1972.) It seems that the symbolic belief attached to events and perceptions is altered in delusion, and this is why the patient does not necessarily act on his delusions. The delusional atmosphere is not an essential prerequisite for a delusional intuition, as the latter may occur apparently *de novo*.

Some writers have not tried to explain delusions, because they find them totally incomprehensible and they consider that they are directly due to an abnormality of the brain (Schneider, 1949). Bleuler concentrated on the *alteration in affect* as primary rather than delusional atmosphere or perception. He considered that heightened affect loosens the capacity to form associations and thus facilitates the arrival of a delusion. At the beginning of his schizophrenic illness, there is extreme affect, perhaps in the form of anxiety or ambivalence, which the patient cannot express.

Kretschmer (1927) stressed the importance of the underlying personality. He described the *sensitive premorbid personality* occurring in a person who retains *affect-laden complexes* and has a limited capacity for emotional self-expression. Such a person is driven painfully by, for example, powerful sexual feelings, but he has great difficulty in communicating his passion and relating to other people. He is very much aware of social constraints and is rigidly controlled by his superego. Such a person, somewhat rigid, narrow-minded and suspicious in his views, readily forms *sensitive ideas of reference*. A *key experience* may occur in his life circumstances, and quite suddenly these ideas become structured as *delusions of reference*.

A girl was always shy, reticent and sensitive at school. Quite often, she was reluctant to go to school. She was meticulous in her attention to personal neatness and cleanliness. After leaving school, she remembered vividly several occasions as a child when she had felt humiliated. At the age of 18, when she was working in a factory, she was in the women's cloakroom brooding because her boyfriend had told her that he was leaving her for someone else. She heard one of the other women say, 'Ugh, doesn't she smell?' Immediately, she applied the statement to herself and to explain her boyfriend's behaviour. From then onwards, she was convinced that she smelt unpleasant all the time, although she could smell nothing herself. This delusion dominated her life, prevented her mixing and caused her great distress. This development of a delusion (*Sensitiver Beziehungswahn*) from sensitive ideas of reference, as the sequel to a *key experience*, is sometimes seen at the onset of schizophrenia but is not common. The key experience, as demonstrated in this case, has two important qualities. First, it has particular appropriateness to the patient's areas of conflict as sensitive ideas of reference. Second, it occurs at a time of marked emotional turmoil and distress, so that the psychic ground is prepared for a catastrophic event.

Attempts have been made to find all delusions understandable in terms of the person's internal experience or social background. Westphal considered that if one knew all about the patient, the change in his view of himself and the belief that he had become noticeable in some way would explain the delusion (Fish, 1967). Freud's (1907) theories on the development of delusions also attempted to make them ultimately understandable through the mechanisms of denial, projection and so on. Other authors have claimed that delusions are understandable in a social context. Laing (1961) considered the flight into madness as a necessary defence against a highly destructive family – not only understandable, but admirable, and even worth emulating.

When four different psychological theories were appraised to explain paranoid phenomena, a basis of *shame-humiliation* was found to be the most consistent (Colby, 1977). Winters and Neale (1983) consider that existing theories of delusional thinking develop two main themes: *motivational* and *defect*. The motivational theme explains the arrival of a delusion to explain unusual perceptual experience or to reduce uncomfortable psychic states. Defect implies some fundamental cognitive-attentional deficit resulting in delusion.

Cognition and reasoning in delusion

The formation, elaboration and persistence of delusional beliefs are probably an expression of numerous causal influences converging; each exerts a different influence in the evolution of the belief (Roberts, 1992). The process of reasoning in order to come to conclusions about one's situation in the outside environment appears to be altered in those experiencing delusions. A 'jump-to-conclusions style' has been demonstrated in deluded subjects when asked to perform a probabilistic reasoning task (Huq *et al.*, 1988). This was confirmed by Garety *et al.* (1991) in showing that 41 per cent of deluded subjects but only 4 per cent of controls reached a conclusion on the basis of only one item of information. A common cause in abnormality of information processing has been proposed for those subjects with abnormal reasoning and abnormal perception; failure to make use of knowledge, previously acquired, of regularities in the world, resulting in over-reliance on information immediately present, may be a factor in delusion formation (Garety, 1991). This model emphasizes the deviant nature of the thinking process that is associated with delusions in patients with schizophrenia. In Garety's model, judgemental processes involved in delusion formation include (a) prior expectation that may be modified by emotion; (b) current information that we have at our disposal, such as the information reaching us by way of our perceptions; and (c) the nature of our information processing bias or style. In this model, if perceptual abnormalities predominate the role of deviant information processing mechanisms will be underemphasized. In other words, when delusions are secondary to hallucinations reasoning should remain intact. The advantage of this model is that it highlights the varying routes to delusion formation.

Attribution in delusion

An alternative psychological explanation for delusion comes from *social attribution theory*. Kaney and Bentall (1989, 1992) found that deluded patients made excessively external, stable and global attributions for negative events ('The fact that I broke my leg proves yet again that the Wetherby freemasons are getting at me.') and excessively internal, stable and global attributions for positive events ('Everyone smiles and nods when they see me because I have been sent by God to communicate with people about evil and I have a letter from the Pope as proof.'). Deluded subjects were unwilling to attribute negative events of which they were the victim to their own cause; also, in judging the behaviour of other people they were reluctant to attribute negative events to the victims themselves. These and other studies suggest that persecutory delusions have a function in protecting the individual from low self-esteem (Bentall, 1993).

Deluded subjects were considered to evaluate their own causal statements in a distinctive manner, and this difference from depressed subjects was greater than the differences in the causal statements themselves; that is, the difference between deluded and other subjects in internality for positive and negative events does not reflect differences in the causal statements of these subjects but rather differences in their attributions about their attributions (Kinderman *et al.*, 1992). Once again, delusions are linked both to personal meaning and to boundaries of self. This investigation of attributional style was further extended using obvious and opaque tests of attributional style. Deluded subjects attributed negative outcomes to external causes in the obvious or transparent tests but a more covert testing to internal causes; this further supported the hypothesis that persecutory delusions function as a defence against underlying feelings of low self-esteem (Lyon *et al.*, 1994). This psychological exploration is further supported by the clinical study that follows.

Delusion and meaning in life

Roberts (1991) has developed the thesis that delusions, in the context of schizophrenic illness, may not themselves be an affliction or illness but an adaptive response to whatever initiates the psychotic break. A group of chronically deluded subjects was compared with previously deluded patients now in remission and with two non-patient groups. Persecutory delusions were common in both patient groups, but grandiose and erotic delusions and delusions of special knowledge were mostly found in the currently deluded group. The chronically deluded group scored much higher than the remitted patients for positive meaning in life, and much lower for depression and suicidal intention. They had a very high level of perceived purpose and meaning in life. It is considered that for some the formation of delusions is adaptive in combating purposelessness, loneliness, sense of inferiority, hopelessness, isolation and painful awareness of broken relationships and provides a new sense of identity, a clearer sense of duty and responsibility, an experience of freedom, protection from past hurts, and a change from fear, worry, depression and boredom towards feeling lively, enthusiastic, interested and peaceful. One patient described this: 'I've had a great time. I've got this one great thought in my mind that I am Jesus – that's enough ... nothing hurts me now, I need nothing now'.

CONTENT OF DELUSIONS

Delusions are, of course, infinitely variable in their content, but certain general characteristics commonly occur. Unlike the *form*, which is dictated by the type of illness, the *content* is determined by the emotional, social and cultural background of the patient: Napoleons are now rare in mental hospitals; schizophrenia sufferers from traditional societies may describe their thoughts as being interfered with by the spirits of their ancestors rather than by television. As computers and the Internet increasingly affect all aspects of our lives, we are beginning to have described by those with mental illness delusions of control concerning the Internet (Catalano *et al.*, 1991).

Delusions of persecution

This is the most frequent content of delusion. It was distinguished from other types of delusion and from other forms of melancholia by Lasègue (1852). People who believe delusionally that their lives are being interfered with from outside more often feel this to be harmful than beneficial. A variant on the usual beliefs of persecution or malevolent intent are delusions of prejudice: the patient or victim believes that he is being slighted, overlooked, passed over in favour of someone else. The interfering agent in delusions of persecution may be animate or inanimate, other people or machines; it may be systems, organizations or institutions rather than individuals. Sometimes, the patient experiences persecution as a vague influence without knowing who is responsible.

Persecutory delusions occur in many different conditions: in schizophrenia, in affective psychoses of manic and depressive type and in organic states both acute and chronic. The affect associated with the belief of persecution may vary from an inappropriate indifference and apathy in schizophrenia to stark terror, as commonly seen in delirium tremens.

Manic patients with persecutory delusions show gross overactivity and flight of ideas in attempting to express and deal with their beliefs. In depression, the persecutory delusions take on the characteristic colouring of the dominant mood state. Persecutory overvalued ideas are a prominent facet of the *litigious* type of paranoid personality disorder.

Morbid jealousy and delusion of infidelity

Morbid jealousy, a disorder of *content* described by Ey (1950), may be manifested in various forms, for example as delusion, overvalued idea, depressive affect or anxiety state. The feeling of jealousy, coupled with a sense that the loved object 'belongs to me' and, therefore, 'I belong to the other', is part of normal human experience; it is of social value in marital relationships for preserving the family. Various terms have been used to describe abnormal, morbid or malignant jealousy. Kraepelin used the term *sexual jealousy*. Enoch and Trethowan (1979) have considered it important to distinguish psychotic jealousy from other types, and this is dependent on the demonstration of a *delusion of infidelity*. It is sometimes difficult to distinguish understandable jealousy from that which is delusional.

Mullen (1997) classified morbid jealousy with *disorders of passion,* in which there is an overwhelming sense of entitlement and a conviction that others are abrogating the subject's rights: 'The morbidly jealous believe that they are the victims of an infidelity that has deprived them of the fealty which is their due and they are driven to expose this disloyalty, reassert their control and punish the transgression'. The other two categories are the querulant, who are indignant at infringements of rights, and the erotomanic, who are driven to assert their rights of love.

Delusion of infidelity, that is, when the subject unreasonably believes him or herself to be the victim of their partner's unfaithfulness, may occur without other psychotic symptoms. It has been described by Todd and Dewhurst (1955) and by Mullen (1990). This is identifiably delusional when the belief of the spouse is based on delusional evidence. Such delusions are resistant to treatment and do not change with time. A patient was very concerned that his wife was being unfaithful with numerous people, including his boss, her general practitioner and others. Four years later, despite various treatments, his belief was unchanged, but he said, 'I don't blame her now. She is much younger than I am and everyone does that sort of thing'. Delusions of jealousy are common with alcohol abuse; for instance, Shrestha *et al.* (1985) found sexual jealousy to be present in 35 per cent of alcoholic men and 31 per cent of women. As jealousy appeared to be justified in some cases, *morbid jealousy* was considered to be present in 27 per cent of men and 15 per cent of women. Delusional jealousy, often associated with impotence, also occurs in some organic states, for example the punch drunk syndrome of boxers (chronic traumatic encephalopathy; Lishman, 1997) following multiple contrecoup contusion. Quite frequently, the spouse, wearied by continued accusations of infidelity, does form another sexual involvement, which may result in an acute exacerbation in the mental state of the patient and further marital conflict.

The sexual content of the delusion is obvious; however, Enoch (1991) regards the nature of the relationship between the two partners as the key aspect of the condition. Jealousy is directed towards the sexual partner. The deluded person is very attached to, and often emotionally utterly dependent on, the other; he may have a misplaced sense of owning her completely. The victim is often much more sexually attractive than the deluded partner, for instance a young wife or a sociable and popular husband. The deluded person may have been promiscuous in the past and therefore resignedly expects his spouse to show similar behaviour. He may have become impotent and projected the blame for his failure on to her. He may have homosexual fantasies directed towards the men with whom he claims his wife is consorting. Morbid jealousy arises with the belief that there is a threat to the exclusive possession of his wife, but this is just as likely to occur from conflicts inside himself, his own inability to love or his sexual interest directed towards someone else as from changing circumstances in his environment or his wife's behaviour. Husbands or wives may show sexual jealousy, as may cohabitees and homosexual pairs. Jealousy is particularly prominent in these latter two types of relationship, because the insecurity of a liaison not sanctioned by convention or law is especially likely to germinate suspicion. Crimes of violence are notoriously associated with morbid jealousy; violence is more often vented on the partner than on the supposed rival, most often by men on women. Morbid jealousy makes a major contribution to the frequency of wife battering and is one of the commonest motivations for homicide (Mullen, 1990).

Delusions of love

The delusions associated with loving and being loved are quite different from the behavioural and affective abnormalities of *nymphomania*, the situation of a woman characterized by morbid or uncontrolled sexual desire, and *satyriasis*, the male equivalent of excessive sexual activity. Both these latter conditions exist initially in the opinion of an external commentator – the doctor.

Approximately twice as many schizophrenic patients had sexual preoccupations in the mid-twentieth century as compared with in the mid-nineteenth century (Klaf and Hamilton, 1961). *Erotomania* was described by Sir Alexander Morrison (1848) as being:

> “ characterized by delusions . . . the patient's love is of the sentimental kind, he is wholly occupied by the object of his adoration, whom, if he approach it is with respect . . . the fixed and permanent delusions attending erotomania sometimes prompt those labouring under it to destroy themselves or others, for although in general tranquil and peaceful, the patient sometimes becomes irritable, passionate and jealous.

Erotomania is commoner in women than in men, and a variety has been called 'old maids' insanity' by Hart (1921), in which persecutory delusions often develop. These have sometimes been classified as paranoia rather than paranoid schizophrenia; these delusional symptoms sometimes occur in the context of manic–depressive psychosis (Guirguis, 1981). Trethowan (1967) demonstrated the social characteristics of erotomania, relating the patient's previous difficulties in parental relationships to the present erotomania.

A variation of erotomania was described by, and retains the name of, de Clérambault (1942). Typically, a woman believes a man, who is older and of higher social status than she, is in love with her. The victim has usually done nothing to deserve her attention and may be quite unaware of her existence; sometimes he is a well-known public figure quite remote from the patient. In a case of the author's, the victim was a previous employer of the patient. She believed that he was the father of her child (although at another time she agreed that there had been no sexual relationship with her employer).

She also believed that he was sending her money, and she would write letters thanking him for his generosity and affirming her gratitude for the evidence of his love (Sims and White, 1973).

In a series of 16 erotomanic cases, Mullen and Pathé (1994) tried to distinguish between those cases in which there is a morbid belief in being loved and those with morbid infatuation. They found that in most cases both notions were described: a mixture of being loved and loving in return.

Delusional misidentification

Delusional misidentification syndromes include a number of discrete but related syndromes that have in common the concept of the double. These syndromes include *Capgras'* syndrome (Capgras and Reboul-Lachaux, 1923), *Frégoli's* syndrome (Courbon and Fail, 1927), the syndrome of *intermetamorphosis* (Courbon and Tusques, 1932) and the syndrome of *subjective doubles* (Christodoulou, 1978).

Capgras' syndrome is regarded by Enoch and Trethowan (1979) as 'a rare, colourful syndrome in which the person believes that a person, usually closely related to him, has been replaced by an exact double'. It is a specific delusional misidentification of a person with whom the subject usually has close emotional ties and towards whom there is a feeling of ambivalence at the time of onset. The belief, in Capgras' syndrome, has the full characteristics of delusion (Enoch and Trethowan, 1979). The basic concept of this syndrome is prominent in all cultures, hence the delusion is universal (Christodoulou, 1991). Like other delusions, *delusion* describes the form; the content is culture-dependent. A recent patient believed his mother had been replaced by an impostor after falling through a time warp to a parallel universe, and this explained the horrible things that had happened in the past 3 weeks.

Frégoli's syndrome is the delusional misidentification of an unfamiliar person as a familiar one, even though there is no physical resemblance. The syndrome of intermetamorphosis is the delusional belief that others undergo radical changes in physical and psychological identity, culminating in a different person altogether. The syndrome of subjective doubles is the delusional belief in the existence of physical duplicates of the self, and these duplicates are usually thought to have different psychological identities (see Moselhy and Oyebode, 1997, for review).

In a series of cases reviewed by Berson (1983), 55 per cent (70 patients) were unquestionably diagnosed as suffering from schizophrenia, and a further eight patients (totalling 61 per cent) were probably schizophrenic; 13 per cent were suffering from manic–depressive psychosis and 24 per cent were considered to have an organic diagnosis. Of 133 patients, 57 per cent were female; the age range was from 12 to 78, with a mean of 42.8 years. Majority opinion would not favour denoting this as a separate disease but rather as a symptom that colours the clinical state and dominates the symptomatology. The four different varieties of delusional misidentification have in common psychopathologically the form of a delusion. Capgras' syndrome, when it occurs in schizophrenia, is based on a delusional percept (Sims, 1986). In Capgras' syndrome, there is no outward change in the appearance of the object, and there is no false perception, for the patient often admits that the double exactly resembles the original

(Enoch and Trethowan, 1979), but careful questioning usually reveals that there are distinguishing stigmata. Sometimes patients will say, 'I know that it is not my mother because she would never stand like that' or 'this person moves too slowly to be my father'.

The ambivalence towards the object of misidentification may be expressed in the history, with a clear account of both negative emotions, such as hostility, fear or contempt, and affection and dependence. On those few occasions when an object, rather than a person, is wrongly identified, that object has important emotional connotations for the patient, for example home or a letter from a relative. The objects of misidentification in Berson's review of 133 patients comprised 60 spouses and 2 lovers; on 29 occasions, a child or children; 40 parents; 24 siblings; 13 therapists; 4 grandparents; 3 in-laws; 2 neighbours; 2 domestics; and 1 each of fiancé, cousin, stepson, employer and priest. On eight occasions, the self was misidentified either solely or with other evidence of the syndrome; on two occasions, animals, and eight times inanimate objects were misidentified. Thus, for 31 per cent of occasions, the delusional misidentification refers to a marital partner, and for 46 percent to a first-degree relative; in only 4 per cent was the misidentification of the patient him- or herself.

There is growing evidence that delusional misidentification syndromes are associated with organic disorders, including dementia, acquired brain injury, epilepsy and cerebrovascular accidents in 25 to 40 per cent of cases, and neuroimaging studies reveal association with right hemisphere abnormalities, particularly in the frontal and temporal regions (Edelstyn *et al.*, 1999). Furthermore, neuropsychological investigations have consistently shown impairments of face processing in delusional misidentification syndromes (Edelstyn *et al.*, 1996; Ellis *et al.*, 1993; Oyebode *et al.*, 1996). These findings underpin the assumption of right hemisphere abnormalities in delusional misidentification syndromes, because the right hemisphere is implicated in face processing and recognition.

Grandiose delusions

Primary grandiose delusions occur in schizophrenia. The patient may believe himself to be a famous celebrity or to have supernatural powers. He may believe himself to be involved in some very special and secret mission about which he has not yet been fully briefed but in anticipation of which he is waiting with excitement for the dénouement. Beliefs of this sort are sometimes called delusions of special purpose and are of the form of delusional intuition.

Expansive or grandiose delusional beliefs may extend to objects. So sometimes a psychotic patient demonstrates delusions of invention in which, for example, he builds a machine that he believes to have special capabilities, considering himself to be a creative prodigy. Secondary grandiose delusions, or delusion-like ideas, occur in manic states. A patient said that there was no life on Mars because 'if there had been I would have been able to get in touch by telepathy using my great genius'. He evinced no evidence of true passivity experiences. A manic patient, mentioned above, believed that she was descended from the royal Stuart line and therefore was actually in some way Mary,

Queen of Scots. She invited the Queen and the Prime Minister to a party in her student flat because she thought they would be honoured to be invited: 'It is only fair that they should have an invitation'. The expansive affect of mania can be very clearly seen to render this delusion understandable.

Religious delusions

Religious delusions are common. However, they formed a higher proportion of all delusions in the nineteenth century than in the twentieth century: three times as many schizophrenic patients of both sexes had religious preoccupation in the nineteenth century (Klaf and Hamilton, 1961). Decision as to whether beliefs are delusional or not must rest on the principles described above; that is, on the way the belief is held and the evidence produced in its support. Because a religious belief is very bizarre and at variance with those held by the interviewer, it does not necessarily make it a delusion. Religious delusions may be grandiose in nature, for example a patient who believed that she was an emissary of God to the Birmingham Housing Department. They may also be secondary to depressive mood, as in the patient of Emil Kraepelin (1905) quoted at the beginning of Chapter 20: 'I cannot live and I cannot die, because I have failed so much, I shall bring my husband and children to hell'.

The religious nature of the delusion is seen as a disorder of content dependent on the patient's social background, interests and peer group. The form of the delusion is dictated by the nature of the illness. So religious delusions are not caused by excessive religious belief, or by the wrongdoing that the patient attributes as cause, but they simply accentuate that when a person becomes mentally ill his delusions reflect, in their content, his predominant interests and concerns.

Sometimes, it can be difficult to make the distinction between religious delusion and the experience of an unusual religious belief or practice. Psychiatric morbidity would be suggested by the following (Sims, 1992).

- Both the subjective experience and the observed behaviour conform with psychiatric symptoms, that is, the self-description of this particular experience is recognizable as being the symptomatology of a known psychiatric illness – it has the form of delusion.
- There are other recognizable symptoms of mental illness in other areas of life: other delusions, hallucinations, disturbance of mood, thought disorder and so on.
- The lifestyle, behaviour and direction of personal goals of the individual subsequent to the event or religious experience are consistent with the natural history of mental disorder rather than with a personally enriching life experience, compatible with the conditions in which delusions occur.

Delusions of guilt and unworthiness

Such delusions are common in depressive illness. They often lead to suicide and, rarely, to homicide, when the killing of a close relative may be followed by the patient's suicide (see Chapters 18 and 20). Affective illness may be followed by the killing of children by depressed mothers or the killing of their wife or sometimes also children by husbands; suicide may follow immediately or later (Higgins, 1990).

The beliefs about guilt may totally dominate the patient's thinking. An elderly woman spent the day rushing round the house wringing her hands and telling her worried family that she was wretched, worthless and only deserved to die. She told her married daughters that they were illegitimate and that the house she lived in was not hers but stolen, and she told her husband of 30 years' standing that they were not legally married. When it was suggested to her that she come into hospital, she assumed that she would be killed on arrival, and she asked whether this could take place there and then so that she could receive her just deserts.

Delusions of poverty and nihilistic delusions

Delusions of poverty are common in depression; an elderly patient believed that 'the nurses' had been systematically raiding her purse and that she was destitute. *Cotard's syndrome* contains features typical of psychotic depression in the elderly: nihilistic and hypochondriacal delusions that are often bizarre, dramatic and tinged with grandiosity; depressed mood with either agitation or retardation and a completely negative attitude. According to Griesinger (1845), 'the patient confuses the subjective change in his own attitude to outside things . . . the real world seems to the patient to have disappeared completely, or to be dead'. This was graphically depicted by Cotard (1882):

> " I would tentatively suggest the name 'nihilistic delusions' (délire de negations) to describe the condition of the patients to whom Griesinger was referring, in whom the tendency towards negation is carried to its extreme. If they are asked their name or age, they have neither – where were they born? They were not born. Who were their father and mother? They have no father, mother, wife or children. Have they a headache or pain in the stomach, or any other part of the body? They have no head or stomach and some even have no body. If one shows them an object, a rose or some other flower they answer, 'that is not a rose, not a flower at all'. In some cases negation is total. Nothing exists any longer, not even themselves.

The central character in Patrick McGrath's novel *Spider* said, 'I was contaminated by it, it shrivelled me, it killed something inside me, made me a ghost, a dead thing, in short it turned me bad'. Elsewhere, the same character says, 'a single pipe takes water from my stomach . . . and this pipe alone drops through the void and connects to the thing between my legs that hardly resembles a formed male organ at all anymore' (McGrath, 1990). Sometimes delusions of persecution and negation coexist, and the more prominent are the nihilistic delusions the more severe is the depression. In general, nihilistic delusions are a depressive form of self-blame, while in persecutory delusions the blame is cast elsewhere. Nihilistic delusions are the reverse of grandiose delusions, in which oneself, objects or situations are expansive and enriched; there is also a perverse grandiosity about the nihilistic delusions themselves. Feelings of guilt and hypochondriacal ideas are developed to their most extreme, depressive form in nihilistic delusions.

Hypochondriacal delusions

A very depressed man said that he was full of water, that there was nothing else inside him, and that he could not pass water but that if he did that would be the end of him. He could not drink or the water would flood the room. Other less striking hypochondriacal beliefs and delusions occur in depression, and Schneider (1920) has considered that locating the experience of depression as a sensation in a bodily organ is equivalent to a 'first-rank symptom' of depressive psychosis (see Chapter 18). An elderly woman with depression, who had had a mitral valve replacement for rheumatic heart disease, said that she felt worthless and hopeless and described her physical functions as 'nothing is working'.

Hypochondriacal delusions may also occur in schizophrenia and have the characteristics of other schizophrenic ideas. They are more likely to be given a persecutory than a nihilistic explanation. Thus, a patient believed that his bodily functions were being interfered with by rays emitted from a planet and that this was part of a plot to control his thoughts and behaviour. Hypochondriacal delusions are discussed further in association with hypochondriasis in Chapter 15; however, other features of hypochondriasis, such as bodily preoccupation, disease phobia and conviction of the presence of disease with non-response to reassurance, are in fact more common than delusion (Pilowsky, 1967). Facial pain is described in Chapter 17 and other delusion-like ideas and overvalued ideas of the body in Chapter 15. Delusions concerning the patient's origins are sometimes described and have some affinity to hypochondriacal delusion. The patient believes, on delusional evidence, that he is not his parent's child, or perhaps that he is of royal birth, part animal or supernatural. Alternatively, he may believe that he does not exist and was never born.

Hypochondriacal delusions are commonly associated with delusional disorder in ICD-10 (previously known as paranoia; World Health Organization, 1992). Munro (1988) has described *delusional disorder* as an encapsulated monodelusional disorder with several subtypes, such as erotomanic, grandiose, jealous, persecutory, somatic and unspecified; the concept has developed from the older term *paranoia* (Munro, 1997). He has described the somatic type as *monosymptomatic hypochondriacal psychosis* and, of 50 cases, the three main groups were:

- delusions of body odour and halitosis
- infestation delusion (insects, burrowing worms or foreign bodies under the skin)
- delusions of ugliness or misshapenness (dysmorphic delusions).

In a factor analysis of the features of delusional disorder, four independent factors were identified, suggesting considerable heterogeneity of the condition (Serretti *et al.*, 1999). The first factor incorporated core depressive symptoms, which may be either a depressive syndrome reactive to stresses deriving from delusional ideation or a comorbid mood disorder, or both. Other factors were hallucinations, delusions and symptoms of irritability.

The complaint was always presented with great intensity, and patients were utterly convinced of the physical nature of the disorder. Hypochondriacal delusions may also occur with administration of drugs, both prescribed drugs and those of abuse.

Koro (Lapierre, 1972) is an unusual condition that has been described as an example of hypochondriacal delusion. This view is probably incorrect. The features of koro include (a) the belief that the penis is shrinking into the abdomen; (b) the belief that when the penis disappears into the abdomen, death will ensue; and (c) extreme anxiety accompanying this belief. Yap (1965) describes this as a culture-bound depersonalization syndrome and considers it to be a manifestation of acute anxiety associated with folk beliefs concerning sexual exhaustion. It has occurred in epidemic proportions among Malays in Singapore (Gwee, 1963) but has also been described in individual cases in a French Canadian (Lapierre, 1972), in a West Indian and a Greek Cypriot (Ang and Weller, 1984) and in an Englishman (Berrios and Morley, 1984). Oyebode *et al.* (1986) have shown in a single case study that this belief is accompanied by real shrinkage as measured by plethysmography. This suggests that the belief is based on physiological changes that are likely to be due to anxiety. In essence, the penile change is similar to tachycardia, hyperhidrosis or other features of sympathetic arousal associated with anxiety.

A group of patients who in some respects are intermediate between those suffering from somatic delusions and delusions of infestation are those who were described by Videbech (1966) as suffering from chronic olfactory paranoid syndromes; these have also been referred to as having 'olfactory reference syndrome' (Pryse-Phillips, 1971). Characteristically, these patients have a fixed and unalterable belief that they smell but do not have hallucinations or other olfactory experience. It is usually seen in the context of sensitive, paranoid personality development. There is a severe phobic reaction, with the behaviour of other people interpreted as finding their smell offensive and aversive.

Delusions of infestation

These have been described by Hopkinson (1970) and by Reilly (1988). In *Ekbom's syndrome* (Ekbom, 1938), the patient believes that he is infested with small but macroscopic organisms. The patient's experience may take the form of a tactile hallucinatory state, a delusion or an overvalued idea. The aetiology is also variable. It is probably most common as a symptom of circumscribed hypochondriasis in affective psychosis, along with other depressive symptoms, but it also occurs in paranoid schizophrenia, in monosymptomatic hypochondriacal psychosis (delusional disorder), in organic brain syndromes or with neurotically determined conditions. This topic is reviewed by Berrios (1985) and by Morris (1991).

Patients have believed that they had a spider in their hair, worms and lice beneath the skin or infestation with various insects. The delusion may be accompanied by other depressive delusions or overvalued ideas of being dirty, guilty, unworthy or ill. These delusions may also occur in schizophrenia, in which condition they characteristically take on a bizarre character and are accompanied by other schizophrenic symptoms. A 49-year-old mother of four children, one of whose sons had developed a schizophrenic illness, complained of recurrent pain in her vagina that she explained as being caused by a parasite that had migrated from her stomach, where it had been responsible for epigastric pain diagnosed earlier as hiatus hernia (McLaughlin and Sims, 1984). She described the parasite as wandering through her bloodstream and as having been responsible for various aches and pains she had experienced in the past. She related having passed multiple small red worms and worm casts in her faeces and, on one occasion, a 2-inch green frog.

Delusions of infestation may occur in organic states with tactile hallucinations, in delirium tremens during alcohol withdrawal and in cocaine addiction. They may be described in cerebrovascular disease, in senile dementia and in other brain disease, and they have been ascribed to disorder of the thalamus. Overvalued ideas and delusion-like ideas of infestation sometimes occur in people with personality disorder of anankastic or paranoid type with no psychotic illness.

Characteristically, these ideas occur in patients aged over 50 years. Typically, those with delusions of infestation have always had a particular concern for personal cleanliness. Sometimes, the condition is precipitated by a skin disease and becomes a delusional elaboration of existing tactile symptoms. It has been suggested that the symptom develops in stages: first, abnormal cutaneous sensation; then an illusion develops; and, finally, the fully formed delusion of infestation occurs. As mentioned above, delusional infestation is now viewed as one form of delusional disorder, in particular being a subtype of monosymptomatic hypochondriacal psychosis.

Communicated insanity

Lasègue and Falret (1877) described 'la folie à deux (ou folie communiquée)'. Occasionally, a delusion (delusional intuition) is transferred from a psychotic person to one or more others with whom they have been in close association, so that the recipient shares the false belief: the principal acquires the delusion first and is dominant, the associate becomes deluded through association with the principal. This situation, in which partners accept, support and share each other's beliefs, has been called the *psychosis of association*. The associate is usually socially deprived or disadvantaged, mentally or physically.

Gralnick (1942), in a review of the English literature on *folie à deux*, subdivided the condition into four possible relationships between principal and associate.

- In *folie imposée*, the delusions of a mentally ill person are transferred to someone who was not previously mentally ill, although characteristically the victim has some social or psychological disadvantage. Separation of the pair is often followed by remission of symptoms in the associate.
- *Folie communiquée* occurs when a normal person suffers a contagion of his ideas after resisting them for a long time. Once he acquires these beliefs, he maintains them despite separation.
- *In folie induite*, a person who is already psychotic adds the delusions of a closely associated person to his own.
- *Folie simultanée* describes a situation in which two or more people become psychotic and share the same delusional system simultaneously. It has been considered that the principal is always psychotic (Soni and Rockley, 1974), but the associate may or may not be psychotic.

However, the validity of this classification has been questioned. It is also not of any particular clinical value, and the psychopathological differences are questionable (Hughes and Sims, 1997).

In a case report of a family affected with folie à quatre (Sims *et al.*, 1977), the initially referred patient believed that a large industrial concern had put 'bugging' devices in the walls of his brother's house. He claimed that employees of the firm had been following him everywhere and interfering with his own house. His wife believed this story initially and produced supposedly corroborative evidence. A year later, following his in-patient treatment, she no longer accepted the plot and she believed her husband to be mentally ill. She was a very anxious person who had previously received psychiatric treatment and came from a family in which three members had suffered from Huntington's chorea. When the patient's brother was visited at home, it was found that he, and the sister who lived with him, both believed in the plot and were both currently receiving treatment for a schizophrenic illness in which first-rank symptoms were present.

Folie à deux demonstrates how the content of belief is dictated by social and environmental circumstances, but the precise form of the symptoms varies according to the nature of the illness. Thus the non-psychotic victim of folie imposée will show delusion-like ideas, overvalued ideas or misinterpretations but will not show 'true' delusions or delusional percept.

An interesting variation on folie imposée was described by Aldridge and Tagg (1998). This was the case of a 7-year-old boy who had presented with spurious psychotic symptoms induced by living in isolation with his mother, who suffered from acute schizophrenia. Initially, he was withdrawn, uncommunicative and ritualistic, with delayed development. At school, he was fearful of toys and teachers, crouching under a table, and was ritualistic concerning timekeeping and toileting, during which he would remove all his clothing and reverse into the toilet. His only speech was to repeat the clock time in a ritualistic way. Foster placement was made with a single mature woman, experienced with children, and after a year this abnormal behaviour had disappeared and he had made progress consistent with his mild degree of learning disability.

Delusions of control

These delusions, otherwise known as passivity or made experiences, are discussed with disorder of thinking in Chapter 9.

REALITY OF DELUSIONS

The degree to which delusions influence the reality of the world inhabited by a patient is most probably best judged by how far patients act on their beliefs. Patients with schizophrenia do not always act on their delusions, but quite frequently they do so act. A man who believed that American battleships were sailing down the main street of Birmingham, United Kingdom (100 miles from the sea), had the refined social conscience to report this to the police! Persons holding delusions of morbid jealousy are potentially very dangerous: extreme physical violence and murder not uncommonly occur in this context. The patient with depressive delusions of guilt and unworthiness may well act on them by killing himself.

Although there is a growing literature casting doubt on whether delusions are false beliefs or not (see above), what is inescapable is the fact that patients do often act on the content of these beliefs. For practical purposes, the content of a delusion is important because it yields information about the likely behaviour of a patient. In other words, the content of delusions acts to motivate behaviour, to give reason to action and to justify conduct; that is, it has predictive power. For this reason alone, the content of delusion is relevant to clinical practice. Hemsley and Garety (1986) have commented on 'the lack of action consequent with apparently sincerely held beliefs' while, paradoxically, forensic psychiatric studies have generally found that psychotic symptoms, especially delusions, are frequently a major factor resulting in the offence (Taylor, 1985). Buchanan (1993) has reviewed the descriptions of situations in which patients act on their delusions. He considers that for affective illnesses, both delusional belief and action may be consequent on the abnormal mood state. In other circumstances, action can be seen as being caused by a combination of 'belief' and 'desire' triggered by factors such as 'noticings': belief clearly is influenced by occurrence of delusion; desire corresponds to concepts such as motivation, drive and inclination; noticing is influenced by the perceptual and cognitive changes of the psychotic state. Taylor *et al.* (1998) conclude for an investigation into violence in a high-security hospital population, 'as symptoms were usually a factor driving the index offence, treatment appears as important for public safety as for personal health'. The conclusion here is that delusions, like normal beliefs, do not necessarily result in action. They may be expressed yet not influence behaviour in any discernible way. But, like normal beliefs, they may motivate behaviour in a way that is comprehensible given the content of the belief.

In general, violent behaviour in response to delusions is not common; however, in a sample of 83 consecutively admitted deluded subjects, some aspect of the actions of half of them was congruent with the content of their delusions (Wessely *et al.*, 1993). When acting on the delusions was described by the subjects themselves, it was associated with being aware of evidence that supported their belief and with having actively sought out such evidence; a tendency to reduce the conviction with which a belief was held when that belief was challenged; and with feeling sad, frightened or anxious as a consequence of the delusion (Buchanan *et al.*, 1993).

ERRONEOUS IDEATION

Overvalued idea

An overvalued idea is an acceptable, comprehensible idea pursued by the patient beyond the bounds of reason. It is usually associated with abnormal personality. Disorders associated with overvalued ideas have been reviewed by McKenna (1984), whose definition of overvalued idea 'refers to a solitary, abnormal belief that is neither delusional nor obsessional in nature, but which is preoccupying to the extent of dominating the sufferer's life'. It is *overvalued* in the sense that it causes disturbed functioning or suffering to the person himself or to others. The background on which an overvalued idea is held is not necessarily unreasonable or false. It becomes so dominant that all other ideas are secondary and relate to it: the patient's whole life comes to revolve around this one idea. It is usually associated with very strong affect that the person, because of his temperament, has great difficulty in expressing.

According to McKenna, the term was introduced by Wernicke (1906), who distinguished it from obsession, in that it was not experienced subjectively as 'senseless', and from delusion. Jaspers considered that delusion is qualitatively different from normal belief, with a radical transformation of the meaning attached to events and incorrigible to an extent quite unlike normal belief. An overvalued idea, on the contrary, is an isolated notion associated with strong affect and abnormal personality and similar in quality to passionate political, religious or ethical conviction. For Jaspers, then, overvalued ideas are 'convictions that are strongly toned by affect which is understandable in terms of the personality and its history'. Furthermore, Jaspers says, 'they are isolated notions that develop comprehensibly out of a given personality and situation'. Fish considered there was frequently a discrepancy between the degree of conviction and the extent to which the belief directed action. But the patient with an overvalued idea invariably acted on it, determinedly and repeatedly; it is almost carried out with the drive of an instinct, like nest building. In many respects, these definitions attempt to locate overvalued ideas somewhere between normal beliefs and delusions. Overvalued ideas differ from delusions in that they arise comprehensibly from what we know about the person and his situation. They are more like passionate political, religious or ethical convictions than normal beliefs. This suggests that there is something about the tenacity of the conviction that distinguishes these overvalued ideas from normal beliefs, yet the degree of conviction and incorrigibility is less than that of delusions.

McKenna lists the disorders of content commonly associated with the form of overvalued idea. These are represented in Table 8.1. Not in all cases of each of these conditions is the psychopathology an overvalued idea, for instance morbid jealousy may be delusional and hypochondriasis may occur secondary to depressed mood. However, when an overvalued idea is found it is usually associated with abnormal personality.

Morbid jealousy is often manifested as an overvalued idea. A husband was terrified that his wife was being unfaithful to him. He checked on her every movement, interrogated her repeatedly, examined her underwear, employed detectives to follow her and misinterpreted any innocent contact she had with

Table 8.1 Disorders with overvalued ideas

Content of disorder	Abnormality of personality	Reference(s)
Paranoid state: querulous or litigious type	Abnormality of personality is usually present with overvalued ideas in all these conditions	Jaspers (1959), Kraepelin (1905)
Morbid jealousy		Ey (1954), Shepherd (1961)
Hypochondriasis		Merskey (1979), Pilowsky (1970)
Dysmorphophobia		Hay (1970), Munro (1980)
Parasitophobia (Ekbom's syndrome)		Hopkinson (1973)
Anorexia nervosa		Crisp (1980), Dally (1969)
Transsexualism		Huxley *et al.* (1981)

(After McKenna, 1984, with permission.)

other men. On examination, he was not deluded, but the importance he attached to investigating and maintaining his wife's fidelity, and the time taken to do this, was excessive and destroyed his family life and lost him his job.

The form of the abnormal idea in many of the disturbances of body image, for example *dysmorphophobia* and *transsexualism*, is usually an overvalued idea. A person with *paranoid personality* disorder became involved in a protracted lawsuit because a farmer ploughed across a public right of way. It is reasonable that hikers get annoyed when a footpath is destroyed, but this person took reasonable irritation to extreme lengths and constructed a mantrap to eliminate the farmer. His enthusiasm for footpaths had become an overvalued idea. Clearly, there is a connection with delusion, especially secondary delusion, in which the individual has come to believe, because of circumstances and the nature of his personality, that people are against him and deliberately frustrating him.

Paranoid ideas and syndromes

In psychiatry, the word *paranoid* is taken to mean 'self-referent' and is not limited to *persecutory*; all delusions are delusions of reference in that they relate to the patient himself. A person will not form a delusional belief concerning 6-inch men on Mars unless he himself is significantly implicated in some way. So a paranoid delusion is a delusion of self-reference, not necessarily persecutory in nature. A paranoid personality disorder is that type of abnormal personality in which the person's reaction to other people is unduly self-referent; paranoid state (see Chapter 23) includes those mental states in which self-referent phenomena are conspicuous, that is, *delusion-like ideas of reference* or *overvalued ideas* predominate. A patient, all of whose delusions are grandiose in nature and none of them persecutory, may still be suffering from *paranoid* schizophrenia.

Although primary delusions are characteristic of schizophrenia, secondary delusions (delusion-like ideas) occur in a number of conditions, for example manic–depressive psychosis in both manic and depressive phases, epilepsy and other organic psychosyndromes, acute drug intoxication, various alcoholic states and, of course, schizophrenia. The term *paranoid* originally was synonymous with delusional insanity. Kraepelin (1905) used the term more specifically to describe the condition in which there are delusions but no hallucinations. The personality, mood state and volition of the patient, in Kraepelin's description, are well preserved.

Overvalued ideas are commonly found associated with personality disorders of paranoid or anankastic type. So *paranoid state* is a collective term for a number of conditions in which the *content* is unduly self-referent but the *form* of the idea has not been precisely delineated. If the bizarre idea is a primary delusion (and there would normally be first-rank symptoms also present to corroborate this), then the patient is probably suffering from paranoid schizophrenia. If the delusion is secondary in nature, another psychosis is the likely diagnosis. If the form of the idea is not delusional but better described as an overvalued idea, the paranoid symptoms are probably associated with personality disorder. Clarification of the *form* is necessary for adequate diagnosis, which in its turn is useful for assessment of prognosis and planning appropriate treatment.

REFERENCES

Aldridge S and Tagg G (1998) Spurious childhood psychosis induced by schizophrenia in the parent. *Advances in Psychiatric Treatment 4*, 39–43.

Ang PC and Weller MPI (1984) Koro and psychosis. *British Journal of Psychiatry 145*, 335.

Bentall RP (1993) Cognitive biases and abnormal beliefs: towards a model of persecutory delusions. In David AS and Cutting JC (eds) *The Neuropsychology of Schizophrenia*. Hove: Lawrence Erlbaum.

Berner P (1991) Delusional atmosphere. *British Journal of Psychiatry 159* (suppl. 14), 88–93.

Berrios GE (1985) Delusional parasitosis and physical disease. *Comprehensive Psychiatry 26*, 395–403.

Berrios GE (1996) *The History of Mental Symptoms: Descriptive Psychopathology Since the Nineteenth Century*. Cambridge: Cambridge University Press.

Berrios GE and Morley SJ (1984) Koro-like symptoms in a non-Chinese subject. *British Journal of Psychiatry 145*, 331–4.

Berson RJ (1983) Capgras' syndrome. *American Journal of Psychiatry 140*, 969–78.

Brockington I (1991) Factors involved in delusion formation. *British Journal of Psychiatry 159* (suppl. 14), 42–5.

Buchanan A (1993) Acting on delusion: a review. *Psychological Medicine 23*, 123–34.

Buchanan A, Reed A, Wessely S, *et al.* (1993) Acting on delusions II: the phenomenological correlates of acting on delusions. *British Journal of Psychiatry 163*, 77–81.

Capgras J and Reboul-Lachaux J (1923) L'illusion des sosies dans un délire systematique chronique. *Bulletin de la Societé Clinique de Médicine Mentale 11*, 6–16.

Catalano G, Catalano MC, Embi CS and Frantel RL (1991) Delusions about the Internet. *Southern Medical Journal* 92, 609–10.

Christodoulou GN (1978) Syndrome of subjective doubles. *American Journal of Psychiatry 135*, 249–51.

Christodoulou GN (1991) The delusional misidentification syndromes. *British Journal of Psychiatry 159* (suppl. 14), 65–9.

de Clérambault GG (1942) *Les psychoses passionelles. Oeuvre psychiatrique*. Paris: Presses Universitaire.

Colby KM (1977) Appraisal of four psychological theories of paranoid phenomena. *Journal of Abnormal Psychology 86*, 54–9.

Cotard J (1882) Nihilistic delusions. In Hirsch SR and Shepherd M (eds) *Themes and Variations in European Psychiatry* (transl. Rohde M, 1974), pp. 353–74. Bristol: John Wright.

Courbon P and Fail G (1927) Syndrome d'illusion de Frégoli et schizophrenie. *Bulletin de la Societé Clinique de Médecine Mentale 15*, 121–4.

Courbon P and Tusques J (1932) Illusion d'intermétamorphose et de charme. *Annals Médicopsychologique 90*, 401–5.

Crisp AH (1980) *Anorexia Nervosa: Let Me Be*. London: Academic Press.

Cutting J (1985) *The Psychology of Schizophrenia*. Edinburgh: Churchill Livingstone.

Dally P (1969) *Anorexia Nervosa*. London: Heinemann.

Eagles JM (1983) Delusional depressive in-patients, 1892–1982. *British Journal of Psychiatry 143*, 558–63.

Edelstyn NMJ, Riddoch MJ, Oyebode F, Humphreys GW and Forde E (1996) Visual processing in patients with Fregoli syndrome. *Cognitive Neuropsychiatry 1*, 103–24.

Edelstyn NMJ, Riddoch MJ and Oyebode F (1999) A review of the phenomenology and cognitive neuropsychological origins of the Capgras syndrome. *International Journal of Geriatric Psychiatry 14*, 48–59.

Ekbom K (1938) Praeseniler Dermat-zooenwahn. *Acta Psychiatrica Scandinavica 13*, 227–59.

Ellis HD, de Pauw KW, Christodoulou GN, Papageorgiou L, Milne AB and Joseph AB (1993) Responses to facial and nonfacial stimuli presented tachistoscopically in either or both visual fields by patients with the Capgras delusion and paranoid schizophrenics. *Journal of Neurology, Neurosurgery and Psychiatry 56*, 215–9.

Enoch D (1991) Delusional jealousy and awareness of reality. *British Journal of Psychiatry 159* (suppl. 14), 52–6.

Enoch MD and Trethowan WH (1979) *Uncommon Psychiatric Syndromes*, 2nd edn. Bristol: John Wright.

Ey H (1950) Jalousie morbide. In *Etudes Psychiatriques*, vol. II. Paris: de Bronwen.

Ey H (1954) *Etudes Psychiatriques*, vol. II. Paris: Desclée.

Fish F (1967) *Clinical Psychopathology*. Bristol: John Wright.

Freud S (1907) Delusions and dreams in Jensen's gradiva. In *Standard Edition of the Complete Psychological Works*, vol. IX (transl. Strachey J, 1959). London: Hogarth Press.

Garety P (1991) Reasoning and delusions. *British Journal of Psychiatry 159* (suppl. 14), 14–8.

Garety P, Helmsley DR and Wessely S (1991) Reasoning in deluded schizophrenic and paranoid subjects: biases in performance on a probabilistic inference task. *Journal of Nervous and Mental Disease 179*, 194–201.

Gogol N (1972) *Diary of a Madman and Other Stories* (transl. Wilks R). London: Penguin.

Gralnick A (1942) Folie à deux: the psychosis of association. A review of 103 cases and the entire English literature. *Psychiatric Quarterly 16*, 230–63.

Griesinger W (1845) *Mental Pathology and Therapeutics* (transl. Robertson CL and Rutherford J, 1882). New York: William Wood & Co.

Gruhle HW (1915) Self-description and empathy. *Zeitschrift fuer Gesundheitswesen Neurologie und Psychiatrie 28*, 148.

Guirguis WR (1981) Pure erotomania in manic–depressive psychosis. *British Journal of Psychiatry 138*, 139–40.

Gwee AL (1963) Koro – a cultural disease. *Singapore Medical Journal 4*, 119–22.

Hamilton M (1978) *Fish's Outline of Psychiatry*, 3rd edn. Bristol: John Wright.

Hart B (1921) *The Psychology of Insanity*. Cambridge: Cambridge University Press.

Hay GG (1970) Dysmorphophobia. *British Journal of Psychiatry 116*, 399–406.

Hay GG (1983) Feigned psychosis – a review of the simulation of mental illness. *British Journal of Psychiatry 143*, 8–10.

Hemsley DR and Garety PA (1986) The formation and maintenance of delusions: a Bayesian analysis. *British Journal of Psychiatry 149*, 51–6.

Higgins J (1990) Affective psychoses. In Bluglass R and Bowden P (eds) *Principles and Practice of Forensic Psychiatry*. Edinburgh: Churchill Livingstone.

Hopkinson G (1970) Delusions of infestation. *Acta Psychiatrica Scandinavica 46*, 111–9.

Hopkinson G (1973) The psychiatric syndrome of infestation. *Psychiatrica Clinica 6*, 330–45.

Hughes TA and Sims ACP (1997) Folie à deux. In Bhugra D and Munro A (eds) *Troublesome Disguises: Underdiagnosed Psychiatric Syndromes*. Oxford: Blackwell Scientific.

Huq SF, Garety PA and Hemsley DR (1988) Probabilistic judgements in deluded and non-deluded subjects. *Quarterly Journal of Experimental Psychology* 40A, 801–12.

Huxley PJ, Kenna JC and Brandon SC (1981) Partnership in transsexualism, part II. The nature of the partnership. *Archives of Sexual Behaviour 10*, 143–60.

Jaspers K (1959) *General Psychopathology* (transl. Hoenig J and Hamilton MW, 1963). Manchester: Manchester University Press.

Kaney S and Bentall RP (1989) Persecutory delusions and attributional style. *British Journal of Medical Psychology 62*, 191–8.

Kaney S and Bentall RP (1992) Persecutory delusions and the self-serving bias: evidence from a continuing judgement task. *Journal of Nervous and Mental Disease 180*, 773–80.

Kendler KS, Glaser WM and Morgenstern H (1983) Dimensions of delusional experience. *American Journal of Psychiatry 140*, 466–9.

Kinderman P, Kaney S, Morley S and Bentall RP (1992) Paranoia and the defensive attributional style: deluded and depressed patients' attribution about their own attributions. *British Journal of Medical Psychology 65*, 371–83.

Klaf FS and Hamilton JG (1961) Schizophrenia: a hundred years ago and today. *Journal of Mental Science 107*, 819–27.

Kraepelin E (1905) *Lectures on Clinical Psychiatry*, 3rd edn (transl. Johnstone T, 1917). New York: W. Wood.

Kretschmer E (1927) The sensitive delusion of reference (transl. Candy J). In Hirsch SR and Shepherd M (eds) (1974) *Themes and Variations in European Psychiatry*. Bristol: John Wright.

Laing RD (1961) *The Self and Others*. London: Tavistock.

Lapierre YD (1972) Koro in a French Canadian. *Canadian Psychiatric Association Journal 17*, 333–4.

Lasègue C (1852) cited by Cotard J (1882) Du délire des négations. *Archives de Neurologie Paris 4*, 152–70, 282–96.

Laségue C and Falret J (1877) La folie à deux (ou folie communiquée). *Annales Médico-psychologique 18*, 321 (transl. Michaud R, 1964), supplement to *American Journal of Psychiatry 121*, 4.

Lishman WA (1997) *Organic Psychiatry: the Psychological Consensus of Cerebral Disorder*, 3rd edn. Oxford: Blackwell Scientific.

Lyon HM, Kaney S and Bentall RP (1994) The defensive function of persecutory

delusions: evidence from attribution tasks. *British Journal of Psychiatry 164*, 637–46.
McGrath P (1990) *Spider*. London: Penguin.
McKenna PJ (1984) Disorders with overvalued ideas. *British Journal of Psychiatry 145*, 579–85.
McLaughlin JA and Sims ACP (1984) Co-existence of Capgras and Ekbom syndromes. *British Journal of Psychiatry 145*, 439–41.
Mellor CS (1991) Delusional perception. *British Journal of Psychiatry 159* (suppl. 14), 104–7.
Merskey H (1979) *The Analysis of Hysteria*. London: Baillière Tindall.
Morris M (1991) Delusional infestation. *British Journal of Psychiatry 159* (suppl. 14), 83–7.
Morrison A (1848) *Cases of Mental Disease*. London: Longman & S. Highley.
Moselhy H and Oyebode F (1997) Delusional misidentification syndromes: a review of the Anglophone literature. *Neurology, Psychiatry and Brain Research 5*, 21–6.
Mullen P (1990) Morbid jealousy and the delusion of infidelity. In Bluglass R and Bowden P (eds) *Principles and Practice of Forensic Psychiatry*. Edinburgh: Churchill Livingstone.
Mullen PE (1997) Disorders of passion. In Bhugra D and Munro A (eds) *Troublesome Disguises: Underdiagnosed Psychiatric Syndromes*. Oxford: Blackwell Scientific.
Mullen PE and Pathé M (1994) The pathological extensions of love. *British Journal of Psychiatry 165*, 614–23.
Munro A (1980) Monosymptomatic hypochondriacal psychosis. *British Journal of Hospital Medicine 24*, 34–8.
Munro A (1988) Monosymptomatic hypochondriacal psychosis. *British Journal of Psychiatry 153* (suppl. 2), 37–40.
Munro A (1997) Paranoia or delusional disorder. In Bhugra D and Munro A (eds) *Troublesome Disguises: Underdiagnosed Psychiatric Syndromes*. Oxford: Blackwell Scientific.
Oyebode F, Jamieson R, Mullaney J and Davison K (1986) Koro – a psychophysiological dysfunction? *British Journal of Psychiatry 148*, 212–4.
Oyebode F, Edelstyn NMJ, Patel A, Riddoch MJ and Humphreys GW (1996) Capgras syndrome in vascular dementia: recognition memory and visual processing. *International Journal of Geriatric Psychiatry 11*, 71–3.
Pilowsky I (1967) Dimensions of hypochondriasis. *British Journal of Psychiatry 113*, 89–93.
Pilowsky I (1970) Primary and secondary hypochondriasis. *Acta Psychiatrica Scandinavica 46*, 273–85.
Porter S and Williams C (1997) Psychiatric dilemmas – surgery and the Mental Health Act (1983). *Journal of the Royal Society of Medicine 90*, 327–330.
Pryse-Phillips W (1971) An olfactory reference syndrome. *Acta Psychiatrica Scandinavica 47*, 485–509.
Reilly TM (1988) Delusional infestation. *British Journal of Psychiatry 153* (suppl. 2), 44–6.
Roberts G (1991) Delusional belief systems and meaning in life: a preferred reality. *British Journal of Psychiatry 159* (suppl. 14), 19–28.
Roberts G (1992) The origins of delusion. *British Journal of Psychiatry 161*, 298–308.
Schneider K (1920) The stratification of emotional life as the structure of the depressive states. *Zentralblatt fuer die gesamte Neurologie und Psychiatrie 59*, 281.
Schneider K (1949) The concept of delusion 'Zum Begriff des Wahns'. *Fortschritte der Neurologie-Psychiatrie 17*, 26–31 (transl. Marshall H). In Hirsch SR and Shepherd M (eds) (1974) *Themes and Variations in European Psychiatry*. Bristol: John Wright.
Schneider K (1957) Primary and secondary symptoms in schizophrenia. *Fortschritte der Neurologie-Psychiatrie 25*, 487–90 (transl. Marshall H). In Hirsch SR and Shepherd M (eds) (1974) *Themes and Variations in European Psychiatry*. Bristol: John Wright.
Serretti A, Lattuada E, Cusin C and Smeraldi E (1999) Factor analysis of delusional disorder symptomatology. *Comprehensive Psychiatry 40*, 143–7.
Shepherd M (1961) Morbid jealousy: some clinical and social aspects of a psychiatric symptom. *Journal of Mental Science 107*, 687–753.
Shrestha K, Rees DW, Rix KJB, Hore BD and Faraghere B (1985) Sexual jealousy in alcoholics. *Acta Psychiatrica Scandinavica 72*, 283–90.
Sims ACP (1972) The English Hospital, Tangier 1883–1908. *Medical History 16*, 285–90.
Sims ACP (1986) The psychopathology of schizophrenia with special reference to delusional misidentification. In Christodoulou GM (ed.) *The Delusional Misidentification Syndromes*. Basel: Karger.
Sims ACP (1991) Delusional syndromes in ICD-10. *British Journal of Psychiatry 159* (suppl. 14), 46–51.

Sims ACP (1992) Symptoms and beliefs. *Journal of the Royal Society of Health 112*, 42–6.
Sims ACP and White AC (1973) Co-existence of the Capgras and de Clérambault syndromes – a case history. *British Journal of Psychiatry 123*, 635–8.
Sims ACP, Salmons PH and Humphreys P (1977) Folie à quatre. *British Journal of Psychiatry 130*, 134–8.
Soni SD and Rockley GJ (1974) Socio-clinical substrates of folie à deux. *British Journal of Psychiatry 125*, 230–5.
Spitzer M (1994) The basis of psychiatric diagnosis. In Sadler JZ, Wiggins OP and Schwartz MA (eds) *Philosophical Perspectives on Psychiatric Diagnostic Classification*. Baltimore: Johns Hopkins University Press.
Stoddart WHB (1908) *Mind and its Disorders*. London: Lewis.
Taylor PJ (1985) Motives for offending among violent and psychiatric men. *British Journal of Psychiatry 147*, 491–8.
Taylor PJ, Leese M, Williams D, Butwell M, Daly R and Larkin E (1998) Mental disorder and violence. *British Journal of Psychiatry 172*, 218–26.
Todd J and Dewhurst K (1955) The Othello syndrome. *Journal of Nervous and Mental Disease 122*, 367–74.
Trethowan WH (1967) Erotomania – an old disorder reconsidered. *Alta 2*, 79–86.
Trollope A (1869) *He Knew He Was Right*. London: Strahan.
Videbech T (1966) Chronic olfactory paranoid syndromes. *Acta Psychiatrica Scandinavica 42*, 183–212.
Walker C (1991) Delusion: what did Jaspers really say? *British Journal of Psychiatry 159* (suppl. 14), 94–103.
Wasik M (1990) Insanity, diminished responsibility and infanticide: legal aspects. In Bluglass R and Bowden P (eds) *Principles and Practice of Forensic Psychiatry*. Edinburgh: Churchill Livingstone.
Wernicke C (1906) *Fundamentals of Psychiatry*. Leipzig: Thieme.
Wessely S, Buchanan A, Reed A, *et al.* (1993) Acting on delusion 1: prevalence. *British Journal of Psychiatry 163*, 69–76.
West DJ and Walk A (1977) *Daniel McNaughton: His Trial and the Aftermath*. Ashford: Headley Brothers.
Winters KL and Neale JM (1983) Delusions and delusional thinking in psychotics: a review of the literature. *Clinical Psychology Review 3*, 227–53.
World Health Organization (1992) *The ICD-10 Classification of Mental and Behavioural Disorders: Clinical Description and Diagnostic Guidelines*. Geneva: World Health Organization.
Yap PM (1965) Koro – a culture-bound depersonalization syndrome. *British Journal of Psychiatry III*, 43–50.

Disorder of the Thinking Process

9

> “With time and years the individual becomes so lazy in public life that he is not even capable of writing any more. On such a sheet of paper, one can squeeze many letters if one is careful not to transgress by one 'square shore'. In such fine weather one should be able to take a walk in the woods. Naturally, not alone, but with a girl. At the end of the year one always renders the annual accounting. The sun is now in the sky yet it is not yet 10 o'clock. *Eugene Bleuler (1857–1939)*

This chapter is concerned with disorder of thinking, and the next chapter with disorders of language. Thinking and thought processes are little understood. Although there is increasing interest in the subject by cognitive neuroscientists, their primary focus of study misses what is of interest to the clinical psychopathologist, namely the subjective experience of thinking, particularly as it relates to abnormalities of thinking. Cognitive neuroscientists are interested in the nature of problem solving; in the various kinds of reasoning, including analogical, inductive and deductive; and in the nature of logic and belief formation. These are all important subjects and can be impaired in psychiatric disorders. However, the process that makes these aspects of thinking possible the unique relationship of the subject to his own thoughts, the experience of thoughts flowing coherently and the effortless yet goal-driven dimension of thinking thoughts that underpin problem solving and reasoning, is poorly understood and researched. Admittedly, it is difficult to study the subjective aspects of thinking, and mostly one is concerned with objective phenomena of psychic life – what Jaspers (1962) calls 'performance'.

There are two distinct aspects in studying disorder of thinking: the patient's subjective awareness of his own disturbed thinking patterns and the manifestation of abnormal thinking he betrays in his speech (Chapter 10). This latter is the expression of thought and determines what the observer may deduce about the patient's thinking. We need to enquire also about the experience of thinking in the patient's description of his subjective psychological processes. *Formal thought disorder*, from the subjective, phenomenological standpoint, is abnormality in the mechanism of thinking described by the patient introspecting into his own processes of thought; that is, the patient describes in his own words a process of thinking that is clearly abnormal to the outside observer.

TYPES OF THINKING

The process of thinking was divided by Fish (1967) into the following three types:

- undirected fantasy thinking – dereistic – autistic thinking
- imaginative thinking
- *rational* or conceptual thinking.

These three types have slightly different implications for psychopathology, the description and categorization of morbid processes. They can be considered as *functions* of thinking; that is, they are the necessary mechanisms for thinking to take place but are not themselves manifest in the phenomena. We can contrast those phenomena, which are the products of the *performance* of thinking, the percept or the idea, with the functions that do not become explicit.

Fantasy thinking

This may be of short duration, for example the daydream before going to sleep, or it may become an established way of life. Jaspers quotes Montaigne: 'Plutarch says of people who waste their feelings on guinea-pigs and pet dogs, that the love element in all of us, if deprived of any adequate object, will seek out something trivial and false rather than let itself stay unengaged. So the psyche in its passions prefers to deceive itself or even in spite of itself invent some nonsensical object rather than give up all drive or aim'.

Fantasy has an important function in the way we all carry out our everyday activities, for instance we model our speech and behaviour in imagination before an important encounter or event, and afterwards we rehearse our performance in fantasy to evaluate it and assess whether we could have done better (imaginative thinking, see p. 155). In order to be able to harness our imagination constructively, we require the capacity for undirected fantasy and the learned skill to structure thoughts. Fantasy also allows a person to escape from or deny reality, or alternatively to convert reality into something more tolerable and less requiring of corrective action. A girl aged 20, who had a very deprived childhood and walked the city streets at night as a prostitute, listened to a vicar broadcasting on local radio. She started to send him and his wife flowers and cards, made contact with them and began to call them 'Mum' and 'Dad'. When questioned by the police one night, she gave their names as next of kin and said they really were her parents.

Shy, reserved people, not suffering from mental illness, may use dereistic thinking to compensate for the disappointments of life. Bleuler (1911) saw this isolation from the real world into autistic thinking as characteristic of the schizophrenic: 'The very common preoccupation of young hebephrenics with "the deepest questions" is nothing but an autistic manifestation'. Fantasy, especially in some with neurotic traits, may develop from the stage of being deliberate and sporadic into an established mode; the person comes to believe the contents of his fantasy, which becomes subjectively real and accepted as fact. Freud, in his later writings, considered that this was so in some of the accounts he received from women of an incestuous relationship with their father during childhood (Jones, 1962). However, in his early writings he had considered that they had experienced actual sexual assault but had used unconscious mechanisms to repress this knowledge (Isräels and Schatzman, 1993; Webster, 1995). Various types of experience come into the category of acting out fantasy, such as *pathological lying* (pseudologia fantastica), *hysterical conversion* and *dissociation* (somatic and psychological dissociative symptoms) and the *delusion-like ideas* occurring in affective psychoses. These last types can be understood as arising from the patient's affective and social setting.

Fantasy is usually understood to be the creation of images or ideas that have no external reality. However, fantasy thinking may also reveal itself in the denial of external events. The observations on which the psychodynamic explanation of *ego defence mechanisms* have been described are relevant in this context. The slip of the tongue, or the 'forgetting' of the emotionally laden word is not accidental; it is a form of self-deception. The obvious, significant, but unpleasant, object of perception may be 'overlooked', and this often reveals fantasy denial. Fantasy thinking denies unpleasant reality, even though the fantasy itself may also be unpleasant. This rearranging or transformation of reality is shown by neurotic patients habitually and all people occasionally. Jonathan Swift commented on it thus: 'When man's fancy gets astride of his reason; when imagination is at cuffs with the senses; and common understanding, as well as common sense, is kicked out of doors, the first proselyte he makes is himself' (Swift, 1667–1745).

Imaginative thinking

The term *imagination* covers psychological states such as fantasy (see above), the generation of novel ideas and the creative outputs that constitute art or discoveries in science. There are at least three components of imagination: mental imagery, counterfactual thinking and symbolic representation. Mental imagery refers to the ability to create image-based mental representations of the world. Counterfactual thinking refers to the capacity to disengage from reality in order to think of events and experiences that have not occurred and may never occur. Symbolic representation is the use of concepts or images to represent real world objects or entities (Roth, 2004). This is, of course, the basis of language, art and mathematics.

A facet of this type of thinking that comes from a psychoanalytic theoretical stance is the concept of *maternal reverie* (Bion, 1962). The mother, while in the situation, both physical and mental, of 'holding the baby' (Winnicott, 1957), has a capacity for reverie or daydreaming on the baby's behalf; this usually concerns the future happiness and achievements of the baby. Bion would regard this as a necessary factor in the healthy development of the self-sensation of the baby; when maternal reverie breaks down, for example in puerperal depression, the baby experiences this as distress. The process of maternal reverie is clearly analogous in some ways to the prayers of a religious person on another's behalf.

Rational or conceptual thinking

Problem solving and reasoning are two key aspects of rational thinking. Problem solving is defined as the set of cognitive processes that we apply to reach a goal when we must overcome obstacles to reach that goal, and reasoning is the cognitive process that we use to make inferences from knowledge and to draw conclusions. These aspects of thinking are distinct but related, so that reasoning can be involved in problem solving (Smith and Kosslyn, 2007). Strategies for problems involve the use of heuristics, that is, rules of thumb that usually give the correct answer. Typically, reasoning involves analogies, induction or deduction. Analogic reasoning involves the application of solutions to already known problems to new problems with similar characteristics. For example, if you lose the keys to your locked briefcase, you can apply the knowledge that sharp-ended implements can be used to open padlocks to this new problem. Inductive reasoning depends on the use of specific known instances to draw an inference about unknown instances. Commonly, this is formulated as generalizing from a single instance to all instances or from some members of a category known to have a given property to other instances of that category. This is known as category-based induction. An example is 'my cat has four legs', therefore 'all cats have four legs'. Deductive reasoning involves an argument in which if the premises are true, the conclusion cannot be false. This is usually studied by way of syllogism: (a) all Martians are green, (b) my father is a Martian, (c) my father is green.

Problem solving and reasoning both require the capacity to form concepts. This is the capacity for abstraction, the ability to theorize about the world, and it includes the categorization of objects or events in the world and the clarification of the concepts that determine the category or class under investigation.

THE PROCESSES OF DISORDERED THINKING

A model of associations based on Jaspers

In this model of thinking (psychological performance), thoughts (psychological events) can be seen to flow in an uninterrupted sequence so that one or more *associations*, with resulting further psychological events, may arise from each thought. The sequence of thoughts, with the associations linking them, forms the framework of this model, which is represented diagrammatically in Figure 9.1.

The mass of possible associations resulting from a psychic event is called a *constellation*. There are an enormous number of possible associations, but thinking usually proceeds in a definite direction for various immediate and compelling reasons. This consistent flow of thinking towards its goal is ascribed to the *determining tendency* (Jaspers). The idea of *associations* is not intended to imply that one psychological event evokes another by an automatic, unintelligent, non-verbal reflex, but that the thought, which may be expressed verbally or not, is a concept that results in the formation of a number of other concepts, one of which is given prominence by operation of the determining tendency. This model is conjectural but has some value in allowing description of the abnormalities of thinking and speech that occur in mental illness.

We are subjectively aware of our thought process being a stream or a flow. To develop the metaphor, thoughts are capable of acceleration and slowing, of eddies and calms, of precipitous falls, of increased volume of flow, of blockages. This analogy should not be taken too far, as it is without neurophysiological basis, but it is useful for examining certain abnormalities and is based on subjective experience.

Acceleration of thinking

Acceleration of flow of thinking occurs as *flight of ideas*. In this, there is a logical connection between each of two sequential ideas expressed. However, the goal

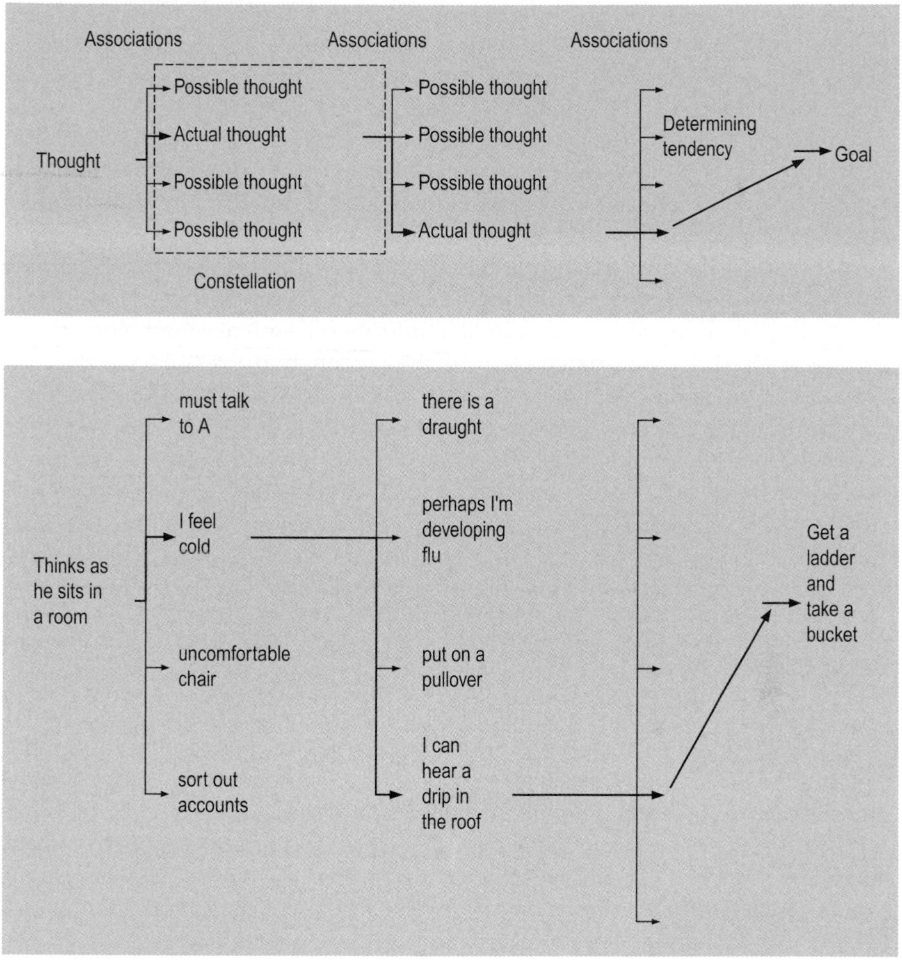

Figure 9.1 Model of association.

of thinking is not maintained for long. It is continuously changing because of the effect of frivolous affect and a very high degree of distractibility. The determining tendency is weakened, but associations are still formed normally. The speed of forming such associations, and therefore of the pattern of thought, is grossly accelerated. This is demonstrated in Figure 9.2.

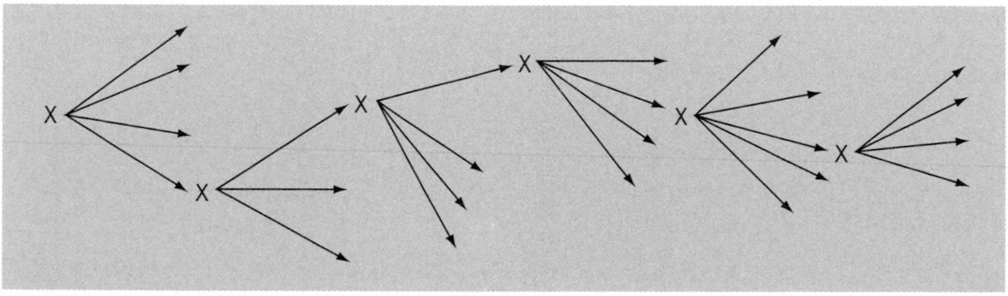

Figure 9.2 Abnormal flow of thinking: flight of ideas.

Here is an example of such flight of ideas from a female manic patient aged 45. She said, 'They thought I was in the pantry at home... Peekaboo ... there's a magic box. Poor darling Catherine, you know, Catherine the Great, the fire grate, I'm always up the chimney. I want to scream with joy... Hallelujah!' Discussing the transcript of this conversation when her mental state had improved, the patient found it quite easy to point out the logical bridges in her thinking between each pair of statements, but there was no sense of building up an argument from the first to the final statement.

Markedly different from manic flight of ideas with pressure of speech and multiple but linked associations is the *confusion psychosis* described by Fish (1962). In this, thinking is disordered while mood and psychomotor activity are unimpaired. In the excited form of this, incoherent pressure of speech is prominent, the context of which is out of keeping with the situation. There may be transient, almost playful, misidentifications of people; fleeting ideas of reference; and auditory hallucinations. In the inhibited state of confusion psychosis, there is poverty of speech, almost mutism. There may also be perplexity, ideas of reference, ideas of significance, illusions and hallucinations – auditory, visual or somatic. This is usually a cycloid psychosis in its presentation, and other features of manic–depressive psychosis may be present.

Retardation

In retardation (such as occurs in depression), thinking, although goal-directed, proceeds so slowly, with such morbid preoccupation with gloomy thoughts, that the person may fail to achieve those goals. The patient is likely to show little initiative and to begin neither planning nor spontaneous activity. When asked a question, he will ponder over it, but as no thought comes to him he makes no response. Eventually, after considerable delay, the answer usually comes. He has difficulty in making decisions and in concentration; there is loss of clarity of thought and poor registration of those events he needs to remember. In terms of the model of the flow of thinking, there is in retardation a poverty in the formation of associations; see Figure 9.3.

Depression, although usually associated with retardation of thought, may occur with *agitation*; there may be a complex situation with impaired concentration from retardation and a subjective experience of restless, anxious thoughts. Thus, Sutherland (1976), a middle-aged psychologist describing his own mental illness, said,

> " I contemplated throwing myself off the cross-Channel ferry... We arrived in Naples ... and my friends ... were upset by my condition while feeling powerless to help ... whilst the others sat at the table I rolled around moaning

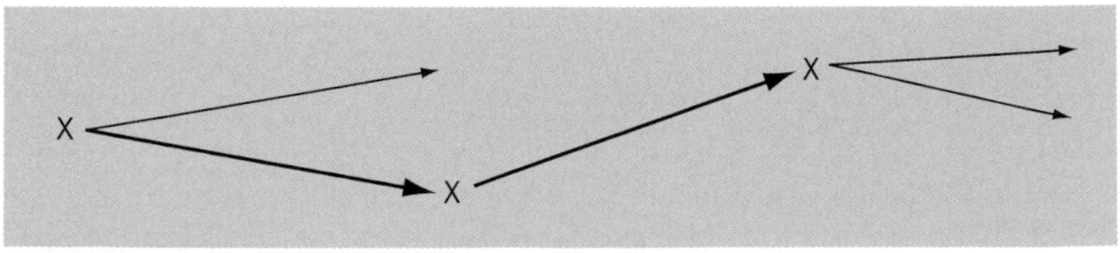

Figure 9.3 Retardation.

> in the dust. I revisited many of the places I had once loved: the Museo Nazionale with its magnificent mosaics pillaged from Pompeii, Pompeii itself and Capri. None of them evoked a spark of interest – I stared listlessly and uncomprehendingly at the pictures in the museum with harrowing thoughts still racing in my mind. I could not guide the children round Pompeii, since I could not concentrate sufficiently to follow the plan. Capri had lost its beauty and charm. I could not even giggle at the vulgarity of the interior of Axel Munthe's villa though the beauty of the formal garden and the magnificent view of the island and the sea from the belvedere evoked a slight response. The phrase 'see Naples and die' echoed through my mind: I was convinced I would never return alive to England, let alone ever revisit Naples.

This possible combination of depressed affect and accelerated activity can be seen to conform quite readily with Kraepelin's (1904) description of *mixed affective states.*

Circumstantial thinking

In both flight of ideas and retardation, affect influences the speed of thinking: it dictates which idea takes precedence and can also distort judgement. In *circumstantial thinking,* the slow stream of thought is not impeded by affect but by a defect of intellectual grasp, a failure of differentiation of the *figure ground.* This is the disorder of perception in which the most distinct percept – the *figure* – cannot be clearly separated from the less distinct – the *ground.* Characteristically, this occurs in epileptic patients, and it is seen in other organic states and in mental retardation. A somewhat similar process occurs with obsessional personality, but here the excess of detail is introduced anxiously to avoid any possible omissions: *i*'s are dotted, *t*'s crossed to such an extent that the process of reaching a goal is substantially impaired. On being asked a question, circumstantial thought is shown by the patient in a reply that contains a great welter of unnecessary detail, obscuring and impeding the answer to the question. All sorts of unnecessary associations are explored exhaustively before the person returns to the point. His whole conversation becomes a mass of parentheses and subsidiary clauses. He even has to explain and apologize for these digressions before he can get back to moving towards the goal. However, the determining tendency remains, and he does eventually answer the question. Circumstantial thinking is represented diagrammatically in Figure 9.4.

Interruption to the flow of thought

There are many ways in which the continuity of flow of thinking may be disturbed. Carl Schneider (1930) has described some of these abnormalities: *verschmelzung* (fusion, literally 'melting'), *faseln* (muddling), *entgleiten* (snapping off), *entgleisen* (derailment). These processes (and others) occur together to give the patient a feeling of confusion and bewilderment. He is likely to complain of feeling bemused, to be lacking in concentration and to be slightly apprehensive of he knows not what. He cannot precisely describe his altered thinking and consequent changes in speech.

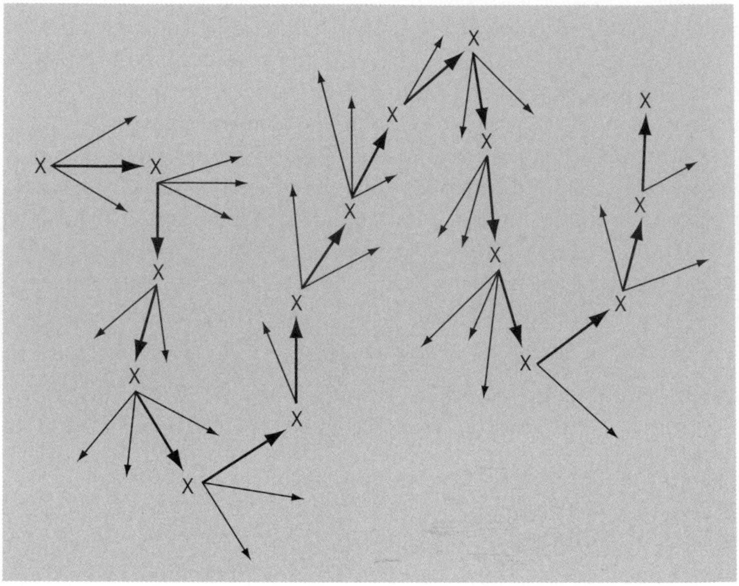

Figure 9.4 Model of circumstantial thinking.

In *derailment* (Figure 9.5), there is a breakdown in association so that there appears to be an interpolation of thought bearing no understandable connection with the chain of thoughts: 'The traffic is rumbling along the main road. They are going to the north. Why do girls always play pantomime heroes?' Such an excerpt from the speech of a patient with schizophrenia contains no meaningful connections, even to the patient himself. With derailment, the subject is unable to link the ideas and describes a change in his direction of thinking.

With *fusion*, there is some preservation of the normal chain of associations, but there is a bringing together of heterogeneous elements. These form links that cannot be seen as a logical progression from their constituent origins towards the goal of thought. A female patient with schizophrenia, aged 38, wrote as follows.

> " Two men are controlling the brain through telethapy [*sic*] or by means of ways of the spirit who open and closes the back channels of my brain releasing words and holding back the truth, by no means will I speak but will answer only to written questions by means of writing, knowing full well the channels of my

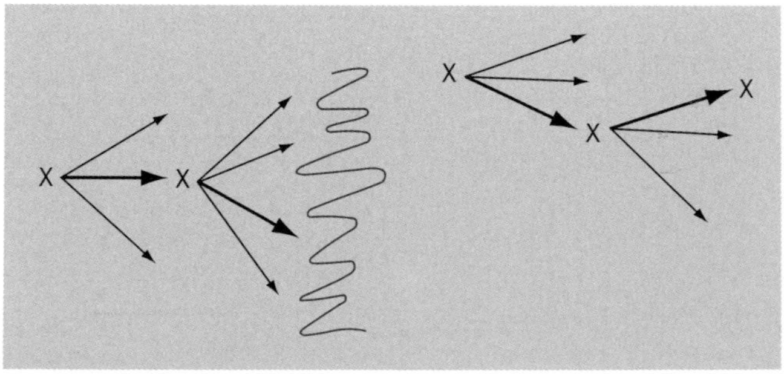

Figure 9.5 Model of derailment.

> brain is filtering and only half of what is the truth, also I knowing I am being read not only by a few but many very clever people but not at all acceptable they make people believe that I am some kind of miracle which I am not, I only hold the name Holyland which came to me by marrying Alfred Holyland, only by doing this do they wish to make some false stories of me coming from some special place which I have not.

Fusion is demonstrated at the beginning of this excerpt, where she says that the brain is controlled 'by means' and then this word becomes associated with 'ways'. 'Telethapy' – not the same as telepathy – is a neologism. There are also examples of passivity. 'Channels' and 'means' are used as stock words, that is, they are used more often in her conversation than their normal meaning could suggest, and they take on for her a greater range of meaning than usual. It is difficult to represent this diagrammatically, and I hope the result in Figure 9.6 is not misleading.

Schneider's *mixing* or *muddling* implies a grossly disordered amalgam of the constituent parts of a single thought process and represents extreme degrees of fusion and derailment. The resultant speech disorder has been called *drivelling*.

Thought blocking

Snapping off is the experience a schizophrenic patient has of his chain of thought, quite unexpectedly and unintentionally, breaking off or ceasing. It may occur in the middle of sorting out a problem or even in mid-sentence. It is not caused by distraction by other thoughts and, on introspecting, the patient can give no adequate explanation for it; it simply occurs. It is otherwise described as *thought blocking*, a somewhat misleading term. The patient may explain it in terms of *thought withdrawal*: 'My thinking stopped because the thoughts were suddenly taken out of my head'. Figure 9.7 shows a model of thought blocking.

Changes in the flow of thinking

Two further abnormalities of the flow of thought are *crowding of thought* and *perseveration*.

Crowding of thought occurs in schizophrenia. The patient describes his thoughts as being passively concentrated and compressed in his head. The associations are experienced as being excessive in amount, too fast, inexplicable

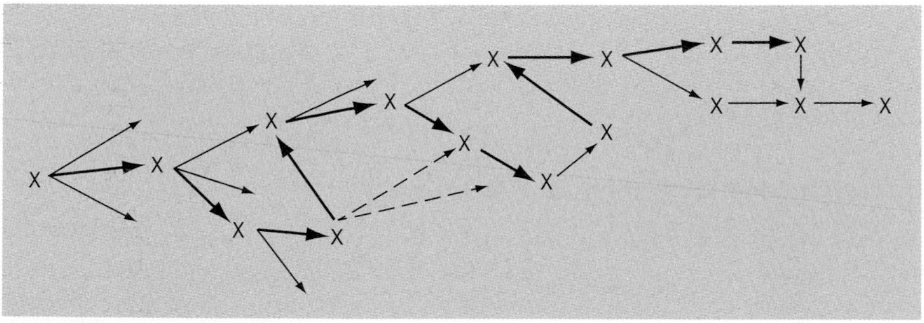

Figure 9.6 Model of fusion.

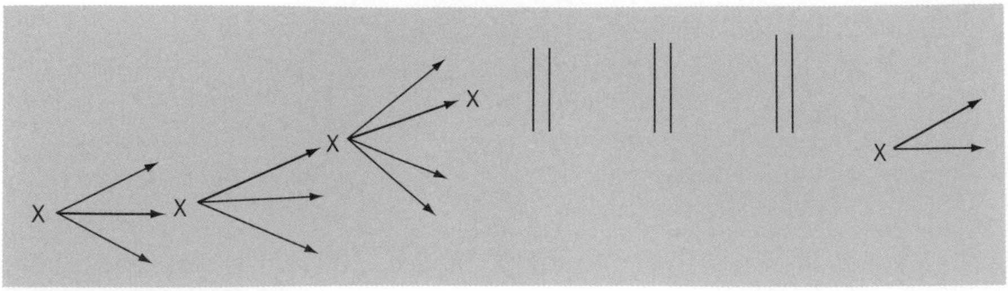

Figure 9.7 Model of thought blocking.

and outside the person's control. The patient may even locate his thinking anatomically as being 'crowded into the back of my head' or elsewhere. It becomes a headlong chase or dance of thoughts and has some of the characteristics of flight of ideas, but it also shows a schizophrenic quality of passivity, being controlled from outside.

Perseveration (Chapter 5) is mentioned here as a disturbance of the flow of thinking. It is characteristically an organic symptom. The patient retains a constellation of ideas long after they have ceased to be appropriate. An idea from that constellation which occurred in a previous sequence of thought is given in answer to a different question. In perseveration, a correct response is given by the patient to the first stimulus, for example 'Where do you live?' – 'Rowley Regis'. However, any subsequent stimuli that demand different responses may get this same, by now inappropriate, first response, for instance 'What is the capital of France?' – 'Rowley Regis', 'Who lives at home with you?' – 'Rowley ... my son and his wife'.

DISTURBANCE OF JUDGEMENT

A *judgement* is a thought that expresses a view of reality. The word is used here in the sense of 'in my judgement, such and such takes place'. To assess whether it is disturbed or not, one needs to measure it against objective fact. This can be difficult, perhaps requiring consultation with an expert in the same field as the patient. Assessment of faulty judgement is not made solely on the basis of that particular belief or argument but on taking the whole of the person's behaviour and opinions into account. A man's claims to be a figure of royalty persecuted by the Marxists could, in fact, be true. But the opinion that his judgement was disturbed would be confirmed if he had suddenly become convinced about his royalty when a psychiatric nurse had commented to him about the tattoos on his arm, or if he were also found to be hoarding pebbles and dead spiders in an old tobacco tin. Delusions are, of course, a disturbance of judgement. Various forms of thought disorder and intellectual deficit may also result in disturbance of judgement.

Disturbance of judgement and delusion

Primary delusions are not synonymous with incorrigible false beliefs, because individuals or groups of people may hold such latter ideas within the context of their culture: some individuals were prepared to burn others for believing that the earth was round. It is necessary to look at the nature of the belief and the evidence and social pressures for believing it. How is it that such a demonstrably false idea should be believed without even the rational doubtings that accompany the abstract convictions of a normal person?

The thinking or psychological performance required to produce a delusion is quite independent of intelligence. It occurs in clear consciousness with no signs of organic disturbance of the brain. Judgement in other areas of life apart from the delusion can be preserved, and the very ingeniousness the patient uses to explain and defend his delusional belief demonstrates that his essential capacity to think logically is largely intact. A schizophrenic delusion is not a simple defect of reasoning; its development cannot be understood solely in terms of the patient's real life experience. For instance, not all those with delusions of persecution have any first-hand experience of being persecuted. It is an assumption about the world the patient inhabits, which he does not create by a process of logical conscious thought from premises distorted by emotion. The starting points of his thinking are already 'deluded', and his logic elaborates from this basis.

We can understand why the belief should be within that particular context (associated with his mother; related to interplanetary travel), but we cannot explain how the *form* of a primary delusion should have occurred. This is a fundamental distinction from delusion-like ideas (secondary delusions), which occur, for example, in affective psychoses. In these latter, we can see the *content* being progressively influenced by the changing mood state so that, eventually, the false belief becomes a logical development from the extreme abnormality of mood.

Although it is usual to describe delusions as disorders of thought content, it is important to be aware that primary delusions are not merely to be understood in this way. The whole process of thought in primary delusion is disordered, not just the content. If an idea were formed on delusional grounds – 'I knew that my wife was unfaithful immediately I saw the bulb had gone out' (Chapter 8) – but the notion itself was not false nor unacceptable to the person's peer group (his wife subsequently admitted to being unfaithful), it would still be a delusion because the notion was formed on delusional evidence. There is a difference between *delusion* and *overvalued ideas* in that, although both may be held with absolute conviction, the latter is a reasonable, possibly even true, belief but is dominating conscious thought to an unreasonable extent.

Concrete thinking

Abnormal processes of thinking in schizophrenia and organic states may result in a literalness of expression and understanding. Abstractions and symbols are interpreted superficially without tact, finesse or any awareness of nuance; the patient is unable to free himself from what the words literally mean, excluding the more abstract ideas that are also conveyed. This abnormality is described as *concrete thinking*. The term was first introduced by Goldstein (1936). It is usually tested for by proverb interpretation or by other psychological tests, but it is well acknowledged that these tests are unreliable. However, it is recognizable clinically, often quite dramatically. For example, a female patient with schizophrenia came into the room for interview and promptly took her shoes off, saying, 'I always like to keep my feet on the ground when I'm talking'. Another patient with long-term schizophrenia was observed by his doctor walking sideways along the hospital corridor. When asked why he was walking like that, he said that it was 'because of the side effects'. And another patient said, 'I was starting to feel high and I didn't want to fly off, so I've tied these dumb-bell weights round my ankle'.

Concreteness is useful in making the psychopathological distinction between the disturbed thinking of the patient with schizophrenia and the description of internal experience of a person with strong religious beliefs. Watson (1982) has regarded some religious experiences as being similar in nature to the symptoms of schizophrenia. There do also appear to be some important differences.

- Religious experiences are usually regarded by the believer as being metaphorical or 'spiritual', while with schizophrenia the experience is concrete and physical. For the religious person, the physical boundaries of self are not invaded. In fact, the paradox the Christian describes is that he is a 'freer' person, more independent of external influences than previously, when Christ 'lives in him'.
- Religious experiences provoke sustained meaningful, goal-directed activity, whereas the behaviour that results from schizophrenic experience is often unreasonable in that it does not follow logically from the experience, is bizarre in flouting popular customs, is concrete in making spiritual values physical and tends to trivialize the sublime. A patient with schizophrenia read 'if thy right hand offend thee, cut it off' and attempted just that, producing a long and permanent scar on his wrist.
- Schizophrenic delusions and hallucinations are associated with a loss of ego boundaries and are based on delusional evidence, but there is no change in the boundaries of self in other areas of his experience for the religious believer, and his belief is based on his source of religious authority.
- Religious beliefs are held alongside the possibility of religious doubts; in this, they are like other abstract concepts. Schizophrenic delusions and hallucinations are accepted without doubt, reminiscent of concrete reality; one does not have doubts about the existence of the chair one sits on.

Psychological theories of thinking in schizophrenia

There are a number of psychological theories that attempt to explain thinking in patients with schizophrenia. These theories are hampered by the fact that there are no satisfactory general theories of thinking. There are now consistent findings of deficits in attention, working memory, recognition memory and executive functions in schizophrenia. These empirical findings are yet to be integrated into a coherent theory that explains the observed and self-reported thinking abnormalities in schizophrenia.

Over-inclusive thinking

The difference between the concrete thinking of organic psychosyndromes and that occurring in schizophrenia was described by Cameron (1944), who considered that in schizophrenia the patient is unable to preserve conceptual boundaries. This he called *over-inclusive thinking*: ideas that are only remotely related to the concept under consideration become incorporated within it in the patient's thinking. Thus, when asked 'What of the following are essential parts of a room: walls, chairs, floor, a window?', the over-inclusive person with schizophrenia might include 'chair'. This feature of over-inclusiveness can be seen in many aspects of schizophrenic thinking, and questionnaires have been devised to test for it, particularly involving sorting tests. The lack of adequate connection between two consecutive thoughts is called *asyndesis*.

The concrete thinking of schizophrenia, however, could not be distinguished from that of other psychotic and neurotic patients (Payne *et al.*, 1970), and it was found to be associated with intelligence. Over-inclusive thinking occurred only in about half of the patients with schizophrenia tested, usually those who were more acutely ill. The other half, usually suffering from more chronic illness, showed much more marked *retardation*. McGhie (1969) found that Payne's tests of over-inclusiveness did not select schizophrenia from some other diagnoses, for example those with obsessional or manic thought disorder, and Gathercole (1965) considered that these tests demonstrated *fluency of association* rather than over-inclusive thinking.

A young man, who had suffered from schizophrenia for several years, was known to have been abusing drugs recently. To the doctor's enquiry 'What drugs have you been using?', he replied 'LSD, health foods and marijuana'. This is an example of over-inclusive thinking. However, it was volunteered spontaneously; he might well have given an entirely correct response to a formal questionnaire that did not touch on significant areas of his experience.

It has been suggested by Chen *et al.* (1995) that there may be a *broadening of category boundary* (for example 'furniture') with preservation of internal category structure in patients with schizophrenia. This results in related issues that are actually outside the category being processed by the patient in a way that is similar to those within it.

Aggernaes (Aggernaes *et al.*, 1976) has taken this theory further from the practical and clinical viewpoint. He considers that patients with schizophrenia have not parted from reality; they seem to experience the real world as being real in the same way as normal people do. However, their defect in reality testing results from a diffuse tendency to experience some fantasy items as being real too.

Schizophrenic inattention and abnormality of working memory: effect on performance

McGhie (1969) has concentrated on the disturbance in the function of *attention* in schizophrenic patients: that they are unable to filter and discount sensory data irrelevant to the task being performed. He showed that the performance of schizophrenic patients was very poor compared with that of normal subjects, but they were not prone to distraction by auditory or visual external stimuli in the way that normal people were. Hebephrenic patients especially showed less distraction and also poor perception and recall of visual information. Hebephrenic patients were considered to have an

> “ inability to sweep out irrelevant extraneous information… especially where the situation demanded the rapid processing and short term storage of information. This experience is described subjectively: 'When people talk to me

now it's like a different kind of language. It's too much to hold at once. My head is overloaded and I can't understand what they say. It makes you forget what you've just heard because you can't get hearing it long enough. It's all in different bits that you have to put together in your head – just words in the air unless you can figure it out from their faces.'

The effect of this inattention in ordinary social life was well observed by Morgan (1977) in his description of 3 weeks lived in close proximity to two chronic schizophrenic patients:

"In the case of Vine our relationship remained just the same, but I did perhaps come to understand his disabilities a little better, and this helped. He would keep 'losing his thread', to some extent in talk but even more noticeably in action. For example, although we went through the sequence of routine tests over 500 times together, he never once completed a sequence without having to be reminded of what came next and what remained to be done each time. Vine's other main trouble was a curious one. I would say to him, for example, 'Let's do the tests first and then I'd like you to get on with the washing up', and I would be surprised when his response to this was to dash off to the sink and start clattering the plates. Eventually I made out that he had some defect of attention. He would often jump like a startled rabbit when he realized he was being addressed anyway, and I think that by the time he had recovered and collected himself from that, the first half of my sentence had gone and all he heard was the second half. Certainly I found that by inserting a little preliminary padding, I got a more competent response.

Frith (1992) hypothesizes that the mechanism for delusions of control was also responsible for the thought or language abnormality in schizophrenia. In this scheme, it is a failure of self-monitoring that is responsible for thought or language disorder. Thus the patient is unable to edit out irrelevant or perseverating phrases, and this results in poor communication. There is also the related possibility that the fundamental problem is in planning. In this scheme, the coherence of the patient's thought or language is undermined by the absence of an explicit goal and plan, and furthermore there is intrusion of thoughts that do not fit in with the overall goal, resulting in disorganized thought or language. In summary, patient's with schizophrenia 'are only able to check the accuracy of an utterance *after* [emphasis in original] they have made it. It is therefore difficult for them to avoid producing a string of faulty utterances, even during attempts at repair' (Frith, 1992).

Liddle (2001) defines the disorganization syndrome as consisting of disjointed thought, emotion and behaviour. But the cardinal symptoms are formal thought disorder, inappropriate affect and bizarre, erratic behaviour. He concludes that disorganization is associated with slowed performance in neuropsychological tasks that demand selection between competing responses, or with errors of commission in tasks that require suppression of an inappropriate response. In his view, this suggests that the disorganization found in schizophrenia derives from impairment of the neural circuits responsible for response selection and inhibition. The circuits involved are the ventrolateral frontal cortex, the left superior temporal gyrus and the adjacent inferior parietal lobule. There is also involvement of the anterior cingulate and thalamus.

DISORDER OF CONTROL OF THINKING

Under this heading, we could discuss three different patterns of thinking: passivity of thought, or delusions of control of thinking; obsessions and compulsions, in which the unacceptable thoughts are accepted by the patient as being under his control but are resisted; and the rigid control of thought and intolerance for variation that becomes habitual with the anankastic or obsessional personality. The latter two will be considered in Chapter 19.

Delusions of the control of thought

Control of thinking may be disorganized in that the patient ascribes his own, internal thought processes to outside influences. The subjective disturbance in thinking in schizophrenia is experienced as *passivity*. The schizophrenic experiences his thoughts as foreign or alien, not emanating from himself and not within his control. There is a breakdown in the way he thinks of the boundary between himself and the outside world so that he can no longer accurately discriminate between the two. He may describe passivity of thought, thought withdrawal, thought insertion and/or thought broadcasting; these are *first-rank symptoms* of *schizophrenia* (Schneider, 1959). In Table 9.1, the first-rank symptoms are listed.

Various forms of thought passivity are described. The patient may describe sharing his thoughts with other people: his thoughts being controlled or influenced from outside himself. These *delusions of control* are often associated with delusional explanations of how his thinking could be controlled, for example electronic devices, computers, telepathy. *Thought insertion* is described, in which he believes that his thoughts have been placed there from outside himself.

Table 9.1 First-rank symptoms of schizophrenia and symptoms from the present state examination

First-rank symptom[a]	Equivalent symptom from the present state examination[b]
Delusion	
Delusional percept	Primary delusion
Auditory hallucinations	
Audible thoughts	Thought echo or commentary
Voices arguing or discussing	Voices about the patient
Voices commenting on the patient's action	Voices about the patient
Thought disorder: passivity of thought	
Thought withdrawal	Thought block or withdrawal
Thought insertion	Thought insertion
Thought broadcasting (diffusion of thought)	Thought broadcast or thought sharing
Passivity experiences: delusion of control	
Passivity of affect ('made' feelings)	Delusions of control
Passivity of impulse ('made' drives)	Delusions of control
Passivity of volition ('made' volitional acts)	Delusions of control
Somatic passivity (influence playing on the body)	Delusions of alien penetration

[a]Schneider (1959), [b]Wing et al. (1974).

Correspondingly, he may describe his thoughts being taken away from himself against his will: *thought withdrawal*. This may be given as an explanation for thought blocking when the thoughts stop and the mind suddenly goes completely blank. Thought insertion and withdrawal are first-rank symptoms of schizophrenia. *Thought blocking* is not, as it is difficult to decide whether it is truly thought blocking or some form of retardation or other difficulty with thinking, and blocking is also subjectively similar to epileptic absences. *Thought broadcasting* occurs in schizophrenia when the patient describes his thoughts as leaving himself and being diffused widely out of his control. It also is a passivity experience and of first rank.

A further subjective symptom associated with thought, of first-rank importance, is the experience of *audible thoughts*: hearing one's own thoughts out loud. The patient knows that they are his thoughts, yet he hears them audibly while he is thinking them, just before or just after. This is of course a disorder of perception, an auditory hallucination (Chapter 7).

We have discussed earlier in the chapter fusion, mixing, derailment and crowding of thought, all of which occur in schizophrenia. The resultant confusion causes a loss of ability to think clearly, often described in terms of passivity. The patient may feel that his brain is replaced by cotton wool or convoluted rubber. His thoughts are jumbled, muzzy, vague, blurred: 'I try to part my way through them but they are like treacle and keep on coming back and making me stick'.

First-rank symptoms of schizophrenia

British psychiatry has used for the clinical diagnosis of schizophrenia the empirical list of first-rank symptoms, and these have proved useful in other cultures, for example in Sri Lanka (Chandrasena and Rodrigo, 1979). According to Schneider, the presence of one or more first-rank symptoms in the absence of organic disease can be used as positive evidence for schizophrenia. These symptoms of first rank are not a comprehensive list of the clinical features of schizophrenia, for the changes in affect, volition and motor activity that may occur in the condition are not included at all, and many other types of delusion, hallucination and disorder of thinking occur also in schizophrenia. For a symptom to be regarded as first rank, it must have the following characteristics.

- It must occur with reasonable frequency in schizophrenia.
- It must generally not occur in conditions other than schizophrenia.
- It must not be too difficult to decide if the symptom is or is not present.

There are some symptoms that occur only in schizophrenia but occur too rarely to be of practical use as first-rank symptoms. There are many features that are characteristic of schizophrenia but may also occur in other conditions, for example unspecified auditory hallucinations, poverty of affect, over-inclusive thinking. There are some symptoms that occur only in schizophrenia, but there is too much scope for argument as to whether it is, or is not, this precise symptom for it to be valued as of first rank. An example of this is a *primary delusion*. Some clinicians may regard a particular belief of the patient as primary delusion, while others do not.

Although first-rank symptoms are used as a diagnostic checklist, a patient who shows seven of them is not more schizophrenic than someone who shows three. To elicit them requires considerable clinical experience; they cannot be collected quantitatively by riding past the patient on a bicycle! For a psychiatrist to use them clinically, she must first know them. Second, she must know how this person from this social and racial background is likely to describe any particular first-rank symptom ('my thoughts are controlled by ... television, by ... the spirits of my dead ancestors'). Third, she must ask the appropriate direct questions skilfully, without putting words in her patient's mouth. Fourth, she must be able to interpret the patient's answers and decide whether a first-rank symptom is being described. The whole process requires a dextrous use of the phenomenological method as described in Chapter 1.

There are many practising psychiatrists whose comment at this stage of the discussion of first-rank symptoms would be 'Why bother?' They would also agree that it is often difficult to diagnose schizophrenia; that it is important not to give this unfortunate label to people who do not suffer from the illness; and that it is equally important to treat those who do suffer from it appropriately, effectively and as early in the course of illness as possible.

In clinical practice, the eliciting of first-rank symptoms could best be seen as a means of deciding the degree of certainty that may be attached to the diagnosis. In a patient who shows the general features of schizophrenia (delusion, hallucination, thought disorder, disordered affect, volition, motor activity, behaviour, social relationships, life history), the diagnosis is made but some doubts remain. If first-rank symptoms are found then, in the absence of clear organic pathology, one can reckon that the diagnosis has been confirmed. Some of the first-rank symptoms are found to be less reliable at follow-up than others as indicators of schizophrenia, for example voices heard arguing (Mellor *et al.*, 1981). One of the advantages of first-rank symptoms as a diagnostic tool is that, because of their emphasis on form rather than content, a person who is feigning mental illness is unlikely to produce them. They therefore have a subsidiary use as a method of distinguishing between true and *simulated psychosis*, for example in prisoners. Despite the value of first-rank symptoms indicating schizophrenia when they are present, there are undoubted patients in whom they cannot be elicited; schizophrenia still remains, to some extent, a diagnosis of exclusion (Carpenter and Buchanan, 1994).

Examples of first-rank symptoms

The only type of *delusion* that is regarded as of first rank is a *delusional perception*, that is, a normal perception delusionally interpreted and regarded as being highly significant to the patient (Chapter 8). Examples of delusional percept, and of other first-rank symptoms as follows, are cited by Mellor (1970). Delusional percept is exemplified in the following account.

> “A young Irishman was at breakfast with two fellow-lodgers. He felt a sense of unease, that something frightening was going to happen. One of the lodgers pushed the salt cellar towards him (he appreciated at the same time that this was an ordinary salt cellar and his friend's intention was innocent). Almost before the salt cellar reached him he knew he must return home, 'to greet the Pope, who is visiting Ireland to see his family and to reward them ... because Our Lord is

going to be born again to one of the women... And because of this they (all the women) are all born different with their private parts back to front.' *(p. 18)*

Three types of auditory hallucinations are regarded as being of first rank. These are *audible thoughts, voices heard arguing* and *voices giving a running commentary*. By *audible thoughts* is meant the patient's experience of hearing his own thoughts said out loud. In British usage, the symptom sometimes carries its German name, *Gedankenlautwerden*, or its French, *écho de pensées*. The patient may hear people repeating his thoughts out loud just after he has thought them, answering his thoughts, talking about them having said them audibly or saying aloud what he is about to think so that his thoughts repeat the voices. He often becomes very upset at the gross intrusion into his privacy and concerned that he cannot maintain control of any part of himself, not even his thoughts.

> A 35 year old painter heard a quiet voice with 'an Oxford accent', which he attributed to the BBC. The volume was slightly lower than that of normal conversation and could be heard equally well with either ear. He could locate its source at the right mastoid process. The voice would say, 'I can't stand that man, the way he holds his hand he looks like a poof'... He immediately experienced whatever the voice was saying as his own thoughts, to the exclusion of all other thoughts. When he read the newspaper the voice would speak aloud whatever his eyes fell on. He had not time to think of what he was reading before it was uttered aloud. *(Mellor, 1970: 16)*

Voices heard arguing with each other implies two or more hallucinatory voices quarrelling or discussing with each other. The patient usually features in the third person in the content of these arguing voices. The symptom is not likely to be volunteered spontaneously in this form: the patient does not actually say, 'I hear voices that argue or discuss with each other'. So the symptom has to be cautiously and subtly enquired for.

> A 24 year old male patient reported hearing voices coming from the nurse's office. One voice, deep in pitch and roughly spoken, repeatedly said, 'G.T. is a bloody paradox', and another, higher in pitch, said, 'He is that, he should be locked up.' A female voice occasionally interrupted, saying 'He is not, he is a lovely man.' *(Mellor, 1970: 16)*

Hallucinatory *voices giving a running commentary* on the patient's activities occur and are of first rank. The time sequence of the commentary may be such that it takes place just before, during or after the patient's activities. Again, the symptom is not volunteered spontaneously but may quite often be inferred from the patient's complaints against his voices. For the interviewer, there is always the problem of asking questions in such a way that she is 'let in on the inside'. She is asking questions about perceptions that are quite obvious to the patient. The patient does not know that his particular perception is unique, that other people do not share his perceptual experience. So the interviewer has the difficulty of asking questions about something of which she has no personal experience; the patient has to answer questions that, because of his situation, seem to have no point. The abnormal thing about *voices commenting* is that they should be experienced as perceptions and as coming from outside the self; many normal people have thoughts, recognized as their own and coming from inside themselves, commenting on their actions:

> A 41 year old housewife heard a voice coming from the house across the road. . . . The voice went on incessantly in a flat monotone describing everything she was doing, with an admixture of critical comments. 'She is peeling potatoes, got hold of the peeler, she does not want that potato, she is putting it back, because she thinks it has a knobble like a penis, she has a dirty mind, she is peeling potatoes, now she is washing them.' *(Mellor, 1970: 16)*

Passivity experiences are those events in the realm of sensation, feeling, drive and volition that are experienced as *made* or influenced by others. They have been well described as delusions of control, because the patient's experience of the event being made to occur takes the form of a delusion. The terms *disorders of passivity*, *made experiences*, *delusions of control* and *disorders of personal activity* are, in practice, synonymous and interchangeable. The event is experienced as alien by the patient in that it is not experienced by the patient as his own but inserted into the self from outside. Passivity experiences of thinking occur as thought withdrawal, thought insertion or thought broadcasting. In *thought withdrawal*, it is believed by the patient that his thoughts are in some way being taken out of his mind; he has some feeling of loss resulting from this process. It may be coupled with other thought passivity experiences:

> A 22 year old woman said, 'I am thinking about my mother, and suddenly my thoughts are sucked out of my mind by a phrenological vacuum extractor, and there is nothing in my mind, it is empty.' *(Mellor, 1970: 16)*

In *thought insertion*, he experiences thoughts that do not have the feeling of familiarity, of being his own, but he feels that they have been put in his mind, without his volition, from outside himself. As in thought withdrawal, there is clearly a disturbance in the self-image, and especially in the boundary between what is self and what is not self; thoughts that have in fact arisen inside himself are considered to have been inserted into his thinking from outside.

> A 29 year old housewife said, 'I look out of the window and I think the garden looks nice and the grass looks cool, but the thoughts of Eamonn Andrews comes into my mind. There are no other thoughts there, only his. . . . He treats my mind like a screen and flashes his thoughts onto it like you flash a picture.' *(Mellor, 1970: 17)*

In *thought broadcasting*, the patient experiences his thoughts withdrawn from his mind and then, in some way, made public and projected over a wide area. The explanation he gives for how this can occur will, as usual for the content of a delusion, depend on his background culture and predominant interests:

> A 21 year old student said, 'As I think, my thoughts leave my head on a type of mental ticker-tape. Everyone around has only to pass the tape through their mind and they know my thoughts.' *(Mellor, 1970: 17)*

Obviously, careful enquiry must be made about the nature of 'influence' or 'control'. There is a phenomenological world of difference between the statements 'My thinking is influenced by my parents inasmuch as my thoughts are crowded from the back into the front of my head' – a passivity experience, and 'What I do is influenced by my father in that I ponder what he would do in the circumstances and then do the same' (or 'do the opposite') – not passivity. All passivity experiences are regarded as first-rank symptoms. It is not really of great significance to decide which type of passivity is described – whether it is, for example, passivity of impulse or of volition – but it is important diagnostically to decide whether it is a passivity experience or not. *Passivity of emotion* occurs when the affect that the patient experiences does not seem to him to be his own. He believes that he has been *made* to feel it:

> “ A 23 year old female patient reported, 'I cry, tears roll down my cheeks and I look unhappy, but inside I have a cold anger because they are using me in this way, and it is not me who is unhappy, but they are projecting unhappiness onto my brain. They project upon me laughter, for no reason, and you have no idea how terrible it is to laugh and look happy and know it is not your, but their reaction.' *(Mellor, 1970: 17)*

In *passivity of impulse*, the patient experiences a drive, which he feels is alien, to carry out some motor activity. The impulse may be experienced without the subject carrying out the behaviour. A Jewish woman, aged 55, suffering from schizophrenia said, 'I feel my hand going up to salute, and my lips saying "Heil Hitler" . . . I don't actually say it . . . I have to try very hard to stop my arm from going up . . . they put drugs in my food; that is what makes it happen'. If carried out, the *action* is admitted to be the patient's own, but he feels that the *impulse* that precipitated him into doing it was not his own.

> “ A 26 year old engineer emptied the contents of a urine bottle over the ward dinner trolley. He said, 'The sudden impulse came over me and I must do it. It was not my feeling, it came into me from the X-ray department, that was why I was sent there for implants yesterday. It was nothing to do with me, they wanted it done. So I picked up the bottle and poured it in. It seemed all I could do.' *(Mellor, 1970: 17)*

Similarly, with *passivity of volition* the patient feels that it is not his will that carried out the action.

> “ A 29 year old shorthand typist described her actions as follows, 'when I reach my hand for the comb it is my hand and arm which move, and my fingers pick up the pen, but I don't control them... I sit there wanting them to move, and they are quite independent, what they do is nothing to do with me... I am just a puppet who is manipulated by cosmic strings. When the strings are pulled my body moves and I can't prevent it.' *(Mellor, 1970: 17)*

Somatic passivity is the belief that outside influences are playing on the body. It is not the same as haptic hallucination, but it is a delusional belief that the body is being influenced from outside the self. It may occur in association with various somatic hallucinations. For example, a kinaesthetic hallucination occurred, with a passivity experience given as explanation, by a patient who felt that his hand was being drawn up to his face. He could feel it moving although, in fact, it was motionless. Somatic passivity may also occur in association with a normal percept; these experiences are quite common in schizophrenia.

> "A 38 year old man had jumped from a bedroom window, injuring his right knee which was very painful. He described his physical experience as, 'The sun-rays are directed by U.S. army satellites in an intense beam which I can feel entering the centre of my knee and then radiating outwards causing the pain.' *(Mellor, 1970: 16)*

First-rank symptoms are of general use, diagnostically, in clinical practice, and they have also been adapted for psychiatric research. The method of ascertaining and measuring schizophrenic symptoms, among other symptoms, developed by Wing *et al.* (1974) in their Present State Examination uses first-rank symptoms as a basis for diagnosing schizophrenia. The Present State Examination provides the clinician with a means of ascertaining which symptoms and syndromes are present.

Koehler (1979), in a review of the way different authors describe the presence of first-rank symptoms in the English literature, considered that they were sometimes used in a very narrow and sometimes a very wide sense. He makes the distinction between *alienation* of thought and *influence* of thought, and makes a plea for clear statements on the boundary criteria for first-rank symptoms and the nosological bias attached to the phenomena. From the quoted examples of Mellor above, alienation is necessary; that is, a delusion of control and not just an experience of influence of thought. Similarly, thought broadcasting would be regarded as of first rank when the patient describes this as having occurred outside his control, irrespective of whether these thoughts are shared with others. Thus, this chapter is recommending a narrow use of first-rank symptoms. First-rank symptoms have been employed to establish the diagnosis; they are not necessarily useful prognostically (Bland and Orn, 1980).

This difference between alienation or experience of control and influence can be exemplified by the schizophrenic symptom of *thought insertion*. Thought insertion is more concrete than the insertion of an idea into one's thinking. A normal person may say, 'my mother gave me the idea' or even 'the idea was put into my head by my mother'. Neither of these is thought insertion. The patient experiencing passivity believes that by some concrete process the boundaries of his self involving thinking are so invaded that his mother is actually placing thoughts inside his head (Chapter 13), so that he thinks her thoughts, or perhaps she, is thinking inside him.

REFERENCES

Aggernaes A, Haugsted R, Myschetsky A, Paikin H and Vitger J (1976). A reliable clinical technique for investigation of the experienced reality and unreality qualities connected with everyday life experiences in psychotic and non-psychotic persons. *Acta Psychiatrica Scandinavica 53*, 241–57.

Bion WR (1962) The psycho-analytic study of thinking. *International Journal of Psychoanalysis 43*, 306–10.

Bland RC and Orn H (1980) Schizophrenia: Schneider's first-rank symptoms and outcome. *British Journal of Psychiatry 137*, 63–8.

Bleuler E (1911) *Dementia Praecox or the Group of Schizophrenias* (transl. Zinkin J, 1950). New York: International Universities Press.

Cameron N (1944) Experimental analysis of schizophrenic thinking. In Kasanin JJ (ed.) *Language and Thought in Schizophrenia*. Berkeley: University of California Press.

Carpenter WT and Buchanan RW (1994) Schizophrenia. *New England Journal of Medicine 330*, 681–90.

Chandrasena R and Rodrigo A (1979) Schneider's first rank syndromes: their prevalence and diagnostic implication in an Asian population. *British Journal of Psychiatry 135*, 348–51.

Chen EYH, McKenna PJ and Wilkins A (1995) Semantic processing and categorization in schizophrenia. In Sims A (ed.) *Speech and Language Disorders in Psychiatry*. London: Gaskell.

Fish F (1967) *Clinical Psychopathology*. Bristol: John Wright.

Fish FJ (1962) *Schizophrenia*. Bristol: John Wright.

Frith CD (1992) The cognitive neuropsychology of schizophrenia. Hove: Lawrence Erlbaum Associates.

Gathercole (1965) A note on some tests of over-inclusive thinking. *British Journal of Medical Psychology 38*, 59–62.

Goldstein K (1936) The modification of behaviour consequent to cerebral lesions. *Psychiatric Quarterly 10*, 586–610.

Israels H and Schatzman M (1993) The seduction theory. *History of Psychiatry 4*, 23–60.

Jaspers K (1962) *General Psychopathology* (transl. Hoenig J and Hamilton MW). Manchester: Manchester University Press.

Jones E (1962) *The Life and Work of Sigmund Freud*. Harmondsworth: Penguin.

Koehler K (1979) First rank symptoms of schizophrenia: questions concerning clinical boundaries. *British Journal of Psychiatry 134*, 236–48.

Kraepelin E (1904) *Lectures on Clinical Psychiatry* (transl. Johnston ET). New York: Hafner.

Liddle PF (2001) *Disordered Mind and Brain: the Neural Basis of Mental Symptoms*. London: Gaskell.

McGhie A (1969) *Pathology of Attention*. Harmondsworth: Penguin.

Mellor CS (1970) First-rank symptoms of schizophrenia. *British Journal of Psychiatry 117*, 15–23.

Mellor CS, Sims ACP and Cope RV (1981) Changes of diagnosis in schizophrenia and first rank symptoms: an 8 year follow-up. *Comprehensive Psychiatry 2*, 184–8.

Morgan R (1977) Three weeks in isolation with two chronic schizophrenic patients. *British Journal of Psychiatry 131*, 504–13.

Payne RW, Hochberg AC and Hawks DV (1970) Dichotic stimulation as a method of assessing the disorder of attention of an overinclusive schizophrenic patient. *Journal of Abnormal Psychology 76*, 185–93.

Roth I (2004) Imagination. In Gregory RL (ed.) *The Oxford Companion to the Mind*. Oxford: Oxford University Press.

Schneider C (1930) *Psychologie der Schizophrenie*. Leipzig: Thieme.

Schneider K (1959) *Clinical Psychopathology*, 5th edn (transl. Hamilton MW). New York: Grune & Stratton.

Smith EE and Kosslyn SM (2007) *Cognitive Psychology: Mind and Brain*. New Jersey: Prentice Hall.

Sutherland NS (1976) *Breakdown: a Personal Crisis and a Medical Dilemma*. London: Weidenfeld & Nicholson.

Swift J (1667–1745) *Tale of a Tub*. London: Dent.

Watson JP (1982) Aspects of personal meaning in schizophrenia. In Shepherd E and Watson JP (eds) *Personal Meanings*. Chichester: John Wiley.

Webster R (1995) *Why Freud Was Wrong*. London: Harper Collins.

Wing JK, Cooper JE and Sartorius N (1974) *The Measurement and Classification of Psychiatric Symptoms: an Instruction Manual for the PSE and Catego Program*. Cambridge: Cambridge University Press.

Winnicott DW (1957) *The Child and the Family: First Relationships*. London: Tavistock Publications.

Disorder of Speech and Language

10

> "To speak is not only to utter words, it is to propositionise. A proposition is such a relation of words that it makes one new meaning. *J. Hughlings (Jackson, 1932)*

It is very obvious that the functions of thinking and speaking overlap and cannot be readily separated from each other; at the same time, they are clearly different. The contents of this chapter cannot be considered in isolation from its predecessor, although it is considering speech and language from a different perspective.

Maher (1972) proposed a model that attempted to demonstrate the link between thinking and the behaviour of speech in language:

> "conceptualizing the relationship between language and thought. The model might be likened to a typist copying from a script before her. Her copy may appear to be distorted because the script is distorted although the communication channel of the typist's eye and hand are functioning correctly. Alternatively, the original script may be perfect, but the typist may be unskilled, making typing errors in the copy and thus distorting it. Finally, it is possible for an inefficient typist to add errors to an already incoherent script. Unfortunately, the psychopathologist can observe only the copy (language utterances): he cannot examine the script (the thought). In general most theorists concerned with schizophrenic language have accepted the first of the three alternatives, namely that a good typist is transcribing a deviant script. The patient is correctly reporting a set of disordered thoughts. As Critchley put it: 'Any considerable aberration of thought or personality will be mirrored in the various levels of articulate speech – phonetic, phonemic, semantic, syntactic and pragmatic'. The language is a mirror of the thought. *(p. 3)*

The script is likened to thought and the typist to language. Most clinicians have taken the view that language closely mirrors thought and see the primary abnormality as the thinking disorder (Beveridge, 1985). Disordered language is then seen as merely a reflection of this underlying disturbance, with diagnosis of thought disorder only possible on the basis of what the patient says. Some of the more recent linguistic theories used for the analysis of schizophrenic speech contradict the primacy of thinking.

The assumption that language directly mirrors thought can be challenged (Newby, 1995). There is a tradition that argues that language itself structures thinking and concepts and determines how the world is understood. This view derives from the works of Edward Sapir (1884–1939) and Benjamin Whorf (1897–1941). In essence, the Sapir–Whorf hypothesis says that language influences cognition. There is very limited empirical support for this view, and Pinker (1994) concludes that 'the representations underlying thinking, on the one hand, and the sentences in a language, on the other, are in many ways at cross-purposes. ... People do not think in English or Chinese or Apache; they think in a language of thought. This language of thought probably looks a bit like all these languages; presumably it has symbols for concepts, and arrangements of symbols that correspond to who did what to whom'. This radical view contradicts the point-to-point relationship between language and thought implicit in Maher's proposition (see above) and the linguistic determinism of the Sapir–Whorf hypothesis.

The relationship between thinking and language is as complicated for organic disorders as for schizophrenia: there can be quite marked disturbance in the use of language with no apparent thought disorder. This is revealed in the rare isolated abnormalities of specific function of language described in this chapter. An understanding of how the healthy person expresses thoughts in language can be achieved only by study of the normal development of language. This is outside the scope of this book but is discussed in relation to perception in Carterette and Friedman (1976).

Language is built up of a number of elements. *Phonemes* are the most basic sounds that are available for use in language, and any particular language, such as English, uses only a limited repertoire of phonemes. The repertoire used in English may share only a limited overlap with that used, for example, in Yoruba. *Morphemes* are produced from phonemes and are the smallest meaningful unit of a word, and combinations of morphemes make up words. A morpheme may be a word such as 'do' or 'un'. *Syntax* (grammar) is the allowable combination of words in phrases and sentences and includes the rules that determine word order. *Semantics* are the meanings that correspond to the words and include the meaning of all possible sentences. *Prosody* refers to the modulation of vocal intonation that influences accents, and also the literal and emotional meanings of words and sentences. The *pragmatics* of language are the ways that language is used in practice. This is a relatively new area of study. It refers to the multiple potential meanings of any utterance, which requires knowledge of context and of the speakers for full interpretation. For example, the sentence 'this room is cold' can have any of several meanings depending on the identity of the speaker, the actual context and who is being addressed. It is perhaps important to distinguish between language and speech for our purpose. Speech is the aspect of language that corresponds to the mechanical and articulatory functions that allow language to be vocalized. Thus, for language to become speech the vocal cords, the palate, the lips and the tongue need to perform a complex and synchronized dance of intricate steps. The dissociation between poorly articulated speech and intact language indicates that these two functions are separate.

Chomsky's theory of language is the most influential (Chomsky, 1986). Essentially, Chomsky argued that language is like an instinct, and furthermore that every 'sentence that a person utters or understands is a brand-new combination of words, appearing for the first time in the history of the universe. Therefore a language cannot be a repertoire of responses; the brain must contain a recipe or programme that can build an unlimited set of sentences out of a finite list of words. The programme may be called a mental grammar' (Pinker, 1994). In addition to this, children rapidly develop these complex grammars without formal instruction. This suggests that they must be innately endowed with a plan common to the grammars of all languages, a universal grammar. How language develops, how word meaning is learned and the neuropsychology of language are all areas of increasing study.

SPEECH DISTURBANCES

This subject is dealt with in textbooks of neurology and has been reviewed by Critchley (1995); it is only summarized here. Many abnormalities, such as paraphasia (see above), have both organic and psychogenic causes; diagnosis will require full medical and psychiatric history and neurological and mental state examination.

Aphonia and dysphonia

Aphonia is the loss of the ability to vocalize; the patient talks only in a whisper. *Dysphonia* denotes impairment with hoarseness but without complete loss of function. It occurs with paralysis of the ninth cranial nerve or with disease of the vocal cords.

Aphonia may also occur without organic disease in *dissociative aphonia*, not uncommon as a presentation among ear, nose and throat outpatients. Such a patient may speak in a 'stage whisper'; phonation may fluctuate according to the response of those the person is addressing.

Dysarthria

Disorders of articulation may be caused by lesions of the brainstem such as bulbar and pseudobulbar palsy. It may also occur with structural or muscular disorders of the mouth, pharynx, larynx and thorax. Idiosyncratic disorders of articulation are sometimes seen in schizophrenia and also, perhaps, with personality disorders consciously produced.

Stuttering and stammering

These have in the past been enquired about in the psychiatric history under neurotic disturbances of childhood, with such behaviour as nail biting. However, psychogenic aetiology has certainly not been proved, and any association with neuroticism may well be secondary to the barriers in communication that stuttering causes.

Logoclonia

This describes the spastic repetition of syllables that occurs with parkinsonism (Scharfetter, 1980). The patient may get stuck using a particular word.

Echolalia

The patient repeats words or parts of sentences that are spoken to him or in his presence. There is usually no understanding of the meaning of the words. It is most often demonstrated in excited schizophrenic states, with mental retardation and with organic states such as dementia, especially if dysphasia is also present.

Changes in the volume and intonation of speech

Many depressed patients speak very quietly with a monotonous voice. Manic patients often speak loudly and excitably with much variation in pitch. Excited schizophrenics may also speak loudly; intonation and stresses on words may be idiosyncratic and inappropriate. None of these modes of behaviour has diagnostic significance. The speed and flow of talk mirrors that of thought and has been dealt with in Chapter 9.

Unintelligible speech

Speech may be unintelligible for several reasons, and most of the abnormalities described here, if taken to extremes, will result in incomprehensibility.

- *Dysphasia* may be so profound that, although syllables are produced, speech is unintelligible.
- *Paragrammatism* (disorder of grammatical construction) and *incoherence of syntax* may occur in several disorders. Recognizable words may be so deranged in their sentences as to be meaningless – *word salad*, as occurs in schizophrenia.

In mania, the speed of association may be so rapid as to disrupt sentence structure completely and render it meaningless, while in depression retardation may so inhibit speech that only unintelligible syllables, often of a moaning nature, are produced.

- Private symbolism may occur in schizophrenia with the use of (a) new words with an idiosyncratic, personal meaning – *neologisms*; (b) *stock words* and *phrases* in which existing words are used with special individual symbolic meaning; or (c) a private language that may be spoken (*cryptolalia*), or written (*cryptographia*).

ORGANIC DISORDERS OF LANGUAGE

Dysphasic symptoms are probably more useful clinically than any other cognitive defect in indicating the approximate site of brain pathology (Lishman, 1997). However, the auditory, visual and motor mechanisms of speech are spread through several different parts of the brain; often, several functions are affected and lesions are usually diffuse, and thus precise brain localization is not often possible. Ninety per cent of right-handed people without any brain damage have speech located in the left hemisphere, and 10 per cent have right hemisphere speech. Among those who are left-handed or ambidextrous, 64 per cent have left-hemisphere speech, 20 per cent right-hemisphere and 16 per cent bilateral speech representation.

Sensory dysphasia

The terms *aphasia* and *dysphasia* are often used interchangeably. However, aphasia implies the loss of language altogether, and dysphasia impairment of, or difficulty with, language. Dysphasia is conventionally divided for classification into *sensory* (receptive) and *motor* (expressive) types. Very frequently, there is a global impairment of language with evidence of impairment of both elements. Table 10.1 summarizes some of the abnormalities that occur with the different aspects of language that are impaired.

Pure word deafness (subcortical auditory dysphasia)

Such a patient can speak, read and write fluently, correctly and with comprehension. He cannot understand speech, even though hearing is unimpaired for other sounds; he hears words as sounds but cannot recognize the meaning even though he knows that they are words. This is therefore a form of *agnosia*

Table 10.1 Impairment of language function with different types of dysphasia

Type	Spontaneous speech-fluent	Comprehension	Repetition	Naming	Reading	Writing
Pure word deafness	+	−	−	+	+	+ (not to dictation)
Pure word blindness	+	+	+	+	−	+
Primary sensory dysphasia	+	−	−	±	−	−
Conduction dysphasia	+	+	−	±	Aloud −, compr.n +	−
Nominal dysphasia	+	+	+	−	±	±
Pure word dumbness	−	+	−	±	+	+
Pure agraphia	+	+	+	+	+	−
Primary motor dysphasia		−	+	−	±, aloud −, compr.n ±	−
Alexia with agraphia	+	+	+	−	−	−
Isolated speech area	−	−	+	−	−	−
Transcortical motor dysphasia	−	+	+	−	Aloud −, compr.n +	
Transcortical sensory dysphasia	+	−	+	−	−	−

Compr.n, comprehension.
(After Lishman, 1997, with permission of Blackwell Scientific.)

(lack of recognition) for the spoken word. The neuropsychiatric implications of this and other symptoms are dealt with more fully in Lishman (1997).

Pure word blindness (subcortical visual aphasia)

This patient can speak normally and understand the spoken word; he can write spontaneously and to dictation but cannot read with understanding (*alexia*). The condition is therefore *agnosic alexia without dysgraphia*. He may have more difficulty with printed than written script. Such a patient will also suffer a right homonymous hemianopia (loss of the right half of the field of vision in both eyes) and an inability to *name* colours even though they can be perceived.

Primary sensory dysphasia (receptive dysphasia)

These patients are unable to understand spoken speech, with loss of comprehension of the meaning of words and of the significance of grammar. Hearing otherwise is not impaired. Consequent on this deficit in the auditory association cortex (*Wernicke's area*), there is also impairment of speech, writing and reading. Speech is fluent, with no appreciation of the many errors in the use of words, syntax and grammar.

Conduction dysphasia could be considered to be a type of sensory dysphasia in which sensory reception of speech and writing are impaired, in that the patient cannot repeat the message although he can speak and write. If he is questioned on the message, he is able to give 'yes' or 'no' answers correctly, thus demonstrating comprehension. There are marked errors of grammar and syntax (*syntactical dysphasia*).

Nominal dysphasia

The patient is unable to produce names and sounds at will. He may be able to describe the object and its function and to recognize the name when presented: a patient described a watch as a 'clock vessel'. Typically, 'empty' nouns such as 'thing' and 'object' are used frequently while 'distinguishing' nouns rarely. Speech is flat, the structure of sentences generally correct and understanding unimpaired.

Jargon aphasia

Speech is fluent, but there is such gross disturbance to words and syntax that it is unintelligible. The intonation and rhythm of speech are retained. This is considered a severe type of sensory dysphasia; there is failure to evaluate the patients' own speech, in that patients are not emotionally disturbed when listening to recordings of their own grossly impaired speech.

Motor aphasia

Pure word dumbness

The patient understands spoken speech and writing and can respond to comments. Writing is preserved but speech is indistinct and cannot be produced at will. There is no local disturbance of muscles required in speaking, and the disability is an apraxia limited to movements required for speech.

Pure agraphia

An isolated inability to write may also occur with unimpaired speech (*agraphia without alexia*); there is normal understanding of written and spoken material. This is the equivalent for writing of pure word dumbness in speech.

Primary motor dysphasia

There is disturbance to the processes of selecting words, constructing sentences and expressing them. Speech and writing are both affected, and there is difficulty in carrying out complex instructions, even though understanding for both speech and writing may be preserved. The patient finds it difficult to choose and pronounce words, and speech is hesitant and slow; he recognizes his errors, tries to correct them and is clearly upset. Gesture may be used to replace verbal communication. Speech is attempted and recognized as spoken words, but words are omitted, sentences shortened and perseveration occurs.

Alexia with agraphia

Visual aspects of language are construed as being more complex than auditory, in that visual schemata are required – 'seeing the written word inside his head', *in addition* to auditory – 'hearing the words in one's head'. In alexia with agraphia, the patient is unable to read or write, but speaking and understanding speech are preserved. Alexia in this condition is similar to that of pure word blindness: the patient cannot understand words that are spelt out aloud, showing that he is effectively illiterate because of disturbance of the visual symbolism of language.

Isolated speech area

Impaired comprehension may occur with slow, hesitant speech in an abnormality in which it is assumed that the anatomical Wernicke's and Broca's areas and the connections between them are intact but connections from other parts of the cortex with this language system are disturbed. Two types, expressive and receptive, are described: *transcortical motor dysphasia* and *transcortical sensory dysphasia*.

Most frequently, of course, with dysphasia, there is a mixture of expressive and receptive elements and the clear syndromes cannot be demonstrated, but their significance is partly theoretical in demonstrating the range of anatomical lesions and the specificity of resultant symptoms. This description has been exclusively concerned with the symptoms; precise description of the anatomical lesions and of associated neurological symptoms is outside our scope. It is important to distinguish the phenomena of dysphasia, perhaps with neologisms and defects of syntax, from the *word salad* of schizophrenia with superficially similar defects of language. *Verbigeration* describes the repetition of words or syllables that expressive aphasic patients may use while desperately searching for the correct word.

Mutism

Mutism, refraining from speech during consciousness, is an important sign in psychiatric illness with an extensive differential diagnosis. Eliciting the history and mental state becomes impossible in a mute patient. All the major categories of psychiatric disorder may manifest mutism: learning disability, organic brain disease (sometimes drug-related), functional psychosis and neurosis and personality disorder. Some more specific causes include depressive illness, catatonic schizophrenia and dissociative disorder. Mutism occurs as an essential element of stupor (Chapter 3), and it is necessary to assess the level of consciousness as part of a full neurological examination for all patients with this sign. If there is no lowering of consciousness, as in functional psychoses and neuroses, it is likely that the mute patient will be understanding everything that is said around him. As well as specific brain disorders, the causes of stupor include general metabolic disorders that also affect the brain, such as hepatic failure, uraemia, hypothyroidism and hypoglycaemia.

SCHIZOPHRENIC LANGUAGE DISORDER

Defective communication in language is the defining characteristic of schizophrenia according to Crow (1997), and it is associated with genetic variation at the time language was acquired by *Homo sapiens*. The schizophrenic patient's use of language and words is different from a normal person's, and this difference is not just caused by delusional beliefs or the interruption of thinking caused by auditory hallucinations. However, the precise nature of this abnormality has so far defied clarification, and this account is provisional; it describes the way some of the phenomena have been viewed but cannot yet fit this into a single explanatory theory. Investigation into language disorder may be ascribed to one of the four models of Table 10.2.

Clinical description and thought disorder

The only unequivocal demonstration of disorder of thinking can be through language. Thought disorder may be revealed in the flow of talk (as in Chapter 9), disturbed content and use of words and grammar, and in the inability to conceptualize appropriately. Critchley (1964) considered that the 'causation of schizophrenic speech affection lies in an underlying thought disorder, rather than in a linguistic inaccessibility'. Some of the ways in which clinicians have categorized schizophrenic thought disorder manifesting in speech are linked in Table 10.3.

The German psychopathological literature on schizophrenic language and speech disorders was concerned with the rules of language dysfunction; it

Table 10.2 Models for investigating language disorder in schizophrenia

Model of language	Technique employed
Concept of thought disorder	Psychiatric: clinical description of schizophrenic speech
Behavioural learning theory	Word association test, multiple choice vocabulary test
Statistical model	The Cloze technique, type:token ratio
Linguistic model	Analysis of syntax, cohesion or propositions

(After Beveridge, 1985, with permission.)

Table 10.3 Categorization of thought disorder in speech	
Clinician	Categorization
Kraepelin	Akataphasia
Bleuler	Loosening of associations
Gardner	Form of regression
Cameron	Asyndesis
Goldstein	Concrete thinking
Von Domarus	Defect of deductive reasoning
Schneider	Derailment, substitution, omission, fusion and drivelling

consistently reported the schizophrenic patient's uncertainty in choosing the correct metaphorical level in communication (Mundt, 1995). Kraepelin (1919) defined *akataphasia* as a disorder in the expression of thought in speech. *Loss of the continuity of associations*, which implied incompleteness in the development of ideas, was the first of the simple functions included among the fundamental symptoms of schizophrenia by Bleuler (1911).

Gardner (1931) considered thought disorder to be a form of *regression*. Cameron (1944), in describing *asyndesis*, considered there to be an inability to preserve conceptual boundaries and a marked paucity of genuinely causal links. He gave the example of a patient who, given these alternatives, completed the sentence 'I get warm when I run because...' with *all* the words: 'quickness, blood, heart of deer, length, driven power, motorized cylinder, strength'. The patient was prone to use imprecise expressions – *metonyms* – and *over-inclusive thinking* because of interpenetration of associations.

Concrete thinking because of an inability to think abstractly was proposed by Goldstein (1944), but this has been challenged by Payne *et al.* (1959). Allen (1984) considers that speech-disordered schizophrenic patients produce evidence of concrete thinking, thinking without inferring and restricted to what is explicitly stated, while non-speech-disordered schizophrenics do not. When the thematic organization of speech was analysed for schizophrenic patients with positive speech disorder (incoherence of speech) or negative speech disorder (poverty of speech), there was no difference found: speech-disordered schizophrenics, positive as well as negative, showed cognitive restriction and produced fewer inferences than non-speech-disordered patients.

A deficiency in the logic of *deductive reasoning* in schizophrenia was suggested by Von Domarus (1944). Some of the abnormalities of thinking expressed in speech observed by Schneider have been discussed in Chapter 9.

An attempt has been made by Andreasen (1979) to classify description of patients' cognitive and linguistic behaviour on the phenomena demonstrated without making inferences for concepts of 'global' thought disorder; these abnormalities occur in both mania and schizophrenia. Some types of thought disorder, such as *neologism* and *blocking*, occurred too infrequently to have diagnostic significance. However, she found high reliability between raters with many types of thought disorder and also discrimination between different psychotic illnesses. Derailment, loss of goal, poverty of content of speech, tangentiality and illogicality were particularly characteristic of schizophrenia. *Derailment* implies loosening of association so that ideas slip on to either an obliquely related, or totally unrelated, theme. *Loss of goal* is the failure to follow a chain of thought through to its natural conclusion. *Poverty of content of speech* includes poverty of thought, empty speech, alogia, verbigeration and negative formal thought disorder; patients' statements convey little information and tend to be vague, over-abstract, over-concrete, repetitive and stereotyped. *Tangentiality* means replying to a question in an oblique or even irrelevant manner. *Illogicality* implies drawing conclusions from a premise by inference that cannot be seen as logical.

Misuse of words and phrases

The schizophrenic patient sometimes shows misuse of words in that he has, in the terminology of Kleist (1914), a defect of word storage. He has a restricted vocabulary and so uses words idiosyncratically to cover a greater range of meaning than they usually encompass. These are called *stock words or phrases*, and their use will sometimes become obvious in a longer conversation in which an unusual word or expression may be used several times. For example, a patient used 'dispassionate' as a stock word, and used it frequently with a bizarre and idiosyncratic meaning in the course of a few minutes' speech. A woman who was delusionally concerned that the police were intruding into her private affairs interspersed her conversation, often bizarrely, with the expression 'confidentially speaking'.

This abnormality appears partly to reflect a poverty of words and syntax and also an active tendency for words or syllables by association to *intrude* into thoughts, and therefore speech, soon after utterance. In the sample of speech in Chapter 9, the following words could be seen as stimuli and responses, by intrusion: 'means' – 'ways', 'opens' – 'closed', 'holding back the truth' – 'by no means will I speak', 'written questions – 'by means of writing', 'miracle' – 'Holyland'. They also appear to be stock words or phrases in that they are used with greater frequency and with a greater range of meaning than is normal and correct.

Words carry a *semantic halo*, that is, their constellation of associations is greater than just the dictionary meaning of the word. A boy aged 16 steals an apple. If I call him 'a trespasser', it has biblical associations; 'a criminal' suggests a greater degree of viciousness than the action merits; 'a delinquent' is readily associated with his youthfulness because of the phrase 'juvenile delinquent'. The constellations of associations in schizophrenic patients are disordered in that they often make apparently irrelevant associations. These may be explained by misperception of auditory stimuli with specific inattention; the actual mediation of associations in patients with schizophrenia may be similar to that in healthy people. This comes some way to explaining why the associations seem appropriate subjectively to the schizophrenic patient himself, as he does not realize that he has misperceived the cue: it seems reasonable to him but is quite irrelevant to the interviewer. To quote Maher, 'What seems to be bizarre is not the nature of the associations that intrude into the utterance, but the fact that they intrude at all' (p. 9).

Among the disorders of words, *neologism* is well recognized. This creation of a new word becomes necessary in schizophrenia to fill a semantic gap. A patient believed that his thoughts were influenced from outside himself by a process of 'telegony'. Although such a word does actually exist, the patient had no notion of this nor what it meant. He created the word to describe a unique experience of his for which no adequate word existed. A 47-year-old male patient with schizophrenia and expansive mood described himself thus: 'I am the triplicate actimetric kilophilic telepathic multibillion million genius' – which does suggest a certain grandiosity!

The unintentional puns of schizophrenia have been explained by Chapman *et al.* (1964). If a word has more than one meaning, it is likely that one usage is *dominant*. For example, the majority of people, in most contexts, would be more likely to use the word 'bay' to refer to an inlet of the sea than to a tree, the noise a hound makes, the colour of a horse, an opening in a wall, the second branch of a stag's horn, an uncomfortable place at which to stand or even, phonetically, a Turkish governor! There is a marked tendency in schizophrenia to show *intrusion* of the dominant meaning when the context demands the use of a less common meaning. Chapman *et al.* (1964) used a sentence such as 'the tennis player left the court because he was tired' and asked schizophrenic patients to interpret its meaning with one of three different explanations: one referring to a tennis court, one to a court of law and one altogether irrelevant. An analysis of responses shows that dominant meanings, here a court of law, intrude into the responses of schizophrenics quite frequently, but intrusion of minor meanings is less frequent.

Maher has described disorder of schizophrenic language in which intrusion occurs through *clang associations* with the initial syllable of a previous word: 'the subterfuge and the mistaken planned *sub*stitutions' (p. 13). This is unlike the clang associations that occur normally in poetry and in humour and also in manic speech, in which the *clang* occurs in terminal syllables. The repetitiveness of speech disorder is also thought to be associated with the intrusion of associations: the normal process of eliminating irrelevant associations does not take place, so that a word in a clause will provoke associations by pun, clang and ideational similarity. When that clause is completed, a syntactically correct clause may then be inserted, disrupting meaning but demonstrably associated with that previous word or idea.

Maher considers that an inability to maintain attention may account for the language disturbances seen in some schizophrenic patients. Disturbed attention allows irrelevant associations to intrude into speech, similar to the disturbance affecting the filtering of sensory input. In this theory, normal coherent speech is seen as the progressive and instantaneous inhibition of irrelevant associations to each utterance, and so the determining tendency proceeds with the active elimination of those associations that are not goal-directed.

Destruction of words and grammar

Alogia is a term used to describe negative thought disorder, or poverty of thoughts as expressed in words. Correspondingly, *paralogia* is used to describe positive thought disorder, or the intrusion of irrelevant or bizarre thought. *Paraphasia* (see p. 187) is a destruction of words with interpolation of more or less garbled sounds. Although the patient is only able to produce this non-verbal sound, it clearly has significance or meaning to him. *Literal paraphasia* is gross misuse of the meaning of words to such an extent that statements no longer make any sense. *Verbal paraphasia* describes the loss of the appropriate word but the statements are still meaningful, for example a patient described a chair as 'a four-legged sit-up'.

Disturbances in the words and their meanings are much more common in schizophrenia than disturbance of grammar and syntax. However, grammar is also sometimes altered; the loss of parts of speech is described as *agrammatism*. Adverbs are occasionally lost, resulting in coarsening and poverty of sentences, a form of *telegramese*. For example, 'rich table is worn; the woman is rich to write; son is also lamentation'. This, as well as showing *stock words* (rich – lamentation), shows loss of parts of speech, for example the indefinite article. The meaning is more disjointed than the grammar. *Paragrammatism* occurs when there are a mass of complicated clauses that makes no sense in achieving the goal of thought. However, the individual phrases are, in themselves, quite comprehensible.

It seems probable that the rules of syntax are preserved in schizophrenia long after a marked disturbance in the use of words, so that, if in the preceding sentence an intrusive association were to replace the word 'rules', the word used would probably, correctly, be a noun. For instance, the patient above might have said in this context 'the *lamentations* of syntax are...'

Psychogenic abnormalities

There is no specific abnormality of language in affective psychosis or the neurotic disorders. However, the prevalent mood influences the flow and choice of words in the former, and neurotic thinking is manifested in the latter, perhaps by greater emphasis in speech on the first person singular.

Manic speech has been analysed, and the speech and number of associations demonstrated in *flight of ideas* and *pressure of talk* is seen in the greater number of *cohesive links* occurring in manic speech. The content of depressive speech is, of course, influenced by the mood state, and so also is the choice of words. Sentences tend to be short and have fewer and simpler associations, with *retardation*.

Hysterical mutism may occur as an abnormal reaction to stress. A man aged 35 had been unable to tolerate the continual nagging from his wife and her two sisters who lived with them. One day, after heavy drinking the previous evening, he smashed his wife's furniture at home and then became mute for 24 hours. He was eventually referred from the accident and emergency department to the psychiatric ward, and speech returned gradually over the next 2 to 3 days without other treatment.

With the phenomenon of *approximate answers* (Chapters 5 and 15), the patient just avoids giving a correct answer to a simple question: 'How many legs has a sheep?' – 'Five'. This is, according to Anderson and Mallinson (1951), 'a false response to the examiner's question where the answer, although wrong, indicates that the question had been grasped'. This symptom may occur in a number of conditions, including hebephrenic schizophrenia (F20.1 in ICD-10; World Health Organization, 1992), in which it is often associated with fatuous mood; dissociative disorder, previously designated hysterical pseudodementia (before making such a diagnosis, the wise psychiatrist thoroughly excludes an organic cause); Ganser's syndrome; and other organic conditions.

Paraphasia is the production of an inappropriate sound in place of a word or phrase. It may be caused by an organic disturbance of speech but is closely mimicked in the situation in which the patient produces a sound, deliberately or unconsciously, to change the topic of conversation. This may be used to avoid a certain subject or because the patient is so preoccupied by internal or external experiences that other questions seem irrelevant.

Pseudologia fantastica is the condition of fluent plausible lying, often associated with histrionic or asocial personality disorders. The patient appears to believe in the fantastic statements. The characteristic picture is of a very isolated person, without family or friends, drifting into the accident and emergency department of a large hospital in a strange city late at night with stories of his own importance and exploits and the unfortunate vicissitudes these have engendered resulting in his need for help. There is considerable overlap with *Münchausen's syndrome* (factitious disorder; see Chapter 15).

Eccentric and pedantic use of words may sometimes be seen in those with *anankastic personality*; obsessionality obtrudes into the choice of words and construction of sentences.

Statistical model of language

The *Cloze* procedure involves deleting words from the transcripts of speech and assessing whether the omitted word can be predicted. Maher considered that, in schizophrenia, the greater the severity of the illness, the greater is the degree of unpredictability of the utterance of language. In normal speech, *a* large *part* of every sentence *could be* omitted without losing *the* meaning. For example, if the words 'a ... part ... could be ... the' were omitted from the last sentence, the meaning would still be obvious; if letters were omitted from words, for instance *nrml spech*, the meaning is still clear. *Predictability* is the ability to predict accurately the missing words; in this sense, schizophrenics are unpredictable in their speech. They are likely to use unexpected words and phrases. In the perception of language, the schizophrenic patient is less able to gain information from the redundancies, both semantic and syntactic, in everyday speech.

A sophistication of the *Cloze procedure* has been investigated by Newby (1998). This involves the following.

- The modified Cloze procedure, in which the nature of the inserted words is noted, such as its part of speech.
- In the reverse Cloze procedure, thought-disordered patients were asked to make sense of a script that had been mutilated by instituting the Cloze procedure, for example by deleting every fourth or fifth word. Patients with schizophrenia performed significantly worse than a control group of orthopaedic patients, with manic–depressive patients intermediate on both modified and reverse Cloze procedures.

Schizophrenic speech is considered less predictable than normal speech, and lack of predictability is more marked with clinically manifest thought disorder (Manschreck *et al.*, 1979). An experiment was carried out on the Cloze procedure, in which raters were asked to assess passages of schizophrenic or normal speech with the fourth or fifth word deleted. With fifth-word deletion, thought-disordered schizophrenic speech was significantly less predictable than normal or non-thought-disordered schizophrenic speech; this latter was no less predictable than normal speech.

Whether schizophrenic speech is really less redundant than normal has been questioned by Rutter (1979), who was able to demonstrate no difference. The view that schizophrenic language can be reduced to such simple mathematical rules has been rejected by Mandelbrot (1965).

The *type:token ratio* is a measure of the number of different words as compared with the total number of words (Zipf, 1935). Maher concluded that the type:token ratio of schizophrenics was lower than for normal subjects. The tendency of schizophrenic patients to repeat certain words and use them in an idiosyncratic way is referred to as the use of *stock words*.

Linguistic approaches to schizophrenia

Various linguistic theories have been applied to schizophrenia. These methods of analysis of schizophrenic language are tentative and do not yet cover the range of abnormalities occurring in the condition. Chomsky (1959) proposed that humans are able to use strings and combinations of words they have never heard before through use of a limited set of integrative processes and generalized patterns. However, Moore and Carling (1982) have labelled Chomskyan linguistics a *container* view of language, separated from the real way users of language apply it to their own meanings and contexts. Individual case studies have used tape-recorded interviews with patients with schizophrenia to demonstrate distinctive abnormalities. However, on closer analysis such abnormalities are often found to occur in the speech of normal people, although less frequently. A further study of bilingual patients showed psychotic symptoms to be present in their native language but absent in their second language. The problem of individual studies is, of course, the extent to which they can be generalized to all patients with schizophrenia.

Syntactical analysis

In two studies of speech analysed for syntax, compared with manic and normal controls patients with schizophrenia showed less complex speech, fewer well-formed sentences, more semantic and syntactic errors and less fluency. Such studies do not, of course, justify the conclusion that differences are due directly to the disease or to thought disorder, nor does it take into account the social context or emotional aspects. However, marked differences are of interest when one considers that the majority of patients with schizophrenia do not show overt disorder of language.

Cohesion analysis

A method of examination of schizophrenic speech has been developed by Rochester and Martin (1979) looking at the links between sentences that occur in discourse. These links are called *cohesive ties*. Schizophrenic patients use fewer of these cohesive ties, and of the five types of tie described they use fewer *reference* ties (connection through meaning) and more *lexical* ties (connected words). For instance, consider the following two sentences.

- 'A commuter and a skier are in a ski lift and *he* looks completely unconcerned.'
- 'Mother needed *independence* she was always *dependent* on my father.'

Sentence 1 shows an *unclear reference*, in that this person with schizophrenia fails to guide the listener as to whom he is describing. In sentence 2, *independence* and *dependent* are lexically tied because of similar derivation. This type of tie is a weaker bond between sentences, and the result of these abnormalities is that they make it more difficult for a listener to follow what the patient is meaning. However, even in the most severe group of schizophrenic speakers, 80 per cent of their speech was still normal. Studies with manic patients have shown more ties than for schizophrenics but also some disruption. Cohesion analysis does not explain all the abnormalities of schizophrenic speech; appropriate ties would still leave much material that is abnormal.

Propositional analysis

This is a form of textual analysis in which the text is broken down into its component propositions, and these are then represented diagrammatically to show the 'mental geometry' (Hoffman *et al.*, 1982). Normal speech is considered to proceed as in a single tree diagram with all branches leading from a single key proposition, but psychotic speech more often breaks the 'rules' of propositional relationships.

Observers, listening to the speech of schizophrenic patients, are often struck with its oddity and deviance. It has been considered by Chaika (1995) that this is not purely a deficit of syntax but more a phenomenon like severe and repeated slips of the tongue, in which the error is a lapse of executive control, a lapse of volition. It has been shown by Morice (1995) that with increasing complexity of syntax there is an increase in the number of errors in the speech of schizophrenic patients; speakers expressing very simple sentences made relatively few errors. One of his patients expressed this: 'and communicating ordinarily I can get lost in the chaos of the language'.

This finding was confirmed by Thomas and Leudar (1995) using the Hunt test, a written test in which subjects produce syntactically complex sentences from simple input phrases. Communication-disordered schizophrenic patients made more errors than non-communication-disordered schizophrenic patients or normal controls, and these errors were more likely to occur with more complex syntactic structures. The patients were therefore thought to have a discrete failure of language processing that was distinct from the more general cognitive disorders of the condition.

Although these methods are still experimental, the patient's use of language and syntax does enable a quantitative method of evaluating the mental state and subjective experience to be developed. Study of language disorder should be an area in which descriptive psychopathology can contribute to psychiatric research.

REFERENCES

Allen HA (1984) Positive and negative symptoms and the thematic organisation of schizophrenic speech. *British Journal of Psychiatry 144*, 611–17.

Anderson WE and Mallinson WP (1941) Psychogenic episodes in the course of major psychoses. *Journal of Mental Science 87*, 383–96.

Andreasen NC (1979) Thought, language and communication disorder. *Archives of General Psychiatry 36*, 1315–30.

Beveridge A (1985) *Language disorder in schizophrenia*. MPhil thesis, University of Edinburgh.

Bleuler E (1911) *Dementia Praecox: or the Group of Schizophrenias*. New York: International University Press.

Cameron N (1944) Experimental analysis of schizophrenic thinking. In Kasanin J (ed.) *Language and Thought in Schizophrenia*. Berkeley: University of California Press.

Carterette G and Friedman MP (1976) *Handbook of Perception Volume VII, Language and Speech*. New York: Academic Press.

Chaika E (1995) On analyzing schizophrenic speech: what model should we use? In Sims ACP (ed.) *Speech and Language Disorders in Psychiatry*. London: Gaskell.

Chapman LJ, Chapman JP and Miller GA (1964) A theory of verbal behaviour in schizophrenia. In Maher BA (ed.) *Progress in Experimental Personality Research*, vol. 1. New York: Academic Press.

Chomsky N (1959) Review of Skinner. *Language 35*, 26–58.

Chomsky N (1986) *Knowledge of Language: its Nature, Origin and Use*. New York: Praeger Publishers.

Critchley EMR (1995) Growth points in the neurology of speed and language. In Sims ACP (ed.) *Speech and Language Disorders in Psychiatry*. London: Gaskell.

Critchley M (1964) The neurology of psychotic speech. *British Journal of Psychiatry 110*, 353–64.

Crow TJ (1997) Is schizophrenia the price that *Homo sapiens* pays for language? *Schizophrenia Research 28*, 127–41.

Gardner GE (1931) The measurement of psychotic age: a preliminary report. *American Journal of Psychiatry 10*, 963–75.

Goldstein K (1944) Methodological approach to the study of schizophrenic thought disorder. In Kasanin JS (ed.) *Language and Thought in Schizophrenia*. Berkeley: University of California Press.

Hoffman RE, Kirstein L, Stopek S and Cicchetti DV (1982) Apprehending schizophrenic discourse: a structural analysis of the listener's task. *Brain and Language 15*, 207–33.

Jackson JH (1932) *Selected Writings of John Hughlings Jackson*. London: Hodder & Stoughton.

Kleist K (1914) Aphasie und Geisteskrankheit. *Munchener Medizinische Wochenschrift 61*, 8.

Kraepelin E (1919) *Dementia Praecox and Paraphasia* (transl. Barclay BM). Edinburgh: Livingstone.

Lishman WA (1997) *Organic Psychiatry: the Psychological Consequences of Cerebral Disorder*, 3rd edn. Oxford: Blackwell Scientific.

Maher BA (1972) The language of schizophrenia: a review and interpretation. *British Journal of Psychiatry 120*, 3–17.

Mandelbrot B (1965) Information theory and psycholinguistics. In Oldfield RC and Marchall JC (eds) (1968) *Language*. London: Penguin Books.

Manschreck TC, Maher BA, Rucklos ME and White MT (1979) The predictability of thought-disordered speech in schizophrenic patients. *British Journal of Psychiatry 134*, 595–601.

Moore T and Carling C (1982) *Understanding Language: Towards a Post-Chomskyan Linguistics*. London: Macmillan.

Morice R (1995) Language impairments and executive dysfunction in schizophrenia. In Sims ACP (ed.) *Speech and Language Disorders in Psychiatry*. London: Gaskell.

Mundt C (1995) Concepts of schizophrenic language disorder and reality assessment in German psychopathology. In Sims ACP (ed.) *Speech and Language Disorders in Psychiatry*. London: Gaskell.

Newby D (1998) 'Cloze' procedure refined and modified: 'modified Cloze', 'reverse Cloze' and the use of predictability as a measure of communication problems in psychosis. *British Journal of Psychiatry 172*, 136–41.

Newby DA (1995) Analysis of language: terminology and techniques. In Sims ACP (ed.) *Speech and Language Disorders in Psychiatry*. London: Gaskell.

Payne RW, Matussek P and George EI (1959) An experimental study of schizophrenic thought disorder. *Journal of Mental Science 105*, 627–52.

Pinker S (1994) *The Language Instinct*. London: Penguin Books.
Rochester S and Martin J (1979) *Crazy Talk. A Study of the Discourse of Schizophrenic Speakers*. New York: Plenum Press.
Rutter DR (1979) The reconstruction of schizophrenic speech. *British Journal of Psychiatry 134*, 356–9.
Scharfetter C (1980) *General Psychopathology: an Introduction*. Cambridge: Cambridge University Press.
Thomas P and Leudar I (1995) Syntactic processing and communication disorder in first onset schizophrenia. In Sims ACP (ed.) *Speech and Language Disorders in Psychiatry*. London: Gaskell.
Von Domarus E (1944) The specific laws of logic in schizophrenia. In Kasanin JS (ed.) *Language and Thought in Schizophrenia*. Berkeley: University of California Press.
World Health Organization (1992) *The ICD-10 Classification of Mental and Behavioural Disorders: Clinical Description and Diagnostic Guidelines*. Geneva: World Health Organization.
Zipf GK (1935) *The Psychobiology of Language*. Boston: Houghton Mifflin.

Disorder of Intellectual Performance

> "'Funny', said George. 'I used to have a hell of a lot of fun with 'im. Used to play jokes on 'im 'cause he was too dumb to take care of 'imself. But he was too dumb even to know he had a joke played on him. I had fun. Made me seem God damn smart alongside of him. Why, he'd do any damn thing I tol' him. If I tol' him to walk over a cliff, over he'd go. That wasn't so damn much fun after a while. He never got mad about it, neither. I've beat the hell outa him, and he coulda bust every bone in my body jus' with his han's, but he nevera lifted a finger against me'. George's voice was taking on the tone of confession. 'Tell you what made me stop that. One day a bunch of guys was standin' around on the Sacramento River. I was feelin' pretty smart. I turns to Lennie and says: "Jump in". An' he jumps. Couldn't swim a stroke. He damn near drowned before we could get him. An' he was so nice to me for pullin' him out. Clean forgot I told him to jump in. Well, I ain't done nothing like that no more'. *John Steinbeck (1937)*

WHAT IS INTELLIGENCE?

Intellectual performance is an absolute prerequisite for sociable functioning in all human activities. *Intelligence* is used in both everyday and technical conversation; everyone understands the word but finds it difficult to define, and it conveys various nuances of meaning for different people and in differing contexts. Binet, in introducing his method of measuring human abilities, considered that intelligence was a *general capacity* for judgement, comprehension and reasoning that could be manifest in many different ways (Binet and Simon, 1905). Other psychologists, such as Thurstone (1938), considered that intelligence comprises several specific abilities that are mutually independent, and a method was introduced for testing these separate *primary abilities*.

Thinking involves the use of rational, problem-solving mental activity: the application of intelligence. Defective intellect is found in learning disability (mental retardation, F70–79 in ICD-10, mental handicap, mental subnormality; World Health Organization, 1992) and in organic mental states, especially in the progressive intellectual impairment of dementia. A person's intelligence is his *permanent* capacity of psychic performance, 'the individual's totality of abilities, those instruments of performance and purpose available to him for adaptation to life' (Jaspers, 1959).

Perception, registration and retention of memory, mental alertness and physical health and adequate motor functions such as speech and writing are not the same as, but are all prerequisites for, the expression of intelligence. Thus sensory functioning, full consciousness and orientation, the capacity for attention and concentration all contribute. For intellectual performance, motivation, drive and the appropriate affective set are necessary. Different thought processes occur *as components of* intelligence, including apperception, abstraction, forming associations and combining them, judgement and logical deduction.

In dementia, there are defects in these qualities that directly and necessarily impair intellectual function. However, the defect is not fundamentally one of intelligence, which may have been normal or above average before the illness, but lies in *intellectual function*, with the sensory apparatus, with registration, with retention of memory or with the motor aspects of speech.

Lack of knowledge is not the same as low intelligence, although the two are often found together. Sometimes, quite a detailed range of knowledge in a small field of interest is compatible with below-average intelligence (*idiot savant*), and there have been notable examples of this with outstanding abilities for number and calculation, musical performance and three-dimensional draughtsmanship combined with severely impaired functional intelligence. On the contrary, those who come new to interviewing and assessing the mental state often expect much more general knowledge and information from those of *normal* intelligence than is actually possessed.

Similarly, memory impairment is not a *specific* deficiency of learning disability. What the individual understands can be remembered reasonably well, such as a threatening episode or a friendly person. On formal tests of memory, performance is likely to be impaired in parallel with other intellectual functions.

Since the concept of intelligence was defined by Binet, there has been argument as to whether intelligence is a unitary factor or a constellation of related abilities such as mathematical ability, verbal facility, quick grasp of situations, aptitude for abstract reasoning, a faculty for extracting the essential elements of a problem, a facility for turning events to one's own advantage and so on. What these skills and abilities have in common is the capacity of the person to think in a purposeful way so that he adapts to new elements in his environment. This adaptation and skill in learning could be applied equally to pearl diving or playing chess. Intelligence, then, implies the capacity to lead one's life, to cope with and to master the external environment. This is much broader than the score on a psychometric test.

General capacity for understanding and reasoning may be contrasted with *primary abilities*. These latter would include, according to Thurstone, verbal comprehension, word fluency, number, space, memory, perceptual speed and reasoning (Thurstone, 1938). However, there does seem to be a unitary general factor of intelligence (g), as proposed by Spearman (1927), in addition to these specific abilities.

Creativity is a different type of ability requiring *divergent* thinking, and this requires, to some extent, different tests for its measurement.

Inheritance and intelligence

From studies of different degrees of relationship, it is clear that genetic determinants are important for intelligence. However, the enormous significance of environmental factors is also of great importance, both subculturally, for instance in situations of social deprivation, and also transculturally, with differences between people of different ethnic groups and in different parts of the world. The mean correlation between the intelligence measurement as intelligence quotient (IQ) of parents and their biological children is 0.50; between identical twins, 0.90; and between parents and adopted children, 0.25. The influence of heredity is very strong, but even in these relationships the environment clearly also plays a considerable part.

There is also a hereditary basis for many of the specific causes of mental handicap (Heaton-Ward and Wiley, 1984), such as those conditions with chromosomal abnormalities and those related to individual genes. Chromosomal abnormalities include disorder of both autosomes, for instance Down's syndrome, which most commonly shows trisomy 21, and of the sex chromosomes, such as Klinefelter's syndrome (XXY), Turner's syndrome (XO; in this condition, mental retardation is rare) and others. Among abnormality of the genes associated with mental handicap, inheritance of the abnormal gene may be dominant, such as tuberous sclerosis (epiloia); recessive, such as microcephaly; or X-linked, such as some forms of hydrocephalus. Further consideration of the genetics of mental retardation is outside the scope of this book.

Measurement of intelligence

Examination for human ability includes *aptitude tests*, which ascertain the capacity to learn, and *achievement tests*, which measure skills, ability and knowledge already acquired. Tests of intelligence have demanded satisfactory levels of *validity*, that is, evidence that they are truly measuring the type of ability of interest to the tester, and *reliability*, that is, they are consistent over time and between raters.

Intelligence testing previously concentrated on the concept of *mental age* but now emphasizes the IQ. Tests such as the Wechsler Adult Intelligence Scale and the Wechsler Intelligence Scale for Children have both *verbal* and *performance* scales. Discrepancy between different abilities tested by these scales is of importance clinically: organic psychosyndromes tend to deplete *performance* score to a significantly greater extent than *verbal* score, as the former is more sensitive to deterioration through brain damage. The verbal scale is highly sensitive, and even the performance scale is to some extent influenced by sociocultural factors. The IQ remains relatively stable in healthy people after the age of 6 years. The British Ability Scales are also used quite widely for assessing intelligence and evaluating problems in children and adolescents (Elliott *et al.*, 1983). Psychologists are now very cautious in using the results of intelligence testing to predict future performance in life activities for the individual, although cohort data are reasonably accurate.

In addition to global assessment of the individual's intelligence, psychometry is useful in looking for specific defects in learning or intellectual grasp suggestive of localized lesions or, at a cruder level, discrepancy between verbal and performance abilities suggesting intellectual impairment due to a global organic process. O'Connor (1976) has discussed whether the intellectual failure in mental retardation is developed hierarchically, for example lack of language resulting in poor thinking and abstracting capacity. He considers that experimental evidence tends to support such theories but is too complex for straightforward interpretation.

IMPAIRED INTELLECTUAL PERFORMANCE

The broad categories of cause of impaired intellectual performance are shown in Table 11.1. Only with irreversible disturbance of brain structure or function is the impairment permanent. Other causes are potentially reversible, and it therefore becomes vitally important to distinguish them from mental retardation or dementia.

Congenital disturbance of cerebral structure and function

Mental retardation of any degree of severity will result in impaired social competence. Brain pathology is demonstrable in most of those with severe mental retardation and is associated with marked effects on memory, language and intellectual performance. The descriptive terms used for the degree of retardation have traditionally been linked to levels of the IQ, and these are summarized in Table 11.2. The diagnostic categories are not based entirely on measures of intelligence but also take account of social and other handicaps; this is especially true for milder degrees of retardation.

Table 11.1 Causes of impaired intellectual performance

Disturbance	Example(s)
Disturbance of cerebral structure or function: congenital or acquired	Mental handicap, dementia
Lack of sensory experience	Blindness, deafness, sensory deprivation
Disturbed contact with reality	Psychosis
Disturbance of affect impairing perception, attention and motivation	Depressive illness

Table 11.2 Mental retardation: ICD-10, F70 to F79

ICD no.	ICD title	Obsolete terms	Retardation range	IQ level
			Dull, normal	85–99
			Borderline	70–84
F70	Mild mental retardation	Feeble-minded, high-grade defect, mild mental subnormality, moron, mild oligophrenia	Mild	50–69
F71	Moderate mental retardation	Imbecile, moderate mental subnormalities, moderate oligophrenia	Moderate	35–49
F72	Severe mental retardation	Severe mental subnormality, severe oligophrenia	Severe	20–34
F73	Profound mental retardation	Idiocy, profound mental subnormality, profound oligophrenia	Profound	0–19

(After World Health Organization, 1992, with permission.)

Intellectual incapacity is the hallmark of mental retardation. However, many other psychiatric symptoms also occur when a person who is mentally retarded has in addition other psychiatric disorders; these are modified, especially in their expression, by the impairment in intelligence and consequent lack of verbal fluency. Psychiatric symptoms such as thought disorder, ideas and experiences of influence and passivity, hallucinations, delusions – especially of complex and systematized content, and ambivalence arising from complex unconsciousness conflict, when they occur at all, are straightforward and lacking in sophistication (Reid, 1982). Abnormalities of mood, such as elation, depression, anxiety and panic, are ascertainable over a broad range of intellectual impairment but are often poorly sustained and subject, in the presence of brain damage, to lability and excitability. With profound retardation, no psychiatric phenomena can be elicited. Abnormalities of behaviour such as hysterical conversion symptoms, self-injury of various types and repetitive acts such as echolalia and stereotypic rituals are relatively common with mild to moderate degrees of retardation. Impaired attention, concentration and memory, and also disorientation, are frequent. Many 'symptoms' that would be construed as evidence of psychiatric morbidity in those not handicapped do not have the same implications for those who are. One cannot rely on verbal descriptions for the presence of symptoms, and this makes accurate serial observations over time of behaviour, posture, gesture, facial expression, social expressiveness and level of activity relatively more important.

Current research does not support a relationship between mental retardation and attentional deficiency (Iarocci and Burack, 1998). *Attention* involves *selective attention*, with the components of filtering, visual orienting, integration and priming, and *sustained attention*. Filtering maximizes the focus on relevant information by minimizing interference from irrelevant information. Visual orienting facilitates the selection process by alerting to new information, helping to monitor surroundings and shifting from internal representation to external object. Integration involves responding to the relations among features rather than to the simple features of a visual image. Priming refers to the influence of prior processing of information on the performance of a new task with different processing demands.

The brain pathology of different syndromes may account for additional psychiatric symptoms. For example, in Down's syndrome there is greatly increased liability to presenile dementia of Alzheimer type; these patients are also more liable to develop affective disorders in adult life. There is no clear evidence that symptoms of schizophrenic or catatonic type are associated with specific forms of retardation. Epilepsy is especially common, occurring in up to 43 per cent of severely and profoundly retarded adults in hospital (Reid *et al.*, 1978), but this was not found to correlate with other behavioural symptoms.

Lack of experience

Lack of exposure to appropriate opportunities for learning will result in impaired intellectual performance (Casey and Bradley, 1982). This results from psychosocial or sensory deprivation. *Critical periods* are important for acquiring specific skills, and if learning has not taken place by the end of that period of time it may not be possible to obtain the skill later. Sensory handicaps for learning would include congenital deafness or blindness. In such situations, there is, of course, no intrinsic defect of intelligence, but some aspects of intellectual performance may be permanently restricted if the sensory defect is not corrected at an early stage or adequate early compensatory training given. This can account for impaired speech and use of language with congenital deafness.

The effect of psychosocial deprivation in lowering mean intellectual performance was demonstrated in the highly contentious issue of relative IQ levels of different ethnic groups in the same society. Children from a socially deprived group, when adopted into more privileged families, may show a 15-point higher mean IQ than children from their original social milieu (Scarr and Weinburg, 1976).

There is now a lot of evidence linking environmental factors, especially the harmful effects of social deprivation, with intelligence; enriched environments have been shown to overcome earlier handicap. For example, low and persistent impairment of intelligence was associated with abuse in 34 patients with *abuse dwarfism* (Money *et al.*, 1983). Relief from this situation resulted in gradual, progressive improvement in IQ over several years.

Acquired disturbance of cerebral structure and function

The clinical picture common to different causes of *dementia* is a progressive disintegration of intellect, memory and personality. From the practical aspect, it is important to distinguish *primary* dementias, which are progressive and untreatable, from those that are *secondary* to some other disease process and may therefore be treatable, at least to the extent of arresting further deterioration (for example hypothyroidism, frontal meningioma). It is usually impossible to diagnose the cause of dementia from signs and symptoms, although there are varying rates in the speed of onset and the pattern of progression of symptoms.

Most commonly, the onset of dementia is insidious, with gradual impairment of memory or other deterioration of intelligence. A previously punctual, efficient and tidy man in his late fifties started arriving late for appointments. He created muddles in his work, became forgetful of current details at home and began to look dishevelled in dress. Occasionally, of course, dementia may be sudden, for instance following unconsciousness from head injury or brain surgery. Deterioration of personality may be the presenting feature, with quite unexpected social blunders from a person of previously impeccable rectitude, for instance an elderly politician who, quite out of character, made a risqué remark to a younger colleague's wife. Sometimes, depressive symptoms are the first noticeable sign superimposed on an intellectual deterioration that is already quite extensive. On occasions, domestic or social circumstances such as the death of the patient's spouse, by giving access to the home to the doctor or social worker, reveal the patient's severely impaired intellectual function.

The intellectual deterioration of dementia is shown in loss of interest in work or hobbies, inability to make decisions, loss of application to the current task, incapacity for persistence and loss of intellectual grasp in complex social situations. Attention and concentration are impaired, and there is a poverty of associations of thought with inability to produce new ideas; the patient is distractible and tires easily. He may react to the challenges of the outside world by keeping rigidly to an absolutely fixed routine of life (*organic over-orderliness*), by reducing his range of activities (*shrinkage of the milieu*) or even by an explosion of anger or acute intense anxiety (*catastrophic reaction*).

Intellectual flexibility is lost, with difficulty in shifting from one frame of reference to another (Lishman, 1997). As there is no capacity to change frames, the subject is limited to responding to the most immediate and recent stimulus. He is unable to grasp the essentials of an argument or situation and cannot exclude from his consideration the inessentials: he is submerged by the detail of circumstances. *Concretization* takes place, in that abstract ideas are interpreted in a concrete way. Judgement is often faulty, and there is limited insight into the nature of his own illness.

Disturbed contact with reality

Liddle (2001) describes three syndromes in schizophrenia: reality distortion, disorganization and psychomotor poverty. Each of these syndromes is associated with cognitive deficits. Reality distortion is specifically associated with impairment of internal monitoring, whereas disorganization is associated with impairments on tasks such as the Stroop test and the choice reaction time. These abnormalities are often present even when there is apparent symptomatic recovery. There is also evidence that there is marked impairment of intellectual function at the outset of schizophrenia. Intellectual function also deteriorates over time, with more marked changes in non-verbal intelligence (Morrison *et al.*, 2006). It is clear that similar neurocognitive deficits are associated with bipolar disorders whether or not symptomatic recovery is apparent (Depp *et al.*, 2007; Green, 2006).

Disturbance of affect

Disturbance of affect may impair perception, attention and motivation and thereby result in apparent deterioration of intellectual performance. This is exemplified by depressive illness. Depressed patients who have previously undergone psychometry, for instance with the Wechsler Adult Intelligence Scale, even though able to give answers on testing may show considerable diminution of score, with marked retardation in completing tasks. On recovery, there is a full return to premorbid intellectual performance. Depressive disorders are difficult to diagnose in those with learning disability (mental retardation), especially with severe or profound disability (Stavrakaki, 1999), and symptoms of irritability, psychomotor agitation, increased behavioural problems and, rarely, loss of adaptive behaviour may reveal underlying depression.

The quality of intellectual appraisal may be substantially altered by disorder of mood, in that disturbed mood may impair the ability to interpret situations. The effect of maternal depression on the cognitive development of the child is an important facet of the association between mood and intelligence. For instance, in a study of 94 women with their first-born children, cognitive functioning of the children was carried out at the age of 4 years (Cogill *et al.*, 1986). Significantly, intellectual deficits were found in those children whose mothers had suffered with depression in the child's first year; marital conflict and a history of psychiatric problems in the father were also linked with lower test scores.

SUBJECTIVE FEELING OF INCAPACITY WITH IMPAIRED INTELLECT

Simply asking someone with learning disabilities to describe his internal subjective cognitive and affective state is even less likely to produce a meaningful response than asking a person of average intelligence. However, there are a number of areas that can be explored with a view to subsequent treatment (Hollins and Sinason, 2000). These include *attachment* to others in the person's domestic environment and the emotional implications of *dependence* and *disability*, *sexuality* and *mortality*. To elicit problems in these sensitive areas, for which the patient may have little language, requires training and considerable skill (Fraser, 1997). The more the emotional life of those with learning disability is explored, the more is revealed.

Subjective feeling has to be inferred obliquely, and it becomes especially apparent through relationships. Understanding is most likely to occur between people who are like-minded, and this includes the approximation of their intellectual capacity or, to quote Proust (1919):

> Save in the case of a few illiterates – high or low, it makes no matter – by whom no difference in quality is perceptible, what brings men together is not a community of views but a consanguinity of minds.

When this process of empathic understanding between two people is inhibited by the presence of mental retardation in one of them, assessment of morbidity becomes more difficult; even dysthymia is rarely reported in mentally handicapped people (Jancar and Gunaratne, 1994). Exploration of psychological processes implies enquiring about the inner world of the mentally retarded person, including his self-concepts and experience of relationship (Bicknell, 1994).

Affect may be distorted, concealed or diminished in its expressions; it would be wrong to assume that it is also not experienced to the same degree. An autistic patient who has good language skills described feelings and the experience of relationships as follows: 'For me, the people I liked *were* their things, and those things (or things like them) were my protection from the things I didn't like – other people' (Williams, 1992).

A feeling of competence in their capacity for performing their normal activities is developed in people successful in any sphere. They form an accurate assessment of what is within their capability to achieve and can gauge what is outside it; they attempt and achieve the possible and rarely have accidents or failures. The feeling of capacity forms a customary association with normal behaviour in the same way that feelings of familiarity invest the objects of perception. The ordinary events and circumstances of each day are tackled with the sense that it will be possible to deal with them. Placed in an entirely new situation, for example a new job in a different town, a person who is normally confident and competent may become anxious, slow and indecisive. His gradual return to efficient action is based on familiarity with the new circumstances, memory of previous coping and the ability to form problem-solving associations. It is characteristic of mental retardation that there is a subjective lack of this feeling of capacity.

What does it feel like to be less capable than normal? What is the phenomenology of mental retardation? There can be no direct answer to these questions, as the person so afflicted does not usually have the words to express himself and he has no experience of normal competence with which to compare his state. However, those who do have language show evidence of a need for esteem and self-esteem, for example the frequent defence by one patient that she is 'high grade' (Kirman and Bicknell, 1975).

Since greater attention has been paid to the feelings and aspirations of learning-disabled people, it has become possible to begin to answer these questions by reading dictated transcripts of autobiographical accounts. A moving and illuminating example is to be found in Craft *et al.* (1985); this is the personal account of Stephen, with a severe mental handicap. He describes his activities, his friends and what he likes. He does not introspect, but he gives a clear impression of emotional and volitional state.

In her thought-provoking account of conducting psychotherapy with mentally handicapped individuals, Sinason (1992) develops the concept of *stupidity* as applied by one individual to another or the victim to himself. What does it do for the individual's self-esteem at the time, and how does it affect his subsequent self-concept and pattern of behaviour to be told, and know that it is true, that one is stupid? And what if this happens not once, but repeatedly, and not by one person, but by everyone?

Sinason deals with the euphemisms of mental retardation, how this human group has been forced to change its name so frequently: 'Embedded in euphemisms are psycholinguistic signs, as to what evokes anxiety, guilty wishes and terror in any society'. So many different areas of the handicapped person can, in fact, reveal the internal subjective state to a sensitive observer. For example, there is a subtle, moral pressure on disabled people, whatever their current emotional state, to smile.

> “Someone afflicted with mental or physical pain has less reason to smile or feel happy than the rest of the population and yet there is a tremendous pressure to insist on signs of pleasure precisely because of that. 'I try to keep him happy', said the mother about her multiply handicapped son. 'Because I brought him into the world with all his difficulties, so if I can't keep him happy what is the point?' Guilt that people exist who have to bear unfair and appalling emotional, physical or mental burdens can be so unbearable that a state of demand is brought about where those in greatest pain are asked to be the happiest. *(Sinason, 1992)*

The subject does not have the ability to analyse his feelings and their causes. Timidity and withdrawal are characteristic of many people with mental retardation; this timidity often alternates with heedless boldness. He is shy with new people and frightened of new experiences, even of ordinary childhood activities like going on a swing or sharing a room with a kitten. At the same time, he is fearless to a reckless extent in other areas of life, for instance playing with bonfires or near busy roads. Both abnormalities of behaviour, timidity and recklessness, can rise from defect in the feeling of capacity.

The combination of unthinking recklessness, lack of awareness of the significance of danger and an inability to devise strategies to reduce risk puts the individual with learning disability in positions of personal physical peril. A young man walked for 12 miles along country roads after leaving his residential home in a bad temper during the night. He was run over by a passing car whose driver had not seen him, and severely injured. When asked later what one should do when one hears a car when walking in the road, he said, 'shout for help'. He did not volunteer any more effective ways of saving himself.

A number of other aspects of attitude and behaviour in mental retardation are associated with this lack of feeling of capacity for normal activities. There is a fear of change, and uncertainty, which may manifest itself in apparent obsessional tidiness. It is, of course, not obsessional in a phenomenological sense of the word, in that there is no resistance. The person demands the curtains be drawn to exactly the same place; he insists on sitting in the same chair; he gets very anxious if members of the family are away from home; he intensely dislikes weeks with bank holidays, when the routine of his daily activities is disturbed; if the traffic system is changed, he may be involved in an accident because he insists on walking along the road in the way he always has.

The concept of mental age is fallacious, because the learning-disabled person does not function like an inquisitive but inexperienced child. His regressed and childlike behaviour, for example sucking his thumb at the age of 12, is not so much a manifestation of infancy as expressing overtly, and without awareness of the social context, the sort of occasional regressive feeling any 12-year-old might experience but would not reveal in public. The normal 12-year-old would usually conceal the wish to regress in behaviour for social reasons; his intellectual grasp of his environment and the social reinforcement he receives from his peers all prevent him from expressing regressive childish behaviour. There is now more attention paid to the subjective experience of those who are handicapped, and there is still a great need for better use of psychopathology and quantified ways of structuring this, as psychiatric disorder is increasingly recognized in those with learning disability, especially mood disorder, schizophrenia and anxiety disorders (Dõsen and Day, 2001). This is likely to result in improvements in the quality of life of these vulnerable people.

REFERENCES

Bicknell J (1994) Psychological process: the inner world of people with mental retardation. In Bouras N (ed.) *Mental Health in Mental Retardation: Recent Advances and Practices*. Cambridge: Cambridge University Press.

Binet A and Simon T (1905) New methods for the diagnosis of the intellectual level of subnormals. *Annals of Psychology 11*, 91.

Casey PH and Bradley RH (1982) The impact of the home environment on children's development: clinical relevance for the pediatrician. *Journal of Developmental and Behavioural Pediatrics 3*, 146–52.

Cogill SR, Caplan HL, Alexandra H, Robson KM and Kumar R (1986) Impact of maternal postnatal depression on cognitive development of young children. *British Medical Journal 292*, 1165–7.

Craft M, Bicknell J and Hollins S (1985) *Mental Handicap: a Multidisciplinary Approach*, p. 5. London: Baillière Tindall.

Depp CA, Moore DJ, Sitzer D, *et al.* (2007) Neurocognitive impairment in middle-aged and older adults with bipolar disorder: comparison to schizophrenia and normal comparison subjects. *Journal of Affective Disorder 101*, 201–9.

Dõsen A and Day K (2001) *Treating Mental Illness and Behavior Disorders in Children and Adults with Mental Retardation*. Washington: American Psychiatric Press.

Elliott CD, Murray DH and Pearson LS (1983) *The British Ability Scales (Revised)*. Windsor: NFER–Nelson.

Fraser W (1997) Communicating with people with learning disabilities. In Russell O (ed.) *The Psychiatry of Learning Disabilities*. London: Gaskell.

Green MF (2006) Cognitive impaiment and functional outcome in schizophrenia and bipolar disorder. *Journal of Clinical Psychiatry 67*, e12.

Heaton-Ward WA and Wiley Y (1984) *Mental Handicap*, 5th edn. Bristol: John Wright.

Hollins SA and Sinason V (2000) Psychotherapy, learning disabilities and trauma: new perspectives. *British Journal of Psychiatry 176*, 12–36.

Iarocci G and Burack JA (1998) Understanding the development of attention in persons with mental retardation: challenging the myths. In Burack JA, Hodapp RM and Zigler E (eds) *Handbook of Mental Retardation and Development*. Cambridge: Cambridge University Press.

Jancar J and Gunaratne J (1994) Dysthymia and mental handicap. *British Journal of Psychiatry 164*, 691–3.

Jaspers K (1959) *General Psychopathology*, 7th edn. (transl. Hoenig J and Hamilton MW, 1963). Manchester: Manchester University Press.

Kirman B and Bicknell S (1975) *Mental Handicap*. Edinburgh: Churchill Livingstone.

Liddle PF (2001) *Disordered Mind and Brain: the Neural Basis of Mental Symptoms*. London: Gaskell.

Lishman WA (1997) *Organic Psychiatry: the Psychological Consequences of Cerebral Disorder*, 3rd edn. Oxford: Blackwell.

Money J, Annecillo C and Kelley JF (1983) Growth of intelligence: failure and catchup associated respectively with abuse and rescue in the syndrome of abuse dwarfism. *Psychoneuroendocrinology 8*, 309–19.

Morrison G, O'Carroll R and McCreadie R (2006) Long term course of cognitive impairment in schizophrenia. *British Journal of Psychiatry 189*, 556–7.

O'Connor N (1976) The psychopathology of cognitive deficit. *British Journal of Psychiatry 128*, 36–43.

Proust M (1919) *Within a Budding Grove* (transl. Scott Moncrief CK and Martin T, 1981). Harmondsworth: Penguin.

Reid AH (1982) *The Psychiatry of Mental Handicap*. Oxford: Blackwell Scientific.

Reid AH, Ballinger BR and Heather BB (1978) Behavioural syndromes identified by cluster analysis in a sample of 100 severely and profoundly retarded adults. *Psychological Medicine 8*, 399–412.

Scarr S and Weinburg RA (1976) IQ test performance of black children adopted by white families. *American Psychologist 31*, 726–39.

Sinason V (1992) *Mental Handicaps and the Human Condition: New Approaches from the Tavistock*. London: Free Association Books.

Spearman CE (1927) *The Abilities of Man: Their Nature and Measurement*. London: Macmillan.

Stavrakaki C (1999) Depression, anxiety and adjustment disorders in people with developmental disabilities. In Bouras N (ed.) *Psychiatric and Behavioural Disorders in Developmental Disability and Mental Retardation*. Cambridge: Cambridge University Press.

Steinbeck J (1937) *Of Mice and Men*. London: Penguin.

Thurstone LL (1938) *Primary Mental Abilities. Psychometric Monographs No. 1*. Chicago: University of Chicago Press.

Williams D (1992) *Nobody Nowhere*, p. 5. London: Doubleday.

World Health Organization (1992) *The ICD-10 Classification of Mental and Behavioural Disorders: Clinical Description and Diagnostic Guidelines*. Geneva: World Health Organization.

Insight

12

> “A man who knows who and what he is, his position in the world, and what the persons and things are around him; who judges according to known, or intelligible rules; and who, if he has singular ideas or singular habits, can give a reason for his opinions and his conduct; a man who, however wrong he may act, is not misled by any uncontrollable impulse or passion; who does not idly squander his means; who knows the legal consequences of his actions; who can distinguish between unseemly and seemly behaviour, who feels that which is proper and that which is improper to utter, according to the circumstances in which he is placed; and who reverences the subject and the ministers of religion; a man who, if he cannot always regulate his thoughts and his temper and his actions, is not continually in the extremes, and if he errs, errs as much from benevolence and hesitation, as from passion and excitement, and more frequently: lastly, a man who can receive reproof, and acknowledge when he has needed correction. *John Perceval (1803–1876),* A narrative of the treatment experienced by a gentleman during a period of mental derangement

The concept of *insight* is much larger than just knowing whether one is ill or not, and if so, having a sensible view regarding treatment. Insight is a profoundly significant human capacity for mental ‘seeing’, seeing with the ‘mind’s eye’, glimpsing what is going on below the surface and also in the minds of other people about us. It involves our capacities for introspection, empathy and communication; not only is it glimpsing ourselves as we really are but also ourselves as others see us, and therefore others as they really are because they go through the same repertoire of mental mechanisms that we do. Even for the most private and internal of insights, social sense, the capacity for relationships, empathy, knowing how our behaviour will affect the emotions and experience of other people is important. Insight is the direct product of knowing ourselves. It is a quality that has been highly valued by most mental health clinicians because a strong link is assumed between having insight and better quality of life (McGorry and McConville, 1999).

Although, in psychiatry, we concentrate mostly on the narrow meaning of insight with regard to mental illness, we need to retain this broader concept. Often, our work with patients involves us having insight into their thinking and behaviour because of our capacity for empathy as fellow human beings and also helping them gain insight into themselves and the roots of their problems.

The relationship between this capacity for insight in a general sense and the practical issues of treatment is very close. A physician suffering from delusional disorder advertised and sold magnets for the medical treatment of arthritis and hay fever. He strongly believed that this form of treatment was of unequalled value for virtually all medical conditions, and he had physically assaulted a pharmacist who had tried to persuade him otherwise. He decried the validity of the whole of psychiatry, 'because I am a scientist and everything has to be proved with evidence'. Because of his lack of insight into his own condition and the nature of his beliefs, it was impossible to initiate treatment. His symptoms persisted long term.

Jaspers (1959) has written about the patient's attitude to his illness under the following headings.

1. Understandable attitudes to the sudden onset of acute psychosis (perplexity, awareness of change).
2. Working through the effects of acute psychoses.
3. Working through the illness in chronic states.
4. The patient's judgement of his illness.
5. The determination to fall ill.
6. The attitude to one's own illness: its meaning and possible implications.

All these points above, and especially 3, 4 and 6, involve the process of insight, the knowledge of oneself with particular reference to illness. A person who becomes seriously and suddenly ill, whatever the nature of the illness, after previously having been unusually fit for many years, is astonished by his change of health status. Such a person is likely to undergo a profound change in self- and body image, from a person who regarded himself as extremely healthy and illness as something that happens to other people to a self who is potentially frail and vulnerable. This can be personally enriching and is not necessarily a wholly negative experience.

INSIGHT IN CLINICAL PRACTICE

So that she can better help her patient with a possible mental illness, the psychiatrist asks specific questions about the patient's opinions concerning his illness. These include his degree of acknowledgement of illness, his attitudes to illness, his understanding of the effects of his illness on his current capabilities and future prospects. All this adds up to the assessment of *insight* into his condition. Insight is not an absolute; it can vary in its impairment with different facets of the condition, for example some limited understanding concerning his unlikelihood to obtain a job compatible with his qualifications but virtually no understanding as to how his psychotic symptoms interfere with relationships. Thus insight is not now considered to be an all-or-none phenomenon, in either clinical evaluation or measurement, but rather a dimensional one, so that subjects can have different levels of awareness into their illness (Surguladze and David, 1999).

All mental illnesses will alter the patient's world view and capacity to cope with circumstances. Assessment of insight measures the awareness of this change by the patient and his ability to adapt to the change. Insight is highly complex as a function. It is the understanding of the individual about his own state of health, capacity and worth; it also relates this assessment of internal state to other people and the world outside. In other words, insight requires both inner and outer orientation. This aspect of insight becomes more apparent, below, in the discussion about the contribution of gestalt psychology to the conceptualization of insight. Insight in gestalt psychology is oriented towards problem solving in the external world, whereas insight in clinical practice is inner-directed.

David (1990) has considered that insight 'is not an "all-or-nothing" phenomenon but is composed of three distinct, overlapping dimensions', namely, the recognition of morbid psychological change, the labelling of this change as deriving from mental illness and the understanding that this change requires treatment that needs to be complied with (p. 798). An assessment schedule was constructed for determining the nature of insight, and quantitative loss of insight correlated with the degree of psychopathology (David *et al.*, 1992).

One of the most frustrating aspects of practising psychiatry is, from the point of view of the treating professional, the apparent inability of patients to recognize that they are mentally ill. Patients, especially those with schizophrenia, often deny that their experiences are abnormal and that they are unwell. The resulting refusal to cooperate with treatment and rehabilitation causes long-term suffering for the patients and their carers. It is this capacity of patients to understand their own illness that is evaluated clinically in *insight*. Like many other concepts, terminological confusion exists, with textbooks describing insight as the patient's capacity to form judgements about their own illness and mental state. In recent years, there has been a resurgence of interest in the concept, with attempts to define it reliably and quantifiably and to study its correlates (Kumar and Sims, 1998).

OVERVIEW OF THE CONCEPT

The attitude of the patient towards his illness has obvious clinical implications, and insight tries to assess the awareness of the patient concerning the impact his illness has had on his life and his capacity to adapt to the changes brought about by the illness. As a function, it is highly complex and has to do with an individual's evaluation of his self and non-self and their relatedness (see Chapter 13). In clinical practice, only certain aspects are given importance, such as the patient's awareness of illness and compliance with prescribed treatment. The assessment of insight assumes more importance in psychosis, as the incongruence between the patient's and others' view of his illness often leads to difficulties with treatment. The convention in psychiatry is that insight is unimpaired in non-psychotic conditions, but it can be seen that a broader view nearer to the lexical definition is relevant when neurotic symptoms hamper the full realization of a person's potential.

Development of the concept

Contributions to the development of the concept of insight derive from psychopathology, gestalt psychology and psychoanalysis. In gestalt psychology, insight is conceived as a sudden, unexpected solution to a problem. According to Markova (2005), the 'suddenness' specifies an abrupt solution to a problem, the 'unexpectedness' refers to the surprise element of the event and the term 'solution to a problem' signals the discreteness of the event in time. In essence, in gestalt psychology, insight is by definition related to a specific task, a problem that stands in need of solution in the external world. Furthermore, there has been extensive debate within gestalt psychology about the nature of insight, whether it is a unique human facility that is also a specific cognitive skill. The fact that in gestalt psychology insight refers to a problem in the external world distinguishes it from the concept of insight in clinical practice. In clinical practice, insight focuses on understanding of changes or happenings within an individual.

For Jaspers (1959), typically the patient's attitude to his illness involves 'an awareness of illness' in which the patient 'expresses a feeling of being ill and changed, but there is no extension of this awareness to all his symptoms nor to the illness as a whole. It does not involve any objectively correct estimate of the severity of the illness nor any objectively correct judgement of its particular type'. For Jaspers, 'only when all this is present and there has been a correct judgement of all the symptoms and the illness as a whole according to type and severity, can we speak of *insight* [emphasis in original]'. Thus, for Jaspers insight becomes manifest only when the patient is able to turn away from the content of his psychic experiences towards making a judgement about it and inquiring into its causes and reasons. Lewis' (1934) definition of insight as 'a correct attitude to morbid change in oneself' (p. 333) is a restatement of Jaspers' description of insight. Freud (1981) used the term *insight* to denote knowledge of illness but, on the whole, in psychoanalytic therapy the development of a deeper awareness of self is considered to be the goal of treatment. This is another way of saying that in psychoanalysis insight refers to knowledge and understanding of one's unconscious mental processes. This is a more complex notion of insight, because it involves the patient acquiring understanding of the unconscious motivations of his behaviour and, in the light of Freud's structure of the mind, it suggests a degree of depth of understanding.

David (1990) has proposed that insight is composed of the three overlapping dimensions described above. It has been suggested that parallels can be drawn between the loss of insight in psychiatric patients and the loss of awareness of disease of parts of the body in certain neurological conditions. In cortical blindness, left-sided hemiplegia following stroke and amnesic syndrome, lack of awareness of disease is well recognized. The term *anosognosia* was coined by Babinski (1857–1932) to refer to the unawareness or denial of hemiplegia seen in patients following a stroke. There is a difference, though, between the lack of insight seen in psychiatry and the lack of awareness seen in neurological disease. In psychiatry, lack of insight is often attended by a wider loss of judgement beyond merely the symptoms or their implications for the patient. In neurological cases, the lack of awareness is focused on a discrete disability. Nonetheless, even though the lack of insight in psychiatry and lack of awareness of disease in neurology are not identical, it may be that comparisons may point to possible neurobiological bases that they share in common.

There are certain philosophical problems when we consider insight in patients with psychosis. People without any psychiatric illness vary in their ability to know themselves and the consequences of their personalities. Because at least some conceptualizations of psychosis rely on the lack of insight as a defining feature, discussion concerning the concept can become circular. Added to this is the fact that varying degrees of insight can occur and that non-verbalization of insight may be different from the lack of it. Yet another problem is that a possibly specious model in which a 'normal' part of the mind is capable of passing judgement on the 'abnormality' of another part has to be accepted.

Measurement of insight

Earlier attempts to measure insight centred on its role in psychodynamic therapies. Tolor and Reznikoff (1960) developed a test using hypothetical situations based on common defence mechanisms and found a correlation with intelligence. This test was used by Roback and Abramowitz (1979), who found a correlation in those with schizophrenia between greater subjective distress and better behavioural adjustment. The validity of this test, for general clinical work, is affected by the concept of insight being based on psychodynamic rather than psychopathological features.

Any reliable and valid measure of insight in clinical practice should be based on the following four assumptions:

- insight is complex and multidimensional
- cultural factors need to be taken into account
- the level of insight can vary across the many manifestations of mental illnesses
- information about the nature of a person's illness from situations other than the interview should be taken into account (McGorry and McConville, 1999).

McEvoy *et al.* (1989a) developed a questionnaire to measure insight, defined as the patient's awareness of the pathological nature of his experiences and also his agreement with the treating professionals about the need for treatment. The Insight and Treatment Attitudes Questionnaire (ITAQ) is a validated 11-item, semistructured interview that generates a score from 0 (no insight) to 22 (maximum insight). Using this questionnaire, they found no correlation with aspects of acute psychopathology.

The Schedule for Assessment of Insight in Psychosis was published in 1992 (David *et al.*), in which, apart from the recognition of mental illness and compliance with treatment, the ability to relabel unusual mental events as pathological was also included. There were seven items with a maximum possible score of 14 and an additional item on hypothetical contradiction.

The Scale to Assess Unawareness of Mental Disorder (Amador and Strauss, 1993) is a much more comprehensive scale with six general items and four subscales, from which 10 summary scores can be calculated. Other scales available are the Global Insight Scale (Greenfield *et al.*, 1989) and the self-reported Insight Scale for Psychosis (Birchwood *et al.*, 1994). The scale by Markova and Berrios (1991) is more directed to evaluate aspects of self-awareness and less to clinical definition of insight with regard to illness.

Other approaches have been to use the 'lack of insight and judgement' item of the Positive and Negative Syndrome Scale (PANSS; Kay *et al.*, 1987) as a single global measure of insight, and the use of psychopathology vignettes. McEvoy *et al.* (1993) used vignettes that cast specific psychopathological features in everyday language to judge whether patients demonstrated these features and the degree to which they attributed them to mental illness. They found that patients failed to acknowledge negative symptoms and failed to view positive symptoms as evidence of mental illness.

From earlier impressionistic assessments of a global nature, measurement of insight has more recently progressed to the use of operationalized definitions and standardized instruments. Although the different instruments might be measuring different aspects of a complex phenomenon, there is at least the freedom to choose one to suit specific clinical or research aims. There is an inverse correlation between insight, the severity of psychopathology and positive affective disturbance (Sanz *et al.*, 1998).

Schizophrenia

It is not really surprising that most of the research work on the clinical correlates of insight has been on patients with schizophrenia. McEvoy *et al.* (1989a) reported that insight as measured by the ITAQ did not correlate with either the severity of acute psychopathology or the changes in psychopathology with treatment. They speculated whether the mechanisms underlying the production of positive symptoms and disturbed insight were independent and whether the latter was more resistant to the effective use of neuroleptic medication. David *et al.* (1992) found that the 'total insight score' in their study had a moderate inverse correlation with the Present State Examination (Wing *et al.*, 1974) total score, which was an indication of the global severity of the illness. Both David *et al.* (1992) and McEvoy *et al.* (1989b) found that, as a group, involuntary (that is compulsorily admitted) patients have less insight. Overall, it does appear that the relationship between poor insight and aspects of psychopathology is not linear but complicated by other factors, including compliance with treatment.

INSIGHT AND COGNITIVE IMPAIRMENT

It has often been speculated that poor insight may have a neurological basis. Lysaker and Bell (1994) found that subjects with impaired insight performed more poorly than subjects with unimpaired insight on the Wisconsin Card Sorting Test (WCST). They used the PANSS item of 'lack of insight and judgement' to measure insight. This item had been shown by factor analytic studies to be a member of the component composed of symptoms of cognitive impairment such as cognitive disorganization, poor attention, stereotyped thinking and poor abstract thinking. However, using a different methodology, Kemp and David (1996) failed to show a relationship between insight and neuropsychological deficits. It is possible that chronicity of the illness could be an additional variable, which predisposes to cognitive impairment. David *et al.* (1992) had found a relationship between aspects of insight and intellectual performance. Cuesta *et al.* (1995) failed to show any relationship between insight and poor performance on the WCST. However, the study did not use any of the standard rating scales to measure insight. In another study, Upthegrove *et al.* (2002) showed that impaired digit span as a measure of working memory was significantly associated with insight as measured by a standardized measure. However, on balance, the issue of whether cognitive deficits underlie poor insight is still unresolved. As in other clinical situations, the relationship may not be a straightforward one, as other variables, such as the chronicity of illness, may be involved.

Outcome

McEvoy *et al.* (1989c) found that patients with good insight were significantly less likely to be rehospitalized and tended to be more compliant with treatment 30 days after discharge; the overall relationship between insight and outcome closely approached statistical significance. Their measure of 'after-care environment', which aimed to reflect the degree to which others' efforts were helpfully invested in maintaining the patient in treatment, was not related to insight. Amador and Strauss (1993) also found their measures of insight to be correlated with the course of the illness.

Related to the issue of prognosis and outcome is compliance with treatment. The relationship between poor insight and poor compliance with treatment has been shown by Bartko *et al.* (1988), Lin *et al.* (1979) and McEvoy *et al.* (1989c). The balance of evidence seems to be that higher levels of awareness of having an illness are associated with better medication compliance and clinical outcome (Amador *et al.*, 1991) in schizophrenia. However, there is a risk of circularity of logic, in that some of the measures of insight are based on definitions of insight that include non-compliance. Moreover, compliance with prescribed treatment is a much more complex phenomenon affected by social factors and beliefs about health and sickness (Bebbington, 1995). It is also possible that the relationship between compliance and different aspects of insight may be different. David *et al.* (1992) found that treatment compliance was not strongly related to the ability to recognize one's own delusions and hallucinations and to relabel them as abnormal.

It is interesting that patients may comply with treatment, even though they do not believe themselves to be ill, if the social milieu is conducive (McEvoy *et al.* 1989b, c). The role of health beliefs and illness representation in determining compliance with treatment is recognized, but how these interact with insight to influence treatment compliance has yet to be studied. The domains of illness representation are identity (the label of the disease), causes (explanatory models), timeline (onset and anticipated duration), control (belief that self can influence outcome) and consequences (functional as well as other consequences) (Brownlee *et al.*, 2000). What is obvious is that insight is not the only determinant of care seeking and treatment adherence. McEvoy *et al.* (1993) proposed that insight would improve with attempts at psychosocial rehabilitation. This was further studied by Lysaker and Bell (1995) on a sample of patients with the diagnosis of schizophrenia or schizoaffective disorder. Earlier, Lysaker *et al.* (1994) had found insight as measured by the item on PANSS to be correlated with poor levels of work quality and participation in rehabilitative programmes. In their study reported in 1995, patients enrolled in vocational rehabilitative programmes were found to have improved insight after 5 months. This improvement was more for patients with comparatively fewer cognitive deficits, echoing their earlier findings regarding a relationship with cognitive impairments. However, the lack of a control group limits the generalizability of the findings. It does seem an interesting suggestion that vocational rehabilitation can favourably affect insight in the absence of cognitive impairment. McEvoy *et al.* (1993) have proposed that enhanced self-esteem from rehabilitation may underlie improvement in insight.

Bipolar disorders

Ghaemi *et al.* (1995) studied insight in acutely manic patients using the ITAQ and found that improvement in insight did not correlate with recovery from other symptoms. However, as in schizophrenia, poor insight was correlated with involuntary admission. Swanson *et al.* (1995) used the case vignette method to study insight in two groups of patients with schizophrenia and mania. They found a qualitative difference between mania and schizophrenia, in that patients with schizophrenia but not mania had a reduced awareness of features of their illness. However, although the manic patients were aware of their symptoms, they did not agree that these emanated from a mental illness. Amador *et al.* (1994) and Michalakes *et al.* (1994), on the other hand, found no significant difference between schizophrenic and manic patients on measures of insight. The former found that severely manic patients were similar to schizophrenic patients on scores of insight, whereas depressed and schizoaffective patients had more insight. More studies are required to elucidate aspects of insight in non-schizophrenic populations.

Criticisms of the concept

The recent resurgence of interest in insight has had its share of criticism. Medical anthropologists have criticized the concept of insight for failing to recognize that people can have various culturally shaped frameworks to explain their illnesses, all possibly valid. From this point of view, the concept of insight is 'eurocentric and essentially arrogant' (Perkins and Moodley, 1993), as it dictates that patients should, apart from agreeing that they are mentally ill and requiring treatment, also agree to reconstruct their experiences within the terms and concepts of western psychiatry. Johnson and Orrell (1995) have reviewed work by social scientists on cultural and social variations in lay perceptions of mental illness and argue that these would influence insight. Social and cultural backgrounds influence perceptions of stigma from mental illness and the congruence of the patients with western medical views of mental illness. The ability to relabel mental phenomena as abnormal may be less influenced by social factors when compared with beliefs about the causation of mental illness. Although there are very few studies in this area, evidence seems to be emerging that social and cultural factors are important in the diagnosis of poor insight. For example, differences in the ethnic background of the psychiatrist and the patient appear to influence the judgement of the former about insight (Johnson and Orrell 1996).

Aetiology of impaired insight

Attempts to explain the causation of poor insight have focused on three hypotheses (Amador *et al.*, 1991; Lysaker and Bell, 1994). The first two focus on putative psychological mechanisms. It has been suggested that refusal to take prescribed medication, implying poor insight, is a wilful preference for the experience of psychotic phenomenology over drug-induced normality. The second formulation suggests that patients deny illness at a psychological level to help them cope with normal life as they recover from a psychosis. A third explanation suggested that poor insight may have something to do with cognitive impairment, drawing on similarities with neurological conditions such as anosognosia. As mentioned earlier, studies have found a significant correlation between impaired performance on the WCST and poor insight, suggesting that cognitive impairments resulting from frontal lobe deficits may underlie poor insight in schizophrenia.

REFERENCES

Amador XF and Strauss DH (1993) Assessment of insight in psychosis. *American Journal of Psychiatry 150*, 873–9.

Amador XF, Strauss DH and Yale SA (1991) Awareness of illness in schizophrenia. *Schizophrenia Bulletin 17*, 113–32.

Amador XF, Flum M and Andreasen NC (1994) Awareness of illness in schizophrenia and schizoaffective and mood disorders. *Archives of General Psychiatry 51*, 826–36.

Bartko G, Herzog I and Zador G (1988) Clinical symptomatology and drug compliance in schizophrenic patients. *Acta Psychiatrica Scandinavica 77*, 74–6.

Bebbington PE (1995) The context of compliance. *International Clinical Psychopharmacology 9* (suppl. 5), 45–50.

Birchwood M, Smith J and Drury V (1994) A self-report insight scale for psychosis; reliability, validity, and sensitivity to change. *Acta Psychiatrica Scandinavica 89*, 62–7.

Brownlee S, Leventhal H and Leventhal EA (2000) Regulation, self-regulation, and construction of the self in the maintenance of physical health. In Boekartz M, Pintrich PR and Zeidner M (eds). *Handbook of Self-regulation*. San Diego: Academic Press.

Cuesta MJ, Peralta V and Caro F (1995) Is poor insight in psychotic disorders associated with poor performance on the Wisconsin card sorting test? *American Journal of Psychiatry 152*, 1380–2.

David AS (1990) Insight and psychosis. *British Journal of Psychiatry 156*, 798–808.

David AS, Buchanan A, Reed A and Almeida O (1992) The assessment of insight in psychosis. *British Journal of Psychiatry 161*, 599–62.

Freud A (1981) Insight: its presence and absence as a factor in normal development. In Solint AJ, Eissler RS and Freud A (eds) *The Psychoanalytic Study of the Child*, vol. 36. New Haven: Yale University Press.

Ghaemi SN, Stoll AL and Pope HG (1995) Lack of insight in bipolar disorder: the acute manic episode. *Journal of Nervous and Mental Disease 183*, 464–7.

Greenfield D, Strauss JS and Bowers MB (1989) Insight and interpretation of illness in recovery from psychosis. *Schizophrenia Bulletin 15*, 245–52.

Jaspers K (1959) *General Psychopathology* (transl. Hoenig J and Hamilton MW, 1963). Manchester: Manchester University Press.

Johnson S and Orrell M (1995) Insight and psychosis: a social perspective. *Psychological Medicine 25*, 515–20.

Johnson S and Orrell M (1996) Insight, psychosis and ethnicity: a case-note study. *Psychological Medicine 26*, 1081–4.

Kay S, Fiszbein A and Opler L (1987) The Positive and Negative Syndrome Scale (PANSS) for schizophrenia. *Schizophrenia Bulletin 13*, 261–76.

Kemp R and David A (1996) Psychological predictors of insight and compliance in psychotic patients. *British Journal of Psychiatry 169*, 444–50.

Kumar TM and Sims ACP (1998) Insight and its measurement in relation to psychosis. *Psychiatry Update 1*, 13–8.

Lewis A (1934) The psychopathology of insight. *British Journal of Medical Psychology 14*, 332–48.

Lin IF, Spiga R and Fortsch W (1979) Insight and adherence to medication in chronic schizophrenics. *Journal of Clinical Psychiatry 40*, 430–2.

Lysaker P and Bell M (1994) Insight and cognitive impairment in schizophrenia: performance on repeated administrations of the Wisconsin card sorting test. *Journal of Nervous and Mental Disease 182*, 656–60.

Lysaker P and Bell M (1995) Work rehabilitation and improvements in insight in schizophrenia. *Journal of Nervous and Mental Disease 183*, 103–6.

Lysaker P, Bell M and Milstein RM (1994) Insight and treatment compliance in schizophrenia. *Psychiatry 57*, 289–93.

McEvoy JP, Apperson LJ and Appelbaum PS (1989a) Insight in schizophrenia: its relationship to acute psychopathology. *Journal of Nervous and Mental Disease 177*, 43–7.

McEvoy JP, Applebaum PS and Apperson LJ (1989b) Why must some schizophrenic patients be involuntarily committed? The role of insight. *Comprehensive Psychiatry 30*, 13–7.

McEvoy JP, Freter S and Everett G (1989c) Insight and the clinical outcome in schizophrenia. *Journal of Nervous and Mental Disease 177*, 48–51.

McEvoy JP, Freter S, Merritt M and Apperson LJ (1993) Insight about psychosis among outpatients with schizophrenia. *Hospital and Community Psychiatry 44*, 883–4.

McGorry PD and McConville SB (1999) Insight in psychosis: an elusive target. *Comprehensive Psychiatry 40*, 131–42.

Markova IS (2005) *Insight in Psychiatry*. Cambridge: Cambridge University Press.

Markova IS and Berrios GE (1991) The assessment of insight in clinical psychiatry: a new scale. *Acta Psychiatrica Scandinavica 86*, 159–64.

Michalakes A, Skatas C and Charalambous A (1994) Insight in schizophrenia and mood disorders and its relation to psychopathology. *Acta Psychiatrica Scandinavica 190*, 46–9.

Perceval J (1840) A narrative of the treatment experienced by a gentleman during a state of mental derangement to explain the causes and the nature of insanity. In Bateson G (ed.) *Perceval's Narrative: a Patient's Account of his Psychosis, 1830–1832*. London: Hogarth Press.

Perkins R and Moodley P (1993) The arrogance of insight? *Psychiatric Bulletin 17*, 233–4.

Roback HB and Abramowitz SI (1979) Insight and hospital adjustment. *Canadian Journal of Psychiatry 24*, 233–6.

Sanz M, Constable G, Lopez-Ibor I, Kemp R and David AS (1998) A comparative study of insight scales and their relationship to psychopathological and clinical variables. *Psychological Medicine 28*, 437–46.

Surguladze S and David A (1999) Insight and major mental illness: an update for clinicians. *Advances in Psychiatric Treatment 5*, 163–70.

Swanson CL, Freudenreich O and McEvoy JP (1995) Insight in schizophrenia and mania. *Journal of Nervous and Mental Disease 193*, 752–5.

Tolor A and Reznikoff M (1960) A new approach to insight: a preliminary report. *Journal of Nervous and Mental Disease 130*, 286–96.

Upthegrove R, Oyebode F, George M and Haque MS (2002) Insight, social knowledge and working memory in schizophrenia. *Psychopathology 35*, 341–6.

Wing JK, Cooper JE and Sartorius N (1974) *Measurement and Classification of Psychiatric Symptoms*. Cambridge: Cambridge University Press.

Section Four

SELF AND BODY

The Disordered Self

13

> Often, when I was alone, I sat down on this stone, and then began an imaginary game that went something like this: 'I am sitting on top of this stone and it is underneath'. But the stone also could say 'I' and think: 'I am lying here on this slope and he is sitting on top of me'. The question then arose: 'Am I the one who is sitting on the stone, or am I the stone on which he is sitting?' This question always perplexed me, and I would stand up, wondering who was what now. *Jung (1963)*

> The self was never meant to be a solid object like a stone, a horse, or a weed, nor even a concept to be considered as semantically tantamount to changes in blood flow or test scores. Of course, patients with disordered minds do sport hurting, afflicted and cursing selves but not as they do carcinomas or broken legs. Their selves live in the same realm as do their virtues, vices, beliefs and aspirations, and that is where they should remain. *Berrios and Markova (2003)*

Ego and self

The *self* is a construct that has changed in meaning and significance since the inception of Hellenistic philosophy (Berrios and Markova, 2003). From the mid-nineteenth century onwards, various concepts about the self have found their way into psychiatry such that in contemporary psychiatry there is reckoned to be some disturbance in the way one thinks about and estimates oneself; this, of course, differs according to the nature of the illness. There is, however, no consensus on what exactly it means to be a self. There is a plurality of conceptions, including the ecological self, the interpersonal self, the extended self, the private self and the conceptual self among many (Zahavi, 2003). In this chapter, the terms *ego* and *self* are used more or less interchangeably. *Ego* has the advantage of being a technical term and therefore more circumscribed in its meaning; this is also a disadvantage when it is simply oneself as usually understood and subjectively experienced that is being referred to.

Freud's use of the word *ego* echoes Nietzsche (1901):

> of *reason*. It is *this* which sees everywhere deed and doer; this which believes in will as cause in general; this which believes in the 'ego' as being, in the ego as substance, and which *projects* its belief in the ego-substance on to all things.

Freud (1933) described ego as standing 'for reason and good sense while the id stands for the untamed passions'. The ego:

> has been modified by the proximity of the external world with its threat of danger. ... The poor ego has to serve three severe masters and does what it can to bring their claims and demands into harmony with one another. These demands are always divergent and often seem incompatible. No wonder that the ego so often fails in this task. Its three tyrannical masters are the external world, the super-ego and the id. *(Freud, 1933)*

Self-concept and body image

The body is unique in that it is experienced from both *inside* and *outside*; that is, both as *subject* and *object*. There is a way in which I am subjectively aware of my own body that is different from how I experience a block of wood. But I am also aware that my body is an object in the world, to be viewed and even acted on by others. For most of the time, we are not aware of our body but, for example in extreme anxiety, pain and sexual excitement, there is an awareness of physiological systems or organs as objects: 'my heart banging, my finger throbbing'. For the rest of the time we assume the parts of the body to be integrated, and this integrated body, for practical purposes, coincides with and is coterminous with the 'self' of which we are not separately aware and which we take for granted. It is through our body that we have contact with the world outside our self: movements of the body relate us to external space.

Many different terms are used to describe the way a person conceptualizes himself. Neurologists, neuropsychiatrists, psychoanalysts and psychologists have used variously the terms *body schema*, *body concept*, *body cathexis*, *body image* and *perceived body*. They describe approximately the same thing but with different nuances. For example, *self-concept* tends to refer to the fully conscious and abstract awareness of oneself, while *body image* is more concerned with unconscious and physical matters and includes experiential aspects of body awareness. Sometimes self-concept is the same as body concept, and at other times conscious self is conceptualized as being independent of its 'cage', the body. The *body schema* implies a spatial element and is more than, and usually bigger than, the body itself. For instance, if you imagine yourself on your way to work, automatically included within your schema of yourself are your clothes and your spectacles, if worn. The body schema changes with changing circumstances. When I drive my car, I incorporate within my concept of my physical size the width of my car, so that I am unlikely to attempt to drive through a doorway or up a flight of steps. Spectacles, a cigar, the carpenter's screwdriver, the blind man's stick all contribute to that person's concept of his *self* in a particular situation. *Cathexis* implies the notion of power, force, libido – perhaps analogous to electrical charge: the self that makes things happen!

Social aspects are obviously important. A man with shoulder-length hair is not usually so endowed through neglect; more likely, it represents a deliberate choice – how he sees himself in his social setting. It accords with his chosen peer group and also distinguishes him from those from whom he would wish to be disassociated. Critchley (1950) has commented on 'that curious emotional state usually known as being in love', in which there is 'a compulsive trend in two body-images of opposite sex towards propinquity and contiguity, eventually culminating in a total fusion or merger'. As a phenomenologist, one could take exception to Critchley's misuse of the term *compulsive*. According to Schilder (1935), body images are never isolated; they are always encircled by the body images of others. Body images are more closely bound together in the erogenous zones and are social in nature. Our body image and the way other people see us are not exclusively dependent on each other. A person sees himself and forms his self-image in a social setting. He sees himself in relation to other people; his view of himself is not totally dependent on, but importantly influenced by, how another individual sees him. It is also determined by how he *believes* that people might see him.

The development of body image has been neatly summarized diagrammatically by Bahnson (1969). He considers that self-image is changeable and amorphous. At any one time, the individual perceives only a small sample from a gallery of possible self-images. In Figure 13.1, the manner in which '*phenomenological selves* are superimposed on each other like the layers of an onion' is demonstrated. Different aspects of self-image develop as the person increases the scope and complexity of his relationships. The term *ego* is not phenomenologically describable, and there has been argument that the self cannot observe itself; that is, a thing and what observes that thing cannot be the same. However, it is the nature of *self* and *ego* to be experienced as either subject or object: a small nuisance like a mouth ulcer can make me feel uncomfortable (subjectively); I can describe what a person with a mouth ulcer experiences (objectively).

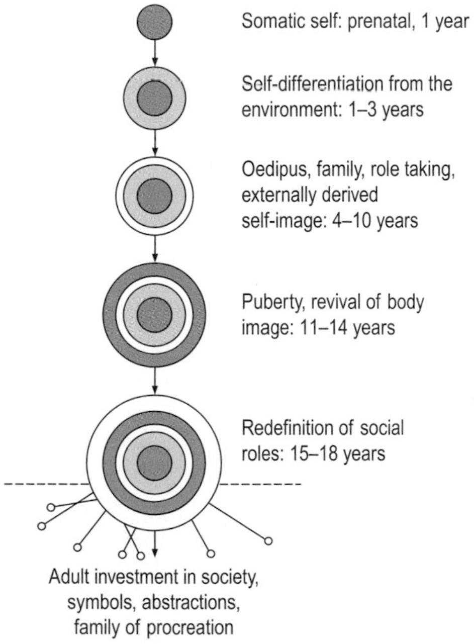

Figure 13.1 Developmental phases of the self-image.

Self-image and non-verbal communication

In a social relationship, a person expresses views he has about himself: his words, and the way he says them, convey how he views his relationship with the other person and also how he sees himself, for example the shopkeeper 'talking down' to a child. Probably more important than this verbal manner of expressing, often unconscious, views on how we see ourselves is *non-verbal communication*. All gestures and postures, movements of the face and pauses in our conversation convey meaning to the person we are talking to; partly, this is also a comment on the way we see ourselves.

'The central core of self image consists for a person of his name, his bodily feelings, body image, sex and age. For a man the job will be central – unless he is suffering from job alienation. For a woman, her family and her husband's job may also be important' (Argyle, 1975). The gender discrimination of that statement is now dated, but it emphasizes that for different people there are varying aspects that form the essential concept of self. Non-verbal aspects of communication are important in sending and receiving information about the personality. The role in society one has adopted and the group with which one identifies are intentionally conveyed and therefore display self-image. These include 'age, sex, race, social class, rank, occupation, school or college attended, nationality, regional origins, religious group and family connections' (Argyle, 1975). These attributes of the person are often deliberately displayed, but there are other characteristics that will be received non-verbally by observers even when the person has no intention of revealing them, for example temperament, personality traits such as introversion, intellect, beliefs and values and past experiences.

Non-verbal communication expresses the attitudes of a person, according to Argyle, for the following reasons.

- There is in some areas of human concern a lack of language or 'verbal coding', for example shape is more readily expressed with the hands than verbally. Describing personality, our own or another's, or commenting on personal relationships is more easily done non-verbally. A person will attempt to communicate non-verbally his or her own physical attractiveness, role and attitude towards the other person.
- Non-verbal signals are more powerful: actions speak louder than words. For a schoolteacher, beckoning may be more likely to result in action than a verbal order.
- Non-verbal signals are less censored and therefore more likely to be genuine. If conflicting messages are given verbally and non-verbally, the non-verbal signal is accepted as truthful.
- Some messages, because of social censorship, cannot be made explicit in a social setting and therefore cannot be verbalized but can be conveyed non-verbally by appropriate posture, gesture and movement in space. For example, by facial expression and turning away, a person might suggest without making it explicit 'I do not like you and am bored with speaking to you'.
- Verbal messages are punctuated and emphasized non-verbally, for example the pause at the end of a phrase or the cadence of voice used. These embellishments add meaning to the actual words used.

A person interacts with others by the use of language. However, non-verbal signals are also important in expressing meaning and conveying feelings. The *ego* talks with the body as well as with words.

Awareness of the body

We have an awareness of our self and an awareness, which overlaps with this but is slightly different, of our bodies. What is this sense of body image or awareness? According to Head and Holmes (1911), the *body schema* is formed as the composite experience of sensations. Schilder (1935) developed further the importance of perceiving sensations in forming the body schema: 'the picture of our own body which we form in our mind, that is to say, the way in which the body appears to ourselves'. Freud (1933) also was concerned with body image in the development of personality: 'the ego is firstly the body ego'. Clearly, abnormality of body image may be the result of abnormal sensations, but this is not always so. For instance, the abnormality of body image of an amputee is directly because of the physical damage, but a hypochondriacal patient may have no abnormal sensations yet believe he has cancer. In transsexualism, a person will have a normal sensory experience of his body but says that he hates his body and especially his penis; he may feel that he is actually a woman trapped inside a male body (Morris, 1974). His disturbed body image is not a result of disturbed sensation; there is a conflict between ego (the way he experiences himself and the gender he ascribes to it) and body image. The distinction made for convenience between this chapter and Chapter 15, between self-awareness and awareness of the body, is artificial.

The body image can be altered through enhancement, diminution (or ablation) or distortion. It incorporates more than just the body, except perhaps for those few occasions when a person is both unclothed and conceptualizing himself as naked: tailors have long tried to persuade us that 'clothes make the man'. Certainly, they are an effective means of non-verbal communication. Clothes give us some insight into the way a person sees himself (or herself) and also in the way he (or she) proposes to interact with other people. A person complements his mood and his social role of the moment in his choice of clothes. He wears clothes, as a ship hoists a flag, for signalling, and particular clothes are worn to convey a message to someone who can read it. A medical student wears a suit for an oral examination, a woman undoes the top button of her blouse on leaving the office for lunch. As the patient comes into a doctor's consulting room, he starts to give information about himself from his appearance before either of them utters a word. A person whose clothes are chosen for him, as in mental hospitals in the past, presents a peculiarly bleak and meaningless appearance; this aspect of his body image is expressionless and conveys nothing of himself.

DISORDERS OF SELF

In descriptive psychopathology, one uses the term *ego disorders* or *disorders of self* to describe the abnormal inner experiences of *I-ness* and *my-ness* that occur in psychiatric illness. These may occur in the patient's state of *inner awareness* irrespective of any changes he may show in his attitude to, or experience of, the world outside himself. Jaspers (1959), with characteristic clarity, described self-awareness, that is, the ability to distinguish I from *not I*, as having four formal characteristics. Scharfetter (1981, 1995, 2003) added a fifth dimension of *ego-vitality* to the list and has made a case for its inclusion based on factor analysis. Previously, this characteristic was incorporated within the awareness of activity, which subsumed 'being' and 'existing' with other present participles. Thus, we now have the following characteristics of self-awareness.

- *The feeling of awareness of being or existing* (ego vitality): I know that I am alive and exist, and this is fundamental to awareness of self.
- *The feeling of awareness of activity* (ego activity): I know that I am an agent who initiates and executes my thoughts and actions.
- *An awareness of unity* (ego consistency and coherence): at any given moment, I know that I am one person.
- *Awareness of identity* (ego identity): there is continuity in my biography, physiognomy, gender, genealogical origin, etc.; I have been the same person all the time.
- *Awareness of the boundaries of self* (ego demarcation): I am distinct from other things and beings and can distinguish what is *myself* from the *outside world*, and I am aware of the boundary between self and non-self.

The disorders of inner experience in which these characteristics are disturbed are now explored in more detail. We will deal with these five functions described by Jaspers and Scharfetter in order.

Disorder of being or ego vitality

I never have to ask myself the question as to whether I exist. It is an assumption that I make with unquestioning certainty. I am so sure of this that it does not even come on to the agenda of doubts and uncertainties. My only knowledge that everything else exists is based on the premise that I do.

Being: the patient's experience of his very existence may be altered: 'I do not exist; there is nothing here' or 'I am not alive any more' or 'I am rotting'. This is the core experience of *nihilistic delusions*, which may occur in affective psychoses (Chapters 8 and 18). Less pronounced nihilistic ideas (not delusions) are experienced as *depersonalization*, an alteration of the way one experiences oneself, which is accompanied by a feeling of an alteration or loss of significance for self: 'I feel unreal, a bit woozy, as though I can't be quite certain of myself any more'.

Disorder of activity

I do something and know that I am doing it. Everything I do, in everything I experience, through every event that impinges on me, I am aware that the experience has the unique quality of *being mine*. 'It was incredible. I pinched myself to make sure it was really happening to me' expresses the relationship we experience between awareness of reality and activity. It is in our actions, including our thinking, that we reinforce ourselves concerning our existence.

Moving may show abnormality, for example in the passivity experience or delusions of control of patients with schizophrenia (see below). Schreber described several examples of this experience: 'The difficulties which were put in my way defy description. My fingers are paralysed, the direction of my gaze is changed in order to prevent my finding the correct keys, the tempo is quickened by making the muscles of my fingers move prematurely: all these were and still are daily occurrences' and 'the bellowing-miracle when my muscles serving the processes of respiration are set in motion by the lower God (Ariman) in such a way that I am forced to emit the bellowing noises'.

Memorizing and *imagining* may be changed in that the patient with depression feels he is unable to initiate the act of memory or fantasy; or, alternatively, a schizophrenic patient feels that this activity when it occurs is not initiated by him but from outside himself. A depressed patient said, 'my memory has gone, I have no thoughts, I cannot think at all'.

Willing may be altered, for example the schizophrenic patient who no longer experiences his will as being his own. Commonly, neurotic patients describe an inability to initiate activity, a feeling of powerlessness, of being ground down in the face of life's vicissitudes.

Some of these abnormalities of experience of one's own activities are closely associated with mood, for example the feeling of the depressed patient who believes that he is incapable of doing anything at all: the alteration of self-concept is directly linked to the mood state. Sometimes, however, it is not the affect associated with the change of activity but the belief about the initiation of the activity that is changed. These are the passivity experiences (made experiences), which are discussed in more detail with other first-rank symptoms of schizophrenia in Chapter 9.

Disorder of singleness or ego consistency and coherence

In health, a person is integrated in his thinking and behaviour so that he does not have to be aware of his feeling of unity. He just assumes that he is one person, and he knows his limitations and capabilities. This assumption of unity may be lost in some conditions. In *dreams*, one sometimes sees oneself, even perhaps with some surprise, in the drama. In some forms of transcendental meditation, by carrying out repetitive monotonous acts the subject enters a *self-induced* trance in which he can observe himself carrying out the behaviour. 'Self' is both the observer and also the object of observation (see Box 13.1).

Autoscopy (heautoscopy)

According to Fish (1967), 'in this strange experience the patient sees himself and knows that it is he. It is not just a visual hallucination because kinaesthetic and somatic sensation must also be present to give the subject the impression that the hallucination is he'. This very rare perceptual experience may involve several of the modalities of sensation, for example touch as well as vision. However, disturbance in visual perception is an essential feature; it is an abnormality of seeing. The loss of *feeling of familiarity* for oneself is prominent; 'self' is viewed quite dispassionately and objectively. In autoscopy, the abnormal perceptual experience is especially associated with disorders of the *parietal lobe*. A patient who had a lesion of the brain occasionally 'saw' himself standing at his left side and felt 'crowded' by this person. Lukianowicz (1958) has defined

Box 13.1 Disorders of singleness

There has been considerable confusion in psychiatric writing between:

- autoscopy, heautoscopy or phantom mirror image (synonyms)
- the double phenomenon, doppelgänger (also synonyms)
- dual, double or multiple personality.

There is not usually confusion in distinguishing between these and:

- delusional misidentification, Capgras' syndrome
- *double orientation*, the situation in which an individual appears to live in two worlds simultaneously – a psychotic world and the real world; for a confused patient on a psychogeriatric ward, he believes both that this man visiting him is the doctor and also the parson come to marry him to his young wife.

it thus: 'Autoscopy is a complex psychosensorial hallucinatory perception of one's own body image projected into the external visual space'.

In practice, these phenomena can be extremely difficult to identify. The following description by a 37-year-old, intelligent man with a history of epilepsy, receiving treatment with phenobarbitone, is considered an example of autoscopic pseudohallucination. The patient held his head rigidly with apparent torticollis to the right. If he rotated it to the left, there was marked head nodding, but not if he turned it further to the right.

> " I'm standing outside myself on the left hand side but only when I'm sitting down . . . it comes in short episodes for about 30 seconds . . . my true self loses all its senses as all the senses are in my hallucinatory self . . . the true self is just a shell without any senses . . . the hallucinatory self can see the true self and the whole surroundings, and it seems to me as though the hallucinatory self is looking at me and at other things in the room from a position standing to the left hand side of me, and everything is in the right perspective. If it was occurring now, the hallucinatory self would see you more full face and from higher up than I see you now because it is standing . . . I can't see it or hear it but it can see the side of my head. It seems to be there. I know that it isn't me as such. It's like having a dream and you know that it is a dream. I thought it was a dream but it has occurred when I am fully waking. It seems as clear as a nightmare at the time but I know afterwards that it is a figment like a very vivid dream but more real than a dream. I would not see a fleck of dust on my cheek or something like that. The other one is not a different personality.

When this experience occurred, the patient felt all sensation was in the 'hallucinatory self', including hearing, seeing and feeling cold: 'I felt cold on the back of the hallucinatory self'. There had been no experience of taste or smell. There had been an experience of affect.

> " I was talking to a representative. The hallucinatory self felt sorry for this man because he looked abnormal. It had no feelings for the real self. He looked abnormal because I had stopped talking and a glazed expression had come into my eye.

A bizarre example of autoscopy was reported by Ames (1984): the self-shooting of a phantom head. This patient was suffering from schizophrenia. He described seeing and hearing a voice from another head that was set on his own shoulders, attached to his body and trying to dominate his own head. He described himself as having two heads but believed that the other head was actually that of his wife's gynaecologist, whom he believed to be having an affair with her. The voice from the second head was that of the gynaecologist, and there were also the voices of Jesus and Abraham around him, conversing with each other and talking about his having two heads. The patient tried to remove the other head by shooting six shots at it and through his own palate, causing extensive damage to his brain. Ames labelled this condition the 'phenomenon of perceptual delusional bicephaly'.

It is important to reserve autoscopy for a *perceptual* disturbance of self-image: 'seeing one's self' (Lukianowicz, 1958). In a comprehensive review, Damas Mora *et al.* (1980) widen the definition considerably to 'the experience of duplication of one's real self'. However, this would include three forms: heautoscopic depersonalization, which is similar to the doppelgänger or experience of the double described below; heautoscopic hallucination (specular hallucination), which is the form described above; and heautoscopic delusion, a rare form when the subject has a fixed delusional belief in his separate concrete existence but has no complementary perceptual experience (delusion of subjective doubles). It is considered best to retain the word 'autoscopy' (heautoscopy) to refer to the perceptual form of heautoscopic hallucination. However, as Damas Mora *et al.* have pointed out, many subjects clearly have doubts about the reality of their vision, and it may then be a visual pseudohallucination. Autoscopic depersonalization, awareness of one's self, is now described under the term *doppelgänger*.

The double phenomenon: doppelgänger

The 'double' or *doppelgänger* phenomenon is an awareness of oneself as being both outside, alongside, and inside oneself: the subjective phenomenon of *doubling*. In the discussion that follows, the description is of a symptom or phenomenon and not a syndrome or diagnosis; the experience occurs with different conditions or with no mental disorder at all. It is cognitive and ideational rather than being necessarily *perceptual*. However, it may also have a perceptual component. It has nothing in common phenomenologically with *Capgras' syndrome* (Chapter 8), which is a delusional misidentification in which the patient believes that someone he knows well has been replaced by an impostor who looks identical. The delusion in Capgras' syndrome is that, although he agrees that the person looks exactly like the person he purports to be, he is actually an impostor falsely simulating the real person.

Having an awareness of one's double may be perceptual, delusional or, more commonly, a variety of *depersonalization*; these *forms* are phenomenologically distinct. There is a North European myth, shared by several countries, that someone may see his *double* ('wraith', 'fetch') shortly before his death, and it has therefore become a sinister omen (Todd and Dewhurst, 1962). These authors present interesting historical material to substantiate the link between perceptual doppelgänger and death. The usual legend is that, as the person lies dying, his wraith floats before his eyes and he sees himself performing all the most disreputable and reprehensible actions of his life; they are paraded before him as he expires.

As a clear hallucination, *seeing* one's double is rare (autoscopy), but the vague feeling of being beside oneself, alongside oneself or having another self (the soul double) is quite common. Jaspers (1959) has stated:

> Heautoscopy is the term used for the phenomenon when someone vividly perceives his own body as a double in the outer world, whether as an actual perception or as an imaginary form, as a delusion or as a vivid physical awareness. There have been patients who will actually speak with their doubles. The phenomenon is not at all uniform.

He gives four examples, one of whom is suffering from an organic condition, two from schizophrenia and one whose condition is definitely not organic, and then goes on to write:

> We can see that we are dealing with phenomena that are really not the same although they are superficially similar. They may occur in organic brain lesions, in deliria, in schizophrenia and in dream-like states, never at least without a mild alteration in consciousness; day-dreaming, intoxication, dream-sleep or delirium. The similarity consists in the fact that the body-schema gains an actuality of its own out in external space.

It would seem that Jaspers is here describing two separate phenomena: *autoscopy* and the *double phenomenon*.

Jaspers' first example of the double came from Goethe – to quote Jaspers quoting Goethe:

> Goethe (in Drang and Verwirrung) had seen Frederika for the last time and was riding to Drusenheim when the following happened: 'In my mind's eye not with my physical eyes, I saw myself distinctly on the same road riding towards myself. I was dressed as I had never been before in grey and gold. Immediately I shook myself out of this dream the figure went' . . . 'the strange phantom gave me a certain peace of mind at that moment of parting'. What is noteworthy in the episode is the dreamy state, 'the mind's eye' and the satisfaction derived from the meaning of the apparition – he was riding in the opposite direction back to Sesenheim – he will return.

Despite Menninger-Lerchental's (1932) title of the relevant paper, 'A hallucination of Goethe', this was certainly not a hallucination; it is described as 'in my mind's eye'. It is not organic, neither is it psychotic; it is, in fact, a description of fantasy (Sims, 1994). It would seem that there could be six possible psychopathological explanations for the phenomenon of non-organic, non-psychotic doubling.

- *Fantasy*: as in this description by Goethe of daydreaming.
- *Depersonalization*: 'while talking we may notice that we are talking rather like an automaton, quite correctly maybe, but we can observe ourselves and listen to ourselves' (Jaspers, 1959).
- *Conflict*: 'Two beings live within my breast where reason struggles with passion' (Jaspers, 1959).

- *Compulsive ideas*: repetitive, self-produced and self ascribed, resisted.
- *Double personality*: alternating states of consciousness.
- Being in two, *being doubled*: 'When both chains of psychic events so develop together that we can talk of separate personalities, each with their own peculiar experiences and specific feeling – associations, and each perfectly alien and apart from the other' (Jaspers, 1959).

These experiences are not wholly distinct from each other and they do overlap; however, there are phenomenological differences between them that are important.

Patients describe experiencing their 'true' self and their 'other' self: their *self* as, unfortunately and realistically, they have to accept themselves; their *ideal self* that they would wish to be; their reticent and submissive self that suffers; and a hostile and accusing self that derides and punishes them. This contrast is a popular literary subject, and it then becomes richly embellished by fantasy. Unlike a psychotic experience, one easily identifies with the victim of his own double, for example Dostoevsky's Golyadkin in *The Double* (1846), who is perpetually humiliated and misunderstood. This double is not clearly described in perceptual terms; he just exists, and the story describes his exploits, the way in which he makes life intolerable for the polite and law-abiding civil servant who is the original. This symptom appears to be neurotically produced, in that the sufferer is unable to resolve the conflicting claims of different parts of his own personality and, rather than accepting that he contains within himself opposed forces, he personifies these aspects and sees himself as having two or more different selves.

This neurotic conflict of the double has also been extensively used in literature, when the two aspects of one personality may be portrayed as different but closely related people who become very involved with each other in a destructive way, for example the brothers James and Henry in Robert Louis Stevenson's *The Master of Ballantrae* (1889). In this story, as in real life, the *victim* is generally conscientious, inhibited, quiet, consistent and moral. He is often respected but unpopular with acquaintances; faithful, but dull in the eyes of women. The *double* (what he feels lies inside himself and wishes he could express) is usually domineering, ruthless, volatile and amoral. In the fantasy of the inhibited subject, this second self is immediately popular with women, but his behaviour soon precipitates calamities that frequently rebound on the victim (these are the reasons the original gives to himself for not indulging these wished-for but dangerous fantasies).

It is of course the anticipation of these disasters that inhibits the real person from acting on his fantasies. The conflicts of an anxious, obsessional person, with profligate fantasies never to be realized, are given expression in these contrasted characters. He wants to break out of the mundane constraints of his orderly life and act in a liberated way, but he feels totally inhibited by the anticipated censure of other people.

The very worst feature of the double for the subject himself is the terrible, inextricable involvement of the double with the subject in trying to mortify him, goad him, provoke him to destroy the double and/or destroy himself. This destructiveness, in severe depressive illness, was described by Styron (1991):

> the sense of being accompanied by a second self – a wraith-like observer, able to watch with dispassionate curiosity as his companion struggles against the oncoming disaster, or decides to embrace it... I, the victim-to-be of self-murder, was both the solitary actor and lone member of the audience... I watched myself in mingled terror and fascination.

Multiple personality (dissociative identity disorder)

In dissociative (hysterical) states, so-called dual and multiple personalities have been described (Abse, 1982; McDougall, 1911; Prince, 1905). Slater and Roth (1969) comment:

> A girl who is by turns 'May' and 'Margaret', may be quiet, studious and obedient as May, and unaware of Margaret's existence. When she becomes Margaret, however, she may be gay, headstrong and wilful, and refer to May in contemptuous terms. It seems that these multiple personalities are always artificial productions, the product of the medical attention that they arouse.

The essence of multiple personality is the embodiment of at least two personalities (identities). This phenomenon raises doubts about our natural intuition that an individual human being is indivisible and is an embodied singular person. Prince's account gave a vivid description:

> Miss Christine L Beauchamp, the subject of this study, is a person in whom several personalities have become developed; that is to say, she may change personality from time to time, often from hour to hour, and with each change her character becomes transformed and her memories altered. In addition to the real, original or normal self, the self that was born and which was intended by nature to be, she may be anyone of the three persons. I say three different, because, although making use of the same body, each nevertheless, has distinctly different character: a difference manifested by different trains of thought, by different views, and temperament, and by different acquisitive tastes, habits, experiences, and memories.

In a characteristic case study of multiple personality before the conditions for medical practice in the United States resulted in a proliferation of cases of so-called multiple personality disorder, Larmore *et al*. (1977) described 'a 35 year old white woman of rural Kentucky background' who had made seven suicide attempts, for which she claimed to have no memory. 'Shortly after admission a hypnotic interview was conducted, during which one of the personalities spontaneously revealed herself and gave hints of the existence of other personalities'. Four distinct personalities were identified: *Faith*, 'the primary personality ... known as "the little angel" by personality Alicia ... kind, loving and helpful ... has difficulty in expression ... anger, and in dealing with criticism'; *Alicia*, 'a Satanic agent ... claims control over most of Faith's physiological functions ... manifesting either assaultive or self-destructive behaviour'; *Alicia–Faith*, under the influence of Alicia, 'has only peripheral awareness of Alicia and no knowledge of Faith or Guardian Angel'; *Guardian Angel*, 'first made its appearance following the grandfather's death ... claims to be the protector of Faith'.

There has been a vast outpouring of the psychiatric literature on the subject of multiple personality disorder, based on the diagnostic criteria of DSM-IIIR (American Psychiatric Association, 1987) but often lacking in psychopathological precision. This has been well summarized by Fahy (1988).

> Recently there has been a dramatic rise in the number of case reports of multiple personality disorder (MPD). . . . A review of the recent literature reveals a poverty of information on reliability of diagnosis, prognosis, or the role of selection bias. It is argued that iatrogenic factors may contribute to the development of the syndrome. There is little evidence from genetic or physiological studies to suggest that MPD represents a distinct psychiatric disorder.

Abse states that 'one-way amnesia' is usual for multiple personality; that is, personality A is amnesic for the other personality B, but the second, B, can discuss the experiences of A. Usually, A is inhibited and depressed and B is freer and more elated. The forms of multiple personality seen in practice are usually:

- simultaneous partial personalities
- successive well-defined partial personalities
- clustered multiple partial personalities.

When such patients have been treated in psychotherapy, ingenious explanations are often given by patient and by therapist for the appearance of the additional personalities. Although this remains a disputed area, an authoritative opinion from Merskey (2000) states:

> In this author's view there is no place for the diagnosis of multiple personality disorder in psychiatry, and the important question is how such a diagnosis managed to achieve so much prominence in professional circles in North America, although generally not elsewhere.

Lability in the awareness of personality

The loss of unity of self in schizophrenia was exemplified by a patient who described how, every night, he became a horse and trotted down Whitehall. At the same time as this was happening in his mind, he also believed he was in Whitehall watching the horse. This type of symptom has been called *lability in the awareness of personality* and was described by Bonhoeffer (1907) as occurring in paranoid psychosis.

Disorder of identity

I am who I was last week or 30 years ago; I am who I will be next week or in 10 years' time. This truism, which we can claim without hesitation, is by no means certain for some people suffering from schizophrenia or from organic states, from neuroses or from depression, or even for some healthy people in abnormal situations (see possession state, below). This disorder of self-awareness is characterized by changes in the identity of self *over time*.

A person who feels threatened in his job and is afraid of redundancy is not likely to function well, because of his feeling of impermanence. A *feeling of continuity* for oneself and one's role is a fundamental assumption of life, without which competent behaviour cannot take place. In health, we have no doubts about the continuity of ourself from our past into our present. However, patients with schizophrenia sometimes deny that they have always been the same person. Characteristically, this takes the form of a *passivity experience*, and the patient claims that at some time in the past he *has been* completely changed from being one person to another, whom he now is. Jaspers (1959) gives an account of a patient who said,

> " When telling my story I am aware that only part of my present self experienced all this. Up to 23rd December 1901, I cannot call myself my present self; the past self now seems like a little dwarf inside me. It is an unpleasant feeling; it upsets my feelings of existence if I describe my previous experiences in the first person. I can do it if I use an image and recall that the dwarf reigned up to that date, but since then his past has ended.

This complete alteration in the sense of identity is exclusively psychotic; there is a break in the sense of identity of self, and there is a subjective experience of someone completely different, although still described as oneself, 'taking over'.

A feeling of loss of continuity, which is, however, of lesser intensity than the psychotic change described above and without its element of passivity, may be experienced in health and in neuroses and personality disorders. The person knows that both people, before and after, are truly himself, but he feels very altered from what he was. This may occur following an overwhelmingly important life situation or during emotional development without an outside event. For example, an adolescent may quite suddenly feel in the course of a week 'as if' he is quite a different person. It should be stressed that the sense of reality is never lost to the extent that he actually believes himself to be a different person. In the non-psychotic, it is more that thoughts and feelings do not seem to be in keeping with himself as he has come to accept himself.

In the next chapter, a man is described as developing long-term depersonalization after experiencing massive stress at work, culminating in an extremely harassing journey in which he was the car driver. Afterwards, his wife said that he was never again like the man she had married, 'but like his (non-existent) twin brother'. She said that, whereas previously he was incisive, was quick-thinking and made the decisions in the family, now he lacked self-confidence and she had to do everything. Neither partner was in any doubt that he was the same person, but his whole demeanour had changed *as if* he had become someone similar but not identical.

The feeling of loss of continuity contributes to the inertia of the person with schizophrenia and the apathy of the depressive. Lack of a clear sense of identity from the past continuing into the future is a strong disincentive to concerted activity. The schizophrenic patient, as part of disturbance of passivity, may have doubts about his continuity from the past to the present; the depressive, secondary to disorder of mood, often sees no continuation into the future: 'everything is bleak, there is nothing to look forward to'.

A part of the sense of continuity of self is accepting that the changes in one's total state at present are *due to illness*. This is the characteristic usually described in the mental state examination under the term *insight* (David, 1990). The individual recognizes that he is still the same person but that his current change in subjectivity is due to the intervening process of illness. This has been discussed further in Chapter 12.

Possession state

This is classified in ICD-10 under dissociative (conversion) disorders (F44) – trance and possession disorders (F44.3) (World Health Organization, 1992). However, although the trance or altered state of conscious awareness is a prerequisite, possession state does not necessarily occur in the context of dissociative or hysterical disorder. It can occur in normal, healthy people in unusual situations, either as a group phenomenon (mass hypnosis) or individually; such a case is described below. There is a *temporary* loss of both the sense of personal identity and full awareness of the surroundings. The person acts as if he has, and believes himself to have been, taken over by another – a spirit, a force, a deity or even another person. The difference between those conditions that constitute disorder and those that may be considered as being within a cultural or religious context alone is that the former are unwanted, cause distress to the individual and those around and may be prolonged beyond the immediate event or ceremony at which it was induced.

Possession of a young, entirely healthy woman with a husband and three children by two 'goddesses' was witnessed in Sri Lanka. The woman had become a *varama*, a healer with special powers, about 2 years previously, when she 'saw' her deceased father-in-law, who came to her and said that she would have supernatural power to help other people and her own family. Her husband had become addicted to *arak*, a local spirit, and his drinking had by then brought the family into extreme economic hardship. After this experience, she offered her services as a healer and solver of domestic difficulties to her village, and several people consulted her each day at home, where she had devoted one tiny room to a sanctuary and another to a waiting room. With her husband blowing a buffalo horn repeatedly and herself chanting, she induced a trance in herself in which she spoke with different voices as either one of two female deities giving advice to her clients, which her husband interpreted. The villagers had found her ministrations to be helpful, it gave useful occupation to her delinquent husband and she had completely solved her own family's financial problems through the gifts she received for services rendered.

A different case, with psychiatric disorder present, was that of a 37-year-old Sri Lankan housewife who believed herself to be possessed by her long-dead grandmother; on three occasions she had gone into a trance, lost contact with the outside world and seen the image of her grandmother coming close to her and trying to squeeze her neck. These episodes were described with fear and distress. She showed symptoms of depressive illness, with poor sleep, early morning wakening, loss of appetite and weight, anergia, fatigue and feeling low in mood; she had been abandoned by her mother when 7 years old.

Wijesinghe *et al.* (1976) surveyed a semiurban population of 7653 people in Sri Lanka and identified 37 subjects, 9 male and 28 female, with 'possession trance states', showing altered state of conscious awareness, behaviour for which the subject did not acknowledge responsibility and amnesia for the period of the trance. Episodes, often lasting about 30 minutes, were usually precipitated either by emotional stress or culture-bound stimuli such as witnessing an exorcism ceremony. During trance, subjects were most often restless with rhythmic trembling of the trunk and exaggerated gesturing, speech was aggressive and commanding and, typically, mood was angry; most often, the possessing spirit was that of a close but dead relative. In females especially, as the condition continued they were increasingly likely to become permanent adepts. These authors regarded only one of their subjects as suffering from schizophrenia, although 17 of 37 manifested active psychiatric disorder, mostly neurotic in nature.

Jaspers (1959), in writing about disorders of self-awareness, concerned himself with disorder of content as well as of form. In discussing states of possession, he commented on the rare condition of *lycanthropy*, the patient believing that he has been transformed into an animal, literally a wolf. Koehler *et al.* (1990) have reviewed this work and have shown that Jaspers differentiated between states of possession presenting with an altered consciousness and states of possession in which consciousness remains clear; the former were usually dissociative (hysterical) in origin, while the latter were more often associated with schizophrenia. This emphasizes the importance for psychiatric diagnosis in assessing psychopathological form. In the few published case reports of lycanthropy, it is usually associated with a belief of possession by the devil.

Near-death experience

Another alteration of the self-awareness of identity is usually described in psychologically normal people in highly abnormal situations. The near-death experience has occasionally been described by those who are dying or have undergone a life-threatening experience. This subject has been reviewed by Roberts and Owen (1988). Like pseudohallucinations of bereavement, which have already been described, near-death experience in survivors may be quite frequent but is not usually discussed openly for fear of being thought insane.

The most prominent clusters of symptoms seem to be depersonalization, increased alertness and various descriptions of 'mystic consciousness'. Out-of-body experience with autoscopy was frequent, as was passage of consciousness into a foreign region or transcendental experience.

Disorder of the boundaries of self or ego demarcation

By this is meant the disturbance in knowing where *I* ends and *not I* begins. Abnormality is not confined to schizophrenia. For example, in lysergic acid diethylamide intoxication the feeling of impending ego dissolution associated with the feeling of self 'slipping away' with considerable anxiety has been described (Anderson and Rawnsley, 1954). One subject put this as:

> “I was being disorganized . . . the world around was looking very distorted indeed . . . things were pretty rocky so I decided to sit back quietly for a moment and reassure myself by returning to my own private inner world. As soon as I introspected in this manner I felt to my dismay that 'I' myself was somehow disturbed. The central core of the personality, the ego, the sense of personal identity, was itself fluctuating and, for want of a better phrase, dissolving.

Another subject said, 'If anyone present went out of the room it felt as though I were being deprived of something. I became smaller – definitely felt vulnerable'.

Boundaries of self in schizophrenia

In schizophrenia, the sense of invasion of self appears to be fundamental to the nature of the condition as it is experienced; many but not all *first-rank symptoms* have in common permeability of the barrier between the individual and his environment, loss of ego boundaries (Sims, 1993). There is a merging between *self* and *not self*; this is clearly portrayed in Figure 13.2, painted by a young schizophrenic patient. The patient is not aware of the disturbance being one of ego boundaries; he describes a problem only inasmuch as 'other people are doing things to me, events are taking place outside myself'. The external observer finds a blurring or loss of the boundaries of self that is not apparent to the patient himself.

All *passivity experiences* falsely attribute functions to *not self* influences from outside, which are actually coming from inside the self. This is also true for disorders of the possession of thought, such as thought insertion and thought withdrawal. Thought broadcasting obviously involves private thoughts becoming public without the consent or action of the patient. This is another example of a breakdown in the normal boundaries of what is self and non-self. Other experiences, such as *auditory hallucinations*, rely on the patient ascribing internally generated activity, that is, internal speech, to external agencies.

Passivity, *delusion of control*, is discussed in Chapter 9. The subjective experience of passivity is a disorder of the distinction between what is and what is *not*

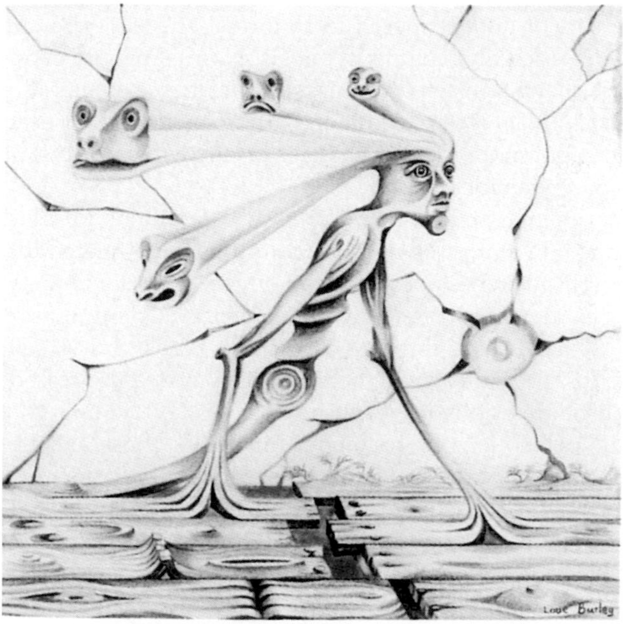

Figure 13.2 Picture by a young schizophrenic patient.

self. Sensations, emotions, impulses and actions that in objective reality come from inside the self are ascribed to *not self*.

Other alterations to boundaries

In states of *ecstasy*, there are also disturbances in the boundaries of self (Chapter 18). The participant might describe feeling at one with the universe, merging with nirvana, experiencing unity with the saints, identifying with the trees and flowers or a oneness with God. Ecstasy states occur in normal people and in those with personality disorder, as well as in sufferers from psychoses. This alteration in awareness of the boundaries of self is different from that of schizophrenia described above. In ecstasy, it is an *as if experience*, and it is mediated affectively.

The phenomenon described by Jung in himself with which this chapter begins is a lack of definition of the boundaries of self. However, there was no loss of reality judgement; it was a game, and Jung did in fact know what was himself and what was the stone. In psychosis, this ability to discriminate is lost. A schizophrenic patient said, 'I am invaded day and night. I have no more privacy since television came inside me'. Another patient believed that while he was in a hospital ward he was helping other patients because he permeated the medical staff and thereby assisted them in their work.

CLINICAL RANGE OF DISORDERS OF SELF

Alterations in the awareness of oneself occur over a very wide spectrum of states of mind and mental illness. They occur in normal people in certain normal life experiences, for example in association with exhaustion, hunger, thirst, ecstasy, acute but appropriate anxiety, sexual arousal, hypnagogic states and dreams. They also occur in normal people in abnormal circumstances, for example in divers or pilots exposed to abnormal effects of pressure or gravity, in sensory deprivation and during hypnosis. Normal people taking drugs may also experience changes in self-awareness. Some degree of alteration amounting to mild *depersonalization* is very common with many drugs, for example tricyclic antidepressants, but more marked changes occur with cannabis, mescaline and lysergic acid diethylamide.

In abnormal mental states, there are many conditions in which awareness of self is changed. In almost all neurotic conditions and related disorders, complaints about self-awareness occur. For example, in acute anxiety state, hypochondriacal disorder, dissociation with conversion symptoms and anorexia nervosa, disturbance of self-image is prominent. In psychosis, self is disturbed as part of the loss of reality judgement. For instance, a depressed patient may describe nihilistic delusions in which he believes 'everything is finished', and he ascribes the perceptions he has about himself to those beliefs: 'I am dead'. Schizophrenic patients are likely to show misinterpretation or alteration of self-perceptions with delusional elaboration. There is a very wide range of abnormalities of perception, both of the self and of parts of the body, occurring with organic states (Chapter 15).

It is, of course, an artificial distinction we make between *self-image* and *body image*, as the self is perceived as the body and *my own body* is experienced as altogether different from *body in general*. The subjective experience of disturbance in self-image is called depersonalization; this is extremely variable in its nature, and its form is related to the underlying psychiatric condition. It is discussed in Chapter 14.

Self-image in neurosis

The neurotic person, irrespective of type of neurosis, is very concerned with himself and how others see him (Chapter 22). He often feels extremely vulnerable to the harmful effects of his bad relationships with others, to exaggerated symptoms in his own body and to the destructive effects of his own neurotic thinking. This results in an all-pervading sense of subjective anxiety that influences all his planning and all his contacts with people. He feels very much alone and different; he feels threatened by 'them', whom he regards as being able to cope normally. This is well exemplified by the quotation from C. Day Lewis with which the next chapter starts. This leads him to think of himself as being absolutely unique, and this uniqueness demands all his attention so that he has great difficulty in thinking of the well-being of others.

This concern with self-image is akin to the idea of *narcissism*; it has the three qualities of total absorption with self, an all-pervading fear of loss of self and an anxiety in relationships that leads to a withdrawal from close personal contact. This disturbance of the thinking of the neurotic individual is neither intellectual nor perceptual; it is restricted to the cognitive and attitudinal realm of self-image and evaluation of personal relationships.

Panic attacks occur in situations either when the individual is stressed in terms of his personal resources to meet threatening objects or circumstances, or when tested in his competence to establish human relationships as an equal. Panic then becomes a withdrawal from this challenge and a demonstration of lack of capacity to cope. Pathological anxiety is very frequent with all neurotic disorders, not only anxiety states.

REFERENCES

Abse W (1982) Multiple personality. In Roy A (ed.) *Hysteria*. Chichester: John Wiley.

American Psychiatric Association (1987) *Diagnostic and Statistical Manual of Mental Disorders*, 3rd edn, revised. Washington: American Psychiatric Association.

Ames D (1984) Self-shooting of a phantom head. *British Journal of Psychiatry 145*, 193–4.

Anderson EW and Rawnsley K (1954) Clinical studies of lysergic diethylamide. *Monatsschrift fuer Psychiatrie und Neurologie 128*, 38–55.

Argyle M (1975) *Bodily Communication*. London: Methuen.

Bahnson CB (1969) Body and self-images associated with audio-visual self-confrontation. *Journal of Nervous and Mental Disease 148*, 262–80.

Berrios GE and Markova IS (2003) The self and psychiatry: a conceptual history. In Kircher T and David A (eds) *The Self in Neuroscience and Psychiatry*. Cambridge: Cambridge University Press.

Bonhoeffer K (1907) *Klinische Beiträge zur Lehre von den Degenerationspsychosen. Alt's Samml*, vol. 7, Halle: Marhold.

Critchley M (1950) The body image in neurology. *Lanceti*, 335–41.

Damas Mora JMR, Jenner FA and Eacott SE (1980) On heautoscopy or the phenomenon of the double: case presentation and review of the literature. *British Journal of Medical Psychology 53*, 75–83.

David AS (1990) Insight and psychosis. *British Journal of Psychiatry 156*, 798–808.

Dostoevsky F (1846) *The Double* (transl. Garnett C, 1913). London: Heinemann.

Fahy TA (1988) The diagnosis of multiple personality disorder: a critical review. *British Journal of Psychiatry 153*, 597–606.

Fish FJ (1967) *Clinical Psychopathology*. Bristol: John Wright.

Freud S (1933) New introductory lectures on psychoanalysis. In *Standard Edition of the Complete Works of Sigmund Freud*, vol. XXII (transl. Strachey J, 1964). London: Hogarth Press.

Head H and Holmes G (1911) Sensory disturbances from cerebral lesions. *Brain 34*, 102–254.

Jaspers K (1959) *General Psychopathology* (transl. Hoenig J and Hamilton MW from the German, 7th edn, 1963). Manchester: Manchester University Press.

Jung CG (1963) *Memories, Dreams, Reflections*. London: Collins Routledge & Kegan Paul.

Koehler K, Ebel H and Vartzopoulos D (1990) Lycanthropy and demonomania: some psychopathological issues. *Psychological Medicine 20*, 629–33.

Larmore K, Ludwig AM and Cain RL (1977) Multiple personality – an objective case study. *British Journal of Psychiatry 131*, 35–40.

Lukianowicz N (1958) Autoscopic phenomena. *Archives of Neurology and Psychiatry 80*, 199–220.

McDougall W (1911) *Suggestion*. Encyclopaedia Britannica.

Menninger-Lerchental E (1932) Eine Halluzination Goethes. *Zeitschrift fuer die Gesamte und Neurologie und Psychiatrie 140*, 486–95.

Merskey H (2000) Conversion and dissociation. In Gelder MG, López-Ibor JJ and Andreasen NC (eds) *New Oxford Textbook of Psychiatry*. Oxford: Oxford University Press.

Morris J (1974) *Connundrum*. London: Faber & Faber.

Nietzsche F (1901) *The Will to Power* (transl. Kaufmann W and Hollingdale RJ, 1968). New York: Vintage Books.

Prince M (1905) *The Dissociation of a Personality*. New York: Longman.

Roberts G and Owen J (1988) The near-death experience. *British Journal of Psychiatry 153*, 607–17.

Scharfetter C (1981) Ego-psychopathology: the concept and its empirical evaluation. *Psychological Medicine 11*, 273–80.

Scharfetter C (1995) *The Self-experience of Schizophrenics: Empirical Studies of the Ego/Self in Schizophrenia, Borderline Disorders and Depression*. Zurich: private publication.

Scharfetter C (2003) The self-experience of schizophrenics. In Kircher T and David A (eds) *The Self in Neuroscience and Psychiatry*. Cambridge: Cambridge University Press.

Schilder P (1935) *The Image and Appearance of the Human Body: Studies in the Constructive Energies of the Psyche*. London: Kegan Paul.

Sims ACP (1993) Schizophrenia and permeability of self. *Neurology, Psychiatry and Brain Research 1*, 133–5.

Sims ACP (1994) Myself and my other self: the 'double phenomenon' in neurotic disorder. In Sensky T, Katona C and Montgomery S (eds) *Psychiatry in Europe: Directions and Developments*. London: Gaskell.

Slater E and Roth M (1969) Personality deviations and neurotic reactions. *Clinical Psychiatry: Mayer-Gross W, Slater E and Roth M*, 3rd edn. London: Baillière Tindall & Cassell.

Stevenson RLB (1889) *The Master of Ballantrae*. London: Collins.

Styron W (1991) *Darkness Visible*. London: Jonathan Cape.

Todd J and Dewhurst K (1962) The significance of the Doppelgänger (hallucinatory double) in folk-lore and neuropsychiatry. *Practitioner 188*, 377–82.

Wijesinghe CP, Dissanayake SAW and Mendis N (1976) Possession trance in a semi-urban community in Sri Lanka. *Australia and New Zealand Journal of Psychiatry 10*, 135–9.

World Health Organization (1992) *The ICD-10 Classification of Mental and Behavioural Disorders: Clinical Description and Diagnostic Guidelines*. Geneva: World Health Organization.

Zahavi D (2003) Phenomenology of self. In Kircher T and David A (eds) *The Self in Neuroscience and Psychiatry*. Cambridge: Cambridge University Press.

Depersonalization

14

> "But could you lift his blue, thick gaze and pass
> Behind, you would walk a stage where endlessly
> Phantoms rehearse unactable tragedy.
> 'In free air captive, in full day benighted,
> I am as one for ever out of his element
> Transparently enwombed, who from a bathysphere
> Observes, wistful, amazed, but more affrighted,
> Gay fluent forms of life weaving around,
> And dares not break the bubble and be drowned.' *C. Day Lewis (1948)*

DEFINITIONS AND DESCRIPTIONS

Depersonalization is the term used to designate a peculiar change in the awareness of self, in which the individual feels as if he is unreal (Sedman, 1972). It is best to reserve the use of the word to this *as if* feeling rather than the experience of unreality that occurs in psychosis. The *as if* prefix is used by the patient to denote that he is not using words literally (how could he know what it would be like not 'fitting into the world', as all his experience has been in the world?). He is expressing uncertainty and painting a picture, and 'as if' is the best way he can do it. This *as if* experience is an extremely common *symptom*, occurring, for example, on careful enquiry in 30 per cent of all new consecutive psychiatric outpatient referrals in an unpublished series of mine. It has been considered that, after depression and anxiety, depersonalization is the most frequent symptom to occur in psychiatry (Stewart, 1964).

Schilder (1928), whose classical monograph in 1914 was a turning point in the study of depersonalization, wrote:

> "To the depersonalized individual, the world appears strange, peculiar, foreign, dream-like. Objects appear at times strangely diminished in size, at times flat. Sounds appear to come from a distance. The tactile characteristics of objects likewise seem strangely altered. Patients characterize their imagery as pale, colourless and some complain that they have altogether lost the power of imagination. The emotions likewise undergo marked alteration. Patients complain they are capable of experiencing neither pain nor pleasure; love and hate have perished with them. They experience a fundamental change in their personality, and the climax is reached with their complaints that they have become strangers to themselves. It is as though they were dead, lifeless, mere automatons.

Depersonalization has been defined by Fewtrell (1986) as a subjective state of unreality in which there is a feeling of estrangement, either from a sense of self or from the external environment.

A more comprehensive definition has been given by Ackner (1954). Positive features are:

- depersonalization is always subjective; it is a disorder of experience
- the experience is that of an internal or external change characterized by a feeling of strangeness or unreality
- the experience is unpleasant
- any mental functions may be the subject of this change, but affect is invariably involved
- insight is preserved.

Excluded from depersonalization are:

- the experience of unreality of self when there is delusional elaboration
- the ego boundary disorders of schizophrenia
- the loss or attenuation of personal identity.

An even more comprehensive description is given in Sierra and Berrios (2001). The symptoms are listed in Box 14.1.

The relationship between depersonalization and various theoretical aspects of self-perception in phenomenology has been reviewed by Mellor (1988), who discusses the influences of Jaspers (1959), Mayer-Gross (1935), Schilder (1920) and Schneider (1958) on the concept. Mellor comments on the frequency of the condition and the variety of different psychiatric illnesses with which it may be associated. It may occur with organic psychosyndromes, especially temporal lobe disorders, cannabis use (Matthew *et al.*, 1993), hysterical dissociation and depressive illness, and less commonly with other conditions.

Although the symptom has been described for longer, the term was used by Heymans (1904) and by Dugas and Moutier in 1911. The earliest theories

Box 14.1 Components of depersonalization

- Emotional numbing
- Changes in body experience
- Changes in visual experience
- Changes in auditory experience
- Changes in tactile experience
- Changes in gustatory experience
- Changes in olfactory experience
- Loss of feelings of agency
- Distortions in the experiencing of time
- Changes in the subjective experience of memory
- Feelings of thought emptiness
- Subjective feelings of an inability to evoke images
- Heightened self-observation

(After Sierra and Berrios, 2001, with permission.)

implicate the sensory system, but loss of mood and loss of feelings were also prominent in early descriptions (Sierra and Berrios, 1997). Frequently, depersonalization is accompanied by the symptom of *derealization*, a term used by Mapother (1935) to denote a similar change in the awareness of the external world. Depersonalization and derealization often go together, because the ego and its environment are experienced as one continuous whole. However, in Mayer-Gross' cases, about a quarter of patients had depersonalization without derealization and 15 per cent had only derealization. The less a patient takes himself for granted, the more unfamiliar and alien does the world around him become (Scharfetter, 1980). A young female patient said:

> " I felt as if I didn't fit into the world. ... When I saw the moon, I felt I couldn't cope. One day it wasn't there and the next it was. I saw it and it upset me and I went to pieces. ... I felt I did not want to be alive because I was not related to anything. I just seemed totally out of everything and I started to cry. I couldn't cope with the hurt and the pain. I felt I never would feel part of anything.

It is important to realize that depersonalization, the experience, like other non-psychotic phenomena, occurs in healthy, normal people. Some people may have feelings of 'not being quite themselves ... looking in on themselves from the outside' and so on, without provocation. Others may have such experiences at times of powerful emotional stimuli or life crisis of any valence: extreme happiness, falling in love, the loss of bereavement or intense fear or anger. The actual self-description of depersonalization is similar in normality to that of mentally ill people describing the symptom.

There is one particular feature described by patients and not occurring in the depersonalization that healthy people, especially children, may experience spontaneously in states of fatigue, after prolonged sleep deprivation or under sensory deprivation. This is the patient's description of the experience being intensely unpleasant (Ackner, 1954). It may subjectively be much the worst symptom in an affective, reactive illness. A young married woman said, 'I feel very weird in my head. I have a great deal of torment. My mind will not leave me alone. It's the surroundings; I cannot get my mind to myself. I felt as though I was going to fall over. I feel as if I'm lost in a fog. I just feel as if I'm not in my head. I feel numb'.

The symptom is described in a number of different ways, and it is often impossible to make a distinction between depersonalization and derealization: 'everything seemed to be going away from me'. The four qualities of the experience of self described in Chapter 13 may each be involved in the description of symptoms, although always with this *as if* character: activity, singleness, identity (continuity) and boundaries or definition. There is virtually always other evidence of disturbance of mood present: depression or anxiety or both. Coupled with this is a feeling of loss of self-esteem as a very prominent symptom: 'I feel unreal, flat, not properly there, less of a person, as though I can't go and get stuck in'; that is, the feeling of unreality about oneself or one's environment has implications for lack of competence in relationships. The patient not only feels unreal but also 'detached'; there is a barrier to normal communication.

At this point, it is important to emphasize the distinction between depersonalization as a symptom, occurring associated with many psychiatric conditions or no disorder at all, and depersonalization as a syndrome (F48.1, depersonalization – derealization syndrome, in ICD-10, World Health Organization, 1992; or 300.6, depersonalization disorder, in DSM-IV, American Psychiatric Association, 1994). In their detailed description of the symptoms of depersonalization disorder, based on classical descriptions from authors in the nineteenth and early twentieth centuries, Sierra and Berrios (2001) have listed the following four symptoms as most prevalent for diagnosis: emotional numbing, changes in visual perception, changes in the experience of the body and loss of feelings of agency. There are features of the disorder that are additional to the symptom itself.

Thus these symptoms are sometimes included with a description of depersonalization but, for the sake of clarity, should be separated and regarded as different psychopathological phenomena. Disturbances of body image or schema, disorder of subjective time sense, hypochondriacal preoccupation, *déjà vu* phenomena or metamorphopsia (the distortion of visually perceived objects) may be described by the same individual and may occur as symptoms of depersonalization syndrome. Langfeldt's (1960) inclusion of schizophrenic passivity experiences within the term depersonalization is confusing, and these experiences should be excluded from depersonalization, both as a symptom and as a disorder.

Subjective experience of depersonalization

Depersonalization is difficult for the doctor to portray; more important, it is extraordinarily difficult also for the patient to describe. He often prefaces his attempts at description by embarrassed statements such as 'sometimes I think I must be going mad' or 'you will think me very peculiar when I tell you this doctor, but...' Then follows a halting and perplexed list of disjointed, unpleasant experiences that the patient feels to be unique and for which he is unable to construe metaphors that satisfy him. Because of his failure in description, he believes that others will find these symptoms either bogus or clear evidence of imminent madness, so he omits them from his initial account even though such symptoms are very common among psychiatric patients and cause enormous suffering. Depersonalization is the symptom the patient has when he experiences himself as being altered or deficient within his inner space; derealization is its equivalent in his outer space, with regard to things outside himself. Because there is no definite and easily ascertained boundary containing self, it is not always easy to decide whether the disorder is depersonalization or derealization. Neither is this important: they merge and overlap and are often simply included within the term *depersonalization*.

There is always a change in mood with depersonalization: the patient loses the *feeling* of familiarity he has for himself or for the world outside himself. He may describe himself as feeling like a puppet: hollow, detached and strange; on the outside; uninvolved with life; not himself; like a ghost, not solid; a stranger to himself. He experiences a loss of emotion. Similarly, with derealization he may describe his environment as flat, dim in colour, smaller, distant, cloudy, dreamlike, still, 'nothing to do with me' and also lacking in emotional significance.

Depersonalization is so common, and to the patient so obscure and unpleasant, that, whenever the description of symptoms is interrupted by the patient's baffled hesitancy, he should be questioned with possible depersonalization symptoms in mind. His relief at finding someone prepared to listen, and even perhaps understand, is often enormous. Schilder (1935) has described these symptoms thus:

> “In a case of depersonalization the individual feels completely changed from what he was previously. This change is present in the ego (self) as well as in the outside world and the individual does not recognize himself as a personality. His actions appear to him as automatic. He observes his actions and behaviour from the point of view of a spectator. The outside world is foreign and new to him and is not as real as before.

Schilder is using the word *personality* to refer to the whole person, not only personality in the modern sense of the word. This changed awareness of self and its relationships with the environment is always experienced as being intensely unpleasant.

The localization of this symptom to an individual organ is called *desomatization*. There are many different possible parameters in the awareness of different organs: changes of size or quality, for example appearing large or tiny, or empty, or detached or filled with water or foam. The patient may have a feeling of his legs being weightless, of floating or of simply being unfamiliar. Koro, a culture-bound disorder described by Yap (1965), is sometimes described as an example of depersonalization. It is probably best to regard this condition as a culture-specific manifestation of acute anxiety in which the patient believes his penis is shrinking and fears that it will ultimately disappear.

Change of feeling concerning the body or depersonalization may be associated with distortion of time sense, when the passage of time appears altered in some way: ‘time, both past and present, seems quite unreal to me, as if it had never happened and was never going to happen’. People with depersonalization are in doubt about just what is troubling them; they may preface their description with *‘as if’*, and it is this element of uncertainty that occurs in the depersonalization of both healthy and neurotic people and differentiates them from the delusions about the self occurring in psychoses. *Deaffectualization* has been used to describe the consistent loss of the capacity to feel emotion, so that the person seems unable to cry, love or hate (Anonymous, 1972).

A patient says, ‘I am going mad inside my head’; on further questioning, he is describing finding his own mental processes to be strange. The feeling of familiarity that occurs when a person perceives previously known objects (opening the front door at home and looking inside) also occurs when one introspects into one’s own thinking (remembering or *fantasizing* my front hall). I know what is there in my thoughts; I know what I will think about any particular object, because it is unlikely to be very different from what I thought about it last time. I also know, in general terms, what I will think about myself because of past experience. It is this assumed certainty that disappears; the loss of familiarity of oneself occurring in depersonalization, or of outside self in derealization, is similar to the abnormality of the feeling of familiarity occurring in *jamais vu* (when there is no sense of previously having seen a well-known object) and its opposite, *déjà vu* (when an unfamiliar object or experience seems to be familiar). This association between the subjective experiences in depersonalization and *déjà vu* phenomena and their common origins in alteration in the feeling of familiarity has been known since the work of Heymans at the beginning of the last century (Sno and Draaisma, 1993).

Like other aspects of self-experience, depersonalization has social and situational aspects. Frequently, the person feels that he is less able to accept himself, his personality, his behaviour than other people accept their own. He considers that his feelings about himself, his loss of reality, is unique. This is a barrier to his giving an account of his symptoms, and this in its turn is a barrier to communication in all areas of life. He feels himself to be different, isolated and ostracized. Depersonalization is an experience within an individual, but it has considerable social consequences.

It frequently occurs in attacks that may be of any duration from seconds to months. Typically, in depersonalization disorder the altered state lasts for a few hours, in temporal lobe epilepsy for a few minutes and in anxiety disorder for a few seconds. Improvement is usually first manifested in a gradual increase in time free from symptoms rather than a reduction in the symptoms themselves when present.

Onset may be insidious and with no known initiating cause, or it may be in response to provocation. A middle-aged man who described his depersonalization 'like something supernatural – my body separated from me – a lost feeling' vividly recalled his first attack at the age of 11, when undergoing anaesthesia for the reduction of a fracture. Subsequent attacks felt similar despite the absence of provocation. He had also experienced attacks of sleep paralysis since the age of 25 and had discovered that by keeping himself awake until very tired he would fall asleep more quickly and thus avoid it. Another man was severely stressed by his quite unreasonable working conditions, hours of work, unsympathetic employer and difficult car journeys in the course of his work. Early one winter morning, he had an appalling journey through fog, along crowded motorways blocked by accidents, and finally suffered a lapse of recall for 24 hours in which he remembered nothing of driving to another town, registering himself into a hotel, ordering a meal, hanging up his clothes tidily and going to bed. His next memory was arriving at a local hospital the next day. He remained depersonalized for years subsequently, and his wife described this as 'he's not the man I married; it's like his twin brother'.

Depersonalization is frequently situational, both in its original cause and in its repeated provocation. Many policemen who were involved in a major disaster at a football ground described depersonalization among other symptoms of post-traumatic stress disorder, sometimes lasting for years subsequently (Sims and Sims, 1998). One man described feeling 'switched off. ... I felt I wasn't on this planet any more'. Because depersonalization occurs at times of great stress, it may occur in the perpetrator of antisocial behaviour, for example violent crime, as well as in the victim. Rix and Clarkson (1994) give an account of a man who savagely assaulted his wife with a large spanner: 'It was as if it was a dream or a nightmare. I realized later what I had done but at the time it was as if I wasn't there'. It was considered that depersonalization in this case was linked to dissociation, that although it represented a change in the individual's self-experience it did not affect his volition or intent.

Although, in these two cases, depersonalization was associated with dissociation, this is not a common association, and depression and anxiety much more frequently occur alongside depersonalization. In DSM-IV (American Psychiatric

Association, 1994), depersonalization is classified as a dissociation disorder. This is misleading psychopathologically, as the two experiences, depersonalization and dissociation, are quite different as described by the patient and observed by the doctor, and not necessarily associated. They may occur in the same patient, although usually at different times. More frequently, they do not occur together. Depersonalization, as a symptom, is more frequently associated with both depression and anxiety than with dissociation. Putnam *et al.* (1996) have shown that depersonalization does not lie on a continuum with dissociation. Neither does it occur with any greater frequency with chronic dissociative disorders such as dissociative identity disorder, formerly multiple personality disorder in DSM-IV (Ross, 1997).

Self-induced episodes of depersonalization, as an unpleasant symptom, have been recorded following particular patterns of behaviour. Thus Kennedy (1976) described self-induced depersonalization persisting as a complaint after transcendental meditation and yoga.

ORGANIC AND PSYCHOLOGICAL THEORIES

Theories accounting for the occurrence of depersonalization, including organic, psychological, psychoanalytic and those linking it with schizophrenia, were reviewed by Sedman (1970). Depersonalization is regularly cited as a common symptom associated with organic states, especially temporal lobe epilepsy (Sedman and Kenna, 1965). This is based on the contention of Mayer-Gross (1935) that depersonalization is a *preformed functional response* of the brain, that is, a non-specific mechanism resulting from many different influences on the brain, occurring in an idiosyncratic way in individuals in a similar manner to epileptic fits or delirium. He was, in this, following the neurophysiological hierarchical concepts of Hughlings Jackson (1884), who considered that the highest levels of cerebral function were lost first, leaving uninterrupted the activity of lower levels.

Organic theories purporting to account for depersonalization would suggest that alteration of consciousness acts as a release mechanism. However, Sedman (1970), in reviewing the literature, showed that, even in various forms of organic psychosyndromes, the incidence of depersonalization phenomena was similar to that found in the general population, at between 25 and 50 per cent; in more severe chronic organic psychosis, the rate was lower. From a variety of studies, no quantitative relationship had been demonstrated between the degree of *torpor* (that is, the stage on the continuum from full alertness to unconsciousness) and the development of depersonalization. On studying the performance of depersonalized subjects on psychosomatic tests, there did not appear to be evidence to support a specific relationship between clouding of consciousness and depersonalization. There appeared to be many individuals who, despite various types of assault on their brains, never developed depersonalization.

From this information, Sedman (1970) concluded that:

> “there may well be a *built in* preformed mechanism in approximately 40 per cent of the population to exhibit depersonalization; that the factors which initiate such a response are not specifically those associated with clouding of consciousness; or where clouding of consciousness appears to be playing a part it may well be the presence of another common factor that is more relevant.

Thus, the relationship between depersonalization and brain pathology remains unclear. Depersonalization is certainly not pathognomonic of organic diseases; in fact, there is no organic or psychotic abnormality in the vast majority of sufferers.

The state of increased alertness observed in depersonalization is considered by Sierra and Berrios (1998) to result from activation of prefrontal attentional systems and reciprocal inhibition of the anterior cingulate, leading to experiences of 'mind emptiness' and 'indifference to pain'. The lack of emotional colouring, reported as feelings of unreality, would be accounted for by a left-sided prefrontal mechanism with inhibition of the amygdala.

Depersonalization is sometimes associated with self-induced organic states. Thus, it occurs following the ingestion of alcohol or drugs, especially psychotomimetics such as lysergic acid diethylamide (Sedman and Kenna, 1964), mescaline, marijuana (Szymanski, 1981) and cannabis (Carney *et al.*, 1984), and with sensory deprivation. It is also described as a side effect with prescribed psychotropic drugs such as the tricyclic antidepressants, but because of the common association between depersonalization and depression it is difficult always to attribute cause.

DEPERSONALIZATION: NEUROTIC OR PSYCHOTIC?

Sometimes, there has been considerable confusion as to whether depersonalization can be distinguished from the disorders of self-image described in Chapter 13 as occurring in schizophrenia. In fact, passivity experiences have even been described as a variant of depersonalization. However, Meyer (1956), as cited by Sedman (1970), has distinguished schizophrenic ego disturbances from depersonalization on phenomenological grounds; that is, on the description by the patient of his own internal experience. It is, of course, well recognized that true depersonalization symptoms do occur in schizophrenic patients, especially in the early stages of the illness, alongside definite schizophrenic psychopathology.

Depersonalization is commonly described in manic–depressive disorder; however, the symptoms occur only in the depressive phase and there are no references to depersonalization occurring in mania (Sedman, 1970). Anderson (1938) considered that *ecstasy states* occurring in manic–depressive disorders were the obverse of *depersonalization* and that, while the former occurred in mania, the latter occurred with depression. Sedman (1972), in an investigation of three matched groups, each of 18 subjects with depersonalization and depressive and anxiety symptoms, considered that the results stressed the importance of depressed mood in depersonalization, while anxiety seemed to carry no significant relationship.

Many other authors have stressed the close association between the symptoms of depersonalization and anxiety. For instance, Roth (1959, 1960) described the *phobic anxiety depersonalization syndrome* as a separate nosological entity, but saw it as a form of anxiety neurosis on which the additional symptoms are superimposed in a particular group of individuals. He considered depersonalization to be more common with anxiety than with other affective disorders, for example depression. The phobic symptoms are usually agoraphobic in nature. The patient, most often female, married and often in the third decade of life, has a great fear of being conspicuous in an embarrassing way in public, for example fainting or being taken ill suddenly on a bus or in a supermarket. Fear of leaving the house unaccompanied develops from this, so that the patient is frightened of being at a distance from familiar surroundings without some supporting figure to whom she can turn. She may be unable to go out of the house at all, even with her husband. She may feel panicky on her own at home and so keeps her child off school, a potential precipitating factor in subsequent school refusal.

The symptom of dizziness is a very common complaint and frequently results in referral to ear, nose and throat departments. Fewtrell and O'Connor (1989) discuss two possible models for the relationship of this condition to depersonalization: one that dizziness and depersonalization are the same experience described differently; the other, a bipolar hypothesis, proposes that the two experiences form opposite ends of a dimension describing disturbed *self–outside world* relationships.

Depersonalization symptoms are commonly described in association with agoraphobia, other phobic states, panic disorder, various types of depressive condition, post-traumatic stress disorder and other non-psychotic conditions. It may also appear as the isolated syndrome, and Davison (1964) has described episodic depersonalization in which other aetiological factors are not prominent. The *International Classification of Diseases* (World Health Organization, 1992), as mentioned above, describes the distinct category of depersonalization–derealization syndrome:

> “ a disorder in which the sufferer complains that his or her mental activity, body and/or surroundings are changed in their quality so as to be unreal, remote or automatized. *(p. 171)*

However, symptoms of depersonalization are commonly found in association with many varied neurotic conditions and, in practice, the different neurotic syndromes are not mutually exclusive but overlap in their symptomatology (Sims, 1983).

Certain personality types are more regularly associated with complaint of depersonalization and may therefore be regarded as predisposing; anankastic or obsessional personality disorder, in particular, has been implicated. Such personalities are:

> “ characterized by feelings of personal insecurity, doubt and incompleteness leading to excessive conscientiousness, checking, stubbornness and caution. There may be insistent and unwelcome thoughts or impulses which do not attain the severity of an obsessional neurosis. There is perfectionism and meticulous accuracy and a need to check repeatedly in an attempt to ensure this. Rigidity and excessive doubt may be conspicuous. *(World Health Organization, 1977)*

Introversion, as measured on the Eysenck Personality Inventory, is also found to be associated with greater frequency of depersonalization symptoms (Reed and Sedman, 1964). When symptoms are present, the neuroticism score on this scale is also raised but returns to normal levels on recovery.

In psychoanalytic theory, depersonalization has taken on a rather different meaning, and therefore there are different explanations for its origin. Psychoanalysts have been less concerned with describing the phenomena than the underlying concept of the alienation of the ego. For example, in the work of the existentialist school, as typified by Binswanger (1963), there is discussion of the *depersonalization of man*.

> "This depersonalization has by now gone so far that the psychiatrist (even more than the psychoanalyst) can no longer simply say, 'I', 'you', or 'he' wants, wishes etc. the only phrases that would correspond to the phenomenal facts. Theoretical constructs dispose him, rather, to speak instead of my, your, or his Ego wishing something. In this depersonalization we see at work that aspect of psychiatry's founding charter that is most at odds with every attempt to establish a genuine psychology. An explanation of this baleful influence need go no further than the clearly recognized task that psychiatry, since Griesinger, has set itself – namely, to create a psychology that, on the one hand, serves to bring a reified functional complex into relation with a material 'organ' but that, on the other hand, allows this organ itself to be divided into and understood in terms of its functions.

This clearly is quite a different sense of the word than the phenomenological, with which this chapter has been concerned.

The distressing experience of depersonalization, with a feeling of unreality, remains central to the description of the disordered self. The disturbance that causes this may be organic or environmental, psychotic or existential. Concern about the experience of self and of the environment most commonly occur together.

REFERENCES

[Anonymous] (1972) Depersonalisation syndromes [leading article]. *British Medical Journal 4*, 378.

Ackner B (1954) Depersonalization I. Aetiology and phenomenology II. Clinical syndromes. *Journal of Mental Science 100*, 838–72.

American Psychiatric Association (1994) *Diagnostic and Statistical Manual of Mental Disorders*, 4th edn. Washington: American Psychiatric Association.

Anderson EW (1938) A clinical study of states of 'ecstasy' occurring in affective disorders. *Journal of Neurology and Psychiatry* 1, 1–20.

Binswanger L (1963) Being-in-the world. In *Selected Papers of Ludwig Binswanger* (transl. Needleman J, 1975). London: Basic Books.

Carney MWP, Bacelle L and Robinson B (1984) Psychosis after cannabis abuse. *British Medical Journal 288*, 1047.

Davison K (1964) Episodic depersonalisation: observations on seven patients. *British Journal of Psychiatry 110*, 505–13.

Day Lewis C (1948) The Neurotic. In *Poems 1943–1947*, pp. 76–77. London: Cape.

Dugas L and Moutier F (1911) *La Depersonalisation*. Paris: Felix Alcon.

Fewtrell WD (1986) Depersonalization: a description and suggested strategies. *British Journal of Guidance and Counselling 14*, 263–9.

Fewtrell WD and O'Connor KP (1989) Dizziness and depersonalization. *Advances in Behaviour Research and Therapy 10*, 201–18.

Heymans G (1904) Eine Enquête über Depersonalisation und 'Fausse Reconnaisance'. *Zeitschrift fuer Psychologie 36*, 321–43.

Jackson JH (1884) Croonian lectures on evolution and dissolution of the nervous system. In Taylor J (ed.) (1958) *Selected Writings of John Hughlings Jackson*, vol. II, pp. 3–120. London: Staples Press.

Jaspers K (1959) *General Psychopathology*, 7th edn. (transl. Hoenig J and Hamilton MW, 1963). Manchester: Manchester University Press.

Kennedy RB (1976) Self-induced depersonalization syndrome. *American Journal of Psychiatry 133*, 1326–8.

Langfeldt G (1960) Diagnosis and prognosis of schizophrenia. *Proceedings of the Royal Society of Medicine 52*, 595–6.

Mapother E (1935) cited by Mayer-Gross (1935).

Matthew RJ, Wilson WH, Humphreys D, Lowe JV and Weithe KE (1993) Depersonalization after marijuana smoking. *Biological Psychiatry 33*, 431–41.
Mayer-Gross W (1935) On depersonalisation. *British Journal of Medical Psychology 15*, 103–22.
Mellor CS (1988) Depersonalisation and self-perception. *British Journal of Psychiatry 153* (suppl. 2), 15–9.
Meyer JE (1956) Studien zur Depersonalisation. *Psychiatrie et Neurologie(Basel) 132*, 221–32.
Putnam FW, Carlson EB, Ross CA, *et al.* (1996) Patterns of dissociation in clinical and non-clinical samples. *Journal of Nervous and Mental Disease 11*, 673–9.
Reed GF and Sedman G (1964) Personality and depersonalisation under sensory deprivation conditions. *Perceptual and Motor Skills 18*, 659–60.
Rix KJB and Clarkson (1994) Depersonalisation and intent. *Journal of Forensic Psychiatry 5*, 409–19.
Ross C (1997) *Dissociative Identity Disorder: Diagnosis, Clinical Features and Treatment of Multiple Personality*. New York: John Wiley.
Roth M (1959) The phobic anxiety–depersonalization syndrome. *Proceedings of the Royal Society of Medicine 52*, 587–95.
Roth M (1960) The phobic anxiety–depersonalization syndrome and some general aetiological problems in psychiatry. *Journal of Neuropsychiatry 1*, 292–306.
Scharfetter C (1980) *General Psychopathology: an Introduction*. Cambridge: Cambridge University Press.
Schilder P (1920) *Medizinische Psychologie* (transl. Rapaport D, 1953, as *Medical Psychologie*). New York: International Universities Press.
Schilder P (1928) Depersonalisation. In *Introduction to Psychoanalytic Psychiatry. Nervous and Mental Disease Monograph* series 50.
Schilder P (1935) *The Image and Appearance of the Human Body: Studies in the Constructive Energies of the Psyche*. London: Kegan Paul.
Schneider K (1958) *Clinical Psychopathology*, 5th edn (transl. Hamilton MW). New York: Grune & Stratton.
Sedman G (1970) Theories of depersonalisation: a reappraisal. *British Journal of Psychiatry 117*, 1–14.
Sedman G (1972) An investigation of certain factors concerned in the aetiology of depersonalisation. *Acta Psychiatrica Scandinavica 48*, 191–219.
Sedman G and Kenna JC (1964) The occurrence of depersonalisation phenomena under LSD. *Psychiatrie et Neurologie (Basel) 147*, 129–37.
Sedman G and Kenna JC (1965) Depersonalisation in temporal lobe epilepsy and the organic psychoses. *British Journal of Psychiatry 111*, 293–9.
Sierra M and Berrios GE (1997) Depersonalization: a conceptual history. *History of Psychiatry 8*, 213–29.
Sierra M and Berrios GE (1998) Depersonalization: neurobiological perspectives. *Biological Psychiatry 44*, 898–908.
Sierra M and Berrios GE (2001) The phenomenological stability of depersonalization: comparing the old with the new. *Journal of Nervous and Mental Diseases 189*, 629–36.
Sims ACP (1983) *Neurosis in Society*. Basingstoke: Macmillan.
Sims A and Sims D (1998) The phenomenology of post-traumatic stress disorder: a symptomatic study of 70 victims of psychological trauma. *Psychopathology 31*, 96–112.
Sno HM and Draaisma D (1993) An early Dutch study of déjà vu experiences. *Psychological Medicine 23*, 17–26.
Stewart WA (1964) Panel on depersonalization. *Journal of the American Psychoanalytic Association 12*, 171–86.
Szymanski HV (1981) Prolonged depersonalization after marijuana use. *American Journal of Psychiatry 138*, 231–3.
World Health Organization (1977) *International Statistical Classification of Diseases, Injuries and Causes of Death*, 9th revision. Geneva: World Health Organization.
World Health Organization (1992) *The ICD-10 Classification of Mental and Behavioural Disorders: Clinical Description and Diagnostic Guidelines*. Geneva: World Health Organization.
Yap PM (1965) Koro – a culture-bound depersonalisation syndrome. *British Journal of Psychiatry 111*, 43–50.

Disorder of the Awareness of the Body

15

> "Beside fear and sorrow, 'sharp belchings, fulsome crudities, heat in the bowels, wind and rumblings in the guts, vehement gripings, pain in the belly and stomach sometimes after meat that is hard of concoction, much watering of the stomach, and moist spittle, cold sweat.' *Robert Burton (1577–1640),* The Anatomy of Melancholia
>
> To some, ill health is
> a way to be important,
> Others are stoics,
> a few fanatics,
> who won't feel happy until
> they are cut open. *W.H. Auden (1969)*

The body is the physical manifestation of the individual being. It is the material, corporeal interface with the external world. The world is experienced through the body's senses. The body, also, is itself experienced as an object. The physicality of the body is ever present: there is density, mass, movement, action, speed, position, heat, cold and various degrees of touch, pain and so on. Since Descartes (1596–1650), the relationship between mind and body has stimulated much investigation and discussion. Descartes' original claim was that the mind and body are distinct and different; furthermore, that the mind can exist without the body. There are other theories that attempt to account for the nature of mind and body. Materialist theories propose that the body is all there is, and variations of these theories account for mind in different ways, whereas idealist theories make the opposite claim that the mind is all that exists. The fact that many descriptions of mood, cognition, volition and other psychological functions are expressed in physical terms – 'a heavy heart', 'bone-headed', 'guts and determination', 'a pain in the neck' – underlines the inextricable relationship between mind and body. It also emphasizes the degree to which bodily metaphors are used to express feelings. Whether these metaphors originally derive from the physical manifestations of emotional distress or whether the language, that is, the metaphor, structures the experience is a moot point. What is clear is that there is no ready division between the subjective experience of self and of body. A 10-year-old girl put this relationship thus: 'You feel better if you've done your homework; if you haven't you get a horrible pain in your stomach'. In order to form a cohesive framework for conceptualizing the disorders of self and the very diverse abnormalities of body image, one needs to apply the methods of descriptive psychopathology (Sims, 1988). In Chapter 13, the nature of self and the pathology of the experience of self were discussed. In this chapter, disorders of the awareness of body are discussed.

CLASSIFICATION

Cutting (1997) gives a good outline for the classification of disorders of awareness of the body, which has been adapted for this chapter (Table 15.1). There are disorders of beliefs about the body including beliefs of illness, disease and death (see below). In this group are also the disorders of dissatisfaction with the body, which occurs in eating disorders. These dissatisfactions with the body are best understood as arising from negative cognitive evaluations, that is, beliefs about the body. Next, there are disorders of bodily function, including the loss of sensory, motor or cognitive function that occurs in the dissociative disorders. There are disorders of the experience of the physical characteristics of the body. These include disorders of the experience of the size, shape, structure or weight of the body. When size is affected, the body may feel smaller (*microsomatognosia*) or bigger (*macrosomatognosia*). These experiences can affect either the whole body or part of it such as the limbs or head. The shape can be experienced as misshapen: 'My lower jaw is twisted and my teeth no longer close properly' or 'My left arm is shrunken and gnarled, a bit like a tree trunk'. When the structure of the body is affected, often it is the internal organs that are the focus of concern: 'I assert therefore that on my body, particularly on my bosom, there are present the properties of a nervous system corresponding to a female body and I am certain that a physical examination would confirm this'

Table 15.1 Classification of disorders of awareness of the body

Classification	Details
Beliefs about the body	
Illness and disease	Hypochondriacal symptoms
Body dissatisfaction	Real and ideal body weight discrepancy
Function of the body	
Sensory deficits	For example dissociative sensory loss (blindness)
Experience of physical characteristics of the body	
Size	Microsomatognosia, macrosomoatognosia and body image disturbance
Shape	'My jaws are misshapen.'
Colour	Skin colour may be experienced as lighter
Structure	'My lungs are connected to my abdomen.'
Weight	Feelings of lightness or heaviness
Experience of emotional value of the body	
Anosognosic overestimation	Exaggeration of body's strength
Misoplegia	Hatred of body part
Dysmorphophobia	Feeling of ugliness or defect of body or one of its parts
Experience of sensory awareness of the body and the world	
Palinaptia	Persistence of sensation beyond the duration of contact with stimuli
Exosomesthesia	Cutaneous sensation in extrapersonal space
Alloaesthesia	Experience of sensation on contralateral side to stimulation

(After Cutting, 1997, with permission of Oxford University Press.)

and 'Food and drink taken simply poured into the abdominal cavity and into the thighs, a process which however unbelievable it may sound, was beyond all doubt for me as I distinctly remember the sensation' (Schreber, 1955). Changes in the experience of weight can involve a sense of either heaviness or lightness.

There are complex disorders of the sensory experience of the body that almost exclusively derive from neurological lesions. *Palinaptia* is the experience of tactile sensation outlasting the stimulus, so that an object held in the hand continues to be perceived well after it has been discarded. Stacy (1987) reports a case of a patient with biparietal lesions who could feel her toothbrush in her hand 15 minutes after putting it away. The palinaptic experience occurred in the setting of astereognosis and palpatory apraxia. The palinaptia can be conceived as a complex haptic hallucination. *Exosomesthesia* is the 'displacement of cutaneous sensation into extrapersonal space' (Shapiro and Fink, 1952; Shapiro *et al.*, 1952). This is a curious condition in which the individual experiences direct cutaneous touch sensation as an object in the room that is distal from them being touched.

> " If the palm of his hand was in contact with some object (bed, table, book) and the dorsum of that pricked with a pin, the patient insisted that the bed or table had been touched and not his hand. This phenomenon could be elicited only from the hand and only when the palm was in contact with some object.

This unusual phenomenon can be experimentally induced, and it has been suggested that the body image, despite its appearance of durability and permanence, is a transitory internal construct that can be altered by the stimulus contingencies and correlations that are encountered (Ramachandran and Hirstein, 1998).

> " It is even possible to 'project' tactile sensations onto inanimate objects such as tables and shoes that do not resemble body parts. The subject is asked to place his right hand below a table surface (or behind a vertical screen) so that he cannot see it. The experimenter then uses his right hand to randomly stroke and tap the subject's right hand (under the table or behind the screen) and uses his left hand to simultaneously stroke and tap the table in perfect synchrony... After 10–30 s, the subject starts developing the uncanny illusion that the sensations are now coming from the table and that the table is now part of his body.

Alloaesthesia is a neurological condition following right-sided vascular lesions of the putamen that is characterized by a sensory stimulus on one side of the body being perceived on the contralateral side. It can also occur following spinal cord lesions such as cervical tumours, cervical disc herniation and multiple sclerosis (Fukutake *et al.*, 1993; Kawamura *et al.*, 1987).

The value attached to the body can be disturbed. This disturbance can vary from strong, positive overvaluation of the body or its parts to a devaluation of the body extending to dislike or hatred of the body. In right-sided hemiparesis, patients can sometimes maintain that their weak arm is in fact stronger and more useful than before. This is referred to as *anosognosic overestimation* (Cutting, 1997). The opposite can be the case in *dysmorphophobia* (see below), wherein subjective feeling of ugliness or imagined defect is the principal focus of the patient's negative valuation. *Misoplegia* is the hatred of a limb and is associated with left-sided parietal lesions (Cutting, 1997).

DISORDERS OF BELIEFS ABOUT THE BODY (BODILY COMPLAINT WITHOUT ORGANIC CAUSE)

Classification of these disorders is difficult, partly because the symptoms are obscure in origin and partly because there are different theoretical bases for the words used. For example, *conversion hysteria* was used as a term that referred to the presumed unconscious conversion of an unacceptable affect into a physical symptom. *Hypochondriasis* refers to a concern with symptoms and with illness that the outside observer regards as excessive; the same amount of concern or complaint associated with pathology that the doctor regards as justifying it would not be deemed hypochondriacal. *Dysmorphophobia* is a phenomenological term and refers to the subjective experience of dissatisfaction with bodily shape or form.

In ICD-10 (World Health Organization, 1992), these disorders are classified under 'somatoform disorders' (F45), which include both somatization disorder and hypochondriacal disorder, and 'dissociative (conversion) disorders' (F44), which include dissociative motor disorders, convulsions, anaesthesia and sensory loss. Unfortunately, *dysmorphophobia* is entered under hypochondriacal disorders (F45.2). All these come within the general category of 'neurotic, stress-related and somatoform disorders' (F4). Eating disorders (F50) are a category of 'behavioural syndromes associated with disturbances and physical factors' (F5), but disorder of body image is almost always manifest. Artefactual illness (factitious disorder) is listed under 'other disorders of adult personality and behaviour' (F68); this condition presents with physical symptoms.

In DSM-IV (American Psychiatric Association, 1994), the conditions discussed in this chapter are described under 'somatoform disorders' and 'factitious disorders'. Somatoform disorders include *body dysmorphic disorder* (300.70), *somatization disorder* (300.81), *conversion disorder* (300.11), *pain disorder* associated with psychological factors (307.80), *hypochondriasis* (300.70), and *undifferentiated somatoform disorder* (300.81). Placing conversion disorder in an entirely different diagnostic category from *dissociative disorders* (hysterical neuroses, dissociative type), which logically belong together, is an example of the arbitrary and inappropriate division of symptoms into bodily and psychological. The *gender identity disorders* form a logical association with other disturbance of body image and identity such as dysmorphophobia; however, for the sake of convenience they are dealt with separately with other psychosexual disorders in Chapter 16 (see Figure 15.1).

Hypochondriasis

Hypochondriasis describes that awareness in which the person takes undue account of the symptomatic component of his sensorium. It is a symptom, not a disease. There are many different modes of expression: minor pain and discomfort dominate his life and occupy his attention; he may have unreasonable fears about the likelihood of developing serious illness, and feels a need to take excessive precautions; he may misinterpret benign blemishes as having sinister

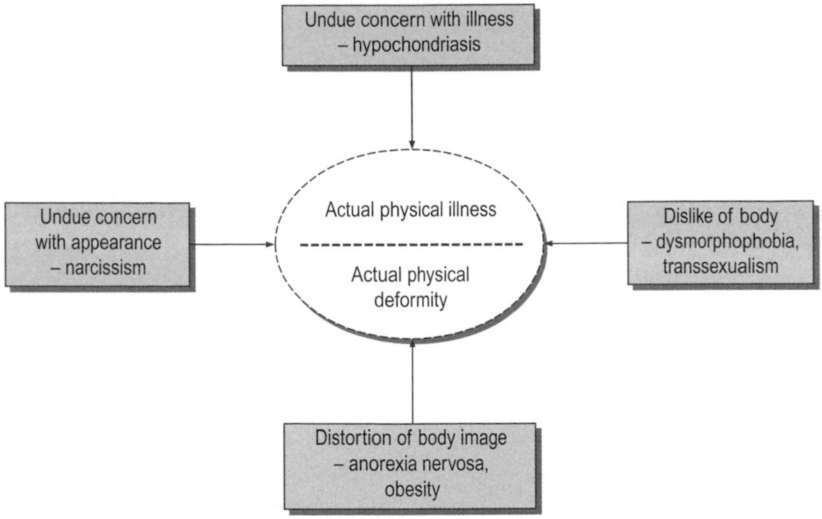

Figure 15.1 Disorders of bodily complaint.

pathological significance. These expressions of dissatisfaction may occur on their own or in any combination, and they can affect any bodily system or psychological process. Hypochondriacal symptoms are very common and usually transient. Only a minority come to medical attention, and only a selected atypical proportion of these are seen by psychiatrists.

There is a distinction between illness fears, when there are no bodily symptoms, and fears and distress associated with bodily symptoms. This shows the overlap between illness phobias (unreasonable fear of developing illness) and hypochondriasis (preoccupation with symptoms). There is often difficulty in diagnosis when a person with demonstrable physical pathology complains excessively about his symptoms; his complaints appear to be out of proportion to the anticipated suffering and disability of the illness. Necessary and entirely routine medical examination and investigation tend to reinforce the patient's symptoms. Somatic symptoms without organic pathology are extremely common and may result from misunderstanding the nature and significance of physiological activity aggravated by emotion (Kellner, 1985). The mechanisms underlying hypochondriacal symptoms include misinterpretation of normal bodily sensations; conversion of unpleasant affect, especially depression, into physical symptoms; and the experience of autonomic symptoms directly caused by disorder of mood.

Explicit in the identification of hypochondriasis is the condition of the patient himself. Implicit, however, is the doctor who labels his patient *hypochondriacal* and deems him *sick*. In a society that is so conscious of physical health and the external physical appearance, the patient may have to shout hypochondriacally because the doctor will only listen organically. What the symptoms communicate to other people is an important component of all disorders of bodily awareness; concentration on the subjective aspects of symptoms should not detract from their social implications. Hypochondriasis is not uncommonly an iatrogenic condition induced by the doctor's failure to listen to his patient's story and inability to give appropriate weight to psychological aspects contributing to symptoms.

What is hypochondriasis?

By derivation, the word *hypochondrium* refers to the anatomical area below the rib cage (Figure 15.2) and hence dysfunction of the liver or spleen. Such words as *atrabilious* or *melancholia* refer to the black bile that was considered to be associated with hypochondriacal complaint and depressed mood. A better synonym is the word *valetudinarian*, derived from *valetudo* – the state of health. Kenyon (1965) has defined hypochondraisis as morbid preoccupation with the body or state of health.

Is hypochondriasis a separate condition – a symptom or a syndrome, a noun or an adjective? In the older psychiatric classifications, and also surprisingly in both ICD-10 (World Health Organization, 1992) and DSM-IV (American Psychiatric Association, 1994), hypochondriasis or hypochondriacal disorder is given a separate designation. However, in ICD-10 and in the more detailed rubric of DSM-IV, hypochondriacal disorder (F45.2 in ICD-10) forms one category of somatoform disorders. In ICD-10, somatoform disorders are part of 'neurotic, stress-related and somatoform disorders' (F40 to F48); it is used adjectivally to describe one type of neurotic disorder. This conforms to some extent with Fischer-Homberger's dictum (1972) that hypochondriasis of the eighteenth century is equivalent to neurosis of the twentieth century. Hypochondriasis is not unitary as a condition but a disorder of content rather than of form. The content is the excessive concern with health, either physical or mental. The form of the condition may be very variable. *Hypochondriacal* is best retained as description rather than as a discrete disease entity (Kenyon, 1976).

Hypochondriasis and somatization are both somatoform disorders. Whereas the patient with hypochondriacal disorder is preoccupied with symptoms, their significance and the probability of having serious illness, the patient with somatization disorder (F45.0 in ICD-10) presents with multiple, recurrent and

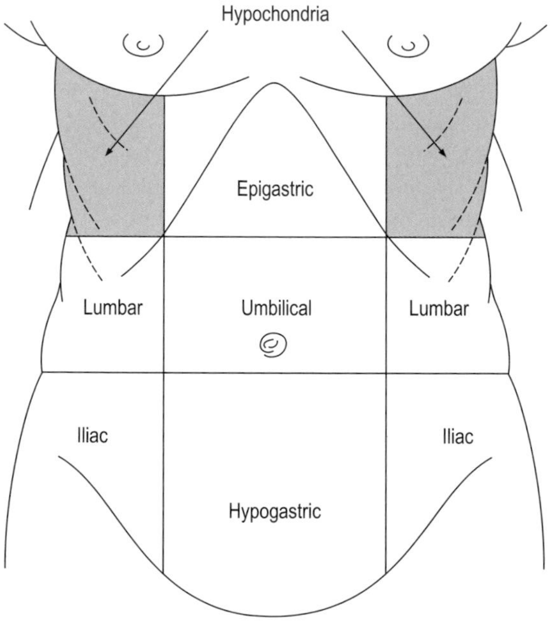

Figure 15.2 The hypochondrium.

changing physical symptoms in many different bodily systems, usually present for many years before referral to a psychiatrist. Using appropriate psychological measuring instruments, Hollifield *et al.* (1999) were able to show that patients in primary care manifesting hypochondriacal responses or high somatic concern (that is, somatization) had a worse perception of their own health and used more health services than control subjects, even though the latter suffered from the same level of chronic medical disorders. Somatization contributed even more to negative health perception and service utilization than did hypochondriasis.

Barsky and Klerman (1983) have considered that the word hypochondriasis is used to describe four quite distinct concepts.

- It describes a psychiatric syndrome characterized by physical symptoms disproportionate to demonstrable organic disease, fear of disease and the conviction that one is sick, preoccupation with one's body and pursuit of medical care.
- Hypochondriasis is seen psychodynamically as a derivative of aggressive or oral drives or as a defence against guilt or low self-esteem.
- It results from a perceptual amplification and augmentation and a cognitive misinterpretation of normal bodily sensations.
- It is socially learned illness behaviour to which the philosophy and practice of the medical profession lends support.

Only the first of these is psychopathological in nature.

These concepts are not alternatives but are all present to a different extent in the individual sufferer. Some individuals use a *somatic style* to describe perception of internal discomfort.

Appleby (1987) points out that closer examination reveals a descriptive triad of the patient being convinced that he has a disease, fearing the disease and being preoccupied with his body. He emphasizes that the patient needs to understand his symptoms before any improvement can be expected.

The diagnostic categories used in ICD-10 are summarized in Table 15.2. In hypochondriasis, 'the essential feature is a persistent preoccupation with the possibility of having one or more serious and progressive physical disorders'.

Bridges and Goldberg (1985) have assessed somatic presentation of psychiatric disorder in primary care in a series of 500 inceptions to illness among 2500 attenders. Their operational criteria for *somatization* were as follows.

- *Consulting behaviour*: seeking medical help for somatic manifestations and not presenting psychological symptoms.
- *Attribution*: the patient considers somatic manifestations to be caused physically.
- *Psychiatric illness*: psychiatric diagnosis justified by psychiatrists.
- *Response to intervention*: the research psychiatrist is of the opinion that treatment of the psychiatric disorder would benefit somatic symptoms.

These authors consider that somatization is a common mode of presentation of psychiatric illness and partly explains the failure of family doctors to detect psychiatric disorders in primary care.

When hypochondriacal symptoms were assessed in medical outpatients using a self-report questionnaire, structured interview and perusal of medical records,

Table 15.2 Somatoform disorders in ICD-10

Code	Disorder	Definition
F45.0	Somatization disorder	(a) At least 2 years of multiple and variable physical symptoms for which no adequate physical explanation has been found. (b) Persistent refusal to accept the advice or reassurance of several doctors that there is no physical explanation for the symptoms. (c) Some degree of impairment of social and family functioning attributable to the nature of the symptoms and resulting behaviour.
F45.2	Hypochondriacal disorder	For a definite diagnosis both of the following should be present. (a) Persistent belief in the presence of at least one serious physical illness underlying the presenting symptom or symptoms, even though repeated investigations have identified no adequate physical explanation, or a physical preoccupation with a presumed deformity or disfigurement. (b) Persistent refusal to accept the advice and reassurance of several different doctors that there is no physical illness or abnormality underlying the symptoms.
F45.3	Somatoform autonomic dysfunction	Definite diagnosis requires all of the following. (a) Symptoms of autonomic arousal such as palpitation, sweating, tremor, flushing, which are persistent and troublesome. (b) Additional subjective symptoms referred to a specific organ or system. (c) Preoccupation with and distress about the possibility of a serious (but often unspecified) disorder of the stated organ or system, which does not respond to repeated explanation and reassurance by doctors. (d) No evidence of a significant disturbance of structure or function of the stated system or organ.
F45.4	Persistent somatoform pain disorder	(a) The predominant complaint is of persistent, severe and distressing pain, which cannot be explained fully by a physiological process or a physical disorder. (b) Pain occurs in association with emotional conflict or psychosocial problems that are sufficient to allow the conclusion that they are the main causative influences. (c) The result is usually a marked increase in support and attention, either personal or medical. (d) There is no other psychiatric illness or psychophysiological mechanism which could explain the symptom.

(From the World Health Organization, 1992, with permission.)

the DSM-III criteria for hypochondriasis were found to be consistent (Barsky *et al.*, 1986). Disease conviction and fear, bodily preoccupation and somatic symptoms were intercorrelated and also correlated with depressive symptoms.

Trying to distinguish between organic and psychological elements of disease or between mental and physical illness is a fruitless task based on an outmoded and misleading linguistic distinction (Kendell, 2001). Psychological conflict may be mediated via physical illness, and a physical illness results in psychosocial sequelae. Both somatic and psychological symptoms occur, and it is perfectly possible for a patient to have a hypochondriacal reaction to a clearly defined organic illness. Stoeckel (1966) regarded the following as being the features of hypochondriasis: bodily complaint, attitudes and beliefs about the body, concerns about illness and the act of complaining to the doctor or complaining too often.

A patient who regards himself as having symptoms of illness communicates this to relatives and also to the doctor in a tacit request for both help and labelling (Parsons, 1951). In order to come to medical attention, the person has to carry out a particular set of actions, that is, undertake illness behaviour (Mechanic, 1962, 1986). Illness behaviour is an important determinant of association between physical and mental illness (Benjamin *et al.*, 1984). Kennedy (1980) suggested that doctors force the *sick role* on their patients so that hypochondriasis becomes a necessary response.

There is overlap between hypochondriasis and dysmorphophobia and other body image disorders. Dissatisfaction with the body may be experienced as narcissism, an absorption with the appearance of the body, or as hypochondriasis, an absorption with symptoms. There may be distortion of the body image without fear of illness as, for example, in anorexia nervosa or gross obesity. There is not necessarily any actual body image disturbance in hypochondriasis.

There are very marked cultural differences in the presentation of symptoms of disordered mood; somatization of emotional distress applies to both anxiety and depression (Rack, 1982). The predominance of description of somatic over mood symptoms in depressive illness has been reported from India, Pakistan, Bangladesh, Hong Kong, the West Indies and various parts of Africa. The reasons for this include the expectations the patient has for what the doctor can do, the use of somatic symptoms as metaphor for distress and the social unacceptability of psychological symptoms. The Bradford Somatic Inventory has been devised for a multiethnic comparison of the frequency of somatic symptoms, their anatomical localization and their association with psychiatric disorder (Mumford *et al.*, 1991). Immigrant populations from Pakistan in the United Kingdom demonstrate more somatic symptoms on the Bradford Somatic Inventory compared with the native population. These symptoms are associated with recognizable anxiety and depression as measured by validated questionnaires (Farooq *et al.*, 1995). It is probable that, in many instances, far from the patient being psychologically dumb, it is rather that the doctor is emotionally deaf. It is like a metaphorical knot in the stethoscope, so that the doctor cannot hear the anxieties of the patient and therefore ignores the psychological and social sources of pain and distress.

Psychopathology of the hypochondriacal patient

The *content* of hypochondriasis is the excessive concern with health, either physical or mental. Possible *forms* of the condition are listed in Box 15.1. These forms for a *content* of concern about cancer can include the following.

- A *hallucinatory* voice may say to the patient, 'you have cancer, you are moribund'.
- A *secondary delusion* associated with affective illness may occur in which the patient unreasonably believes he has cancer; he is quite unable to accept his doctor's reassurance. The belief is understandable in terms of the patient's overall depressed mood state. That such secondary delusions could be

Box 15.1 Psychopathology of hypochondriasis

- Hallucination
- Secondary delusion
- Primary delusion
- Overvalued idea
- Obsessional rumination
- Depressive rumination
- Anxious preoccupation

associated with affective psychoses was clearly described by Cotard (1882): 'she blamed herself and felt guilty. After some months she entertained hypochondriacal delusions, believing that she had no stomach and that her organs had been destroyed; she attributed these beliefs to the effects of an emetic which she had, in fact, been given'. This association of hypochondriacal and nihilistic delusions with depressive psychosis in the elderly has been called Cotard's syndrome.

- The *delusion* may be *primary* in nature. A patient with schizophrenia believed that he had been inoculated under a general anaesthetic with a transmissible cancer because others believed him to be homosexual.
- Hypochondriasis often manifests as an *overvalued idea*. Such a person is constantly worried and concerned about the risk of illness and the need to take precautions in ways that his friends find ridiculous, for instance in the lengths that he will go to avoid a possible carcinogen. He considers it perfectly reasonable that he should take due care to maintain his health, but he agrees that his measures are excessive. He cannot stop himself, night or day, from thinking, worrying and trying to prevent illness. Such an overvalued idea is found reasonable, or at least not alien to the person's nature, but preoccupies the mind to an unreasonable extent that the whole energy and being becomes directed towards this single idea.
- The hypochondriacal idea may take the form of an *obsessional rumination* in which the possibility of a particular illness or a form of words, as 'I have cancer', may recur. This is recognized as being both 'alien to my nature' but also 'coming from inside myself'. It is resisted yet occurs repetitively.
- Without its amounting to a delusion, patients may often have hypochondriacal symptoms of a non-specific nature in the course of a *depressive* illness. It may be possible to reassure them concerning any particular symptom, but this does not make them feel better in their mood nor does it prevent the occurrence of further hypochondriacal symptoms in the form of depressive ruminations.
- In the context of acute or chronic *anxiety*, the patient may be prone to multitudinous worries concerning illness and fears of illness. The normal sensorium is interpreted as symptoms; symptoms are interpreted as serious illness. Most hypochondriacal symptoms occur in relation to anxiety and depression; the other forms of disorder are much less frequent.

The commonest bodily symptoms implicated in hypochondriasis are musculoskeletal; gastrointestinal, including indigestion, constipation and other preoccupation with malfunction; and central nervous system, including headache (Kenyon, 1964). The most commonly affected parts of the body are head and neck, abdomen and chest. In 16 per cent of patients, symptoms are predominantly unilateral, and of these, 73 per cent, according to Kenyon, were left-sided. There was no significant physical abnormality found in 47 per cent of those admitted to a psychiatric ward for hypochondriasis. Pain was prominent in 70 per cent of patients.

Hypochondriasis may be associated with smell; bodily appearance; sexual hypochondria; ear, nose and throat symptoms; and ophthalmological abnormalities (Karseras, 1976) such as *asthenopia,* which includes such complaints as ocular discomfort, aching eyes, soreness, pressure in or around the eyes, tiredness of eyes, grittiness, chronic redness, feelings that the eyes are pushed out on stalks, tightness of the skin across the bridge of the nose or pricking of the skin around the eyes. Photophobia is a common hypochondriacal complaint, as are 'floaters' – muscae volitantes, photopsia and sometimes diplopia.

Hypochondriacal complaint may relate to psychological symptoms and the fear of mental illness. In this context, sleep is often involved, with subjective feelings of sleep not occurring at all, not occurring in sufficient amount or not being of satisfactory quality. Fear of madness and inevitable psychiatric deterioration is commonly associated with acute anxiety disorders and also with depressive illness.

Diagnosis of hypochondriasis from other conditions

Hypochondriasis is an important presentation of depressive illness and was quite clearly recognized by Schiller, for instance, when writing about the illness affecting his pupil Grammont on the 26 June 1780 (Dewhurst and Reeves, 1978):

> “ in my view the ailment is nothing but a case of true hypochondria, that unfortunate condition, wherein one is the lamentable victim of the intimate sympathy between the abdomen and the soul, an illness that afflicts deeply reflective and emotional spirits and the majority of great men of learning.

> “ The close connection between the body and the soul makes it extremely difficult to discover the origin of the complaint and to ascertain whether it originates from the body or the soul. Gradually, a state of physical disorder came to be associated with the derangement of his reason – I dare not offer an opinion on whether there was an underlying organic cause in the abdomen. Then came digestive disturbance, exhaustion and headaches, which, as the effects of a disturbed state of mind, in turn aggravated his mental condition still further.

> “ This led to the terrible state of melancholy into which he fell for some weeks. He despaired of his own strength, often telling me that he was not a human being since he could not think; that he could not see any reason for remaining alive as he had no purpose in life, and other things of a similar nature.

This presentation of depression as somatization often misleads the doctor in primary care into missing the underlying depressive illness. Because of the emphasis on, and rewards accruing from, bodily symptoms in childhood and in many cultures, patients often selectively complain about physical symptoms and minimize the mood disorder and cognitive aspects of depression (Katon *et al.*, 1982). Somatization within depression is regarded as a coping mechanism that protects the individual, for a time, from psychological pain. Culture, childhood experience and the stage of development of the individual's coping mechanism all emphasize this process. This concentration by the individual on the somatic symptoms of depression, with relative under-reporting of emotional and cognitive symptoms, has a profound effect on interactions with healthcare systems because physicians are also somatizers. Diagnosis, investigation and treatment are likely to be influenced by this, at great cost to the individual and the healthcare system. 'Somatization is a metaphor for personal distress.'

Hypochondriacal neurosis is a common diagnosis. ICD-10 ascribes a category to hypochondriacal disorder (F45.2), but in fact hypochondriacal symptoms may occur in all neurotic disorders and neurosis cannot be tidily compartmentalized (Gelder, 1986).

In schizophrenia, hypochondriasis manifests with the bizarre symptomatology associated with that condition. The diagnosis is made on the presence of abnormal *form*.

Hypochondriasis may occur in the context of an organic psychosyndrome. Diagnosis is made by precise assessment of the mental state, looking for the appropriate features. Hypochondriasis and an organic psychiatric state may of course coexist, especially in a person who prior to a dementing illness was prone to somatic symptoms.

In children, hypochondriasis of the parents may be communicated to a child to produce hypochondriacal symptoms in him. This is an extremely common situation, and it is often easy to see how hypochondriasis becomes a type of learned behaviour. Two much rarer conditions have been described. First, the *masquerade syndrome* (Waller and Eisenberg, 1980) occurs in children who have required long-term medical treatment for serious illness; as they improve physically, they manifest hypochondriacal school phobia associated with separation anxiety and use their previous physical disability as a reason for not leaving home and returning to school. Second is *Münchausen's syndrome by proxy*, described by Meadow (1977), in which a parent produces factitious illness in the child – a complaint of haematuria in the child may be caused by the mother placing blood in his urine. This may on occasions be a form of hypochondriasis in the parent, reflecting his or her over-concern for the child's health.

There is overlap between the terms *hysteria* (dissociative conversion) and *hypochondriasis*. This is discussed further in the section on dissociative conversion that follows.

The term *somatization disorder*, mentioned above, is used in ICD-10 to designate a condition with recurrent, multiple and frequently changing somatic complaints of several years' duration, for which medical attention has been sought but which are apparently not due to any physical disorder. The disorder usually begins before the age of 30 years and has a chronic but fluctuating course. Complaints are often presented in a dramatic, vague or exaggerated way. Such individuals receive medical care from a number of physicians, sometimes simultaneously, and complaints are invariably made in many different organ systems. This is synonymous with the condition previously called Briquet's syndrome (De Souza and Othmer, 1984). This condition has also been called multiple complaint syndrome and multiple psychosomatic disorder; it could be considered to be *polysystematic, polysymptomatic, chronic, hypochondriacal neurosis*.

In dealing with hypochondriasis, one is often met with the nagging suspicion that there may be concealed physical illness and, of course, this is usually the fear of the patient. Hypochondriasis and severe physical illness may coexist, and these two diagnoses should not be polarized in terms of either/or.

DISORDERS OF BODILY FUNCTION: DISSOCIATIVE (CONVERSION) DISORDER

Hysteria is an old-fashioned word, the existence and meaning of which has been argued over for centuries (Veith, 1965). Slater (1965) wished to reject the diagnosis of hysteria while retaining the word as an adjective to describe certain types of symptoms and personality. Lewis (1975) summarized this controversy: 'The majority of psychiatrists would be hard put to it if they could no longer make a diagnosis of "hysteria" or "hysterical reaction"; and in any case a tough old word like hysteria dies very hard. It tends to outlive its obituarists'. Dissociative or hysterical symptoms are extremely common, but the primary diagnosis of hysteria or dissociative (conversion) disorder is not. At the beginning of the twenty-first century, hysteria is no longer an acceptable term and therefore the synonym 'dissociative conversion' will generally be used here. Hysteria the concept, if not the word, can be safely predicted to make a comeback at some time in the future.

What is dissociative conversion (hysteria)?

ICD-10 (World Health Organization, 1992) uses the rather clumsy term *dissociative (conversion) disorder* to describe hysteria, while DSM-IV (American Psychiatric Association, 1994) removes the term altogether by fragmenting it into different parts: conversion disorder under *somatoform disorders*, and *dissociative disorders*, a separate generic category; this destruction and division is the worst of all options. Merskey (1979) retained the term 'as a medical issue, to treat patients who have it as subject to illness, and to accept that it is a valid diagnosis embracing ... symptoms'. British psychiatry implemented ICD-9 for diagnosis until 1994 (Bewley, 1979) and subsequently has adopted ICD-10.

The implications that may be drawn from the classification of dissociative conversion (hysteria) are (a) symptoms are psychogenic, (b) causation is thought to be unconscious, (c) symptoms may carry some sort of advantage to the patient and (d) they occur by the mediation of the processes of *conversion* or *dissociation*.

Conversion and dissociation are also common mechanisms of hypochondriacal and psychogenic pain symptoms, although often overlooked. Hysteria is an example of classification being based on psychodynamic formulation, in that *conversion* involves an unacceptable affect or perception of current life circumstances being *converted* into physical symptoms. The symptoms do not carry aetiological implications, but their descriptive use refers to symptoms suggesting neurological disease such as amnesia, paralysis, difficulty in walking and so on (the so-called pseudoneurological or grand hysterical symptoms; Guze, 1970). The question that haunts psychiatrists and other physicians is, of course, how can one be sure that the disturbance is psychogenic?

Conversion implies the behaviour of physical illness without evidence of organic pathology; the patient is not aware of psychogenicity. *Dissociation* implies 'a narrowing of the field of consciousness with selective amnesia. There may be dramatic but essentially superficial changes of personality, at times taking the form of a fugue (wandering state). Behaviour may mimic psychosis, or rather the patient's idea of psychosis' (World Health Organization, 1977). Dissociation can therefore be seen as a form of conversion in which environmental stresses result in illness behaviour in the psychological, rather than the physical, realm. Thus, the symptoms of hysteria may be considered to be motor, sensory (including pain) or psychological.

At 10-year follow-up of patients diagnosed with hysteria at a neurological hospital, many were found to have subsequently developed a serious physical or psychiatric illness, and for this reason the existence of hysteria as a diagnostic category was questioned (Slater and Glithero, 1965). Follow-up of 113 patients diagnosed as hysterical by psychiatrists revealed 60 per cent with evidence of affective disorder and only 13 per cent with a consistent picture of hysteria (Reed, 1975). However, Merskey and Buhrich (1975) carried out a follow-up on patients diagnosed as having motor conversion symptoms at a neurological hospital and a control group of other patients from the same clinical setting. They found a higher rate for organic symptoms at follow-up in the control group. From follow-up studies of neurological or psychiatric patients, when the diagnosis of hysteria has been highly inclusive, other organic and psychiatric conditions have commonly manifested at follow-up, but there are still 15 to 20 per cent who retained the diagnosis of hysteria. Hysteria exists but is much less common than previously thought.

The archaic term *Briquet's syndrome* developed from the concept of hysteria formed by the St Louis group (Guze, 1967; Perley and Guze, 1962); most of these patients had severe personality disorder and showed chronic hypochondriacal rather than dissociative conversion symptoms.

Clinical syndromes of dissociative disorder (hysteria)

For the diagnosis of dissociative disorder to be made, positive psychological features must be present as well as organic features absent; it is important to emphasize the danger of diagnosing dissociation or hysteria for chronic and obscure physical symptoms. Thus for *astasia–abasia* (see Figure 15.3) to be considered dissociative, the symptoms should have psychogenic aetiology; the patient is unaware of this, and the symptoms can be seen to be a way of dealing with stress. If symptoms are clearly consciously produced, deliberate disability, malingering or artefactual illness is present. One may have to distinguish between the symptoms of the original illness, for example head injury, and a secondary hysterical reaction (Sims, 1985).

Ganser's syndrome, and the confused issue of distinguishing between organic and hysterical memory impairment, has been described in Chapter 5. Hysterical *pseudodementia*, a most unsatisfactory term, is sometimes regarded as synonymous with Ganser's syndrome, thus implying the need to exclude organic causation. However, the term *pseudodementia* is also used to describe the cognitive impairment that occurs in old people with affective disorders, especially severe depression, and reflects the clinical concept that the cognitive

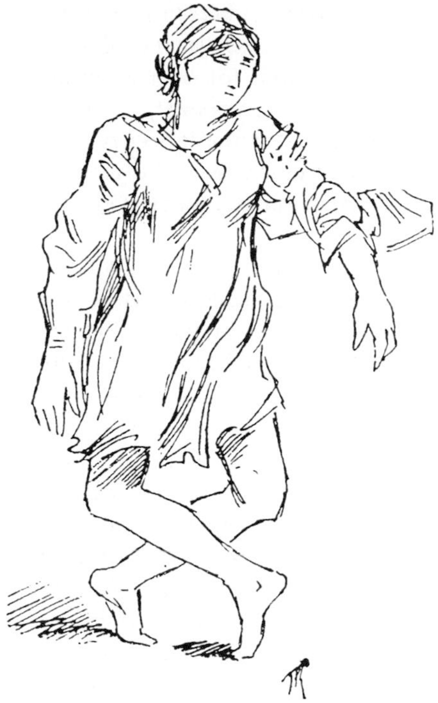

Figure 15.3 Astasia–abasia. (From Merskey, 1979.)

impairment in these cases is secondary to a mood disturbance and that it is also reversible.

Multiple personality disorder, in which the patient assumes in series a number of different personalities, was described by Morton Prince (1905). His patients showed dissociative symptoms, but several of them also showed organic pathology. Sometimes these personalities claimed to know the other personalities in the same person and intensely disliked them, and sometimes they denied all knowledge of them. This topic is discussed with disorders of ego consistency and coherence in Chapter 13.

Epidemic, communicated or *mass* hysteria has been known and described from earliest times, for example the physical symptoms of conversion type associated with the millennialist movements of the Middle Ages (Cohn, 1958), in a closed female community in a French seventeenth century convent (Huxley, 1952) and among Lancashire mill girls (St Clare, 1787). A rather similar epidemic spread through a school in Blackburn 180 years later, with symptoms of over-breathing, dizziness, fainting, headache, shivering, pins and needles, nausea, pain in the back or abdomen, hot feelings and general weakness (Moss and McEvedy, 1966). The spread of such epidemics has been described: they almost always occur in young females; they often start with a girl of high status in her peer group who is unhappy; they tend to occur in largest numbers in the younger children in a secondary school, that is, just after the age of puberty; they appear to affect most severely those who on subsequent testing are found to be the most unstable.

War neurosis, or shell shock, may be dissociative in nature when conversion symptoms occur in the absence of organic disorder. Dissociation or conversion may occur as part of the reaction to severe stress. There are other, transcultural forms of hysteria described, for example *latah* (Yap, 1951). This has a number of different names in slightly different forms in various communities in South-East Asia, but characteristic are hypersuggestibility, automatic obedience, coprolalia and various echo phenomena. It occurs in lower-social class women exposed to sudden overwhelming stress and can be considered an acute catastrophic reaction. 'Such a reaction does not generally occur in the western world except in special stress situations of war, natural disaster or drastic social change' (Kiev, 1972).

It would be unrewarding to list all the possible symptoms that may be of dissociative origin: motor, sensory, pain and alterations in consciousness. With the use of skilled examination and additional neurophysiological techniques, for example in the investigation of dissociative blindness, it is very often possible to demonstrate discrepancy between the severity of symptoms and physiological dysfunction, which may be minimal or absent. The physiological impossibility of dissociation symptoms is well demonstrated in Figure 15.4, which shows the visual field of a patient with dissociation complaining of impaired vision. Pain, in this context, is a contentious issue; it is unwise to diagnose dissociation when the only complaint is of pain. Pain also commonly occurs with depressive illness and, of course, may indicate organic pathology. Disorders of consciousness associated with dissociation include fugues, the Ganser state, dissociative convulsions and multiple personality. Acute dissociative symptoms with a good prognosis are quite common, especially at times of great stress such as during war, after disaster, in hospital emergency departments and with grave physical illness.

It is important to take into account the effect dissociative symptoms have on other aspects of a patient's behaviour and social relationships. Symptoms result in the patient being regarded as *ill* or *disabled*, and this alters the way he or she is perceived both by relatives and friends and by the medical and related professions. There may be long-term physical consequences of dissociative motor symptoms, for example contractures; this is the ultimate mimicry hysteria shows of organic conditions.

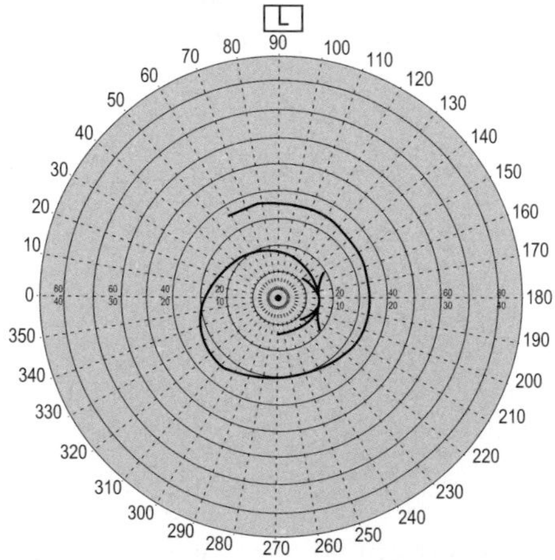

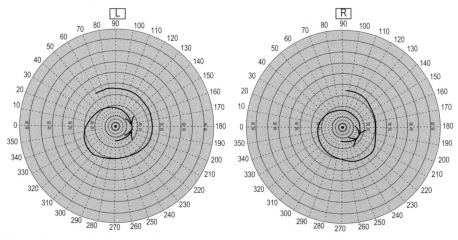

Figure 15.4 Visual fields of a hysterical patient.

Classically, mood in dissociative disorder is described as *belle indifference*. Such mood occurred in a girl aged 20 with severe disability that had entailed her using crutches for the past 2 years. She smiled with sublime resignation at her unfortunate situation, and everyone around her was relieved that she accepted her symptom so stoically! However, some patients with conversion symptoms show higher autonomic arousal than do anxious and phobic patients (Lader and Sartorius, 1968). Patients with dissociative disorders often describe feeling extremely anxious at the time of interview. They may also describe depression, and it is of course important to decide whether depression is the primary diagnosis or not. They may quite frequently manifest anger and hostility towards their relatives and also those treating them, which may be overt or concealed.

In the history of dissociation/hysteria, abnormal sexual behaviour has commonly accompanied other symptoms. This seems less frequent in contemporary accounts, perhaps because the general climate towards sexual expression has become more permissive and therefore sexually provocative behaviour evokes less comment.

Exclusions from the term **dissociation disorder, hysteria**

In considering such an imprecise term as hysteria, it is important to exclude syndromes that are psychopathologically separate. *Histrionic (hysterical) personality disorder* (ICD-10, F60.4; World Health Organization, 1992), previously called hysterical personality disorder, is characterized by shallow, labile affect; seeking for excitement; craving for appreciation and attention; suggestibility and theatricality; over-concern with physical attractiveness; and inappropriate seductiveness. Although dissociation may occur in those with hysterical personality disorder, it may also be superimposed on other personality types, and people with histrionic personalities do not necessarily develop dissociative disorder.

A difficult distinction is between dissociation and *deliberate disability* (Hawkins *et al.*, 1956). This describes mainly young, single women who feign illness and who may engage in behaviour that endangers life; sometimes they are involved in a paramedical profession. A patient, an electrocardiogram technician, presented with repeated admissions for severe hypoglycaemia; it was eventually revealed that these followed self-injection with insulin. Another, a nurse, had burns that failed to heal on parts of her body readily accessible to her right hand. To make a diagnosis of deliberate disability (feigning symptoms or disabilities), it is necessary to demonstrate that the symptoms must have been caused by the conscious, deliberate action of the patient.

Artefactual illness

A variety of different terms have been used to describe this condition. These terms include *artefactual illness, intentional production or feigning of symptoms or disabilities, either physical or psychological* (ICD-10, F68.1; World Health Organization, 1992) and *deliberate disability, Münchausen's syndrome, hospital addiction syndrome* and *factitious disorders* (DSM-IV; American Psychiatric Association, 1994). The term *artefactual* is preferred, as it implies that the illness, lesion or complaint is ultimately the individual's own production. It is important to make the distinction between these terms attempting to describe the same process and *malingering*, which has obvious pejorative implications and should be used only when there is no possibility of doubt; for instance, even when the patient admits to feigning symptoms there is often evidence of psychiatric illness (Hay, 1983). When the term *factitious disorders* was searched for in the *Cumulated Index Medicus* in the 1980s, 100 consecutive titles of articles showed the different terminologies listed in Table 15.3.

Factitious disorder implies that symptoms are not real, genuine or natural but produced by the individual under voluntary control. From external evidence and on the subjective judgement of the observer, illness is considered to be simulated and the behaviour that results in the symptoms to be deliberate and purposeful. When there is a goal that is obviously recognizable with a knowledge of environmental circumstances, then the diagnosis is *malingering* rather than factitious disorder, for instance if symptoms are deliberately produced for compensation or to avoid military service.

> " The essential feature of malingering is the intentional production of false or grossly exaggerated physical or psychological symptoms, motivated by external incentives such as avoiding military duty, avoiding work, obtaining financial compensation, avoiding criminal prosecution, or obtaining drugs. Under some circumstances, malingering may represent adaptive behaviour – for example, feigning illness while a captive of the enemy during wartime. *(American Psychiatric Association, 1994: 683)*

In factitious disorder, there is no apparent goal other than to assume the sick role, and it is therefore regarded as psychopathological rather than in any way as being adaptive. Factitious disorder may present with psychological symptoms, as in Ganser's syndrome or pseudodementia; or it may present with physical symptoms, as in complaints of acute abdominal pain without detectable abnormality at all; it may be self-inflicted, as in the production of abscesses by injection into the skin, or haematuria by deliberate abrasion of the urethra; or it may be an exaggeration of a pre-existing physical condition, such as overdosage of insulin in a known diabetic. Chronic factitious disorder with physical symptoms and repeated presentation at hospital is sometimes known as Münchausen's syndrome or hospital addiction syndrome; it is an important

Table 15.3 'Factitious disorders' in the *cumulated index medicus*: 100 consecutive titles of articles

Term used	Frequency	Term used	Frequency
Factitious (factitial)	38	Fictitious	2
Pseudodementia	27	Pathomimia, pathomimicry	2
Ganser	4	Pseudostigmata	1
Feigned	4	Counterfeit	1
Münchausen	4	Simulated	1
Artefactual	4	Imposter	1
Surreptitious	3	Psychogenic	1
Dematitis artefacta	2	Masquerade	1

Box 15.2 Diagnostic criteria for factitious disorder

- Intentional production or feigning of physical or psychological signs or symptoms.
- The motivation for the behaviour is to assume the sick role.
- External incentives for the behaviour (such as economic gain, avoiding legal responsibility, or improving physical well-being, as in malingering) are absent.

(From American Psychiatric Association, 1994, with permission.)

part of this condition that the patient seeks and achieves hospital treatment by deception. Diagnostic criteria for factitious disorder are shown in Box 15.2.

Narcissism

In classical mythology, Narcissus was punished for his disdain of Echo's admiration by being condemned to fall in love with his own reflection in a pool. An exaggerated concern, amounting to psychiatric symptom, with one's self-image, and especially with personal appearance, is called *narcissism*. This is not used as a diagnostic term in either ICD-10 or DSM-IV, and this is not surprising, as it refers to a symptom and not a condition. However, this self-experience is different from other symptoms of hypochondriasis that have already been described.

The absorption with self and excessive self-love of narcissism arises in the presence of feelings of insecurity about the self: there is felt to be some imminent threat to the body or to the integrity of oneself. The concentration of interest on, and admiration of, himself impairs other interpersonal relationships. The term is mostly used in psychoanalytic psychiatry and is often associated with sexual and gender abnormalities; there is considerable disagreement as to how the term should be used, for instance whether it refers to state or trait (Gottschalk, 1988). It is, strictly, an abnormal attitude to the body rather than an abnormality of body image. The features of this state were described with literary insight in the *Picture of Dorian Gray* by Oscar Wilde (1948).

Narcissism is not a precisely defined state; it is sex-linked and culture-bound. For example, the same qualities of attention to personal appearance that would result in a woman being considered well groomed might be considered narcissistic in a man; perhaps current trends towards uniformity of the sexes are altering this. The term *narcissism* cannot be used in descriptive psychopathology unless the patient himself describes what he considers to be an excessive concern with his own appearance and a consequent inability to relate to other people. Using it indiscriminately about a patient makes it into a pejorative blunt instrument that does not add to one's knowledge of internal state.

Narcissism is not essentially different from hypochondriasis, in that the former is fear of deterioration of bodily appearance, but the processes by which this may occur are seen in illness terms, while hypochondriasis is fear of illness itself. Our social standards for determining which blemishes in appearance are cosmetically acceptable are influenced by general pressures to conform in society and by the availability of medical resources. Thus, in Britain now, any young person, irrespective of his or her financial state, might expect to have a relatively minor deformity of their nose corrected, while in the seventeenth century, Cardinal Richelieu, one of the wealthiest men in Europe, held his eminent public position while suffering offensive anal ulceration and suppurating sores that made his life miserable and eventually killed him (Bailly, 1939).

Narcissism is especially associated with ageing and the fear of growing old. Simone de Beauvoir (1972) described the concern with facial appearance of growing old. This has a lot in common with the overvalued idea of dysmorphophobia; there may also be evidence of depression with narcissism.

DISORDERS OF THE PHYSICAL CHARACTERISTICS AND EMOTIONAL VALUE OF THE BODY (DISLIKE OF THE BODY)

Distortion of body image and dislike of the body are subjectively different experiences. However, they often occur together. It is, for example, usual in anorexia nervosa and with gross obesity to experience both features. It is important in elucidating symptoms to make a distinction.

Dysmorphophobia (body dysmorphic disorder)

There are many people dissatisfied with the way they look and, of course, this does not of itself constitute a psychiatric symptom. However, unreasonable loathing or excessive preoccupation with a disliked feature may result in psychiatric referral. Such people may show generalized disapproval of their appearance, or it may be concentrated on one feature. Dysmorphophobia was first defined by Morselli (1886) as 'a subjective feeling of ugliness or physical defect which the patient feels is noticeable to others, although his appearance is within normal limits'. As the meaning of the term *phobia* has changed in the past century, Berrios (1996) considers that dysmorphophobia is at least as satisfactory as modern equivalents. According to Andreasen and Bardach (1977), the primary symptom of dysmorphophobia is the patient's belief that he or she is unattractive. In both ICD-10 and DSM-IV, dysmorphophobia (body dysmorphic disorder in DSM-IV) is classified as a variety of hypochondriasis.

Dysmorphophobia has been defined, more inclusively, as the primary complaint of some external physical defect thought to be noticeable to other people but, objectively, its appearance lying within normal limits (Hay, 1970). Patients presenting to a plastic surgeon for cosmetic rhinoplasty were examined psychiatrically. They were, as a group, more disfigured than a control group, and they showed some psychological disturbance in that 40 per cent showed disorder of personality. There was, however, no relationship between the degree of deformity and the amount of psychological disturbance. Hay and Heather (1973) commented that when surgery was carried out, those patients with minimal disfigurement did as well as those with more marked defects, both subjectively in description of their self-image and on psychological testing. They considered that the degree of deformity was not of major importance in coming to a decision with regard to operation. Patients reported marked improvement in their appearance 6 months after rhinoplasty, and this was associated with reduction of psychiatric symptom scores (Robin *et al.*, 1988).

Body dysmorphic disorder occurs most frequently in late adolescence; three-quarters of patients are female and most are either single or divorced (Veale *et al.*, 1996). There is frequent comorbidity with mood disorder, social phobia and obsessive–compulsive disorder, and 72 per cent of cases manifested personality disorder, usually of paranoid, avoidant or obsessive–compulsive type. Twenty-four per cent of this group of patients had attempted suicide. In a similar American study, 73 per cent of patients reported excessive mirror checking and 63 per cent attempts to camouflage their 'deformities' (Phillips, 1993). Almost all had severe limitations of their social activities. Most patients had suffered from a major mood disorder, and 17 per cent had made suicide attempts.

Those complaining about their face, and especially their nose, do so in extreme and exaggerated terms despite the deformity often being relatively slight. The dissatisfaction with their appearance and the extent to which they feel others are aware of their disfigurement are quite out of proportion, as are the discomfort and disturbance in function: 'agonizing pain' and 'total inability to breathe'. At the same time, the actual description is often quite imprecise: 'the skin under my eyes joins my nose in a funny way' (Birtchnell, 1988). Because of the extreme degree of reaction they show, they may contemplate radical remedies, for example wishing to have their nose amputated or threatening to kill themselves. Dysmorphophobia is a relatively common disturbance of self and usually takes the psychopathological *form* of an *overvalued idea*.

The complaint of dysmorphophobia is made by the subject in relation to others but not usually based on the opinion of others. So a patient complains of his nose, or the small size of her breasts, and considers that others will regard them as ugly or unattractive. Often, the appearance is well within normal limits, with no deformity, but the patient is convinced that surgery will be beneficial. Patients often present in their late teens or early twenties. There is quite often underlying personality disorder of anankastic or dependent types; there may be depression, of neurotic type, as a reaction to the complaint; and such patients not infrequently talk of, and attempt, suicide.

A female student, aged 20, was referred to the psychiatric clinic following self-poisoning. When asked her problem, she burst into tears and said, describing the small size of her breasts:

> “ Basically there is a big difference between me and other girls. I've always been self-conscious. I used to pad myself. Even my mother made fun of me. I've tried to convince myself I would change physically. I don't feel like a total woman. I have to buy clothes that look ridiculous on top. My present boyfriend I have been going out with for over a year always talks about other girls he has. He went to a dance and danced with another girl, I knew that it was because she was bigger-busted than me. I was always aware of my figure, that I am not attractive... I detest myself, I hate my body... I don't like my boyfriend touching me there, I can't wear nice clothes, I can't make the best of what I already have ... even my little sister of 16 has more than I have ever had.

It is of interest to note that surgery can result in restitution of normal body image. In a study of 11 young women with no other disease and breast size not grossly inappropriate for body size requesting reduction mammoplasty, Hollyman *et al.* (1986) found that after surgery body image had returned to normal; self-confidence, feelings about femininity and sexual attractiveness were also enhanced.

Dysmorphophobia is sometimes described by schizophrenic patients. It may occur as the first symptom as the condition develops, and the clinician should therefore look carefully for suggestive symptoms. It may also be present in the established case and will then show characteristic schizophrenic symptomatology. A 19-year-old African-Caribbean girl, previously diagnosed with schizophrenia, said,

> “The Spirit is a man, he feels warm and moves in me. I can't feel yet. I've got to pray for my new body. I'll have it in March. I will have to look beautiful, I don't feel beautiful at the moment, I don't look nice enough. I'll have a nice face, nice teeth, red eyebrows, red eyes, pupils red and smooth red lips. My skin will be light and I'll have long fair thick hair down to my knees. My voice will be different and I'll have a new tongue. I'll speak many languages. I'll sing too. My brain and my mind will be the same. I'll have long fingernails, a smaller waist, bigger breasts and my legs will be a bit shapelier. My figure will change from 33″ 24″ 35″ to 38″ 18″ 36″.

Transsexualism

This is discussed in more detail in Chapter 16. It is a disorder of content in which the person believes that true gender identity is at variance with biological and physical characteristics. The psychopathological form is usually that of an overvalued idea.

Disturbance of eating and body size

Disturbance of eating occurs with various conditions in which alteration of body image either causes eating disorder or results from it. Three conditions will be discussed: obesity, anorexia and bulimia nervosa. Once again, it is the subjective aspects, the effect on self-image, that concerns us here and not the physical aspects.

Obesity

Obesity has become a major concern in the western world. Both in Europe and in North America, the prevalence of obesity has increased considerably since the mid-1970s. Between 1976 and 1980 in the United States of America, 15 per cent of the adult population aged 20 to 74 were obese, whereas by 2003 to 2004 the prevalence had risen to 33 per cent (Centers for Disease Control and Prevention). These trends are replicated in Europe too (World Health Organization Regional Office for Europe). Obesity is defined as a body mass index of greater than 30 kilograms per metre squared; being overweight is a body mass index of between 25 and 29.9 kilograms per metre squared. There is also concern about the rise of obesity in children. It is now estimated that approximately 17 to 20 per cent of children are obese. The concern about obesity derives from the associated health risks; hyperlipidaemia, insulin resistance, diabetes, hypertension, morbidity and premature death are recognized complications. Thus, there are national and international health programmes to combat the apparent unrelenting rise in the prevalence of obesity.

In discussion of the body image phenomena of obesity, Kalucy (1976) considers that adolescence is the critical stage of development when primary disorders of shape and body experience appear. Obesity in adolescents in diet-conscious western societies results in self-loathing and self-denigration. The presence of any physical deformity at this stage of life is likely to provoke revulsion from the self-image; individuals feel especially physically loathsome with regard to the opposite sex. They may avoid mirrors and any other reminder of their shape. There is also present a distortion of body size in that they often overestimate their size. This is interesting in comparison with anorexia nervosa patients, who also often overestimate their size and whose behaviour of dieting and food rejection may start when they are mildly obese at the time of puberty.

Anorexia nervosa

This is a condition that in the past was misplaced diagnostically; initially, sufferers were usually thought to be physically ill. Marcé (1860), however, considered it to be one form of hypochondriasis. Anorexia nervosa is an illness that occurs mainly in young women; the proportion of male cases seen ranges from one in twenty to about one in ten in different series (Dally and Gomez, 1979) and the proportion of boys is higher in childhood. There is a failure to eat, low body weight and amenorrhoea. It has been considered by Crisp (1975) that the disorder is primarily a *weight phobia*, a fear of increasing body weight, and not only a feeding disorder similar to those of childhood. Prominent is the fear of loss of control; if one eats normally, one will be unable to stop and therefore become fat. As well as an abnormal self-image, there are also abnormal attitudes towards food, gender and sex. How does the patient with anorexia nervosa see herself? It is in part a narcissistic disorder according to Bruch (1965), who has called it 'the pursuit of thinness'. In the definition in ICD-10, body image distortion is one of five essential features: 'There is body-image distortion in the form of a specific psychopathology whereby a dread of fatness persists as an intrusive, overvalued idea and the patient imposes a low weight threshold on himself or herself' (World Health Organization, 1992: 177). The other features are:

- body weight at least 15 per cent below that expected
- weight loss is self-induced
- amenorrhoea
- delayed or arrested puberty.

Anorexia nervosa became more common in the United Kingdom in the latter part of the twentieth century (Kendell *et al.*, 1973). It is much rarer in, for example, India and other developing countries. This apparent difference in prevalence suggests that it may well be linked to social attitudes towards thinness, dieting and slimming. In the western world, slimness is regarded as beautiful, and dieting may become a social norm that acts as a persuasive pressure on an impressionable adolescent female whose body weight has increased a little more than average at puberty. If there are other psychological difficulties and social conflicts, the slimming may get out of control. In other parts of the world, where the aesthetic norms of feminine beauty are based on a fulsome body, the pressure towards thinness is less but the pressure towards obesity may be greater. Even in western society, the prevalence of anorexia nervosa is not uniform within society but rather is determined by gender, age, social economic class and ethnicity.

Patients with anorexia nervosa often deny their thinness and sometimes claim to be too fat. Because of their extreme concern over their physical size and weight, a technique was devised by Slade and Russell (1973) to investigate bodily perception in anorexics. This involved comparing real size in subjects (measured by an anthropometer) and perceived size, which was measured by the observer moving horizontal lights to a distance that the subject estimated as the width across four body regions: face, chest, waist and hips. When compared with an age-matched normal control group, anorexic patients significantly overestimated their own perceived width at all regions, with the face being overestimated by more than 50 per cent. Although actually thinner at chest, waist and hips, anorexic patients saw themselves as fatter than normal women. The body image disturbance could not be accounted for by a general perceptual disorder, as anorexics were fairly accurate at the measurement of width of wooden blocks and also extremely accurate at measuring physical height. They tended to overestimate the width of other people, but not as much as themselves. The body image distortion tended to lessen as patients put on weight, especially if they did so slowly. It was shown that a greater degree of body image disorder held a worse prognosis. Slade and Russell (1973) considered that 'patients with anorexia nervosa show a faulty appreciation of their own body image in the sense that they perceive their bodies as possessing an exaggerated girth'. It was found by Garfinkel *et al.* (1979) that some anorexic subjects tend to overestimate body size and that this overestimate was stable over a year and not affected by weight change.

Experimental work by Button *et al.* (1977) called into doubt the finding that anorexics alone overestimate their size while normal females are more accurate and that disturbance of body perception is variable among anorexics. This finding has now been confirmed in a large meta-analysis by Cash and Deagle (1997). Body image disturbance does not appear to be associated with other features of either anorexia nervosa or bulimia nervosa and does not help to differentiate normal women from patients with eating disorder. Furthermore, attitudinal body dissatisfaction as measured by questionnaires or self:ideal discrepancy best differentiated the patients from the normal controls. Thus, the role of perceptual size estimation inaccuracy, the formal measure of body image distortion, as a diagnostic criterion of anorexia nervosa has to be called into question.

Slade (1988) has also shown that non-anorexic subjects overestimate the dimensions of their body, especially normal females, neurotic subjects, those who are pregnant and patients with secondary amenorrhoea. He has contrasted the use of *full body* techniques (with distorting mirrors, photographs, television images) for investigating this with *part of body* methods (visual size estimation, callipers), and has shown that relatively fixed cognitive attitudes towards body size with the former demonstrate irrational beliefs about body shape, while a more fluid state of the estimation of body size depends more on emotional factors that change over time. He has also shown that the more 'overfat' the individual considers herself to be, the more dissatisfied she will be.

Many recent studies have been carried out on supposedly normal populations. Strauman *et al.* (1991) studied the views of self in a large number of female undergraduates for the factors they described as 'actual:ideal self-discrepancy' and 'actual:ought discrepancy'. They showed that the actual:ideal discrepancy correlated with body shape dissatisfaction. The actual:ought discrepancy was associated with what they described as anorexic-related attitudes and behaviours and actual:ideal discrepancy with bulimic-related attitudes and behaviours. Gustavson *et al.* (1990) investigated body image distortion and showed differences between normal students and those suffering from eating disorders. Moore (1988) surveyed 854 females aged between 12 and 23 years from outpatient clinics; 67 per cent were found to be dissatisfied with their weight and 54 per cent with their shape.

Zellner *et al.* (1989) studied the effects of eating abnormalities and gender on the perception of desirable body shape, using figure drawings by their subjects. They found that women desire to be thinner than they think they are, and that women with eating disorders desire to be thinner than that degree of thinness that they think that men will find attractive. Steiger *et al.* (1989) found that anorexics, but not bulimics, exhibited body image distortion, and that body weight predicted the degree of body image disturbance. Dolan *et al.* (1990) demonstrated differences between white, African-Caribbean and Asian British women for some of the symptoms of eating disorders but no differences for body image disorder.

Supported by these studies is the finding of a clear association between body image disturbance and eating disorder. This is related inversely to weight, that is, the lower the weight the greater the degree of body image abnormality. Thus, in general, those with anorexia are more affected than those with bulimia nervosa.

It does seem that abnormality of self- and body image is universal in eating disorders: 'I eat therefore I am'. There are associations between abnormal eating, especially in anorexia nervosa, and low body weight, with a belief or fear that 'I am too fat' and with a more pervasive denial of self. In attempting to investigate the factors that influence this overestimation of their body size by anorexic and bulimic women, Hamilton and Waller (1993) studied the influence of media portrayal of idealized female bodies. They concluded that eating-disordered women overestimated themselves substantially more after seeing such images than after seeing photographs of neutral objects. Such images in the media do appear to influence female behaviour, at least in some vulnerable people.

Strober *et al.* (1979) assessed perception of body size, subjective experience of body image distortions and differentiation of body concepts by asking adolescent anorexic patients and controls to draw the human figure soon after their hospital admission and 6 months later. Both groups tended to overestimate size at both times, but experiences denoting estrangement from the body, insensitivity to body sensations and weakness of body boundaries were more prevalent in anorexics, and they persisted at high levels after frank symptoms of weight and eating disorder had subsided. There was a greater degree of a more persistent body image distortion in those who vomited. These authors considered that 'defects in body image formation render the anorexic vulnerable to their manifest pathology, which is itself activated by maturational conflicts unique to adolescence'.

The underlying fear of loss of control, and the incessant need for vigilance concerning any calorie that enters the mouth, influences all other areas of the patient's life. Obsessional tidiness and cleanliness may be manifested, and also an attempt to control the behaviour of other people at home. An anorexic patient controlled the behaviour of her parents and twin sister by threatening to starve herself yet further if they would not cooperate. She weighed not only her own food but that of all the other members of the family. Before her illness, she and her sister both weighed about 57 kg, but as her anorexia progressed she insisted on her twin eating her food also, which the patient cooked. As a result, the patient dropped in weight to about 32 kg, while her sister reached 83 kg.

Bulimia nervosa

This condition was first described by Russell in 1979. Although the patient is currently of normal or near-normal weight, there is often a history of anorexia nervosa with weight loss (Fairburn and Cooper, 1984). Body image distortion is also a feature of the condition, with the patient believing herself to be too fat and too heavy.

The characteristic eating disorder is of gross preoccupation with food, with episodic binge eating or gorging. This is frequently countered with self-induced vomiting and other methods of weight reduction such as abuse of drugs, for example laxatives or amphetamine-like drugs, or voluntary starvation. Weight is thus maintained with a fragile stability; sometimes weight loss may reach anorexic proportions, and sometimes there may be mild obesity that is associated with feelings of guilt. The fear of putting on weight and the dominating preoccupation with food is an *overvalued idea*.

There is marked dissatisfaction with the body in bulimia nervosa that is similar to that in anorexia nervosa (Cash and Deagle, 1997). There is evidence that the dissatisfaction with the body derives from cognitive evaluative dissatisfaction and is not dependent on sensory perception, although it may be influenced by mood (Gardner and Bockenkamp, 1996). Various abnormal behaviours may occur, including alcohol abuse, shoplifting (especially involving stealing food) and deliberate self-harm. A variety of serious physical complications may result from rigorous self-induced vomiting or purging.

Underlying factors are particularly centred on doubts concerning femininity (Lacey *et al.*, 1986). Poor relationships with parents, academic striving, parental marital conflict and poor relationships with the patients' own peers also occur. These patients described major life events in the areas of sexual conflict, major changes in life circumstances and experience of loss.

DISORDERS OF THE SENSORY AWARENESS OF THE BODY (ORGANIC CHANGES IN BODY IMAGE)

Disease of, and trauma to, the brain alter the body image in a variety of ways. This is either because of damage of the conceptualized object, for example amputation with phantom limb or blindness necessarily altering the way one perceives oneself, or damage to the process of conceptualization itself, for example section of the corpus callosum. Often, of course, there is scattered damage, as with arteriopathy or multiple sclerosis, and these two features cannot be separated.

The expression *body image* as used in neurology was defined by Critchley (1950) as the mental idea that an individual possesses as to his own body and its physical and aesthetic attributes. Visual sensation, tactile impulses and proprioceptive stimuli contribute to the formation of body image but are not essential; following amputation of a limb, a phantom limb retaining the integrity of the body image occurs in the majority of cases. The body image 'lives on the fringe of awareness and is by no means obtrusive in ordinary circumstances. It is however available and can be brought into consciousness as soon as the stream of attention voluntarily or involuntarily focuses upon it' (Critchley, 1950). Morbid changes in the body image may show enhancement, diminution (or ablation) or distortion. In neurology, the term *body schema* is used for the awareness of spatial characteristics of one's own body, involving current and previous sensory information, while *body experience* is more comprehensive, including psychological and situational factors also (Cumming, 1988). The parietal lobes play a major role, but the somatoaesthetic afferent system and the thalamus are also involved.

Pathological accentuation of body image (Hyperschemazia)

Pain or discomfort causes the affected part of the body to loom large. After dropping a heavy weight on his great toe, a man felt his body to be 'an insubstantial shell around a huge throbbing toe'. Such a description of the painful organ seeming larger in size is frequent following surgery and traumatic injury. Critchley gives several examples of neurological lesions causing enhancement of an organ.

- With partial paralysis of a limb, the affected segment gives the impression of being too heavy and too big, for example with Brown-Séquard paralysis (unilateral lesion of the spinal cord) the side with the pyramidal signs is hyperschematic while the other side, with loss of pain and temperature sensation, is perceived as normal in body scheme.
- Unilaterally, following thrombosis of the posterior inferior cerebellar artery.
- In multiple sclerosis, again unilaterally.

Hyperschemazia may also occur with peripheral vascular disease when the affected limb feels larger and heavier. It may also occur in acute toxic states. Non-organic cases occur with hypochondriasis; in depersonalization states; with dissociation (conversion disorder), for example pseudocyesis; and also, occasionally, in dreams.

Diminished or absent body image (Hyposchemazia, aschemazia)

This may occur when afferent and efferent innervation is lost, for example with transection of the spinal cord the patient may feel sawn off at the waist.

Hyposchemazia may accompany the sensory deprivation of weightlessness, for instance under water. With vertigo, the patient may feel excessively light, as if floating in the air.

Parietal lobe lesions may result in complicated states of diminution of the body image. Critchley (1950) cites a patient with embolism of the right middle cerebral artery:

> 'It felt as if I was missing one side of my body (the left), but it also felt as if the dummy side was lined with a piece of iron so heavy that I could not move it... I even fancied my head to be narrow, but the left side from the centre felt heavy, as if filled with bricks'. At one time he thought that his paralyzed leg belonged to the man in the next bed. His body felt to him half as wide as it should have done. Lying on the left side gave him the sensation that he was 'lying on a void' ... that he was at the extreme edge of the bed and would presently fall off. In the early days he also felt that he had no penis at all. On this account he was clumsy with the urinal and the bed was frequently soiled. His sensations of owning a penis returned quite suddenly one morning in association with an erection, and it afterwards felt quite normal.

In *hemisomatognosia* (hemidepersonalization), which was described by L'Hermitte (1939) and is a unilateral misperception of one's own body, the patient behaves as though the limbs on one side are missing; this may occur as part of an epileptic aura or migraine. *Anosognosia* describes the lack of awareness of disability, which may, for instance, occur with neglect of a hemiplegic limb. *Hemispatial neglect* describes those patients who, when asked to perform a variety of behavioural tasks in space, neglect the hemispace contralateral to their lesion (Cumming, 1988). Gerstmann's syndrome (Gerstman, 1930) comprises finger agnosia, acalculia, agraphia and right–left disorientation.

Again, non-organic conditions such as depersonalization may also show diminution of body image. An anxious and depersonalized patient said, 'I don't feel at all the same person. Sometimes my head feels so numb when I walk to the shops. I feel I've left half my body behind'. This was clearly an *as if* experience.

Distortion of the body image (paraschemazia)

This may occur with enhancement or diminution of the body image. It may occur with the use of hallucinogenic drugs such as mescaline, marijuana and lysergic acid diethylamide. Parts of the body may feel distorted, twisted, separated from the rest of the body or merged with the external environment. With hashish,

> the sensations produced were those of exquisite lightness and airiness... I expected to be lifted up and carried away by the first breeze. ... the walls of my frame were burst outward and tumbled into ruin, and without thinking what form I wore. ... I felt that I existed throughout a vast extent of space. The blood pulsed from my head, sped through uncounted leagues before it reached my extremities; the air drawn into my lungs expanded into seas of limpid ether, and the arch of my skull was broader than the vault of heaven. I was a mass of transparent jelly, and a confectioner poured me into a twisted mould. *(Taylor, 1856)*

Distortion of body image may occur with epileptic aura and also rarely with migraine.

Autoscopy is a related reduplicative phenomenon and may occur in similar circumstances.

Phantom limb

This occurs immediately following the loss of a limb in virtually all patients, and it is particularly common following the traumatic loss of a limb or if there had been a pre-existing painful condition of the limb. The onset appears immediately as the anaesthesia wears off in the majority of cases but may be delayed for up a few weeks in about 25 per cent of cases. The phantom may last for a few days or weeks then gradually fades from consciousness. There are, however, cases that have persisted for decades. As well as occurring with the loss of a limb, this type of distortion of body image is relatively common after surgical removal of an eye, parts of the face, breasts, the rectum or the larynx. There are reports of phantom ulcer pains after partial gastrectomy and of menstrual cramp following hysterectomy. If an amputee experiences a generalized peripheral neuritis involving sensation, paraesthesiae will also occur in the phantom limb. The amputee is aware of the phantom limb in space and also experiences pain in the space conceived as being occupied by the limb.

With time, the limb appears to change in size. The image shrinks, but unevenly, distal joints shrinking more slowly than proximal; this is the so-called telescoping phenomenon. There are several postulated explanations for 'telescoping'. In loss of the upper limb, telescoping is thought to occur because there is over-representation of the hand in the sensory cortex, hence this is the area from which sensation survives longest. There is also the possibility that telescoping occurs because the representation of the limb in the primary somatosensory map changes progressively. The posture of the phantom is often said to be 'habitual', for example partially flexed at the elbow, with forearm pronated. The limb can sometimes feels fixed in an awkward position, and this can cause the patient difficulty, for instance in walking upstairs. The limb may feel twisted and painful.

There is increasing literature on the plasticity of the somatosensory system, using phantom limb as a natural experiment to demonstrate deafferentation following loss of a limb and corresponding reorganization of the somatosensory map (Ramachandran and Hirstein, 1998). Following loss of the upper limb, sensory input from the face and upper arm have been shown to invade the hand territory such that sensory stimulus to the face can be mislocalized in the phantom limb.

Orbach and Tallent (1965) described the body concepts of patients 5 to 10 years after the construction of a colostomy. These patients had a conviction that they had been seriously damaged.

> “They believed that their bodily intactness and integrity had been violated. In common with such beliefs many patients on a fantasy level perceived the operation as a physical or sexual assault. Patients who fantasized the surgery as a sexual assault were supported in this belief by the colostomy stoma, a new opening in the front of the body. Most men regarded this opening as evidence of having been feminized, while women often interpreted it as the addition of

> a second vagina. The bleeding from the stoma reinforced the fantasy of a second vagina because it was interpreted as comparable to menstruation.

In one-fifth of patients, preoccupation about the bodily processes concerned with food intake and elimination

> "was embodied in a replacement concept which attempted to establish equality between intake and evacuation by eating approximately as much as had recently been evacuated. A majority of the remaining patients communicated a sense of confusion about the machinery and functioning of their bodies.

> "When colostomy patients were initially studied and reports published the constriction of activity and of the life space was emphasized. It is now apparent that the constriction is paralleled by a body concept of being damaged and fragile as a consequence of the injury.

Mastectomy also results in relatively severe disturbance in self-concept and body image. A patient described this as 'I will never be like before . . . it is like a hole, like a gap. . . . When I lie on that side, it's like being a man' (Hopwood and Maguire, 1988). Body image problems result not only from the loss of body part or disfigurement but also from the loss of bodily function. The disorder of self-image is frequently associated with depressive symptoms.

Phantom limb pain may be psychologically determined (Parkes, 1976). Forty-six amputees were studied 4 to 8 weeks and 13 months after amputation; a third to a half showed moderate disturbance tending to persist a year later.

Body image disturbance is not necessarily associated with abnormal sensation or perception. The hypochondriac may believe he has cancer although he has no physical symptoms. The transsexual experiences his body normally, but he believes that he is in the wrong body. The narcissist is inordinately concerned with his body; nevertheless, he is quite accurate in his objective quantitative perception of self, that is, he knows how long his nose is or how far he can throw a cricket ball. When sensation is abnormal or even deficient altogether in some modality, for example with blindness or deafness, body image is undoubtedly altered, but this alteration does not in any way imply mental illness; the alteration of body image is usually appropriate to the disability.

CULTURE-BOUND DISORDERS OF BODY IMAGE

Various culturally determined hysterical conditions have been described by Langness (1967). These conditions have in common a sudden, dramatic onset related in time to a psychosocial upset. Manifestations of these conditions are grossly unusual behaviour, volatile mood, transient occurrences of alterations of speech, depersonalization with altered body awareness and symptoms somewhat similar to delusions and hallucinations. The course of these conditions is usually limited to 1 to 3 weeks, but they may recur with further episodes. They appear to be more likely in those predisposed with histrionic (hysterical) personalities. The precise symptoms are often localized to that particular culture and demonstrate how neurotic symptoms in their content comply with the expectations of the society in which they occur. For instance, Adair, writing from Bath in 1786, described how fashion influenced the great and opulent in the choice of their diseases and considered that Queen Anne's nervousness resulted in the transfer of similar symptoms 'to all who had the least pretensions to rank with persons of fashion'.

Some of the culturally localized disorders of awareness of the body are summarized in Table 15.4 (from Kiev, 1972). The variability of such syndromes is immense, but the preoccupation with bodily organs and functions is common to many of them. The bizarre nature of symptoms, for example *koro*, in which there is fear of the penis shrinking into the abdomen, is often explained by a faulty knowledge of human anatomy and physiology that seems naive to doctors practising in Europe. However, it is not generally known how ignorant British patients are concerning the organization and functions of the organs they cannot see. Hospital outpatients were compared with doctors by Boyle (1970) in their understanding of commonly used medical terms. As might be expected, the doctors were consistent in their use of terms, but patients had enormous variation in their understanding of such terms as 'piles', 'least starchy food', 'palpitation', 'jaundice' and 'flatulence'. When asked to detail the surface anatomy of internal organs, for example bladder, kidneys and thyroid gland, the patients showed great variation and were generally quite inaccurate. There are also bizarre anomalies of body image and function occurring in practice in the United Kingdom. A young Lancashire woman working in a mill complained of migrainous headaches and ascribed these to insufficiently heavy periods. This explanation was found to be culturally acceptable to her peers.

Table 15.4 Culture-bound disorders of body image

Disorder	Diagnostic equivalent	Site	Key symptom(s)
Koro	Anxiety state	South-East Asia	Belief that the penis will retract into the abdomen and cause death
Frigophobia	Obsessive–compulsive neurosis	East Asia	Morbid fear of the cold, preoccupation with loss of vitality, compulsive wearing of layers of clothes
Latah	Hysteria	Malaysia	Hypersuggestibility, automatic obedience, coprolalia, echolalia, echopraxia, echomimia, altered consciousness, disorganization, depression and anxiety
Evil eye	Phobic neurosis	Mexico, North Africa	Strong glances are harmful; precautions taken to avoid or counteract evil eye
Voodoo	Phobic neurosis	Haiti	Violation of taboo may result in death
Windigo	Depressive reaction	Canadian Indians	Fear of engaging in cannibalism and of becoming a sorcerer, depression of mood
Amok	Dissociative state	Malaysia	Neuraesthenia, depersonalization, rage, automatism and violent acts

(After Kiev, 1972, with permission of Penguin.)

REFERENCES

Adair JM (1786) *Medical Cautions for the Consideration of Invalids, Those Especially who Resort to Bath*. Bath: Dodsley & Dilly.

American Psychiatric Association (1994) *Diagnostic and Statistical Manual of Mental Disorders*, 4th edn. Washington: American Psychiatric Association.

Andreasen NC and Bardach J (1977) Dysmorphophobia: symptom or disease? *American Journal of Psychiatry 134*, 673–5.

Appleby L (1987) Hypochondriasis: an acceptable diagnosis? *British Medical Journal 294*, 857.

Auden WH (1969) The Art of Healing: In Memoriam David Protech, MD. In *Epistle to a Godson. Collected Poems* (1976), p. 626. London: Faber & Faber.

Bailly A (1939) *The Cardinal Dictator* (transl. Miles H, 1939). London: Jonathan Cape.

Barsky AJ and Klerman GL (1983) Overview: hypochondriasis, bodily complaints and somatic styles. *American Journal of Psychiatry 140*, 273–83.

Barsky AJ, Wyshak G and Klerman GL (1986) Hypochondriasis: an evaluation of the DSM-III criteria in medical out-patients. *Archives of General Psychiatry 43*, 493–500.

de Beauvoir S (1970) *Old Age* (transl. O'Brien P, 1972). London: Andre Deutsch & Weidenfeld and Nicolson.

Benjamin S, Barnes D, Falconer G and Hoare E (1984) The effect of illness behaviour on the apparent relationship between physical and mental disorders. *Journal of Psychosomatic Research 28*, 387–95.

Berrios GE (1996) *The History of Mental Symptoms: Descriptive Psychopathology Since the Nineteenth Century*. Cambridge: Cambridge University Press.

Bewley T (1979) Implementation of the 9th International Classification of Diseases. *Bulletin of the Royal College of Psychiatrists 3*, 188.

Birtchnell SA (1988) Dysmorphophobia – a centenary discussion. *British Journal of Psychiatry 153* (suppl. 2), 41–3.

Boyle CM (1970) Difference between patients' and doctors' interpretation of some common medical terms. *British Medical Journal ii*, 286–9.

Bridges KW and Goldberg DP (1985) Somatic presentation of DSM-III psychiatric disorders in primary care. *Journal of Psychosomatic Research 29*, 563–9.

Bruch H (1965) Anorexia nervosa and its differential diagnosis. *Journal of Nervous and Mental Disease 141*, 555–66.

Burton R (1628) *The Anatomy of Melancholia*. Oxford: Cripps.

Button EJ, Fransella F and Slade PD (1977) A reappraisal of body perception disturbance in anorexia nervosa. *Psychological Medicine 7*, 235–43.

Cash TF and Deagle EA (1997) The nature and extent of body-image disturbances in anorexia nervosa and bulimia nervosa: a meta-analysis. *International Journal of Eating Disorder 22*, 107–25.

Centers for Disease Control and Prevention. Online. Available: http://www.cdc.gov. nccdphp/dnpa/obesity/index.htm

Cohn N (1958) *The Pursuit of the Millennium*. London: Secker & Warburg.

Cotard M (1882) Nihilistic delusions. In Hirsch SR and Shepherd M (eds) (1974) *Themes and Variations in European Psychiatry*. Bristol: John Wright.

Crisp AH (1975) Anorexia nervosa. In Silverstone T and Barraclough B (eds) *Contemporary Psychiatry*. Ashford: Headley Brothers, 150–158.

Critchley M (1950) The body image in neurology. *Lancet i*, 335–41.

Cumming WJK (1988) The neurobiology of the body schema. *British Journal of Psychiatry 153* (suppl. 2), 7–11.

Cutting J (1997) *Principles of Psychopathology*. Oxford: Oxford University Press.

Dally P and Gomez J (1979) *Anorexia Nervosa*. London: Heinemann.

De Souza C and Othmer E (1984) Somatization disorder and Briquet's syndrome: an assessment of their diagnostic concordance. *Archives of General Psychiatry 41*, 334–6.

Dewhurst K and Reeves N (1978) *Friedrich Schiller: Medicine, Psychology and Literature*. Oxford: Sandford Publications.

Dolan B, Lacey JH and Evans C (1990) Eating behaviour and attitudes to weight and shape in British women from three ethnic groups. *British Journal of Psychiatry 157* (suppl. 2), 523–8.

Fairburn CG and Cooper PJ (1984) The clinical features of bulimia nervosa. *British Journal of Psychiatry 144*, 238–46.

Farooq S, Gahir SM, Okyere E, Sheikh AJ and Oyebode F (1995) Somatization: a transcultural study. *Journal of Psychosomatic Research 39*, 883–8.

Fischer-Homberger E (1972) Hypochondria of the eighteenth century – neurosis of the present century. *Bulletin of the History of Medicine 46*, 391–401.

Fukutake T, Kawamura M, Sakakibara R and Hirayama K (1993) Alloaesthesia without impairment of consciousness after right putaminal small haemorrhage. *Rinsho Shinkeigaku 33*, 130–3.

Gardner RM and Bockenkamp ED (1996) The role of sensory and nonsensory factors in boy size estimations of eating disorder subjects. *Journal of Clinical Psychology 52*, 3–15.

Garfinkel PE, Moldofsky H and Garner D (1979) The stability of perceptual disturbances in anorexia nervosa. *Psychological Medicine 9*, 703–8.

Gelder MG (1986) Neurosis: another tough old word. *British Medical Journal 292*, 972–3.

Gerstmann J (1930) The symptoms produced by lesions of the transitional area between the inferior parietal and middle occipital gyri. In Rottenberg DA and Hochberg FH (eds) (1977) *Neurological Classics in Modern Translation*. New York: Hafner Press.

Gottschalk LA (1988) Narcissism: its normal evolution and development and the treatment of its disorders. *American Journal of Psychotherapy 42*, 4–27.

Gustavson CR, Gustavson JC, Pumariega AJ, *et al.* (1990) Body-image distortion among male and female college and high school students, and eating-disordered patients. *Perceptual and Motor Skills 71* (3 part 1), 1003–10.

Guze SB (1967) The diagnosis of hysteria: what are we trying to do? *American Journal of Psychiatry 124*, 491–8.

Guze SB (1970) The role of follow-up studies: their contribution to diagnostic classification as applied to hysteria. *Seminars in Psychiatry 2*, 392–402.

Hamilton K and Waller G (1993) Media influences on body size estimation in anorexia and bulimia: an experimental study. *British Journal of Psychiatry 162*, 837–40.

Hawkins JR, Jones KS, Sim M and Tibbetts RW (1956) Deliberate disability. *British Medical Journal i*, 361–7.

Hay GG (1970) Dysmorphophobia. *British Journal of Psychiatry 116*, 399–406.

Hay GG (1983) Feigned psychosis: a review of the simulation of mental illness. *British Journal of Psychiatry 143*, 8–10.

Hay GG and Heather BB (1973) Changes in psychometric test results following cosmetic nasal operations. *British Journal of Psychology 122*, 89–90.

Hollifield M, Paine S, Tuttle L and Kellner R (1999) Hypochondriasis, somatization, and perceived health and utilization of health care services. *Psychosomatics 40*, 380–6.

Hollyman JA, Lacey JH, Whitfield PJ and Wilson JSP (1986) Surgery for the psyche: a longitudinal study of women undergoing reduction mammoplasty. *British Journal of Plastic Surgery 39*, 222–4.

Hopwood P and Maguire GP (1988) Body image problems in cancer patients. *British Journal of Psychiatry 153* (suppl. 2), 47–50.

Huxley A (1952) *The Devils of Loudon*. Harmondsworth: Penguin.

Kalucy RS (1976) Obesity: an attempt to find a common ground among some of the biological, psychological and sociological phenomena of the obesity/overeating syndromes. In Hill OW (ed.) *Modern Trends in Psychosomatic Medicine 3*. London: Butterworth.

Karseras AG (1976) Psychiatric aspects of ophthalmology. In Howells JG (ed) *Modern Perspectives in the Psychiatric Aspects of Surgery*. London: Macmillan.

Katon W, Kleinman A and Rosen G (1982) Depression and somatization: a review. *American Journal of Medicine 72*, 127–35, 241–7.

Kawamura M, Hirayama K, Shinohara Y, Watanabe Y and Sugishita M (1987) Alloaesthesia. *Brain 110*, 225–36.

Kellner R (1985) Functional somatic symptoms and hypochondriasis. *Archives of General Psychiatry 42*, 821–33.

Kendell RE (2001) The distinction between mental and physical illness. *British Journal of Psychiatry 178*, 490–3.

Kendell RE, Hall DJ, Hailey A and Babigian HM (1973) The epidemiology of anorexia nervosa. *Psychological Medicine 3*, 200–3.

Kennedy I (1980) Unmasking medicine. *The Listener* 600–4, 641–4, 677–9, 713–15, 745–8, 777–9.

Kenyon FE (1964) Hypochondriasis: a clinical study. *British Journal of Psychiatry 110*, 478–88.

Kenyon FE (1965) Hypochondriasis: a survey of some historical, clinical and social aspects. *British Journal of Medical Psychology 38*, 117–33.

Kenyon FE (1976) Hypochondriacal states. *British Journal of Psychiatry 129*, 1–14.

Kiev A (1972) *Transcultural Psychiatry*. Harmondsworth: Penguin.

Lacey JH, Coker S and Birtchnell SA (1986) Bulimia: factors associated with its aetiology and maintenance. *International Journey of Eating Disorders 5*, 475–87.

Lader M and Sartorius N (1968) Anxiety in patients with hysterical conversion symptoms. *Journal of Neurology, Neurosurgery and Psychiatry 13*, 490–5.

Langness LL (1967) Hysterical psychosis: the cross-cultural evidence. *American Journal of Psychiatry 124*, 143–52.

Lewis AJ (1975) The survival of hysteria. *Psychological Medicine 5*, 9–12.

L'Hermitte J (1939) *L'image de notre corps*. Paris: Revue Nouvelle Critique.

Marcé L-V (1860) Note on a form of hypochondriacal delusion consecutive to the dyspepsias and principally characterized by refusal of food (transl. Blewett A and Bottéro A, 1994). *History of Psychiatry 5*, 273–83.

Meadow SR (1977) Münchausen syndrome by proxy. *Lancet ii*, 343–5.

Mechanic D (1962) *Students Under Stress: a Study in the Social Psychology of Adaption*. New York: Free Press.

Mechanic D (1986) The concept of illness behaviour: culture, situation and personal predisposition. *Psychological Medicine 16*, 1–7.

Merskey H (1979) *The Analysis of Hysteria*. London: Baillière Tindall.

Merskey H and Buhrich NA (1975) Hysteria and organic brain disease. *British Journal of Medical Psychology 48*, 359–66.

Moore DC (1988) Body image and eating behaviour in adolescent girls. *American Journal of Disease of Children 142*, 1114–8.

Morselli E (1886) Sulla Dismorfofobia e sulla tafefobia. *Bolletino Accademia delle Scienze Mediche di Genova VI*, 100–19.

Moss PD and McEvedy CP (1966) An epidemic of over-breathing among schoolgirls. *British Medical Journal ii*, 1295–300.

Mumford DB, Davington JT, Bhatnagar JS, *et al.* (1991) The Bradford Somatic Inventory: a multi-ethnic inventory of somatic symptoms reported by the Indo-Pakistan Subcontinent. *British Journal of Psychiatrists 158*, 379–86.

Orbach CE and Tallent N (1965) Modification of perceived body and of body concept. *Archives of General Psychiatry 12*, 126–35.

Parkes CM (1976) The psychological reaction to loss of a limb: the first year after amputation. In Howells JG (ed.) *Modern Perspectives in the Psychiatric Aspects of Surgery*. London: Macmillan.

Parsons T (1951) Illness and the role of the physician: a sociological perspective. *American Journal of Orthopsychiatry 21*, 452–60.

Perley MJ and Guze SB (1962) Hysteria – the stability and usefulness of clinical criteria. A quantitative study based on a follow-up period of 6 to 8 years in 39 patients. *New England Journal of Medicine 266*, 421–6.

Phillips KA, McElroy SL, Kerk PE, Pope HG and Hudson JI (1993) Body dysmorphic disorder: 30 cases of imagined ugliness. *American Journal of Psychiatry 150*, 302–8.

Prince M (1905) *The Dissociation of a Personality*. New York: Longman.

Rack P (1982) *Race, Culture and Mental Disorder*. London: Tavistock.

Ramachandran VS and Hirstein W (1998) The perception of phantom limbs: The DO Hebb lecture. *Brain 121*, 1603–30.

Reed JL (1975) The diagnosis of 'hysteria'. *Psychological Medicine 5*, 13–7.

Robin AA, Copas JB, Jack AB, Kaesar AC and Thomas PJ (1988) Reshaping the psyche: the concurrent improvement in appearance and mental state after rhinoplasty. *British Journal of Psychiatry 152*, 539–43.

Russell GFM (1979) Bulimia nervosa: an ominous form of anorexia nervosa. *Psychological Medicine 9*, 429–48.

St Clare W (1787) Country news. In *The Gentleman's Magazine 57*, 1,268. Cited by Hunter R and Macalpine I (1963) *Three Hundred Years of Psychiatry*. London: Oxford University Press.

Schreber D (1955) *Memoirs of My Nervous Illness* (transl. Macalpine I and Hunter RA). London: Dawson.

Shapiro MF and Fink M (1952) Exosomesthesia: the displacement of cutaneous sensation to extrapersonal space. *Transaction of American Neurological Association 56*, 260–2.

Shapiro MF, Fink M and Bender MB (1952) Exosomesthesia or displacement of cutaneous sensation into extrapersonal space. *Archives of Neurology and Psychiatry 68*, 481–96.

Sims ACP (1985) Head injury, neurosis and accident proneness. In Trimble MR (ed.) *Advances in Psychosomatic Medicine: Neuropsychiatry*. Basel: Karger.

Sims ACP (1988) Towards the unification of body image disorders. *British Journal of Psychiatry 153* (suppl. 2), 516.

Slade PD (1988) Body image in anorexia nervosa. *British Journal of Psychiatry* 153 (suppl. 2), 20–2.

Slade PD and Russell GFM (1973) Awareness of body dimension in anorexia nervosa: cross-sectional and longitudinal studies. *Psychological Medicine 3*, 188–99.

Slater E (1965) Diagnosis of hysteria. *British Medical Journal i*, 1395–9.

Slater E and Glithero E (1965) A follow-up of patients diagnosed as suffering from hysteria. *Journal of Psychosomatic Research 9*, 9–13.

Stacy CB (1987) Complex haptic hallucination and palinaptia. *Cortex 23*, 337–40.

Steiger H, Fraenkel L and Leichner PP (1989) Relationship of body-image distortion to sex-role identifications, irrational cognitions, and body weight in eating-disordered females. *Journal of Clinical Psychology 45*, 61–5.

Stoeckel JD (1966) Hypochondriasis. *International Journal of Psychiatry 2*, 330–1.

Strauman TJ, Vookles J, Berenstein V, Chaiken S and Higgins ET (1991) Self-discrepancies and vulnerability to body dissatisfaction and disordered eating. *Journal of Personality and Social Psychology 61*: 946–56.

Strober M, Goldenberg I, Green J and Saxon J (1979) Body image disturbance in anorexia nervosa during the acute and recuperative phase. *Psychological Medicine 9*, 695–701.

Taylor B (1856) *Putmans' Monthly Magazine 8*, 233.

Veale D, Boocock A, Gournay K, *et al.* (1996) Body dysmorphic disorder: a survey of 50 cases. *British Journal of Psychiatry 169* (suppl. 2), 196–201.

Veith I (1965) *Hysteria: the History of a Disease*. Chicago: University of Chicago Press.

Waller D and Eisenberg L (1980) School refusal in childhood – a psychiatric-paediatric perspective. In Hersov L and Berg I (eds) *Out of School*. Chichester: John Wiley.

Wilde OFFW (1948) *The Picture of Dorian Gray*. London: Unicorn Press.

World Health Organization (1977) *International Statistical Classification of Diseases, Injuries and Causes of Death*, 9th revision. Geneva: World Health Organization.

World Health Organization (1992) *The ICD-10 Classification of Mental and Behavioural Disorders: Clinical Description and Diagnostic Guidelines*. Geneva: World Health Organization.

World Health Organization Regional Office for Europe. *Obesity in Europe*. Online. Available: http://www.euro.who.int/obesity/import/20060220_1

Yap PM (1951) Mental illness peculiar to certain cultures. *Journal of Mental Science 97*, 313–27.

Zellner DA, Harner DE and Adler RL (1989) Effects of eating abnormalities and gender on perceptions of desirable body shape. *Journal of Abnormal Psychology 98*, 93–6.

Disorders of Gender and Sexuality

16

" Transsexualism is something different in kind. It is not a sexual mode or preference. It is not an act of sex at all. It is a passionate, lifelong, ineradicable conviction, and no true transsexual has ever been disabused of it…

" I myself see the conundrum in another perspective, for I believe it to have some higher origin or meaning. I equate it with the idea of soul, or self, and I think of it not just as a sexual enigma, but as a quest for unity. For me every aspect of my life is relevant to that quest – not only the sexual impulses, but all the sights, sounds and smells of memory, the influences of buildings, landscapes, comradeships, the power of love and of sorrow, the satisfactions of the senses as of the body. In my mind it is a subject far wider than sex; I recognise no pruriency to it, and I see it above all as a dilemma neither of the body nor of the brain, but of the spirit. *Morris (1974)*

This chapter attempts only to outline psychopathology associated with disorders of gender and sex. More detailed information, both on symptoms and treatment, are found in textbooks on this topic (Bancroft, 1974, 1989; Feldman and MacCulloch, 1980; Gagnon and Simon, 1967; Rosen, 1979). Because of the emphasis on individual and subjective experience, the social, cultural and relationship aspects are scarcely mentioned in this chapter. Marital dysfunction and disorders of pregnancy and the puerperium are discussed here for convenience: there are often associations in the mind of the sufferers between their present state of conflict and their role as woman, spouse, sexual partner and mother.

Gender describes the lifelong state or category of an organism as regards masculinity and femininity. *Sex* describes its physical manifestation, with an implication of its participation in the appropriate copulatory activity for that gender, male or female. The difference of meaning between the two words *gender* and *sex* has become blurred with usage. The sex of a child is, of course, normally assigned at birth. Mistaken or uncertain assignment at this stage will have serious psychological implications at a later stage. Gender identity is normally established by about the age of 18 months: the child knows that he is a boy and that this is different from being a girl; he begins to learn what are masculine interests and behaviours and to apply them to himself. This begins to occur from the beginning of the establishment of language. This development does not occur in a vacuum; it is strongly reinforced by the parents and by society in general. If there had been faulty assignment at birth, this establishment of gender identity on the ascribed sex overrides the biological sex.

This *core gender identity* is the private view of *own* gender, which the subject retains, and is established very early in life. It is biologically influenced and also strongly socially reinforced. It remains throughout life. The tendency is, once having settled on gender, for subsequent development and social interchange to encourage that gender identity to become more pronounced.

Gender role is the working out of this gender identity in a social milieu, the public aspect of gender. So the little boy plays the role of the man, the father, in his games of pretence and later plays the role in adult life. Gender role is developed on the basis of gender identity but is not fixed or immutable like gender identity. Qualities such as aggressiveness, gentleness and effeminacy may be seen as having gender role connotations, but gender role is on a continuum: a male person with masculine gender identity may play a female gender role either consistently or occasionally. Sexual behaviour, which lies dormant until puberty, is clearly related to gender identity and role but is not wholly dependent on them for its orientation. The pattern of sexual behaviour that becomes established is dictated by the fantasy life, especially masturbation fantasies, of that person based on his previous memories; by the time of life and his physical constitution; and by the availability of sexual outlets, as well as by gender. Cultural norms and patterns establish the framework that limits the possibility for sexual expression.

GENDER IDENTITY DISORDERS

There is in these conditions a lack of congruence between biological sex and gender identity. Gender identity is usually clearly established as male or female in early childhood but, occasionally, there is a feeling of discomfort and inappropriateness about his or her biological sex, with a persistent wish to be of the opposite sex and repudiation of his or her own anatomy. Such people may have involved themselves as children in stereotypical behaviour of the other sex and preferred to cross-dress. The vast majority of such children eventually develop normally in gender identity and sexual behaviour; a few become predominantly homosexual; and very few indeed are eventually, as adults, established in transsexualism.

Psychotic disturbances of gender identity and role are not uncommon manifestations of illness. In fact, with schizophrenia, the disturbance of self-image is global and virtually always affects feelings about sex and gender in some way. Schizophrenic patients often describe delusions and hallucinations with sexual content. They quite often believe that they may be changing sex or that they are homosexual, or they believe that other people believe them to be homosexual. A schizophrenic man aged 32 believed he was changing into a woman because:

> “ I went back for the clock ... everybody seemed to move inside my body the next day ... I started to wind the clock and thought to myself, ‘What time did Tom say that he was going to call for me?’ He was the last one I thought to going into the bedroom with. I couldn’t get him out of my mind. I like the chap but I couldn’t care less about him. My sister said, ‘Don’t forget to bring in the clock’. I don’t know what the clock has got to do with it.

Schreber (1955) described his situation as follows.

> "When the rays approach, my breast gives the impression of a pretty well-developed female bosom; this phenomenon can be *seen* by anyone who wants to observe me *with his own eyes*. I am therefore in a position to offer objective evidence by observation of my body. A brief glance however would not suffice, the observer would have to go to the trouble of spending 10 or 15 minutes near me. In that way anybody would notice the periodic swelling and diminution of my bosom. Naturally hairs remain under my arms and on my chest; these are by the way sparse in my case; my nipple also remains small as in the male sex. Notwithstanding, I venture to assert flatly that anybody who sees me standing in front of a mirror with the upper part of my body naked would get the undoubted impression of a female trunk – especially when the illusion is strengthened by some female adornments... I believe that I have thus furnished proof which must arouse doubt among serious men as to whether what as so far been attributed to hallucinations and delusions is not after all reality.

Depressive delusions may also be associated with gender, and these have characteristic nihilistic or guilt-ridden content.

Transsexualism (gender identity disorder)

In this condition, there is a disturbance of body image with a disorder of core gender identity, a discrepancy between anatomical sex and the gender the person ascribes to himself. In transsexualism, wearing clothing of the opposite sex (transvestism) occurs, usually, as a means of personal gratification without genital excitement. It is much commoner in biological males than in females, but it occurs in both sexes. The sufferer from this anomaly feels he should have been of the other gender, 'a female spirit trapped in a male body' (Morris, 1974), and is quite unconvinced by scientific tests that show him to be indisputably male. In adults, the disturbance is manifested by preoccupation with getting rid of primary and secondary sexual characteristics and the request for hormone therapy or surgery or other means of simulating the required gender (Green, 2000). The strength of this bizarre conviction is described in *Conundrum* by Jan Morris (1974) with literary éclat: 'I was three or perhaps four years old when I realized that I had been born into the wrong body, and should really be a girl ... through each year my every instinct seemed to become more feminine, my entombment within the male physique more terrible to me'. Another transsexual described himself:

> "I know that I am biologically a man but it is all a horrible freak of nature. Really I am a woman and by some accident I have got a male body. I think as a woman and have female feelings and interests, and am only comfortable when wearing women's clothes and in a feminine job. So, genuinely, I am a woman... I am not against homosexuals although I am not one myself. When I have sex with a man, you must remember that I am really a woman.

The transsexual person has succeeded on occasions in persuading his or her partner about the 'mistake' of his body. His belief is an *overvalued idea*, often taken to an extreme degree. He may change his name to a feminine one by deed poll, change the description of sex on his employment card and seek surgery to achieve 'restitution to my rightful appearance'.

Transsexuals describe their feelings about their body as having been present from early childhood: the feeling of comfort and 'rightness' they experienced when wearing their sister's dress, how they 'fell naturally' into female pursuits and interests. The difference of self-image from the biological sex is usually, in their own account, clearly established before puberty. In the development of their condition, a mutually over-dependent relationship with the mother and an absent or abnormal father has often been described. Background family dynamics, of dependence on a dominant mother and a weak or absent father, are by no means universal for transsexual individuals and, of course, may precede entirely normal sexual development.

Many showing transsexualism experience disturbance in their life situation from personality disorder, but transsexualism is also compatible with a stable way of life. A biological female aged 45 had lived for over 20 years as the masculine proprietor of a hardware shop in a small country town. He lived with his sister and brother-in-law and their family and did all the carpentry, plumbing and painting jobs about the house. The family accepted his gender as 'a male person'. His presenting complaint to his doctor was that if he needed to go to a public convenience at a football match, he could not use the male toilet, and he was in danger with the law in the female one. Although he showed no other psychological abnormality at extensive psychiatric interview, at 15-year follow-up he had killed himself.

Transsexual people usually describe difficulties in adjustment at school, and they tend to have jobs below their intellectual capacity. If married, the male transsexual tends to be envious of his wife's femininity, pregnancy and motherhood. He is repelled by his external genitalia, and he repudiates his biological sex. Intense preoccupation with feminine pursuits in male transsexualism is often a caricature of womanhood, a pretentious consciousness of femininity unusual in women. They tend, if biologically male, to have a stereotyped male attitude to what it is to be female: a transsexual with muscular, male physique expatiated on the delights of having silky underwear next to the skin and how 'it is so feminine'; another considered an idyllic existence was to sit at home in the evening knitting woollen baby clothes.

DISORDERS OF SEXUAL PREFERENCE

Most of the descriptive accounts in this area are concerned with the nature of the behaviour rather than the subjective experience of the person who carried out that behaviour. The phenomenologist is concerned with such questions as 'Why did this person carry out this sexual behaviour, and why now?' Interest lies in the current subjective state of the individual and in understanding the background from which it emerged. Most of the answers to the questions will be revealed only on detailed phenomenological enquiry, but often such enquiry is omitted in favour of behavioural analysis and symptomatic treatment.

Figure 16.1 represents graphically a notion of P.D. Scott's concerning the relationship between deviant sexuality and society. The definition of sexual perversion (deviation) ascribed to Scott (1964) and quoted by Wakeling (1979) is as follows.

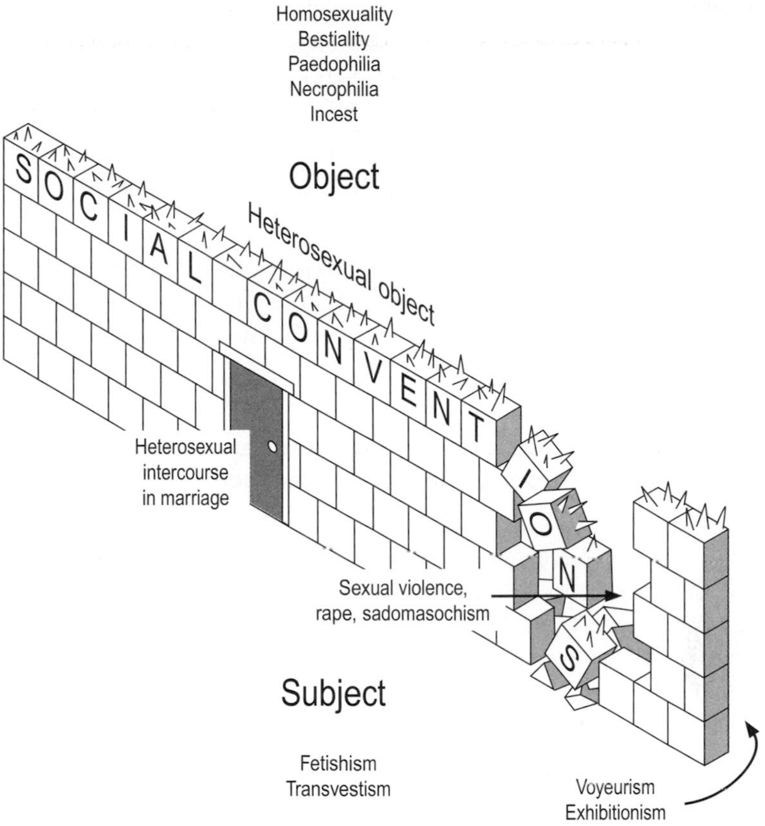

Figure 16.1 Deviant sexual activity.

> "The elements of a comprehensive definition of sexual perversion should include sexual activity or fantasy directed towards orgasm other than genital intercourse with a willing partner of the opposite sex and of similar maturity, persistently recurrent, not merely a substitute for preferred behaviour made difficult by the immediate environment and contrary to the generally accepted norm of sexual behaviour in the community.

The disorders of sexual development and orientation described below are categorized according to the predominant behaviour, but there is overlap between different types of behaviour, and within each type there is much variation in pattern, attitude and sociocultural aspects; most types of behaviour may be heterosexual or homosexual or both. Phenomenological description of self-experience associated with these behaviours varies from the aggressively political stance that theirs is normal behaviour to the extreme of guilt and self-loathing, sometimes culminating in suicide, that may occur with any form of behaviour that the individual himself regards as deviation. Fantasies of domination and destruction are more serious predictors of violent sexual acts than sexual arousal alone; the feature of these behaviours is that violent fantasy is required for sexual excitement.

Masturbation

This is mentioned to demonstrate how what is regarded within the social context as 'deviant' will change in response to alterations of attitude in society. Masturbation in the nineteenth century was not only regarded as sexual deviation but as a substantial cause of serious physical and mental illness, and it was recognized to be a dangerous disease entity in its own right (Engelhardt, 1981). This should make us wary of too readily labelling what we regard as unacceptable as deviant, mentally ill or pathological. Much of the psychopathology, especially anxiety and depression, of those caught in the act of masturbation 100 years ago could be ascribed to the social sanctions and dire consequences attributed to it in the public and medical mind rather than to the act itself.

Disorders associated with sexual development and orientation: specific forms of disorder of sexual preference

Those abnormalities of sexual preference listed in ICD-10 are shown in Table 16.1. These forms of behaviour are statistically abnormal, and as attitudes to sexual behaviour are emotionally charged in society, deviation from the norm, abnormal behaviour, is regarded in a pejorative way: there is a marked social stigma. Subjective experience of deviance in sexual behaviour is determined by the social context. This has been categorized by Gagnon and Simon (1967) into three types.

1. *Normal* deviance, including such behaviour as masturbation, premarital intercourse, homosexuality and oral sex, which have been in the past and are still, in some communities, regarded as deviant.
2. *Subcultural* deviance, for example transsexualism, for which, although the larger society rejects this behaviour as deviant, an accepting subculture can be found.
3. *Individual* deviance, for which no such subculture exists, for instance with exhibitionism or incest. Within this classification, individual deviance is seen to carry a much higher risk of ostracism, alienation and consequent psychiatric symptoms. With changing sexual mores in society, membership of these groups alters with time.

Table 16.1 Disorders of sexual preference in ICD-10

Code	Disorder
F65.1	Fetishism
F65.1	Fetishistic transvestism
F65.2	Exhibitionism
F65.3	Voyeurism
F65.4	Paedophilia
F65.5	Sadomasochism
F65.6	Multiple disorders of sexual preference

(From World Health Organization, 1992, with permission.)

A broadly similar list is found in DSM-IV (American Psychiatric Association, 1994). This includes, as *paraphilias* within the broader category of sexual disorders, exhibitionism, fetishism, frotteurism, paedophilia, sexual masochism, sexual sadism, transvestic fetishism and voyeurism. *Frotteurism* describes recurrent, intense sexual urges and sexually arousing fantasies involving touching and rubbing against a non-consenting person.

Psychological symptoms are common for many different forms of sexual behaviour and are especially related to *feelings about oneself*, such as guilt, shame and disgust, and *problems with relationships*. Concentration on these behaviours, as the predominant sexual activity, will adversely affect a long-term sexual and loving relationship and also tend to distort less intimate, companionable interactions with others.

Bestiality (zoophilia)

This describes any type of sexual intercourse with animals; it is both uncommon and also a criminal offence. By legal definition, it is a form of buggery involving the use of animals as sexual objects (Bluglass, 1990). It is most likely to be indulged in by those of limited intellectual capacity and restricted social outlet for whom access to animals is easy, for example a shy, mentally handicapped adolescent boy living on a farm.

Paedophilia

Paedophilia is defined as 'a perversion in which an adult has a sexual interest in children' (Glasser, 1990) and 'the expressed desire for immature sexual gratification with a prepubertal child' (Mohr *et al.*, 1964). Thus it involves an adult engaging in sexual activity with a child of the same or opposite sex. *Pederasty* is anal intercourse practised by adults with boys. The adult in such activity is guilty of a criminal offence, and physical contact of a sexual kind is regarded as an assault, even though the majority of such actions are not violent in nature. When the child is an older girl (over 12 years), the offender is often a young male, relatively indiscriminate about sexual partners, but neither consistently deviant nor psychiatrically ill. For younger children below the age of puberty, the adult is likely to be substantially older than the child; more consistently interested in sexual activity with children; and more likely to show psychiatric illness such as schizophrenia, manic phase of affective disorder, alcoholism, dementia or mental handicap (Bancroft, 1974). There is frequently history of severe psychosocial deprivation during the perpetrator's own childhood, which often includes sexual abuse. Thus, paedophilia is known to be associated with other psychiatric disorders, notably mood disorders, substance misuse, impulse control disorders and other paraphilias. There is also association with personality disorders such as dissocial personality disorder.

Paedophilia is associated with extreme social disapproval and, despite recent attempts by those involved to establish a clandestine subculture, such people feel themselves to be utterly rejected. Severe depressive reaction is associated with shame and self-loathing; suicide is not uncommon. In prison, such individuals require protection from serious physical assaults by their fellow inmates.

Transvestism

This is the persistent wearing of clothes of the opposite sex. Usually, the cross-dresser is a heterosexual man who carries out the behaviour for the purpose of sexual excitement. However, the term encompasses all types of cross-dressing, from the occasional, solitary wearing of female clothes or more persistent wearing of, for example, one female undergarment, to the regular wearing by a male of entirely female clothing.

Transvestism is carried out for the following reasons or in these contexts.

1. In entertainment or theatre as female impersonators.
2. To provoke heterosexual erotic excitement as part of fetishistic, masturbatory or coital ritual (a man was impotent in intercourse with his wife unless he was wearing high-heeled feminine shoes).
3. Within homosexual relationships, cross-dressing has a symbolic significance. The aim is not to simulate the opposite sex but rather to carry out a burlesque, pointing fun at the image of the opposite sex (Brierley, 1979). There is also the political posture of establishing the right of the homosexual person not to conform with the social conventions of his or her own gender.
4. Exhibitionistic cross-dressing occurs, in which a man dressed partly in female clothes exposes himself to a female person. The intention, again, is not to pass as a female but to frighten the victim and express a hostile sexual message in the context of relationship difficulties with women.
5. Cross-dressing has been used as a device, for example to escape from prison, to serve in a one-sex profession or to gain entry to a harem!
6. Gratification of social role without sexual excitement is the form transvestism takes in transsexualism.

In all these situations, except perhaps 5, it is vastly more common for biological males to wear female clothes than vice versa. However, this could be challenged with the undoubtedly true contention that it is much easier for females to wear male (or nearly masculine) garments without social disapproval. Such well-known behaviour as the cross-dressing of Joan of Arc is exceptional; most abnormalities of sexual preference, of all types, are predominantly male.

Fetishism

Etymologically, this means 'the worship of inanimate objects' (Christie-Brown, 1983), but it implies repeated sexual preoccupation and excitement with non-living objects; these come to take central importance in achieving orgasm. Fetishes may be articles of clothing, perhaps a woman's shoe; substances and textures, for example rubber or shiny black plastic; or even parts of the body, such as hair or nails. To be regarded as deviant, fetishism must be essential for orgasm and causing problems, for instance in the relationship between partners; it may occur within the context of sexual intercourse or masturbation. Fetishism is almost exclusively male.

The sexual behaviour may involve masturbation using the fetish alone, or the fetish may be incorporated within sexual activities involving another person.

Exhibitionism

The main sexual pleasure and gratification is derived from exposure of the genitals to a person of the opposite sex (Snaith, 1983a). This is the commonest of sexual offences; from the victim's point of view, the behaviour is a nuisance but not dangerous. While the behaviour of exhibitionism is predominantly male, the offence of *indecent exposure* is confined to men; this is perhaps more dependent on the cultural context and what it ordains to be illicit, rather than a difference of individual experience between the sexes. The victim of indecent exposure is female, adult or child, and there is often an intention to surprise, shock or even insult the observer. The exhibitionist exposes his genitals and may masturbate while doing so; he may return regularly to the same spot where passers by will see him, and repeat his behaviour persistently despite numerous court appearances and punishments. The compulsive nature of the behaviour is strongly marked in that there is an overriding need to act in the same way, even though the individual himself recognizes the act as senseless and harmful. It is quite exceptional for such people to proceed to any other type of sexual deviation. Such individuals are often passive, inadequate men with problems in relationships and low self-esteem; they may show personality disorder of dependent type.

Voyeurism

In order to achieve sexual excitement, as the preferred or exclusive method, such a person (a 'peeping Tom') repetitively looks at unsuspecting people who are naked, getting undressed or engaged in sexual activity. No other sexual contact with the observed individual is attempted; masturbation may take place during viewing or afterwards while recalling the memory. The voyeur often has fantasies of humiliating or embarrassing the victims with the knowledge that they have been observed.

Sadomasochism

Sexual arousal is in response to the infliction of pain, psychological humiliation or ritualized dominance or submission. Sadism is the infliction of pain or suffering on another for sexual excitement, and masochism the passive experience of being made to suffer to achieve sexual stimulation. The latter often involves submission in various forms of *bondage*, being tied up and constrained, often associated with *flagellation*. Sadomasochistic fantasies, of a mild kind, occur during intercourse or masturbation in both sexes, often within a stable relationship, but more violent fantasies and practices are predominantly or exclusively male in nature. Sadomasochism is quite common among those who are exclusively homosexual; among those who are heterosexual, it may provoke marital breakdown.

Multiple disorders of sexual preference

The various sexual preferences outlined above are not necessarily exclusive to any one individual. Thus a person who shows one form of deviation is more likely to find sexual arousal in another, the most frequent combination being fetishism, transvestism and sadomasochism. Such a person, showing many different abnormalities, is described as having multiple disorders of sexual preference.

Necrophilia

Necrophilia, which is extremely rare, involves achieving sexual excitement through contact with a dead body; it may occur in association with homicide.

Sexual violence: rape

Sexual violence is defined as the infliction of physical injury on another person or threat thereof as part of, or during, sexual interference (Quinsey, 1990).

Rape is sexual intercourse by a male with a female who at the time does not consent. Legally, for the act to be regarded as rape, it must involve vaginal penetration by the penis, and the man must be aged over 14 years.

Buggery refers to anal intercourse and is more commonly homosexual; buggery with violence is endemic in some prison populations, in which it is more an expression of physical domination than sexual gratification.

Heterosexual assault, rape, usually involves physical violence that sometimes is extreme. Violence is usually a more important part of the motivation than sexual excitement. Holmstrom and Burgess (1980) considered that sexual assault had four principal meanings:

- power and control over the victim
- expression of anger or hatred
- in group rape, camaraderie experienced by rapists
- sexual experience, which was never the dominant theme.

On the other hand, the violence of sexual assault is itself found to be sexually stimulating. This was demonstrated in the finding that rapists in prison were found to develop erections during an audible description of rape scenes, while non-rapist prisoners did not (Abel *et al.*, 1978).

Rape victims

In terms of mental symptoms associated with sexual behaviour, the victim of rape should, of course, also be considered. Although the characteristics of rape victims are not entirely dissimilar to other victims of violence or traumatic stress, in the victim's subjective experience this form of violence has different implications. The way it is regarded by the public and dealt with by the police and others often produces feelings of guilt and shame that exacerbate what is already an appalling experience. Rape and its consequences are a significant factor for victims in producing long-term psychiatric morbidity and psychosocial disability.

Childhood sexual abuse predisposes to greater levels of psychopathology in adult life, including substance abuse and suicidal behaviour; the more severe the abuse, the greater the degree of adult morbidity (Mullen *et al.*, 1993). However, the matrix of deprivation and disadvantage in which it usually occurs makes it possible to understand the relationship only within the social context from which it emerged.

Child sexual abuse

Incest refers to sexual relations between family members forbidden by taboos, social mores and the law (Cooper and Cormier, 1990). Under the Sexual Offences Act, 1956, it is an offence for a man to have sexual intercourse with a woman whom he knows to be his granddaughter, daughter, sister (or half-sister) or mother, and it is an offence for a woman over the age of 16 years to permit a man of similar affinity to have intercourse with her by consent (Bluglass, 1979). Incest probably occurs in all social class groups; the mean intelligence of offenders is probably higher than that of other sexual offenders and mental illness is unusual, although a substantial minority of offenders show such abnormalities of personality as being persistently violent and irascible, maladjusted at work, alcoholic and having a previous criminal record. There is also a relatively normal group of otherwise well-adjusted individuals.

Brother–sister and mother–son relationships are rare; father–daughter incest is the most common type, both in fact and to come to court. Now, with large-scale breakdown of marriage and the nuclear family, incest involving stepfather and daughter has become frequent. Bluglass has considered the following to be predisposing factors to incest.

- A man returning home after many years of separation to find an ageing wife and a young daughter, who now seems almost a stranger and also a temptation.
- The loss of a wife by divorce, separation or death, leaving a bereaved father alone with an adolescent daughter who becomes a substitute wife providing love, solace and sexual comfort.
- Gross overcrowding, physical proximity and alcoholism leading to sexual intimacy.
- A lack of social contact outside the family as a result of poverty and geographical remoteness.
- Anxiety associated with a lack of sexual potency.
- Marital disharmony and rejection or a decrease in marital sexual activity.
- Psychopathic characteristics of poor impulse control, aggressiveness and lack of guilt feelings, with or without any of the above factors.

The father may have severe feelings of guilt and depression while the relationship is still continuing and after discovery and sentencing. Such depression will require treatment, and there is considerable risk of suicide. The daughter may also show subsequent psychiatric disability: four out of twenty-six daughters in one study subsequently showed frank psychiatric symptoms, eleven developed character disorder and five frigidity or aversion to sexual relations with their husbands (Lukianowicz, 1972). It is now accepted that sexual abuse during childhood, usually perpetrated by someone in the family home, is a major factor in the subsequent development of adolescent and adult psychological maladjustment and emotional disturbance.

Egodystonic sexual orientation

ICD-10 uses the above term effectively to encompass *egodystonic homosexuality*, in which the individual explicitly states that the sustained pattern of homosexual arousal is unwanted and a source of distress, and there is a desire to acquire heterosexual orientation. There is no comparable group of those with heterosexual behaviours who wish to change their sexual orientation in the opposite direction. Neither is there an example from other species of exclusive homosexual preference; the phenomenon of sexual orientation is uniquely human and is a consequence of multifactorial biological and psychosocial factors (Bancroft, 1994).

Homosexuality is the preference for sexual behaviour with a member of one's own, rather than the opposite, sex, either in fact or in fantasy or in both. There is not necessarily disturbance of gender identity, but some effeminate male homosexuals have conflicts concerning masculinity and femininity (Rosen, 1979). There is often dissonance of gender, in that the gender identity is usually clearly male but the role may be construed by the person himself as female.

It is difficult at present to give a balanced account of homosexuality, as many recent developments in society have tended to polarize and politicize issues. The self-perception of a person as one with homosexual identity is not easy to separate from him seeing himself as a member of a minority group with its own established standards and mores. Attitudes are changing very fast, both within the homosexual community and towards it by those outside. Over recent years, distinctive political and sociological views have developed among those who identify themselves with a wider homosexual community. Acquired immune deficiency syndrome (AIDS) has had an effect both on individuals' feelings about themselves and on the way they are viewed by the larger society. The women's movement and feminism has not only affected the position of female homosexuals in society but also that of males. All these external, social and political influences have tended to obscure individual self-attitudes concerning gender identity and sexual preference.

The factors contributing to male homosexuality have been summarized by Bancroft (1975) as 'push' and 'pull' factors. The push factors involve anxiety about the heterosexual role. This may be based on learned reluctance of involvement in heterosexual contact, incestuous feelings towards the mother, lack of confidence in sexual potency, fear of failure in heterosexual relationships or impaired gender identity with fear of rejection of his masculinity by women. The pull factors include sexual drive, the feeling of need for a one-to-one emotional relationship, self-esteem engendered by the partner's attraction, eroticization of a person who is otherwise a threatening object and material gain. Bancroft stresses that an important determinant of whether a person continues with homosexual behaviour is his ability to tolerate the idea of himself as homosexual; the challenge to his self-esteem may outweigh the positive reinforcement he experiences.

In female homosexuality, there is a definite preference for erotic attraction to another female, commonly implying some physical expression (Kenyon, 1975). Disturbance in gender identity is not usually conspicuous, but gender role may be quite markedly masculine. *Lesbians* more often described disturbance in their early life than heterosexual women, with a poor relationship with a mother who was more likely to have died prematurely or had mental illness. They also described more often poor relationships with their father, disturbed parental marriage and an unhappy childhood. Family attitudes towards sex were less accepting; lesbians had rarely received sex instruction from their mother, and a quarter reported a family history of homosexuality. Lesbians were more likely to have experienced a traumatic heterosexual approach during childhood. More of the lesbian group felt that they were not fully feminine, and their lifestyle and choice of occupation had been more likely to result in proximity and access to other women.

Certainly, since the Kinsey Reports, in which many thousands of Americans were questioned about their sexual behaviour (Kinsey *et al.*, 1948, 1953), it has been realized that there are gradations from exclusive homosexual practice to exclusive heterosexuality, and that there may be a discrepancy between fantasy and practice in the relative proportions. However, Kinsey's original high figures for the prevalence of homosexual practice have been challenged by more recent studies (Gagnon and Simon, 1967); especially, the claim that many people were in the intermediate grades was contradicted, and the distribution was found to be bimodal, with most people claiming to be predominantly either heterosexual or homosexual. Most recent studies show that about 1 to 2 per cent of the population consider themselves to be homosexual (Bancroft, 1989). Homosexuality and heterosexuality are not fixed and immutable: there is the possibility of change in both directions, and this is influenced by environmental/social and internal/psychological factors. A person who has not previously manifested homosexual experience may do so for the first time, even in late middle age, in response to some life crisis, especially if the problem is associated with confidence in himself as a mature and competent adult, or with marital difficulties. A person who has shown homosexual practice for decades may voluntarily change to heterosexual identity initially, and practice subsequently, for example in association with religious conversion (Pattison and Pattison, 1980). The cognitive change precedes behavioural change, which precedes orientation or preference. Because of this possibility of change, it is better to use the word *homosexual* as an adjective rather than as a noun; a person is not *a* homosexual, although he or she may regard him- or herself as having homosexual orientation.

The relationship between homosexuality and psychiatry is highly complex and has become more so over recent years with the addition of a sociopolitical dimension. The vast majority of those whose sexual preference is homosexual will never consult a psychiatrist and will make no long-standing complaint of psychiatric symptoms. There is a need, however, to consider four groups of individuals who may be seen by psychiatrists:

- those with egodystonic sexual orientation
- those whose sexual practice is homosexual and who also have psychiatric symptoms
- those with various problems associated with the human immune deficiency virus (HIV) and AIDS
- those with a disorder of sexual preference that is illegal or not socially sanctioned and takes place in a homosexual context.

Those who do make complaint specifically related to their homosexuality and how this affects their self-concept (egodystonic) are most likely to do so on one or both of two grounds:

- feelings of guilt that they are unable to expunge; this relates to their background social, cultural and religious beliefs about the nature of relationships

- breakdown of relationships; for a variety of reasons, homosexual relationships tend to be brittle, jealousies are intense and severe feelings of loss and abandonment occur frequently when such relationships are severed.

Even if the homosexual population is only 2 per cent of the total, it still represents a large number of people, and it is not surprising therefore that among these there are sufferers from psychiatric illnesses. No excess of those with disorder of personality was found among populations of homosexual people not consulting a psychiatrist. Male homosexuals have been found to be less happy than heterosexual controls (Weinberg and Williams, 1974) and to have more psychosomatic symptoms, more loneliness, lower self-esteem, more depression and suicidal ideas (Bell and Weinberg, 1978). There is therefore a trend towards higher affective morbidity in the homosexual population.

Acquired immune deficiency syndrome

This topic is introduced here as, in the United Kingdom in the 1990s, apart from heroin addicts sharing needles and a few individuals with haemophilia (transfused in the past), the chief effects of this scourge are among the homosexual community. AIDS, which was first described only in 1981, results from infection with a retrovirus, HIV. There may be an initial, transitory infection somewhat similar to glandular fever; persistent glandular lymphadenopathy frequently develops early. AIDS-related complex is usually manifested next, with malaise, loss of weight, diarrhoea and fever. Finally, fully developed AIDS shows one or more of three syndromes:

- pulmonary opportunistic infection
- Kaposi's sarcoma
- AIDS encephalopathy.

The psychiatrist in general adult practice may well encounter one of six different types of presentation associated with AIDS.

- AIDS encephalopathy. This occurs in 40 per cent of established sufferers from AIDS. It progresses to dementia and may be associated with peripheral neuropathy.
- Psychosis associated with AIDS or HIV infection. In a series of five cases, labile affective changes, which were predominantly neither manic nor depressive, and delusions and auditory hallucinations occurred; the symptoms were considered to be functional rather than organic in nature (Halstead *et al.*, 1988).
- Anxiety and depression in established sufferers from AIDS. These symptoms may be very severe and are similar to those seen in others suffering a rapidly fatal condition.
- Anxiety, depression and other psychological symptoms in those who are HIV-positive. Here, there is fear of developing AIDS coupled with fear of transmitting the virus to partners knowing that the subject is potentially infective. There may also be considerable stigma both from the immediate homosexual community and from society, and there may be experience of loss and bereavement following the death from AIDS of close friends and associates.

- Fear of AIDS in those who have been exposed to risk, either through homosexual or heterosexual contact or through needle exchange.
- Fear of AIDS, and a belief that one has contracted AIDS, is also presented to psychiatrists occasionally by those who have not and could not have contracted the condition.

This is necessarily a brief account of an important subject.

The syndrome of fear of AIDS may be very similar, in its psychological symptoms, to the disease itself in the early stages, as anxiety and depression may be prominent in either (Miller *et al.*, 1985). In AIDS, the sufferer feels lethargic, loses appetite and weight and sweats excessively. There is an increasing concern among homosexual men concerning the development of AIDS, and there are some who show a pseudo-AIDS syndrome, of psychogenic cause, that can result in considerable disability. The AIDS epidemic among homosexual men has some of the features of epidemic anxiety: a discrete, vulnerable subculture who communicate both the infection and the mass neurotic anxiety.

> “ The male gay community is gripped with fear of AIDS. There is a widespread folk-myth that ... AIDS has been sent as retribution... The anonymous, and semi-anonymous, nature of much male gay sex – and the extent of recreational sex – means that many gay men simply do not know whether or not they have had sex with someone who is now suffering from AIDS – with someone who has had sex with someone who is now suffering from AIDS – or with ... and so it goes on. *(Macourt, 1985)*

PSYCHOSEXUAL DYSFUNCTION

Symptoms associated with ‘normal’, heterosexual intercourse are extremely frequent; the more the interviewer allows the patient to express him- or herself freely, the more likely they are to be described. Symptoms may be associated with the functions of the genital organs during intercourse (sexual dysfunction), with the subjective feelings during intercourse (sexual difficulties) and with the sexual relationship; of course, these areas overlap.

Sexual dysfunction

For men, this includes erectile and ejaculatory difficulties; for women, inhibition of sexual excitement and problems with orgasm, and also genital pain and discomfort, occur.

Male sexual dysfunction

Lack of, or inhibited, sexual excitement during intended sexual activity is manifested by partial or complete failure to achieve or maintain an erection throughout sexual intercourse (*erectile dysfunction*, previously *impotence*). There may also be *delay* or absence of ejaculation following an adequate phase of sexual excitement. *Premature ejaculation* may take place before the man wishes it and is clearly out of his control (Cooper, 1970). When any of these symptoms or more than one occurs persistently, this would be regarded as dysfunction. This may be responsible for causing further symptoms, such as anxiety and loss of self-esteem, or result from psychological symptoms such as anxiety or fatigue. It can be seen how sexual dysfunction and neurotic illness become a mutually reinforcing vicious circle.

Female sexual dysfunction

In women, inhibited sexual excitement, low interest and low enjoyment (previously *frigidity*) are shown by partial or complete failure to achieve or maintain the lubrication and swelling of the genitalia during the sexual act. There may also be persistent delay or absence of orgasm following normal sexual excitement and activity. Coitus may also be associated with persistent genital pain (*dyspareunia*) or involuntary spasm of the vaginal musculature (*vaginismus*). As in the male, this may both cause further psychological symptoms and result from them.

Sexual difficulties and the sexual relationship

Doctors tend to classify symptoms into the above categories of dysfunction. However, patients regard as more serious in promoting sexual dissatisfaction such difficulties as inability to relax, lack of interest in sex, distaste or revulsion, 'too little foreplay' and 'too little attention after intercourse' (Frank *et al.*, 1978). These symptoms are extremely common. The subjective experience during intercourse, the interaction with the partner and other aspects, such as fantasy, are as important as the purely physical elements involved.

The sexual relationship with the partner is, of course, crucial. One cannot consider, categorize or treat the sexual symptoms of one partner without taking into account the characteristics, attitudes and expectations of the other. If one partner is experiencing either symptoms or dissatisfaction in the sexual relationship, the other partner is likely also to be dissatisfied.

DISORDERS OF PREGNANCY AND THE PUERPERIUM

It remains an enigma why epidemiological studies should regularly show for most mental illnesses a considerable excess of females over males. Biological, social and psychological explanations have been given. There are some disorders specifically associated with female sex, gender and role. Thus, psychological symptoms may be associated with the menarche, with menstruation (Gerrada and Reveley, 1988) with amenorrhoea, with pregnancy and the puerperium and with the menopause. Some of these have been mentioned in Chapter 6. These disorders are discussed only briefly here, and the reader is referred to Snaith (1983b) and Cox (1986).

Disorders of pregnancy

Pregnancy is the most dramatic and rapid change in bodily form that occurs in adult life, and there is a gross and realistic change in body image accompanying it. The subsequent change of role of the woman becoming a mother further accentuates the changing self-image through pregnancy. It is not surprising, therefore, that there are often disturbances such as anxiety, depression, hypochondriasis or hysterical conversion in this process. It is more surprising that these disturbances may affect the husband as well as the wife herself. The abnormality of self-experience when a husband also complains of obstetric symptoms during his wife's pregnancy and parturition is called the *couvade syndrome* (Enoch and Trethowan, 1979).

Pseudocyesis is the occurrence of a false pregnancy. It can occur both in women and in men, although understandably it is much more commonly in women. Hysterical pseudocyesis occurs quite dramatically, with swelling of the abdomen to simulate a full-term pregnancy. This disappears under general anaesthetic, but the muscular spasm producing depression of the diaphragm and lumbar lordosis returns as the patient regains consciousness. Delusions of pregnancy in men have been described in schizophrenia, depressive psychosis, senile dementia, cerebral syphilis and following encephalitis. The delusion remains at the level of a fixed belief without somatic concomitants. Similar delusions of pregnancy occur in psychotic women, sometimes in those who are either postmenopausal or virginal. A most unusual but illustrative example of this condition involved a mother, aged 50, who believed herself to have been pregnant for 10 years; her daughter, who worked as a midwife, had been admitted with phantom pregnancy with other psychotic symptoms but had discharged herself from hospital. Both subjects and all the siblings of the daughter accepted both pregnancies as fact (Milner and Hayes, 1990).

Less exotic but more common symptoms associated with pregnancy are the presence of anxiety and depression. This is not uncommon during pregnancy. It is likely to have been provoked by the pregnancy itself or its associations. Psychotic disturbance may occur during pregnancy but is more common in the puerperium.

Puerperal (postpartum) disorders

Psychiatric involvement in the postpartum period or puerperium includes management and advice for puerperal psychoses, mother–infant relationship disorders, anxiety, obsessional and stress-related neuroses and depression (Brockington, 2000). The terms *postpartum* or *puerperal*, referring to the life epoch, are to be preferred to postnatal, which should logically refer to the baby. The puerperium holds the strongest (relative) risk for psychiatric disorder that has yet been demonstrated (Kendell *et al*., 1987).

Between one-half and two-thirds of women experience a brief episode of lability of mood, tearfulness and irritability, often starting on the third or fourth day after normal delivery. The condition is more common in primigravida and in those who previously suffered premenstrual tension or depressive symptoms before delivery or a previous episode of puerperal depression.

Puerperal psychosis is not a distinct disease entity; affective, schizophrenic or organic psychoses occur but now, with good obstetrics and nutrition and asepsis, 80 per cent of cases are affective. Affective features may occur with schizophrenic psychoses, and altered consciousness and disorientation, with either affective or schizophrenic psychoses, to a greater extent than with non-puerperal disorders. Puerperal psychoses often have a very acute onset and are florid in their symptoms; mania is relatively common among puerperal affective psychoses.

In a few patients, depressive symptomatology of lesser severity may persist for months, or sometimes even for years, after childbirth. This is associated with the changes in lifestyle, looking after a baby, changes in relationships with husband and others and alteration of self-image. It is more frequent in those who have previously experienced affective disorder. Further information on these conditions may be found in Cox (1986).

Couvade syndrome

The couvade syndrome takes its name from a ritual that has been observed in different cultures over many centuries, in which the father of the child to be born mimics the behaviour of his wife through labour. At the onset of her labour, he is put to bed, simulates labour pains and remains 'convalescent' for some days after 'delivery'. It is thought that these rituals may symbolize the father's assertion of paternity or act as decoy to protect the expectant mother from evil. Gross forms of the couvade syndrome are very rare, but minor symptoms in the husband directly associated with his wife's pregnancy are quite common. It has, less frequently, been described in other members of the family. Couvade symptoms in the husband occur from the third month of pregnancy onwards and affect approximately 20 per cent of husbands. They are most frequent in the third and ninth month. Symptoms complained of are very variable and include loss of appetite, toothache, nausea and vomiting (often morning sickness), indigestion, vague abdominal pains, constipation and diarrhoea. The chronological relationship with the wife's pregnancy is more important for making the diagnosis than the nature of the symptoms. Anxiety, tension, insomnia and instability are common complaints, and there is preoccupation with his wife's condition. The symptom can be seen as a *conversion* of the husband's anxiety over his wife's health into somatic symptoms. It is not delusional: the husband with couvade syndrome does not believe himself to be pregnant!

REFERENCES

Abel GG, Barlow DH, Blanchard EB and Guild D (1978) The components of rapists' sexual arousal. In Neale JM, Davison GC and Price KP (eds) *Contemporary Readings in Psychopathology*, 2nd edn, pp. 217–33. New York: John Wiley.

American Psychiatric Association (1994) *Diagnostic and Statistical Manual of Mental Disorders*, 4th edn. Washington: American Psychiatric Association.

Bancroft JH (1974) *Deviant Sexual Behaviour*. Oxford: Clarendon Press.

Bancroft JH (1975) Homosexuality in the male. In Silverstone T and Barraclough B (eds) *Contemporary Psychiatry*. Ashford: Headley Brothers.

Bancroft JH (1989) *Human Sexuality and its Problems*, 2nd edn. Edinburgh: Churchill Livingstone.

Bancroft JH (1994) Homosexual orientation: the search for a biological basis. *British Journal of Psychiatry 164*, 437–40.

Bell AP and Weinberg MS (1978) *Homosexualities. A Study of Diversity Among Men and Women*. London: Mitchell Beazley.

Bluglass RS (1979) Incest. *British Journal of Hospital Medicine 22*, 152–7.

Bluglass RS (1990) Bestiality. In Bluglass R and Bowden P (eds) *Principles and Practice of Forensic Psychiatry*. Edinburgh: Churchill Livingstone.

Brierley H (1979) *Transvestism: a Handbook with Case Studies for Psychologists, Psychiatrists and Counsellors*. Oxford: Pergamon Press.

Brockington I (2000) Obstetric and gynaecological conditions associated with psychiatric disorder. In Gelder MG,

López-Ibor JJ and Andreasen NC (eds) *New Oxford Textbook of Psychiatry*. Oxford: Oxford University Press.

Christie-Brown JRW (1983) Paraphilias: sadomasochism, fetishism, transvestism and transsexuality. *British Journal of Psychiatry 143*, 227–31.

Cooper AJ (1970) Guide to treatment and short-term prognosis of male potency disorders in hospital and general practice. *British Medical Journal i*, 157–9.

Cooper I and Cormier B (1990) Incest. In Bluglass R and Bowden P (eds) *Principles and Practice of Forensic Psychiatry*. Edinburgh: Churchill Livingstone.

Cox JL (1986) *Postnatal Depression: a Guide for Health Professionals*. Edinburgh: Churchill Livingstone.

Engelhardt HT (1981) The disease of masturbation: values and the concept of disease. In Caplan AL, Engelhardt HT and McCartney JJ (eds) *Concepts of Health and Disease*, pp. 267–80. Reading: Addison-Wesley.

Enoch MD and Trethowan WH (1979) *Uncommon Psychiatric Syndromes*. Bristol: John Wright.

Feldman P and MacCulloch M (1980) *Human Sexual Behaviour*. Chichester: John Wiley.

Frank E, Anderson C and Rubinstein D (1978) Frequency of sexual dysfunction in 'normal' couples. *New England Journal of Medicine 299*, 111–5.

Gagnon JH and Simon W (1967) *Sexual Deviance*. New York: Harper & Row.

Gerrada C and Reveley A (1988) Schizophreniform psychosis associated with the menstrual cycle. *British Journal of Psychiatry 152*, 700–2.

Glasser M (1990) Paedophilia. In Bluglass R and Bowden P (eds) *Principles and Practice of Forensic Psychiatry*. Edinburgh: Churchill Livingstone.

Green R (2000) Gender identity disorder in adults. In Gelder MG, López-Ibor JJ and Andreasen NC (eds) *New Oxford Textbook of Psychiatry*. Oxford: Oxford University Press.

Halstead S, Riccio M, Harlow P, Oretti R and Thompson C (1988) Psychosis associated with HIV infection. *British Journal of Psychiatry 153*, 618–23.

Holmstrom LL and Burgess AW (1980) Sexual behaviour of assailants during reported rapes. *Archives of Sexual Behaviour 9*, 427–46.

Kendell RE, Chalmers JC and Platz C (1987) Epidemiology of puerperal psychoses. *British Journal of Psychiatry 150*, 662–73.

Kenyon FE (1975) Homosexuality in the female. In Silverstone T and Barraclough B (eds) *Contemporary Psychiatry*, pp. 185–200. Ashford: Headley Brothers.

Kinsey AC, Pomeroy WB and Martin CE (1948) *Sexual Behaviour in the Human Male*. Philadelphia: Saunders.

Kinsey AC, Pomeroy WB, Martin CE and Gebhard PH (1953) *Sexual Behaviour in the Human Female*. Philadelphia: Saunders.

Lukianowicz N (1972) Incest: part I: paternal incest; part II: other types of incest. *British Journal of Psychiatry 120*, 301–14.

Macourt MPA (1985) *AIDS, gay liberation and pastoral care: a problem concerning the fusion of pastoral care with an emerging ideology in a time of conflict*. Pastoral Studies Conference, University of Birmingham.

Miller D, Green J, Farmer R and Carroll G (1985) A 'pseudo-AIDS' syndrome following from fear of AIDS. *British Journal of Psychiatry 146*, 550–1.

Milner GL and Hayes GD (1990) Pseudocyesis associated with folie à deux. *British Journal of Psychiatry 156*, 438–40.

Mohr JW, Turner RE and Jerry MB (1964) *Paedophilia and Exhibitionism*. London: Oxford University Press.

Morris J (1974) *Conundrum*. London: Faber & Faber.

Mullen PE, Martin JL, Anderson JC, Romans SE and Herbison GP (1993) Childhood sexual abuse and mental health in adult life. *British Journal of Psychiatry 163*, 721–32.

Pattison EM and Pattison ML (1980) 'Ex-gays': religious mediated change in homosexuals. *American Journal of Psychiatry 137*, 1553–62.

Quinsey V (1990) Sexual violence. In Bluglass R and Bowden P (eds) *Principles and Practice of Forensic Psychiatry*. Edinburgh: Churchill Livingstone.

Rosen I (1979) *Sexual Deviation*, 2nd edn. Oxford: Oxford University Press.

Schreber D (1955) *Memoirs of My Mental Illness* (transl. Macalpine I and Hunter R). London: Dawson.

Scott PD (1964) Definition, classification, prognosis and treatment. In Rosen I (ed.) *The Pathology and Treatment of Sexual Deviation*. London: Oxford University Press.

Snaith RP (1983a) Exhibitionism: a clinical conundrum. *British Journal of Psychiatry 143*, 231–5.

Snaith RP (1983b) Pregnancy-related psychiatric disorder. *British Journal of Hospital Medicine 29*, 450–6.

Wakeling A (1979) A general psychiatric approach to sexual deviation. In Rosen I (ed.) *Sexual Deviation*, 2nd edn, pp. 1–28. Oxford: Oxford University Press.

Weinberg MS and Williams CJ (1974) *Male homosexuals: Their Problems and Adaptation*. New York: Oxford University Press.

World Health Organization (1992) *The ICD-10 Classification of Mental and Behavioural Disorders: Clinical Description and Diagnostic Guidelines*. Geneva: World Health Organization.

The Psychopathology of Pain

17

> 'You want to hear of me, my dear? That's something new, I am sure, when anybody wants to hear of me. Not at all well, Louisa. Very faint and giddy.'
> 'Are you in pain, dear mother?'
> 'I think there's a pain somewhere in the room,' said Mrs Gradgrind, 'but I couldn't positively say that I have got it.' *Charles Dickens (1854),* Hard Times

Pain is an unpleasant experience that involves the conscious awareness of noxious sensations, hurting and aversive feelings associated with actual or potential tissue damage (International Association for the Study of Pain, 1994). Since Aristotle, pain has been classified not as a perception but as a mood state, and so excluded from the five senses. It is conceptually a most difficult topic, hard to describe and to categorize; the only aspect that is clear is that it represents a state of subjective suffering of the patient. But what does he mean by 'my pain'? Where is it and what is it? Certainly, the *meaning* of the pain is more than the pain itself, and often it is the reason for the sensation being interpreted as suffering. A patient with soreness of the throat believed herself to have a cancer of the throat; her mother had died of that condition. The relation between symptoms and their meaning is not straightforward. Another person believed herself to be suffering from venereal disease without having been exposed to the risk. But she had previously been successfully treated for Hodgkin's disease. She had no fears concerning her factual, and potentially lethal, illness but only admitted consciously to fearing the impossible.

Among psychiatric patients, the complaint of pain is often associated with diagnostic uncertainty (Anstee and Fleminger, 1977). Ten per cent of patients discharged from a psychiatric unit in a general hospital had an 'uncertain' diagnosis at the time of discharge; nearly one-fifth of these were complaining of pain. At long-term follow-up, nearly half of those complaining of pain remained undiagnosed; of those in whom a diagnosis could by then be made, neuroses and depressive psychoses were commonest, with *atypical facial pain* and physical illness (abdominal neoplasm and coronary disease) less frequent. When pain, without known cause, is the major symptom it is very difficult to apply the usual psychiatric diagnoses.

Phenomenological aspects of the experience of pain are not well charted, although in general medicine this is, above all others, the area in which phenomenology could be most helpful: pain is a subjective experience that occurs only in consciousness (Bond, 1976). The psychiatrist is often confronted with the problem of whether the pain is *physical* or *mental, organic* or *functional, medical* or *psychiatric*, and, of course, the answer for each contrasted pair is often both. We may then be requested to assess how much of the pain is psychogenic, although this is virtually impossible because, following Aristotle, pain is a state of mind, even when there is such an obvious cause as a haematoma under the fingernail.

ORGANIC OR PSYCHOGENIC PAIN?

The transmission of pain results in a subjective, conscious experience. For an account of the anatomical basis for pain and also the physiological and biochemical mechanisms, the reader is referred to Wall and Melzack (1999). There is a threshold for pain: light pressure is perceived as touch, heavy pressure as pain. An explanation for this has been suggested in the *gate control theory* of Melzack and Wall (1965), who considered that painful stimulation through the thin myelinated and unmyelinated fibres results in positive feedback in the substantia gelatinosa; this is transmitted in the lateral spinothalamic tract. However, this gate is under the influence of the higher centres, which can override the local input, as demonstrated by the effect of *attention*: sometimes pain is not felt when attention is directed away from the affected site. Current biochemical theories are also important in accounting for the mediation of pain.

Other theories involve the study of presynaptic and postsynaptic mechanisms in the central nervous system (Nathan, 1980). Electrical stimulation in various sites in the brainstem, including the medulla oblongata, the periaqueductal grey matter and the hypothalamus around the third ventricle, may produce analgesia. Endogenous opiate substances (endorphins) have been discovered to inhibit nerve fibres reporting noxious events. This was initially discovered following electrical stimulation in the periaqueductal grey matter of the brainstem in rats but has subsequently been demonstrated in humans (Bond, 1976). Central nervous system mechanisms for the modulation of pain include descending modulatory control and an increasing number of neurotransmitters, especially serotonin and endogenous opioids; it is almost certainly the interaction of these different systems that is effective in pain modulation (Fields and Basbaum, 1994).

The temptation to regard pain simply as any other sensation creates certain dilemmas. For example, what is the subjective experience of the person who complains of severe pain with no organic pathology detectable, or the person with mild pathology who complains of excruciating pain? How does one assess the person with apparently painful injury who claims he did not notice any pain at the time?

Purely organic, physiological terms, and also psychological, emotional words, have been used. Beecher (1959) believed that pain could be defined and listed many distinguished physiologists and psychiatrists to support his case. However, Merskey (1976) considers that pain is a psychological experience, private to the individual but tending to be described in terms of damage to the body, and so defined pain as 'an unpleasant experience which we primarily associate with tissue damage or describe in terms of such damage, or both'.

Clearly, irrespective of the physical stimulus, psychological factors are enormously important in the appreciation of pain. For example, *psychological analgesia* (educated or natural childbirth in obstetric care), using psychological preparation, explanation and sometimes hypnosis, will result in 5 to 10 per cent of subjects experiencing little or no pain, 15 to 20 per cent experiencing only moderate pain and in the rest pain is not modified but fear and anxiety are diminished (Bonica, 1994). Doctors have frequently, through neglecting subjective evaluation, missed the important distinction between the experience of pain and the physical causes of pain (Noordenbos, 1959). The patient assumes that his pain indicates the presence of physical illness, but pain of various types is a very common symptom in many psychiatric conditions without there being physical pathology.

The experience of psychogenic pain has been associated with particular personality types (Engel, 1959). The most important traits of personality associated with pain are those of anxiousness, depressiveness and the cyclothymic personality at its depressive pole – hysterical, hypochondriacal and obsessional traits (Bond, 1976). Subjects with such personality traits developed to abnormal extent are especially likely to respond to life stresses with pain. Complaints of pain are common with neurotic disorder, especially with chronic anxiety or hysterical traits (Merskey, 1965).

Pain commonly occurs in those patients, usually female, who complain of multiple physical symptoms in many different bodily systems but without evidence of physical disease. Such a conglomeration of symptoms, starting before the age of 30 and often continuing for decades, was described by Perley and Guze (1962). They called this condition *hysteria*, and later the label *Briquet's syndrome* was used (Cloninger *et al.*, 1975; Woodruff *et al.*, 1971); more recently, the term *somatoform disorder* has been applied generically (F45, ICD-10, World Health Organization, 1992; DSM-IV, American Psychiatric Association, 1994). *Somatization disorder* is the subcategory of this, which refers to multiple physical symptoms, in both ICD-10 and DSM-IV. Persistent somatoform pain disorder is described in ICD-10.

> " The predominant complaint is of persistent, severe, and distressing pain, which cannot be explained fully by a physiological process or a physical disorder. Pain occurs in association with emotional conflict or psychosocial problems that are sufficient to allow the conclusion that they are the main causative influences. The result is usually a marked increase in support and attention, either personal or medical. *(World Health Organization, 1992)*

It is important to be very careful in attempting to distinguish pain of physical origin from that which is largely psychogenic: generalizations can be dangerous. However, Trethowan (1988) considers that there are certain important differences between pain of psychiatric and organic origin. These are as follows.

- Pain associated with psychiatric illness tends to be more diffuse and less well localized than pain due to a physical lesion. It spreads with a non-anatomical distribution.
- Pain is complained of as a constant feature. It may become even more severe at times, but it persists unremittingly. Physical pains usually have more definite provocative agents and are relieved by specific measures.
- Psychogenic pain is clearly seen to be associated with an underlying disturbance of mood that appears to be primary in terms of both time and causation.

- It seems to be much more difficult accurately to describe the quality of psychogenic pain. The patient is in no doubt that he is suffering, that the pain is very unpleasant and that he feels he cannot bear it. But in contrast to painful damage to a defined organ, when pain may be described as burning (skin), shooting (nerve) or gripping (heart muscle), the patient with non-organic pain can find no adequate words for description.
- A further addition to this list is the finding of progression of the severity and extent of the pain over time – unusual for a purely physically mediated pain without increased tissue damage (Tyrer, 1986).

PAIN AND HEIGHTENED SENSATION

Generalized increase in sensory input may be experienced as pain. This is exemplified by hyperacousia: the patient complains of noises being uncomfortably loud. There is no objective improvement in his capacity to hear, but the threshold at which sound is perceived as unpleasantly loud is lowered. Noises, even a normal speaking voice, are described as painful to listen to.

With lysergic acid diethylamide, intense pain may be experienced in the limbs, which seem to the sufferer to be twisted or contorted. Similarly, in the early stages of thiamine deficiency there may be increased sensitivity to pain. In these situations, there is an alteration to perception of sensations so that they are experienced as pain.

During consciousness, the person receives countless sensations from all over his body, such as itching, distension, pressure, borborygmi, mild aching, thumping, warmth and so on. These form the *sensorium* of the body image; they make possible the location of self in space. Most of these sensations, for most of the time, escape attention. However, occasionally the person concentrates and may take action to eliminate the sensation – scratch his ear or cross his legs. Attention to such sensations, especially if linked to an unpleasant emotion, may occasion the experience of pain. Noticing the sensation results in fear, and the distress of this emotion is perceived as pain.

This would appear to be the explanation for the *vital feelings* of depression described in Chapter 18. Vital feelings are the localization of depression in a bodily organ, complained of, perhaps as pain, in the head or chest or elsewhere. On further questioning, symptoms are described as being unpleasant, painful pressure or even a feeling of misery and depression in that organ: morbid interpretations of ordinary bodily sensations. The sensation is unpleasant but normal and would be ignored in health. With disorder of affect, the sensation may be morbidly interpreted as due to cancer, tuberculosis or venereal disease. There are, of course, also actual physical changes in depression, for example slowing of peristalsis and decreased gastrointestinal secretions, and these may also provoke unpleasant sensations such as spasm and constipation.

Central pain (thalamic syndrome) is experienced as a spontaneous burning sensation that can be activated by cutaneous stimulation or temperature changes. It can also present as tactile allodynia, cold allodynia or ongoing pain (Greenspan *et al.*, 2004). It is usually intractable and occurs in the setting of cerebrovascular accident, multiple sclerosis, syringomyelia and spinal cord injury. The current hypothesis is that it arises as a result of disruption in the spinothalamic pathways associated with ectopic neuronal discharges and potentially involves adrenergic, GABAergic, glycine and other neurotransmitters (Devulde *et al.*, 2002).

DIMINISHED PAIN SENSATION AND PAIN CRAVING

In certain situations, there is a decrease in the perception of pain. *Pain asymbolia* is a condition in which situations that should give rise to pain do not (Schilder and Stengel, 1931). This condition can occur as a congenital or an acquired disorder. There are at present five recognized hereditary varieties, usually associated with autonomic neuropathies including anhidrosis (Butler *et al.*, 2006). Several mutations of nerve growth factor have been identified (Einarsdottir *et al.*, 2004). Acquired pain asymbolia has been described in patients with vascular lesions, predominantly left-sided and involving the insular (Berthier *et al.*, 1988). These patients show an absent or inadequate response to painful stimuli over the entire body and an inability to learn appropriate escape or protective responses. In patients with schizophrenia and their relatives, there is evidence of elevated pain thresholds and pain tolerance demonstrated by relative insensitivity to finger pressure (Hooley and Delgado, 2001). Self-damage of a gross nature also occurs sometimes in schizophrenia, for example self-castration. In other situations, such as acute drunkenness, there is diminished appreciation due to the central depressant action of alcohol, and opiates similarly are analgesic through their action on the central appreciation of pain.

Attention is also an important factor in the perception of pain. Excitement or aggression, as in footballers or soldiers, may render the subject oblivious to serious injury. When a wound has advantages to the patient, for example enabling a soldier to leave the battlefield, it causes less pain than when the injury is seen as wholly disadvantageous. Various psychological techniques can reduce the experience of pain, including hypnosis, various stratagems in childbirth, placebo medication and, possibly, acupuncture. In dissociation (conversion), there may be localized anaesthesia and analgesia for the affected limb, for example the patient may describe no perception of pinprick sensation.

A blunting and perverting of pain perception is described in severe mental retardation, resulting occasionally in gross self-damage. The patient may bang his head so that there is chronic haematoma formation, bite himself or otherwise harm himself repeatedly, causing permanent damage. Meanwhile, he appears to experience no pain or even discomfort. Self-application of constricting bands has been described in schizophrenic and organically disordered patients (Dawson-Butterworth *et al.*, 1969). These are most often applied to the left arm; despite extensive tissue damage, the patient does not complain of pain.

Self-inflicted harm occurs also in those of disturbed personality without intellectual deficiency. Such behaviour may include skin cutting, wrist slashing, skin burning, self-hitting, severe skin scratching and bone breaking (McElroy *et al.*, 2000). These patients are usually female (Graff and Mallin, 1967), and the behaviour appears to be linked with the desire to relieve tension and alleviate negative emotions. There is empirical evidence that it does relieve negative emotions (Klonsky, 2007). There is also limited evidence that the self-injurious behaviour has several possible goals: as self-punishment, to influence personal relationships, to reduce tendency to dissociation and also to induce intense sensory stimulation (Box 17.1).

Box 17.1 Examples of self-injurious behaviour

When SHE's home alone, she cuts herself, slicing off her nose to spite other people's faces. She always waits and waits for the moment when she can cut herself unobserved. No sooner does the sound of the closing door die down than she takes out her little talisman, the paternal all-purpose razor. SHE peels the blade out of its Sunday coat of five layers of virginal plastic. She is very skilled in the use of blades; after all, she has to shave her father, shave that soft paternal cheek under the completely empty paternal brow, which is now undimmed by any thought, unwrinkled by any will. This blade is destined for HER flesh. This thin, elegant foil of bluish steel, pliable, elastic. SHE sits down in front of the magnifying side of the shaving mirror; spreading her legs, she makes a cut, magnifying the aperture that is the doorway into her body. She knows from experience that such a razor cut doesn't hurt, for her arms, hands, and legs have often served as guinea pigs. Her hobby is cutting her own body.
Elfriede Jelinek (1988), The Piano Teacher

Late at night I went into the bathroom and took the broken pieces of a razor blade which I had kept. I slashed my wrist again and again, as deeply as I could. I knew perfectly well that it would not kill me, not like the times before. They have been something quite different. As my writing to you comes to a close, the pain is so unbearable inside me that a force of such strength has driven me to inflict a physical pain on myself in the hope of appeasing the other.
Sarah Ferguson (1973), A Guard Within

PAIN WITHOUT ORGANIC CAUSE

Unfortunately, pain is an unpleasant feature common to almost all medical settings; it is a frequent complaint in medical, surgical, gynaecological and psychiatric practice. Recalcitrant cases may be referred to a pain clinic, and prominent among such referrals are those in whom no organic basis can be found to account for the complaint of pain (Tyrer, 1985). Pain in the back and in the head and face, particularly, are often found not to be associated with organic lesions. From 3 to 5 per cent of patients, depending on how referrals are made, have measurable psychiatric disturbance.

There are various possible mechanisms to explain the presence of pain without physical disease: autonomic nervous activity may be interpreted and elaborated through fear of possible consequences, normal sensations may be experienced as painful in situations of stress or in fear, relatively minor pain and discomfort of benign cause may be misinterpreted as being more ominous than it really is.

Classification of non-organic pain is complex. As well as occurring without other ICD-10 diagnosis in *persistent somatoform pain disorder* (F45.4), pain also may be conspicuous with hypochondriasis, with somatization disorder and, especially, with depression in mood disorder. In Tyrer's series, two-thirds of those patients without organic cause and with measurable psychiatric disturbance were diagnosed as suffering from major depressive disorder. The remainder had personality disorders, anxiety state, hysteria and drug dependence; paraphrenia and organic brain syndrome also occurred, but rarely (Tyrer, 1985).

Pain without adequate organic explanation is one of the most difficult problems psychiatrists are called on to treat. In a study of patients with pain referred to psychiatrists in a general hospital, the head and neck was the most common site, followed by the back, abdomen, arm or leg, rectum or genitalia and chest (Pilling *et al.*, 1967). Of these medical and surgical patients, in 32 per cent pain was the presenting complaint, and it was considered that these patients 'spoke to their physicians in terms of pain or other organic symptoms rather than anxiety, depression and the like'. In the evaluation of the significance of emotional factors in chronic pain, adequate history and examination, including the assessment of attribution and the relationship with mood state, was found to be most helpful (Tyrer, 1992); the most useful questionnaires were the Hospital Anxiety and Depression Scale (Zigmond and Snaith, 1983) and the West Haven–Yale Multidimensional Pain Inventory (Kerns *et al.*, 1985).

It is, of course, wholly understandable that someone suffering pain should be miserable and that chronic pain or the anticipation of recurrent pain should provoke depression of mood. This is often so much taken for granted that no steps are taken to alleviate the depressed mood if the cause of the pain is obvious. However, if the perception of pain is considered to have two separate contributions – the sensory perception and the investing affect – efforts to relieve the latter, if successful, will produce a global diminution of pain. Pain can be a cause of depression, and in this situation treatment for the depression is appropriate.

There is an association between abdominal pain in childhood and the subsequent demonstration of hypochondriacal symptoms in adult life. Apley (1975) found such children typically to be 'highly strung, fussy and excitable'; to have an increase of such symptoms as fearfulness, nocturnal enuresis, sleep disturbance and appetite difficulties; and to come from 'painful families'.

Pain and loss

The best-known model for this topic is the *phantom limb* pain so often experienced in amputees. Pain is experienced within a limb that is not there; that is, spatially, pain is located outside the patient. However, this is not a hallucination. The person knows full well that he has lost his leg and that the *feeling* of pain is inside himself. The body image takes a very long time to adjust to a change such as an amputation, and it may never fully adjust. Ramachandran and Hirstein (1998) provide a thorough review of the subject. The phantom limb experience occurs almost immediately following the loss of a limb, but the incidence may be higher following atraumatic loss. Phantoms appear immediately in the vast majority of cases, and in the case of amputations as soon as the anaesthetic wears off. The phantom is present for a few days or weeks and gradually fades but may persist for years or even decades in some people. Indeed, some people are able to recall a phantom limb at will after its disappearance.

Phantoms are most common following amputation of an arm or a leg but have been reported following mastectomies or removal of parts of the face;

even internal viscera can produce sensations of bowel movements and flatus. The posture of the limb can become habitual, often partially flexed at the elbow with forearm pronated, and when the phantom fades from consciousness, especially with the forearm, it becomes progressively shorter until the patient is left with just the phantom hand. Perhaps most surprising, children with congenitally missing limbs can experience phantoms. Originally, it was thought that the phantom pain was due to stump neuromas, but given that patients born without limbs can have phantom pain neuromas do not seem necessary for phantom pain to occur. The persistence of central representation of the amputated limb is largely responsible for the phantom illusion and associated pain.

Parkes (1976) has pointed out the importance of viewing amputation in its psychological context, both for understanding the symptoms and for making a prognosis.

Psychogenic facial pain

It has been known for a long time that many patients with chronic pain at a variety of sites do not have abnormal physical signs and do not manifest serious organic illness. *Atypical facial pain* is an especially frequent and intractable example, manifesting no organic signs but causing great suffering; the patient is referred from surgeon to dentist to pain clinic physician to psychiatrist, often without benefit. Such pain has often been associated with depression. Lascelles (1966) described a series of 93 patients suffering from prolonged facial pain, of whom the majority suffered from *atypical depression* with intense fatigue, tension and sleep disorder superimposed on 'obsessive' personality; 53 of these patients responded well to antidepressant therapy.

More recently, Blumer and Heilbronn (1982) have seen chronic, intractable pain without organic cause as being a variant of depressive illness. Garvey *et al.* (1983) investigated the association between headache and depression in 116 patients suffering from major depressive disorder. During a non-depressed period, these patients experienced a similar rate for headache to that of non-depressive control subjects, but they had a markedly increased rate during depressive episodes. Feinmann *et al.* (1984) investigated the efficacy of an antidepressant, dosulepin (dothiepin), in the treatment of psychogenic facial pain. Seventy-one per cent of patients were free of symptoms at 9 weeks, compared with 47 per cent in a placebo group; at a 12-month follow-up, 81 per cent of patients were pain-free. Good prognostic indicators for successful treatment included pain following an adverse life event, minimal previous surgical intervention and freedom from pain after 9 weeks' treatment. Such studies would suggest an association between facial pain without physical signs and depressive illness.

PAIN AND SUFFERING

Pain is an appropriate study for the phenomenologist, in that the external signs may be irrelevant and the subjective experience all important. The chief problem in assessing pain is the extraordinary difficulty a patient has in describing the quality of his pain: the greater the psychogenic component of the pain, the more difficult it is to find the right words to describe it. Sometimes, it seems that pain may be needed as a neurotic solution to a neurotic conflict: for the equilibrium to remain, it is necessary for the pain to be retained. It has been considered by Trethowan (1988) that such a patient 'is not suffering from pain at all. What she is suffering from is suffering'.

An illuminating account of severe depressive illness experienced as pain was given by an eminent general practitioner (Sims, 1993). He experienced an episode of depressive illness as a young man and experienced this as 'physical pain, gnawing at life'. When, several decades later, he suffered myocardial infarction, he recognized the severe pain as being similar in quality and quantity to his previous experience.

There are differences between the person suffering from organically determined pain and the chronic sufferer with multiple symptoms whose pain is considered psychogenic. The latter truly suffers but does not show the physical correlates of severe pain. It seems that the state of suffering in which this person exists finds expression, dons respectability and can only be communicated when it is transformed peripherally into a specific pain. Pain may occur with little suffering, as in the injection of local anaesthetic that, after the small prick, brings relief from a worse pain. Suffering may also occur without pain, but it may also be described as pain, and this may be the nature of many neurotic complaints of pain. This transposition of affect is wholly understandable when one considers the semantics of suffering. Suffering of all non-physical kinds – indignation, humiliation, disappointment – finds expression in pain terms: taking pains, feeling crushed, bruised self-esteem, rubbing salt in the wound, getting one's fingers burnt, searing remarks. It is not just that pain is a metaphor for suffering, but in many situations suffering can be experienced and explained by the sufferer only in *pain* terms.

So the use of pain words can be construed metaphorically, and the neurotic patient may follow this to its logical conclusion and describe concretely the unbearable and humiliating suffering of his daily existence as complaints of localized physical pain. The experience of pain is a physical sensation that takes on an affective component for its expression and interpretation. This affective component – suffering – may occur without physical perception and sometimes still be experienced by the person himself as pain.

REFERENCES

American Psychiatric Association (1994) *Diagnostic and Statistical Manual of Mental Disorders*, 4th edn. Washington: American Psychiatric Association.

Anstee BH and Fleminger JJ (1977) Diagnosis 'uncertain': a follow-up study. *British Journal of Psychiatry 131*, 592–8.

Apley J (1975) *The Child with Abdominal Pains*, 2nd edn. Oxford: Blackwell Scientific.

Beecher HK (1959) *Measurement of Subjective Responses, Quantitative Effects of Drugs*. New York: Oxford University Press.

Berthier M, Starktein S and Leiguarda R (1988) Asymbolia for pain: a sensory–limbic disconnection syndrome. *Annals of Neurology 24*, 41–9.

Blumer D and Heilbronn M (1982) Chronic pain as a variant of depressive disease: the pain-prone disorder. *Journal of Nervous and Mental Diseases 70*, 381–406.

Bond MR (1976) Psychological and psychiatric aspects of pain. In Howells JG (ed.) *Modern Perspectives in the Psychiatric Aspects of Surgery*, pp. 109–39. London: Macmillan.

Bonica JJ (1994) Labour pain. In Wall PD and Melzack R (eds) *Textbook of Pain*, 3rd edn. Edinburgh: Churchill Livingstone.

Butler J, Fleming P and Webb D (2006) Congenital insensitivity to pain – review of a case with dental implications. *Oral Surgery, Oral Medicine, Oral Pathology, Oral Radiology, and Endodontics 101*, 58–62.

Cloninger CR, Reich T and Guze SB (1975) The multi-factorial model of disease transmission. III Familial relationships between sociopathy and hysteria (Briquet's syndrome). *British Journal of Psychiatry 127*, 23–32.

Dawson-Butterworth K, Wallen GDP and Gittleson NL (1969) Self-applied constricting bands. *British Journal of Psychiatry 115*, 1255–9.

Devulde R, Crombez E and Mortier E (2002) Central pain: an overview. *Acta Neurologica Belgica 102*, 97–103.

Dickens C (1854) *Hard Times*. London: Penguin.

Einarsdottir E, Carlsson A, Minde J, *et al* (2004) A mutation in the nerve growth factor beta gene (NGB) causes loss of pain perception. *Human Molecular Genetics 13*, 799–805.

Engel GL (1959) 'Psychogenic' pain and the pain prone patient. *American Journal of Medicine 26*, 899.

Feinmann C, Harris M and Cawley R (1984) Psychogenic facial pain: presentation and treatment. *British Medical Journal 288*, 436–8.

Ferguson S (1973) *A Guard Within*. London: Chatto & Windus.

Fields HL and Basbaum AI (1994) Central nervous system mechanisms of pain modulation. In Wall PD and Melzack R (eds) *Textbook of Pain*, 3rd edn. Edinburgh: Churchill Livingstone.

Garvey MJ, Schaffer CB and Tuason VB (1983) Relationship of headaches to depression. *British Journal of Psychiatry 143*, 544–7.

Graff H and Mallin R (1967) The syndrome of the wrist-cutter. *American Journal of Psychiatry 124*, 36–42.

Greenspan JD, Ohara J, Sarlani E and Lenz FA (2004) Allodynia in patients with post-stroke pain (CPSP) studied by statistical quantitative sensory testing within individuals. *Pain 109*, 357–66.

Hooley JM and Delgado ML (2001) Pain insensitivity in the relatives of schizophrenic patients. *Schizophrenia Research 47*, 265–73.

International Association for the Study of Pain (1994) Classification of chronic pain: descriptions of chronic pain syndromes and definitions of pain terms. *Task Force on Taxonomy*, suppl. 3. Seattle: IASP Press.

Jelinek E (1988) *The Piano Teacher* (transl. Neugroschel J). New York: Weidenfeld & Nicholson.

Kerns RD, Turk DC and Rudy TF (1985) The West Haven–Yale Multidimensional Pain Inventory (WHYMPI). *Pain 23*, 345–56.

Klonsky (2007) The functions of deliberate self-injury: a review of the evidence. *Clinical Psychology Review 27*, 226–39.

Lascelles RG (1966) Atypical facial pain and depression. *British Journal of Psychiatry 112*, 651–9.

McElroy SL, Arnold LM and Beckman DA (2000) Habit and impulse control disorders. In Gelder MG, López-Ibor JJ and Andreasen NC (2000) *New Oxford Textbook of Psychiatry*. Oxford: Oxford University Press.

Melzack R and Wall PD (1965) Pain mechanisms: a new theory. *Science 150*, 971.

Merskey H (1965) The characteristics of persistent pain in psychological illness. *Journal of Psychosomatic Research 9*, 291.

Merskey H (1976) The status of pain. In Hill O (ed.) *Modern Trends in Psychosomatic Medicine 3*, pp. 166–86. London: Butterworth.

Nathan P (1980) Recent advances in understanding pain. *British Journal of Psychiatry 136*, 509–12.

Noordenbos W (1959) *Pain: Problems Pertaining to the Transmission of Nerve Impulses Which Give Rise to Pain*. London: Elsevier.

Parkes CM (1976) The psychological reaction to loss of a limb: the first year after amputation. In Howells JG (ed.) *Modern Perspectives in the Psychiatric Aspects of Surgery*, pp. 515–33. London: Macmillan.

Perley MJ and Guze SB (1962) Hysteria – the stability and usefulness of clinical criteria. A quantitative study based on a follow-up period of 6–8 years in 39 patients. *New England Journal of Medicine 266*, 421–6.

Pilling LF, Bannick TL and Swenson WM (1967) Psychological characteristics of patients having pain as a presenting symptom. *Canadian Medical Association Journal 97*, 387.

Ramachandran VS and Hirstein W (1998) The perception of phantom limbs. The DO Hebb lecture. *Brain 121*, 1603–30.

Schilder P and Stengel E (1931) Asymbolia for pain. *Archives of Neurology and Psychiatry 25*, 598–600.

Sims A (1993) The scar that is more than skin deep: the stigma of depression. *British Journal of General Practice 43*, 30–1.
Trethowan WH (1988) Pain as a psychiatric symptom. In Hall P and Stonier PD (eds) *Perspectives in Psychiatry*. Chichester: John Wiley.
Tyrer S (1985) The role of the psychiatrist in the pain clinic. *Bulletin of the Royal College of Psychiatrists 9*, 135–6.
Tyrer S (1986) Learned pain behaviour. *British Medical Journal 292*, 1–2.
Tyrer S (1992) Psychiatric assessment of chronic pain. *British Journal of Psychiatry 160*, 733–41.
Wall PD and Melzack R (1999) *Textbook of Pain*, 4th edn. Edinburgh: Churchill Livingstone.
Woodruff RA, Clayton PS and Guze SB (1971) 'Hysteria': studies of diagnosis, outcome and prevalence. *Journal of the American Medical Association 215*, 425–8.
World Health Organization (1992) *The ICD-10 Classification of Mental and Behavioural Disorders: Clinical Description and Diagnostic Guidelines*. Geneva: World Health Organization.
Zigmond AS and Snaith RP (1983) The hospital anxiety and depression scale. *Acta Psychiatrica Scandinavica 67*, 361–70.

Section Five

EMOTIONS AND ACTION

Affect and Emotional Disorders

18

> " I wish to inform you that I have received the cake. Many thanks, but I am not worthy. You sent it on the anniversary of my child's death, for I am not worthy of my birthday; I must weep myself to death; I cannot live and I cannot die, because I have failed so much, I shall bring my husband and children to hell. We are all lost; we won't see each other any more; I shall go to the convict prison and my two girls as well, if they do not make away with themselves because they were born in my body. *A patient of Emil Kraepelin (1905)*

Assessing and observing the state of, and changes in, mood is essential in psychiatry but at the same time requires skill. Part of the problem has always been the conceptual confusion and lack of cohesive psychopathological theory that has traditionally been associated with disturbance of affect (Berrios, 1985). In a study of patients with unsolved diagnostic problems at the time of discharge from hospital, atypical psychotic depression was found, at follow-up, to be the condition most frequently responsible for doubt (Anstee and Fleminger, 1977). In another study, depressed affect was a major cause of somatic problems without physical pathology (Brenner, 1979). However, the terms used are not standardized, nor mutually exclusive. Different languages, unlike the names given to physical objects, have an entirely different range of descriptions of mood, so that one is left wondering whether it is just the terms that differ in different cultures or perhaps even the experience of emotion itself. So *Angst* cannot be translated exactly into English with a single equivalent word; neither can *depression* be precisely translated into German. The word *feeling* describes an active experience of somatic sensation, touch, as well as the passive subjective experience of emotion. *Emotion*, according to Whybrow (1997), 'is actually memory and feeling intertwined'. Feelings are also personal convictions, predictive forecasts and social sensibilities. All these nuances of meaning are somewhat different from the associations of the word *mood*.

Traditionally, *feeling* has been used to describe a positive or negative reaction to an experience; it is marked but transitory. *Affect* is a broad term that is used to cover mood, feeling, attitude, preferences and evaluations. In psychiatry, it is customary to limit its use to the expression of emotion as judged by the external manifestations that are associated with specific feelings, for example laughter, crying and fearful appearance. *Mood* is a more prolonged prevailing state or disposition, whereas *emotion* is often used to refer to spontaneous and transitory experience similar to but not identical to feeling, as it need not incorporate the physical accompaniments of the experience. In practice, these terms are used more or less interchangeably, a fact that contributes to much confusion.

Mood describes the state of the self in relation to its environment. There is an enormous range of variation of what could reasonably be called *normal* mood. Pathological mood, that is, mood from which the patient suffers or mood that causes disturbance or suffering to others, also varies very greatly, and the extent to which it is acceptable to others in its expression is different in different social contexts. The clinician has to ask two questions concerning the mood of his patient. First, is the person suffering? Second, is the expression of mood inappropriate in this social setting? Psychopathology of mood is confined to those situations in which there is an affirmative answer to at least one of the questions, and treatment is directed towards improving the mood.

Like other human characteristics, pathology of mood arises in the context of a diathesis. It is the physical constitution that forms the tendency for developing, for example, a prolapsed intervertebral disc; in the mental realm, personality is closely associated with the type, quality and direction of mood. So, a person of cyclothymic personality is more prone to morbid states of elation and excessive activity or taciturn dejection and retardation.

Theories of emotion

The James–Lange theory of emotion was developed independently by William James (1842–1910) and Carl Lange (1834–1900). Simply, it posits that emotions are the result of self-awareness of physical and bodily changes in the presence of a stimulus. William James (1884) wrote:

> “ My theory ... is that the bodily changes follow directly the perception of the exciting fact, and that our feeling of the same changes as they occur is the emotion. Common sense says, we lose our fortune, are sorry and weep; we meet a bear, are frightened and run; we are insulted by a rival, and angry and strike. The hypothesis here to be defended says that this order of sequence is incorrect ... and that the more rational statement is that we feel sorry because we cry, angry because we strike, afraid because we tremble... Without the bodily states following on the perception, the latter would be purely cognitive in form, pale, colorless, destitute of emotional warmth. We might then see the bear, and judge it best to run, receive the insult and deem it right to strike, but we should not actually feel afraid or angry.

This theory was criticized by Walter Cannon (1871–1945) and Philip Bard (1898–1977). Visceral (physiological) responses to stimuli are too slow to account for the rapidity of emotions that arise in the presence of appropriate stimuli. In other words, the timeliness of my awareness of the increased heart rate and dry mouth that occurs when I am in the presence of a hostile lion is inadequate to explain my fear of the lion. Furthermore, the visceral responses to varying stimuli are similar, yet the emotions may be as disparate as fear, surprise, joy and so on. And injection of adrenaline (epinephrine) is accompanied by visceral changes but not necessarily by emotional change. In addition, animals that have spinal lesions continue to experience emotions. Instead, the Cannon–Bard theory argued that emotion has temporal primacy and that any visceral or behavioural change follows the emotion. In this theory, I see a hostile lion and become fearful. My fearfulness provokes the typical physiological response of increased heart rate etc., and the resulting behaviour is that I run off. This theory obviously leaves no room for any cognitive aspect to the origin of emotions.

The other influential theory is Schachter and Singer's (1962) two-factor theory of emotion. The two relevant factors are physiological arousal and cognition. In this theory, an individual is in a given social context, and he responds to this situation with a physiological arousal. The meaning attributed to this arousal is determined by his cognitions. If his appraisal is that the context is threatening then he will feel fear, but if the appraisal is that the situation is funny then the emotion will be a positive one. This theory has obvious implications for the clinical evaluation of disorders of mood. It specifies that the social context is important, that the cognitions of the individual are relevant and, finally, that careful consideration and description of the accompanying emotion is also important.

Basic emotions

Ekman and colleagues (Ekman and Friesen, 1971) have shown that there are six basic emotions that are expressed in the face: anger, disgust, fear, happiness, sadness and surprise. These basic expressions of emotion are universal. Ekman's findings were anticipated by Charles Darwin (1872). It is also the case that the fact that there are universals in facial expressions of emotions does not mean that expressions are universal in every regard. In Ekman's fieldwork in Papua New Guinea among the Fore people, there was little distinction between surprise and fear. Furthermore, it is also true that when people experience strong emotions there are display rules that determine who can show which emotion to whom and when. Cultures also differ on which events are likely to produce particular emotions. This is well exemplified by what food one culture regards as a delicacy and what another regards as revolting. The important point is that the general theme is universal; ingesting something repulsive is a cause for disgust (Ekman, 1998).

Communication of mood

'No man is an Island, entire of itself' (John Donne, 1571–1631), and in no area of life is this more true than that of feelings. Our feelings are very much affected by those around us. They are observable and understandable to other people, and this is not accidental; they are actually signalled as a non-verbal message. The affect itself is not directed towards another person, but the expression of the affect is conveyed both deliberately and unintentionally to others.

One of the most important findings in the past decade has been that of *mirror neurons*. These neurons have been found in primates and birds, and their existence inferred in humans. Mirror neurons fire when an animal performs an action and also when an animal observes the same action performed by another animal. In other words, these neurons mirror the behaviour of another animal. In humans, the relevant neurons are in the premotor cortex and inferior parietal cortex. Rizzolatti and Fadiga (1998) showed that in the macaque monkey there are two distinct groups of neurons in the rostroventral premotor cortex that respond to the observation of grasping objects and grasping actions. The canonical neurons responded specifically to the three-dimensional objects, whereas the mirror neurons responded to the direct observation of the hand actions performed by another animal. Rizzolatti and Craighero (2004) argue that this mirror neuron system underlies imitative learning and is therefore important for the development of human culture and the acquisition of language. More recently, Gallese (2007) proposed that the mirror neuron system is an embodied simulation system wherein we not only see an action, emotion or sensation but form internal representations of these actions, emotions or sensations based on evocations of the same neural systems as when we perform the same actions or experience the same emotions or sensations. Thus, by means of this system, the objectified other becomes for us another experiencing self. In other words, empathy and the capacity to understand another person's emotional state have an already identified basis.

Emotions are communicated non-verbally by different parts of the body, for example by the face (especially the eyes), gesture, posture, tone of voice and general appearance, especially the choice of clothes. While assessing another's affective response, the assessor in part influences it by his own behaviour and disposition. A person who is cheerful on meeting someone else will greet him cheerfully and induce a feeling of cheerfulness, even if transitory, which he then reads as the other person being cheerful also. This has important implications in the way that mood is assessed. It would seem that emotion is evaluated empathically. Without having to go through this elaborate argument in words, the observer says to himself, 'if I felt how I estimate the feelings of that person from his appearance, I would feel very unhappy; he is unhappy'. This is, of course, the empathic method as described earlier, and it takes place spontaneously and without deliberate training. Assessment of others' mood does not need to become verbal to be acted on. It takes place rapidly and is followed by the appropriate behavioural response from the observer.

Classification of pathology of emotions

There is no consensus on how to classify abnormalities of the experience and display of emotions. Cutting (1997) provides a viable framework, which has been adapted for use in this chapter. There are morbid states of the basic emotions, including sadness, happiness, fear, anger, surprise and disgust. These basic emotions can be affected in the intensity, duration, timing, quality of experience, expression and appropriateness to the object or social setting. There are abnormalities of the physiological and arousal mechanisms associated with emotions. Finally, there are abnormalities of the cognitive evaluation of the social world and of the perception of the emotions of others (Box 18.1).

PATHOLOGICAL CHANGES IN BASIC EMOTIONS

Changes in intensity of emotions

Most often in psychiatric practice, subjective description of *change* in the experience of emotion is for the worse – a state of dysphoria, meaning the condition of 'being ill at ease'; more rarely, the patient may describe the onset of ecstasy or euphoria. The subjective experience of change of mood can be quantified approximately and represented graphically as in Figure 18.1, which shows part

Box 18.1 Classification of disorders of emotion

Abnormalities of basic emotions
- Intensity of emotions, including diminution and exacerbation
- Duration, time and quality of experience, including lability of mood, pathological crying and laughing, parathymia and paramimia
- Expression of emotion, including blunting and flattening of affect
- Appropriateness to object, including phobia

Abnormality of physiological arousal
- Alexithymia

Abnormalities of evaluation of social context
- Negative cognitive schemas
- Prosopoaffective agnosia
- Receptive vocal dysprosody

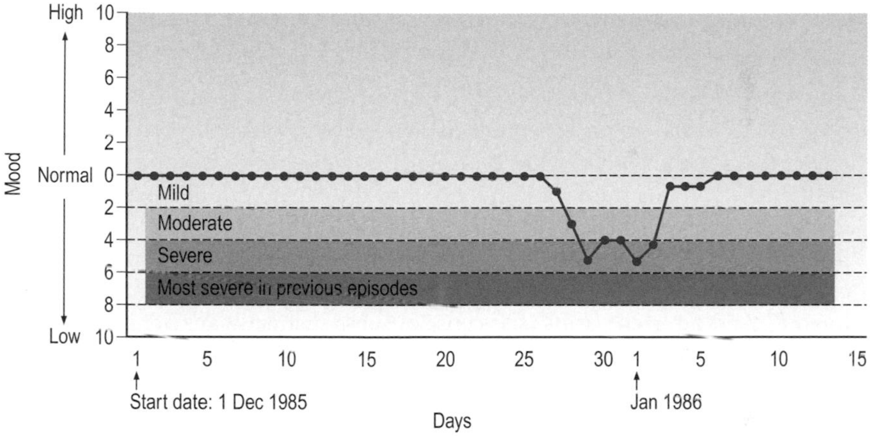

Figure 18.1 Mood chart kept by a depressed patient who had had acute bronchitis.

of a mood chart a previously depressed patient had recorded; he had noticed an association between an acute attack of bronchitis and exacerbation of depressive symptoms.

Diminution of intensity: feeling of a loss of feeling

This is experienced as a loss of feeling, a deficiency that is all-pervasive, affecting all emotions including sadness, joy, anger, fear and so on. The patient resents or does not understand it, suffers very greatly and often feels guilty about the feeling. It is a subjective experience of loss of feelings that were formerly present rather than an objectively observed absence. A depressed young woman said, 'I have no feelings for my children. That is wicked. They are beautiful children'. A person with religious belief may experience this loss of feeling with a religious content: they no longer believe in God. On more detailed eliciting of their subjective experience, they are likely to describe a loss of the feeling of assurance associated with their faith rather than any actual change in the content of their beliefs. This affect occurs particularly in depressive psychosis but also occasionally with personality disorders and schizophrenia. Milder forms are experienced as *depersonalization* or *deaffectualization* (see Chapter 14): the patient complains that his feelings are numbed, diminished, made remote from himself, to which is ascribed the unmelodious word deaffectualization.

Anhedonia

Anhedonia specifically refers to a loss of the capacity to experience joy and pleasure. It is a subset of the diminution of the intensity of emotions. In *anhedonia*, there is a total inability to enjoy anything in life or even get the accustomed satisfaction from everyday events or objects, a 'loss of ability to experience pleasure' (Snaith, 1993). The term was originally introduced by Ribot (1896) and considered to be a prominent symptom of depressive illness by Klein (1974), probably the best clinical marker predicting response to treatment. This would seem to be a fundamental symptom of depressive illness. A highly intelligent and perceptive man suffering from psychotic depression said, 'I have a sort of uncanny feeling. I know what I am reading is amusing but I am not at all amused by it'. The experience was very well described by J.S. Mill (1806–1873):

> " It was the autumn of 1826. I was in a dull state of nerves, such as everybody is occasionally liable to; unsusceptible to enjoyment or pleasurable excitement; one of these moods when what is pleasure ay other times, becomes insipid or indifferent... In this frame of mind it occurred to me to put the question directly to myself, 'suppose that all your objects in life were realized; that all the changes in institutions and opinions which you are looking forward to, could be completely effected at this very instant: would this be a great joy and happiness to you?' And an irrepressible self-consciousness distinctly answered, 'No!' At this my heart sank within me.

Anhedonia is also described as a symptom in schizophrenia, in which it is especially likely to be social – absence of the ability to feel pleasure in relationships (Cutting, 1985).

Exacerbation of emotions: melancholia, mania, ecstasy

In affective disorders, the mood is usually the primary focus of the abnormality. The pathology of mood can be manifest as intensification of sadness or joy. In sadness, this may present as feelings of sadness and gloom, despondency, despair or hopelessness. Often, the actual experience is indescribable but recognized as different in character from normal sadness. In other words, the character is qualitatively different from sadness and akin to physical pain:

> " I was feeling in my mind a sensation close to, but indescribably different from actual pain. *(William Styron, 1990)*

> " It is a positive and active anguish, a sort of psychical neuralgia wholly unknown to normal life. *(William James, 1902)*

William Styron (1990), in his book about his personal experience of depression, argued that the term depression was a weak word for the experience.

> 'Melancholia' would appear to be a far more apt and evocative word for the blacker forms of the disorder, but it was usurped by a noun with a bland tonality and lacking any magisterial presence, used indifferently to describe an economic decline or a rut in the ground, a true wimp of a word for such a major illness... Nevertheless, for 75 years the word has slithered innocuously through the language like a slug, leaving little trace of its intrinsic malevolence and preventing, by its insipidity, a general awareness of the horrible intensity of the disease when out of control.

The positive feeling of joy and pleasure can also be intensified. Jamison (1995) described her personal experience of mania:

> When you're high it's tremendous. The ideas and feelings are fast and frequent like shooting stars and you follow them until you find better and brighter ones. Shyness goes; the right words and gestures are suddenly there, the power to captivate others a felt certainty. There are interests found in uninteresting people. Sensuality is pervasive and the desire to seduce and be seduced is irresistible... But somewhere this changes... Everything previously moving with the grain is now against – you are irritable, angry, frightened, uncontrollable, and enmeshed in the blackest caves of the mind.

It is clear that the positive, joyful aspect of the elevation of mood can quickly turn into a dysphoric sensation that is uncomfortable and unwelcome, yet that is not an aspect of depression. *Euphoria* is a state of excessive unreasonable cheerfulness; it may be manifested as extreme cheerfulness, as described above in mania, or it may seem inappropriate and bizarre. It is commonly seen in organic states, especially associated with frontal lobe impairment.

Heightened states of happiness such as ecstasy sometimes occur in people with mental illness or abnormality of personality. Understandably, most psychiatrists writing about the mood state of ecstasy have described its occurrence in psychotic patients, but with the pattern towards increased numbers of psychiatric outpatient referrals, patients with neurotic disorder giving a previous description of less bizarre ecstatic symptoms are now seen. The patient may describe a calm exalted state of happiness amounting to ecstasy, although this tranquil mood state is relatively uncommon and usually short-lived. In schizophrenia, ecstatic mood may be associated with exalted delusions, for example the chronic patient who sat placidly enraptured on a long-stay ward, knowing herself to be the Queen of Heaven and waiting for a messenger to inform her that she was to take over the rule of the world. Ecstatic states, usually with a histrionic flavour, may occur in dissociative disorder and may be associated with religious stigmata (Simpson, 1984). Bizarre, mass hysterical phenomena, often with religious associations, are usually of this type, for example in the devils of Loudon as described by Aldous Huxley (1952). The social, institutional and group psychological prerequisites for the development of epidemic or mass hysteria (Sirois, 1982) are usually present in these situations, and mismanagement is usually responsible for the development from isolated hysteria in one individual to an epidemic. Ecstasy, solemn elation or excessive exuberant expansiveness may also be seen in epilepsy and in other organic states, for example in general paresis.

Characteristic of ecstasy is that it is self-referent; for example, the flowers of spring 'open for *me*'. There is an alteration of the boundaries of self so that the person may feel 'at one with the universe', or he may 'empty myself of all will' so that 'I am nothing but feelings'. The change in ego boundaries does not usually have the aspect of interference with self that accompanies passivity experiences. In ecstasy, the abrogation of self is experienced as being voluntary. Expert knowledge of the abnormal does not preclude ignorance of the normal, and the psychiatrist can never generalize from the sample of people selectively referred to him to the whole of mankind. This discrepancy can become very obvious in the area of *ecstatic* and *religious experience*. There is a need to acknowledge, take into account, have respect for and use in treatment the patient's own subjective experience in this area (Sims, 1994). The psychiatrist sees a most unrepresentative group of those having some form of religious experience, which has been considered to amount to over 40 per cent of the adult population of the United States of America, more of whom are males than females, more are stable than unstable and more happy than unhappy.

The anthropology of ecstasy (Lewis, 1971) can be traced through Christian and other cultures and makes contact with recognizable mental illness only at a few points. William James (1902), in *The Variety of Religious Experience*, demonstrated the vast extent of the phenomenology of religion and showed how unwise it would be to equate the surprising with the pathological. Accounts vary as to the extent of psychopathology among converts to religious groups and sects; it is probably associated with the nature of the group. Thus Ungerleider and Wellisch (1979) found no evidence of severe mental illness in one study, while Galanter (1982) described evidence of emotional problems among adherents to Divine Light, the Unification Church, Baba and Subud.

Suggestive indicators for establishing a religious experience as probably associated with psychiatric morbidity are:

- the phenomenology of the experience conforms with psychiatric illness
- there are other recognizable symptoms of mental disturbance
- the lifestyle, behaviour and direction of personal goals of the person subsequent to the event are consistent with the natural history of mental disorder rather than with an enriching life experience
- such behaviour is consistent with disorders in the person's personality.

With the following signs, the experience is more likely to be intrinsic to the person's belief and less likely to denote psychiatric illness:

- the person shows some degree of reticence to discuss the experience, especially with those he anticipates will be unsympathetic
- it is described unemotionally with matter-of-fact conviction and appears 'authentic'
- the person understands, allows for and even sympathizes with the incredulity of others
- he usually considers that the experience implies some demands on himself
- the religious experience conforms with the subject's recognizable religious traditions and peer group.

In his clinical practice, the psychiatrist is likely to come across patients describing religious experience; in some patients he will feel this is symptomatic of mental illness, but in others it is clearly intrinsic to the values of the patient and independent of illness even though illness may also be present.

Intensification of fear, anger and surprise

The intensification of fear and anger is described in Chapter 19. These two basic emotions can occur in pure form but can also complicate the intensification of sadness or joy so that is not uncommon for depressed or elated mood to be associated with anxiety or irritability. Morbid surprise is seen in *latah,* a culture-bound disorder described in Malaysia in which there appears to be an exaggerated startle response characterized by a myriad of echo phenomena including echolalia, echopraxia and echomimia. There is also coprolalia, automatic obedience and hypersuggestibility (Bartholomew, 1994). *Hyperekplexia* is a heightened startle reflex that occurs either as a hereditary neurological condition involving the inhibitory glycine receptor or as a symptomatic disorder predominantly of epilepsy in which a surprise stimulus provokes a normal startle response that then triggers a focal, usually frontal lobe, seizure (Meinck, 2006). Late-onset cases, without demonstrable pathology, have been reported in which audiogenic, visual or tactile stimuli trigger myoclonic jerks characterized by eye blinking, head flexion, abduction of the upper arms, movement of the trunk and bending of the knees (Hamelin *et al.*, 2004). In addition, in post-traumatic stress disorder and alcohol withdrawal states the startle reflex can be exaggerated (Howard and Ford, 1992).

Changes in timing, duration and appropriateness to situation

Timing, duration and appropriateness to situation

The timing and duration of emotions are aspects of the emotional expression that determine whether the emotion is appropriate to the context. In pathological grief, the timing and duration may be altered such that the grief is delayed or prolonged. Delayed grief is in essence prolongation of the initial numb phase (see below). Lability of mood involves both a heightening or an intensification of emotions accompanied by an instability in the persistence of emotions that communicates itself to the observer as an inappropriateness to the social context. It can also appear as a shallowness of emotional expression despite being intense, because it is transitory and can seem not to be deeply felt. It is often a sign of brain damage and is seen following frontal lobe injury or cerebrovascular accident.

Pathological laughter or crying is usually an unprovoked emotion that does not have an apparent object. In other words, the emotion is not related to any identifiable social situation. Pathological laughter occurs in epilepsy, in which it is known as gelastic epilepsy, but it may also be associated with acquired brain injury. It is commonly associated with pathological crying, which is also associated with focal brain injury. It is noteworthy that pathological crying occurs as a discrete condition without pathological laughter (Poeck and Pilleri, 1963, quoted in Cutting, 1997).

In schizophrenia, Bleuler (1911) described *parathymia* and *paramimia*. In parathymia, patients react to sad news with cheerfulness or even laughter. These patients may become sad or irritated by events to which others will react with indifference or pleasure. Furthermore, the term parathymia is also used for unprovoked or inappropriate bursts of laughter. This particular aspect of parathymia is similar if not identical to pathological laughter. *Paramimia* refers to the lack of unity between the various modes of expression of emotions:

> “A female catatonic patient approached one of the female attendants whom she liked and told her in the friendliest manner and in her sweetest tone of voice: 'I really would like to slap your face, people like you are usually called s.o.b.s.'

> “A woman patient complained bitterly about her 'voices' and body-hallucinations; her mouth and her forehead manifested disgust, but her eyes expressed happy eroticism. After a few minutes the mouth also assumed the expression of happiness while her forehead continued to appear gloomy and wrinkled.

Abnormalities of expression and appropriateness to object

Blunting and flattening of feeling

The terms *blunting* and *flattening* are used interchangeably to refer to unchanging facial expression, decreased spontaneous movements, poverty of expressive gesture, poor eye contact, affective unresponsivity and lack of vocal inflection (Andreasen, 1979). Thus, the terms refer to a composite of features that are related but are not necessarily part of a unified abnormality. *Blunting* implies a lack of emotional sensitivity, such as that displayed by the girl with schizophrenia who, with obvious relish for the sensational effect, took her visitors up to the bedroom to show them her mother, who had been dead for 48 hours. *Flattening* is a limitation of the usual range of emotion expressed usually by facial but also bodily gestures. The individual does not express very much affect in any direction, although that which is expressed is appropriate in direction. Both blunting and flattening occur in schizophrenia.

Bodily feelings associated with emotion

In the theories of emotion, physiological changes such as palpitations, dry mouth, sweatiness, etc. have a key determining part in the labelling of emotion. These and other changes can be the sole features of emotional disorder in some individuals. The relationships between mood and somatic symptoms have been discussed in Chapter 15. In a number of cultures and languages, depression is considered to have an anatomical location to such an extent that the mood state and the part of the body become synonymous. Melancholia literally means 'black bile'; similarly, in Urdu the word *jee*, meaning self, describes the hypochondrium anatomically and comes to mean depression, that is, depression is a central assault on the well-being of the self. Changes in bodily feeling are important in a number of conditions. Physical illness frequently precipitates a loss of the accustomed sense of well-being. This is subjectively experienced as a generalized lowering of vitality and may be associated with other psychological abnormalities, for instance hypochondriasis or dissociation. In these settings, the expression of emotional disturbance is likely to emphasize the physical rather than the emotional:

> "And thence proceeds wind, palpitation of the heart, short breath, plenty of humidity in the stomach, heaviness of heart and heartache, and intolerable stupidity and dullness of spirits. Their excrements or stool hard, black to some, and little. If the heart, brain, liver, spleen, be misaffected, as they usually are, many inconveniences proceed from them, many diseases accompany ... those frequent wakings and terrible dreams, intempestive laughing, weeping, sighing, sobbing, bashfulness, blushing, trembling, sweating, swooning, etc. *(Burton, 1577–1650,* The Anatomy of Melancholia*)*

Vital feelings was a term used by Wernicke (1906) to describe certain somatic symptoms occurring in the affective psychoses. The word *vital* comes from the concept of the *vital self*, which describes the close relationship of the body to awareness of self, the way we experience our bodies and the impression we consider our physical presence makes on others. So, vital feelings are those that make us aware of our vital self. These are the feelings of mood that appear to emanate from the body itself: localized and somatized affect. For example, depressed patients commonly complain of headache. On more informed enquiry, the patient may say, 'it's not exactly a pain, but more an unbearable feeling of pressure like a tight band around the head', 'a feeling of misery, like a black cloud pressing on my head'. The head is the commonest site for vital feelings, but they may also occur in the abdomen – 'I have a dull feeling in my bowels, they are slowing down and blocking', in the chest – 'it feels like a weight bearing down on my chest, stopping me breathing', in the eyes – 'everything looks black, dark and drab; my eyes are heavy, I cannot see properly' or in the legs – 'my legs are terribly heavy; I cannot walk I feel so exhausted'. They may occur in other regions of the body, for instance the bladder, the feet, the hair and so on. The features that appear to be constant are the association of the localized body sensation with the prevailing depressed mood; the sensation of weight, tension, heaviness, even depression in the particular organ; and a consequent loss of function – 'I cannot think properly ... my bowels are blocked'.

Schneider (1920) considered vital feelings to be of paramount diagnostic significance in depressive illness, equivalent to the first-rank symptoms in schizophrenia, the core of cyclothymic depression and autonomic in origin. He considered these feelings to be common in depression. It would seem that Dupré (1913), writing about what he called *coenestopathic states*, was describing the same symptom: 'Coenestopathic states are, indeed, so common as to figure among the most frequent features of the psychoses'. He described *coenaesthesia* as the 'deep but more or less indefinite awareness that we have of our own bodies and the general tone of functional activity'. Coenestopathic states are 'the distressing feelings which emanate from one or other of the coenesthesic areas ... a change in the normal quality of physical feeling in certain parts of the body'. They are localized, but there is no local pathogenic lesion. Dupré claimed that coenestopathic states were autonomous, not associated with other psychiatric disorders; but, in describing the affects with which they are associated, he appears to describe affective disorders. The mood of depression may be described as a global loss of vitality in which all functions are affected and all performances depressed.

A change in vital feelings does not occur only in depression. The bizarre feelings that a patient with schizophrenia has about his body is a change in the way he expresses himself, often further elaborated by delusions. It should be noted that the term *vital* is used rather differently in *vital anxiety states*. These states have been described (López Ibor, 1966), in which the anxiety is thought to be endogenous, developing relatively acutely in people of stable personality.

The depressive content of what phenomenologists would consider to be vital feelings varies very greatly, for example 'I have turned to stone... I have a feeling of depression in my chest ... it is a pain, a knot, a weight... I have a cloud on my head, a feeling of nothingness'. Burns (1971) commented with regard to respiratory vital feelings, 'A striking feature of the breathlessness described by the patients with depression was its fairly sudden onset and cessation, corresponding exactly with the onset and resolution of the depressive illness'.

Trethowan (1979) considered that lowering of vitality is fundamental to the experience of depressive illness. He described this as 'a lowering of vitality which is all-pervasive and leads to a marked loss of ability of the subject to function as he did before he became ill in terms of both mind and body'.

Feelings attached to the perception of objects

Objects may evoke an emotional response in a normal person, for instance a comfortable feeling of familiarity towards an armchair in which one rests after an energetic walk, or apprehensive dislike towards a dentist's chair. This normal affective response may be exaggerated pathologically. Excessive feelings of fear amounting to terror may remain associated with objects. The objects to which affect is attached may not only be physical, inanimate objects but also thoughts, and patterns of thoughts, and people. The occurrence of certain ideas may regularly be associated with specific pathological emotion, perhaps resulting in phobia (see Chapter 19). Any object of perception may be invested with idiosyncratic affect.

Feelings directed towards people

These may be disturbed in a number of different ways. Affect may be absent or deadened, increased and excessive or distorted. It may also be ambivalent – both loving and hating, rejecting and overprotecting synchronously. A girl described in Chapter 15, suffering from anorexia nervosa, would take great care to cook enormous meals for her twin sister, to whom she was very close; the sister became grossly obese while the patient vanished almost to a skeleton. In answer to remonstrations about feeding her sister, she said, 'I look horrible, so she should look horrible as well'.

Free-floating emotion

This is commonly described in psychiatric disturbance, and in his original description of anxiety neurosis Freud (1895) considered that the condition was characterized by free-floating anxiety. A powerful affect seems to have no goal and is associated with no object. The patient describes himself as feeling generally anxious, not anxious about anything in particular but just anxious. This free-floating anxiety has somatic and psychological concomitants. It may seem to be localized physically in certain areas of the body. Other free-floating affects occur, such as restlessness, tension, gloom, despondency, euphoria, irritability and so on.

ABNORMALITY OF EXPERIENCE AND PHYSIOLOGICAL ACTIVITY

A speculative hypothesis that clinicians have found helpful is the term *alexithymia*, which was coined by Sifneos (1972) to describe a specific disturbance in psychic functioning characterized by difficulties in the capacity to verbalize affect and elaborate fantasies. This was originally introduced to describe psychosomatic disorders occurring in individuals with difficulty expressing their emotions. The link with absence or diminution of fantasy is a consistent finding (Nemiah and Sifneos, 1970). The communicative style shows markedly reduced or absent symbolic thinking so that inner attitudes, feelings, wishes and drives are not revealed; few dreams and a paucity of fantasies are reported (Taylor, 1984). Thinking is literal, utilitarian and concerned with the minutiae of external events. These individuals have great difficulty in recognizing and describing their own feelings and in discriminating between emotional states and bodily sensations. They show a stiff, robot-like existence, 'almost as if they are following an instruction book'; there may be stiffness of posture and lack of facial expression. They show an impaired capacity for empathy in their interpersonal relationships. Alexithymic characteristics have been found especially among patients with psychosomatic disorders, somatoform disorders, psychogenic pain disorders, substance abuse disorders, post-traumatic stress disorder, masked depression, character neuroses and sexual perversions, but these findings have not been consistently replicated.

The Toronto Alexithymia Scale, which is the most widely used measure of alexithymia, has four factors: difficulty in identifying feelings, externally oriented thinking, difficulty expressing feelings and reduced daydreaming (Kirmayer and Robbins, 1993). The two factors difficulty in identifying feelings and difficulty expressing feelings appear to be correlated with somatosensory amplification (Nakao *et al.*, 2002). This provides some validation for the idea that alexithymia is the basis for excessive somatization and that this may be due to undue awareness of discrepant sensations that are then misconstrued as evidence of physical illness.

Somatization in patients with mental disorder can be defined as the selective perception and focus on the somatic manifestations of the disorder with denial or minimization of the affective and cognitive changes (Katon *et al.*, 1982). As a method of expression of emotion, it is frequently reported in transcultural studies, especially in the Indian subcontinent, according to Rack (1982). Murphy and coworkers (1967) studied basic depressive symptomatology in 30 countries and showed how culture changes illness and the way dysphoria is expressed. Bavington (1981), studying depression in a predominantly Pathan culture in Pakistan, found somatization to be expressed in 45 per cent of cases; hypochondriasis was present in 55 per cent, hysterical (dissociative) features in 60 per cent, feelings of guilt in 50 per cent, paranoid ideas in 38 per cent, suicidal thoughts in 75 per cent, diurnal variation in 18 per cent, retardation in 50 per cent and irritability in 80 per cent of depressed patients. Bavington explains these somatic ideas by the presence of vital feelings rather than poverty of language. Mumford (1992) found that patients with psychiatric disorders originating from India and Pakistan typically communicate their distress in terms of somatic symptoms; somatic presentation was common in general hospital settings where psychiatric disorders were often unrecognized and untreated. The use of somatic symptoms and somatic metaphor to communicate emotional distress is found in all languages and cultures. Complaining of emotional dysphoria in terms of somatic symptoms may reflect the limitation of the medical profession in listening to complaints rather than a poverty of language or paucity of verbal expression of the patient.

ABNORMALITIES OF EVALUATION

The relationship between cognitions and emotions is difficult to disentangle. Initially, it was thought that the emotional state determined the associated cognitions. Thus, low mood provoked negative thoughts about the self and the world. However, Beck (Beck 1967; Beck *et al.*, 1979) proposed that a constellation of cognitive errors initiated or maintained depression. These included arbitrary inferences, selective abstractions, overgeneralizations, magnification and minimization. Furthermore, there were cognitive schemas, that is, underlying assumptions about the self, the world and the future, that developed from previous experiences and that habitually influenced how events in the world were appraised and could induce mood change either directly or via disruption in self-esteem. This proposal is line with Schachter and Singer's two-factor theory of emotion, in which cognitions play a central role.

There are also abnormalities of appraisal of the facial or vocal expression of emotions in others. *Prosopoaffective agnosia* refers to the selective deficiency in appreciating the emotional expression displayed in the face of others. This abnormality is distinct from prosopagnosia, in which only recognition of familiar faces is impaired. It is usually associated with acquired brain disease and has been reported in frontotemporal dementia, when it is also associated with impairment of recognition of vocal expression of emotion (Keane *et al.*, 2002); following right thalamic infarct (Vuillemier *et al.*, 1998); and in subjects with right-sided limbic and heteromodal cortical lesions (Weniger and Irle, 2002). It has been reported in autism and Asperger's syndrome, but it is not part of a pervasive impairment of face-processing skills (Hofter *et al.*, 2005). In other words, it occurs in some patients but not in others and dissociates from impairment of face recognition per se.

Receptive emotional dysprosody refers to the selective deficit in recognizing the emotional tone in speech. This is often associated with *expressive emotional dysprosody*, the impairment of the production of emotional tone in speech. Both abnormalities are found in Parkinson's disease (Caekebeke *et al.*, 1991; Pell, 1996).

MANIC–DEPRESSIVE MOOD

Certainly since the writings of Kraepelin, the apparently opposite mood states of mania and depression have been recognized as occurring in the same illness – frequently at different times and stages of the illness in the same patient, more rarely at the same time in the same patient. The affective disorders are now recognized as a very considerable part of psychiatry, with an impressive body of research in most relevant areas (Paykel, 1992). Although depression occurs more frequently than mania in bipolar illnesses, the first attack of mania may occur even after the age of 60 (Shulman and Post, 1980).

Although they are described separately, it is important to realize that these mood states may occur together. Mania and depression are not opposite mood states; they are both pathological, and the opposite of either would be freedom from morbid emotion. Agitation and overactivity may occur with depression, irritability and a feeling of frustration with mania. It is usual for a person to go through a depressive phase before becoming manic, and again on the return from mania before reaching a state of normal mood. A patient, now depressed, having previously been manic, described this: 'The first fine careless rapture has disappeared. I feel more tired and moody'.

Depression of mood

Core experience: psychological and physical

Depression of mood is very common, and depression of such persistence and intensity as to be regarded as illness frequently occurs. There is considerable discussion as to what is the central core of depression. Of course, arguments advocating biochemical, psychodynamic or conditioning factors as initiating causes are not mutually exclusive. Depression affects virtually all physical and psychological functions, for example, using a tachistoscopic method, Powell and Hemsley (1984) were able to show that depression influenced perception.

The word *depression* is a misnomer, as depressive illness may occur without the patient making a complaint of depression as a symptom (*depressio sine depressione*). For this reason, the term *melancholia* may be preferred; although this literally means 'black bile', it has come to be accepted as a medical illness. It was the term used by Lewis (1934) in his classical description of depressive states in a detailed study of 61 cases; this has influenced all subsequent investigation of the condition. However, there is some nosological confusion, as this term is used in DSM-IV (American Psychiatric Association, 1994) to describe just one aspect of *major depressive disorder* (major depressive episode with melancholic features). Melancholia is the preferred term for Whybrow (1997), who considers that it 'better captures the "veritable tempest in the brain" that marks the experience of inner turmoil and confused thinking as harmony and emotion drain away, often to be replaced by a withered imitation of life'.

The subjective symptoms of depression are very variable. The mood varies from indifference and apathy to profound dejection, despondency and despair. *Anhedonia*, the complete inability to experience pleasure, is a constant feature; it is experienced as joylessness and revealed in facial expression, speech, behaviour, lifestyle and the patient's account of personal experience.

A slowing down of the ability to initiate thought or action is noted by the observer as *retardation*. A patient, describing this after recovery, said, 'it feels as if treacle has been poured into my head through your ears'. Psychic retardation is experienced subjectively as an inability to fulfil normal obligations, as loss of coping. The proneness to self-blame often results in the patient describing himself as lazy and good for nothing. There is a catastrophic lowering of self-esteem as a prominent cognitive component.

Agitation and purposeless restlessness add to the discomfort and to the inability of the depressed person to achieve anything. This anxiety and preoccupation with gloomy thoughts impairs concentration. Diurnal variation of mood is often prominent, with the patient feeling at his worst, and perhaps most suicidal, when he wakes early in the morning or, alternatively, somewhat later in the morning. The degree of depression and misery may sometimes successfully be concealed; this is the presentation of *depressio sine depressione* (smiling depression) in a patient who appears not to be depressed in the consulting room but may, much to his doctor's dismay, kill himself. The concealment is probably conscious and may be associated with habitual masking of the expression of emotion or alternatively aimed at avoiding treatment.

Concentration, application and decision making become difficult, painful and sometimes impossible. The person describes difficulty or impossibility in fantasy and recollection of emotion. This is described as loss of memory and loss of feeling. Often, this loss of mental function makes the patient believe he is 'going mad' or 'losing his mind', a sort of mental hypochondriasis. Physical retardation may become the focus for hypochondriacal beliefs about the body: 'I am constipated . . . my bowels are totally blocked'. A very depressed middle-aged woman described her bodily feelings thus: 'I have a feeling like having an injection at the dentist's. My face feels numb, but at the same time painful all over'.

Anxiety is a common concomitant with depression and may completely obscure the latter. In agitated depression, agitation and restlessness are extreme and the patient carries a serious risk of suicide. Histrionic behaviour may also obscure the underlying depressive illness. A patient who was actually profoundly depressed kept picking her skin and pulling her hair, saying, 'look, I can't feel anything when I do this to myself'.

The affect of depression may be localized somatically in vital feelings (see above). It may take the form of profound misery or dejection. There is usually a feeling of loss of capacity, helplessness and a feeling that the patient cannot cope. Absence of feelings is often described, or it may be described as an inexplicable loss of feelings 'that ought to be there'.

Feelings of guilt and unworthiness are prominent in depressive illness of endogenous type. This has long been known, for example Plutarch, in the first century AD, described a person: 'He looks on himself as a man whom the gods hate and pursue with their anger . . . "Leave me," says the wretched man, "me the impious, the accursed, hated of the gods, to suffer my punishment."' (Zilboorg and Henry, 1941). On the other hand, Shepherd (1993) considers that guilt feelings did not feature predominantly in depressive states described in pre-Puritan England. The patient may blame himself for having allowed himself to get into this state of mind. He is full of self-reproach and recrimination for all sorts of peccadilloes from the distant past. For all that goes wrong around him he takes personal blame; this may be of delusional intensity. Using a scale for the evaluation of feelings of guilt, it was possible to identify two separate components: 'delusional' guilt or shame (experienced in relation to one's actions) and 'affective' guilt (a more general feeling of unworthiness) (Berrios *et al.*, 1992). As well as delusions of guilt and unworthiness, hypochondriacal and nihilistic delusions are relatively common in depression, especially when it occurs in the elderly.

Delusions occur in psychotic depression. It is important to make the distinction between a belief about the state of the world coloured by current mood – 'I feel that I must have done something to my brain as I can't think properly', from an actual delusional belief – 'I can't think at all, it is impossible, my brain is dead'. The former is a metaphorical statement, the latter a belief held with conviction. In practice, there is often a grey area between frank depressive delusions and emotionally laden views of the world.

Table 18.1 shows the frequency of symptoms, however slight, in depressive illness that were recorded quantitatively using a rating scale in 239 men and 260 women (Hamilton, 1989). It is seen that anxiety is a frequent symptom in depressive illness.

Suicidal thoughts

'I feel as though I want to destroy myself. There is no point in going on.' Suicidal ideas, ruminations and impulses are common. Alvarez (1971) has written a detailed study of suicide from a literary point of view. He is concerned with the background and the reasons for suicide and attempted suicide in many well-known writers, especially poets. He writes about suicide as 'letting go':

> " I have to admit that I am a failed suicide. ... Seneca, the final authority on the subject, pointed out disdainfully that the exits are everywhere: each precipice and river, each branch of each tree, every vein in your body will set you free. ... Yet despite all that, I never quite made it.

The intertwined threads of artistic creativity, manic–depressive illness and suicide have been explored by Goodwin and Jamison (1990).

Both the muse and madness as the gift of the gods have been a recurring theme from earliest times through such nineteenth century poets as Browning, Shelley, Coleridge and Byron to the modern American poets, among whom there was found to be a very high prevalence of manic–depressive illness and many suicides. In her enlightening study of manic–depressive illness and the artistic temperament, *Touched With Fire*, Jamison (1993) demonstrates differential rates for depressive illness and suicide in poets, artists and other writers and comments on this.

Extreme mood swings are frequent, with enthusiasm and creativity during elation and stark despair when the poet finds him- or herself lacking in inspiration. Poets and also creative musicians (Schumann, Wolf, Rachmaninov, Tchaikovsky, etc.) show this pattern especially frequently, while it is much less common among biographers – and presumably writers of textbooks. In the same way that depression may occur without suicide or suicidal ideas, suicide may be carried out without predisposing pathological depressive mood.

Depression is regarded as the final common pathway leading to suicide (Van Heeringen *et al.*, 2000). These authors imply depression the emotion and not the diagnostic category. They consider that psychological, social and biological

Table 18.1 Frequency of symptoms in depressive illness

Males		Females	
Symptoms	Subjects (%)	Symptoms	Subjects (%)
Depressed mood	100.0	Depressed mood	100.0
Loss of interest	99.6	Loss of interest	98.8
Anxiety, psychic	97.1	Anxiety, psychic	97.8
Anxiety, somatic	87.4	Somatic, general	94.2
Insomnia, initial	83.7	Anxiety, somatic	87.3
Suicide	82.0	Somatic, gastrointestinal	83.5
Somatic, general	82.0	Suicide	80.4
Somatic, gastrointestinal	80.3	Insomnia, initial	77.7
Insomnia, delayed	74.1	Guilt	72.7
Guilt	71.5	Insomnia, delayed	71.9
Insomnia, middle	71.5	Weight loss	68.8
Weight loss	69.0	Agitation	68.1
Agitation	68.1	Insomnia, middle	66.5
Libido	59.8	Libido	49.5
Retardation	52.3	Retardation	43.5
Hypochondriasis	33.1	Hypochondriasis	25.8
Loss of insight	28.0	Loss of insight	21.9
Paranoid symptoms	25.1	Depersonalization	21.1
Obsessional symptoms	13.3	Obsessional symptoms	20.7
Depersonalization	10.9	Paranoid symptoms	13.8
Diurnal variation:	59.4	Diurnal variation:	60.1
worse in morning	61.4	worse in morning	65.5
worse in evening	30.7	worse in evening	25.0
worse in afternoon	7.9	worse in afternoon	9.5

(After Hamilton, 1989, with permission.)

aetiological factors, and the increased rates associated with many psychiatric disorders, are all mediated through hopelessness resulting in suicidal behaviour. This emotion of hopelessness arises from feeling defeated in some important area of life and feeling closed in with no possible escape or rescue. Suicidal behaviour is then a 'cry of pain', an attempt to escape these feelings of entrapment.

Plans for suicide may not be carried out solely because of the degree of *retardation*; occasionally, electroconvulsive therapy may lessen retardation after three or four treatments and thereby increase the risk of suicide, because improvement from depression of mood and lowered self-esteem because of guilt feelings has not yet occurred. Death is often welcomed with a sense of relief. A psychotically depressed patient, when offered admission to hospital, accepted with resignation, 'I will come in and there you will kill me. It is what I deserve'. It is frequently described afterwards by the relatives of suicides that in the days or hours preceding their death they were happier and more tranquil than they had been for a long time.

Homicide of one or more of those close to the patient followed by suicide is a real danger with a small minority of sufferers from depressive illness. A profoundly depressed man felt that life was not worth living, that he had failed completely and that the world was intolerable. The only person he cared for was his 5-year-old son, and he did not want to condemn him to what he anticipated would be a lifetime of misery. He put his son on the handlebars of his bicycle and rode over the quay into the harbour, intending to kill them both. The boy was drowned but the father was rescued, resuscitated and charged with murder. Subsequently, he responded to treatment for his severe depressive illness.

'That internal restlessness'

That Internal Restlessness and Disorder in Man, Which Has Been the Complaint of All Ages was part of the title of James Vere's book (1778) in which restlessness of mood is associated with instinctual conflict in a way that anticipates Freud's theory of anxiety: the resultant conflict from the opposing forces of the superego and id. Mood is a variable expression of the self; it may be a transient feeling reactive to a certain situation or it may be a more long-lasting, sustained, inexplicable mood that is regarded as endogenous.

Internal restlessness also describes the emotions of neurotic disorder: anxiety, irritability and the situational fears of phobic state. These, with obsessional disorders, are discussed in Chapter 19.

Cyclothymia and related conditions

As well as the major episodes of mania and depression occurring in manic–depressive disorder, for which admission to hospital will often be indicated, there are also recurrent and cyclical conditions with episodes of depression and hypomania of mild to moderate severity that rarely lead to hospitalization (Akiskal and Mallya, 1987); the symptoms are manifested as abnormalities of personality, such as cyclothymia, rather than as symptoms of mood disorder. These conditions are common in the general population. These authors would see such conditions as including contributions from the hyperthymic temperament, subaffective dysthymic temperament, irritable temperament and cyclothymic temperament. There are, therefore, soft bipolar spectrum disorders, which are characterized by abrupt biphasic shifts in mood, cognition, behaviour and circadian rhythms.

These conditions are described as cyclothymia (F34.0) in ICD-10 (World Health Organization, 1992) and cyclothymic disorder (301.13) in DSM-IV (American Psychiatric Association, 1994). The patient shows mood swings over many years in both directions, that is, gloom and elation, but severity does not amount to that seen in manic–depressive illness. Disorder of personality should always be considered in the differential diagnosis.

Depression and loss

Any social situation of transition is associated with some disturbance of emotion (Parkes, 1971). Depression is the affect associated with experience of loss. It is not the intention here to enter into theoretical aspects but to discuss the subjective experience. Parkes (1976) has demonstrated how loss of a person, loss of a limb and even loss of a home are stressful in similar ways, and that there is a mental process going on in which the person is 'making real inside the self events which have already occurred in reality outside'. This process is associated with marked psychic pain and unhappiness. An example of depression associated with the threat of loss of a loved object was a taxi driver who owned his own car, which was the only thing he valued in life. During an episode of profound depression, he polished the taxi to perfection, took it into the garage, connected a pipe to the exhaust of the car, started the engine and killed himself.

The dysphoric mood associated with the experience of loss is always exacerbated if there is any sense of guilt or self-blame attached to the circumstances of the loss: 'if only I had called the doctor in to see Mother earlier, I shall never forgive myself'. Byatt (1985) comments about this in relation to crime fiction: 'Detective stories, like the belief in Original Sin, console and comfort men for death, because someone always *is* responsible for bringing it into the world (of the novel) and all our woe goes out with retribution or atonement. One of the many unpleasant aspects of grief is the need to feel responsible or guilty'.

Grief

The immediate experience of loss is shock and numbness. The suddenly bereaved person may say that he cannot believe that it has happened to him. He just feels numb and empty. He may describe depersonalization feelings. There is a tendency to deny that the loss has happened. A woman was referred to a surgeon for a lump in the breast. At operation, the mass was found to be malignant and the breast was amputated. For several days after the operation, she was unable to accept that the painful area under the dressing signified the loss of her breast rather than a minor excision.

Following initial shock and denial come the pangs of grief. This is an acute feeling of loss, with anxiety prominent, as well as grieving – *anxious searching*. The implications of the experience of loss begin to be realized, and this may cause the person feelings of anxiety amounting to panic: 'However am I going to cope without him?' The somatic symptoms of anxiety may be present as well as the psychological.

Three distinct patterns of *morbid grief* have been observed (Lieberman, 1978):

- phobic avoidance of persons, places or things related to the deceased, combined with extreme guilt and anger about the deceased and his death
- a total lack of grieving, with anger directed towards others and over-idealization of the deceased
- physical illness and recurrent nightmares of the deceased.

These patterns have relevance for treatment using the behavioural method of *forced* or *guided mourning*.

When the experience of loss has been accepted as a reality, *depression*, the affect appertaining to loss, occurs. The person feels very low and hopeless, perhaps with the lowering of vitality and apathy of depression. He becomes resigned to his situation but sees no way out: 'there is simply no future for me now'. Not surprisingly, this state is often associated with suicidal ideas and impulses, and there is an increased mortality from suicide and other causes in the 6 months subsequent to bereavement (Parkes *et al.*, 1969).

As the state of grieving is resolved, the person gradually overcomes this despairing hopelessness. There is an attitude of mind that results in reorganization and redirection. He gradually makes decisions and carries out activities that demonstrate his emotional and intellectual acceptance of the loss and intention to continue his life as congenially as possible, although still remembering the loss. This stage of *resolution* may be postponed for many years, as with Queen Victoria's grieving for Prince Albert.

Parkes (1976) discriminates between the subjective experience of *external loss* and *internal change*. The external loss is shown by pining for the lost object. Anxiety following loss occurs both in bereaved people and in amputees and is associated with anxious searching: a bereaved person was walking up and down the street wondering if she would see her husband, whom she knew to be dead. In these circumstances, misperception of strangers as being the lost relative may happen. A man whose father had died some long time before thought he heard his father's voice in another room and then realized it was his son. People return to places associated with the lost person or keep articles that belonged to them sacrosanct.

Internal change, with a sense of mutilation, is common to people with different types of loss. Amputees feel themselves to be badly damaged both in their function and in their self-image. Because a man has lost his leg, he will be unable to carry out his previous activities as before and may feel himself to be less of a man. Similarly, the woman with an amputated arm may prefer a cosmetic but useless prosthesis rather than a more functional hook. She may feel the affront to her self-image of a mutilated arm more than the loss of function. Parkes and Napier (1975) stress the social associations of loss in their discussion of prevention and alleviation of the problems resulting from amputation. Widows also describe a feeling of loss within themselves due to their bereavement; there is, of course, often a real loss of status. Those rehoused often described an internal change on moving: 'something of me went when I left the old home'.

Mania

Mania is a word with a long history. Hare (1981) considers that the early descriptions of intellectual deterioration with excitement were made because of the association with organic deterioration from poor general health during the nineteenth century. As the physical health of the population improved, it was possible to describe separate conditions with different natural histories. However, mania still forms a much higher proportion of affective psychoses occurring puerperally than of affective disorders occurring at other stages of life (Dean and Kendell, 1981).

Mania refers to elation of mood, acceleration of thinking and overactivity. Subjectively, although it may be described as a different state from normal, it is rarely complained of by the patient as a symptom. A young manic in-patient described his internal state thus: 'I feel hypersuffused with experience... I am developing a close secretarial relationship with Camilla Brown (another young patient)... I feel like a rocket with the blue paper lit, standing in a bottle and just ready to take off'. It has become conventional to refer to all but the most severe cases as suffering from *hypomania*. This is unfortunate, as one does not refer to 'hypodepression' and the person using the term *hypomania* often gives the impression that wrong diagnosis is permissible to a greater extent than if the term *mania* had been used.

The early stages of mania may be experienced as enjoyable, even 'wonderful', and an enormous relief from the depression that preceded it. A patient quoted by Whybrow (1997) put it this way: 'In the early stages of mania I feel good – about the world and everybody in it. There's a faster beat; a sense of expectation that my life will be full and exciting'. For this reason, the patient may be reluctant to take medication or to report his condition to his doctor. Later on in manic illness, the patient's experience is usually described as unpleasant and even frightening.

In pure form, it is characterized by excessive cheerfulness, rapid train and association of thought and overactivity. The speed of thinking and the ready ability to form associations results in rapid and apparently sparkling conversation (see Chapter 9). Puns and clang associations abound, for example in a case quoted by Bingham (1841):

> " A fine bold lady, well dressed and well known to the officers of a certain house, 'a regular madwoman', as they called her, was brought thither by her friends. She was no sooner announced than every missile and instrument of attack was carefully removed out of her way. She opened the conference by a familiar address to the physician under whose care she had been before and was going to remain, by saying to him, 'Well, Doctor M(orrison), but I beg pardon, I forgot whom I was speaking to – it is Sir A(lexander). Well, Sir A—, since I had the pleasure of seeing you last, I have been benighted, and you have been knighted'.

REFERENCES

Akiskal HS and Mallya G (1987) Criteria for the 'soft' bipolar spectrum: treatment implications. *Psychopharmacology Bulletin 23*, 68–73.

Alvarez A (1971) *The Savage God: a Study of Suicide*. London: Weidenfeld & Nicolson.

American Psychiatric Association (1994) *Diagnostic and Statistical Manual of Mental Disorders*, 4th edn. Washington: American Psychiatric Association.

Andreasen N (1979) Affective flattening and the criteria for schizophrenia. *American Journal of Psychiatry 136*, 944–7.

Anstee BH and Fleminger JJ (1977) Diagnosis 'uncertain': a follow-up study. *British Journal of Psychiatry 131*, 592–8.

Bartholomew RE (1994) Disease, disorder or deception? Latah as habit in a Malay extended family. *Journal of Nervous Mental Disease 182*, 331–8.

Bavington J (1981) *Depression in Pakistan*. Leeds: Transcultural Psychiatry Society (UK) Workshop.

Beck AT (1967) *Depression: Clinical, Experimental and Theoretical Aspects*. New York: Hoeber.

Beck AT, Rush AJ, Shaw BF and Emery G (1979) *Cognitive Therapy of Depression*. New York: Guilford Press.

Berrios GE (1985) The psychopathology of affectivity: conceptual and historical aspects. *Psychological Medicine 15*, 745–58.

Berrios GE, Bulbena A, Bakshi N, *et al*. (1992) Feelings of guilt in major depression: conceptual and psychosomatic aspects. *British Journal of Psychiatry 160*, 781–7.

Bingham N (1841) *Religious Delusions*. London: Hatchard.

Bleuler E (1911) *Dementia Praecox: or the Group of Schizophrenias*. New York: International University Press.

Brenner B (1979) Depressed affect as a cause of associated somatic problems. *Psychological Medicine 9*, 737–46.

Burns BH (1971) Breathlessness in depression. *British Journal of Psychiatry 119*, 39–45.

Burton R (1628) *The Anatomy of Melancholia*. Oxford: Henry Cripps.

Byatt AS (1985) *Still Life*. London: Chatto & Windus.

Caekebeke JF, Jennekens-Schinkel A, van der Linden ME, Buruma OJ and Roos RA (1991) The interpretation of dysprosody in patients with Parkinson's disease. *Journal of Neurology, Neurosurgery and Psychiatry 54*, 145–8.

Cutting J (1985) *The Psychology of Schizophrenia.* Edinburgh: Churchill Livingstone.
Cutting J (1997) *Principles of Psychopathology.* Oxford: Oxford University Press.
Darwin C (1872) *The Expression of the Emotions in Man and Animals.* London: John Murray.
Dean C and Kendell RE (1981) The symptomatology of puerperal illness. *British Journal of Psychiatry 139,* 128–33.
Dupré E (1913) Les Cénestopathies, Mouvement Médical 3–22 (transl. Rohde M, 1974) In Hirsch SR and Shepherd M (eds) *Themes and Variations in European Psychiatry.* Bristol: John Wright.
Ekman P (1998) Afterword. In Darwin C *The Expression of the Emotions in Man and Animals.* London: Harper Collins.
Ekman P and Friesen W (1971) Constants across cultures in the face and emotion. *Journal of Personality and Social Psychology 17,* 124–9.
Freud S (1895) On the grounds for detaching a particular syndrome from neurasthenia under the description 'anxiety neurosis. In *Standard Edition of the Complete Psychological Works of Sigmund Freud,* vol. III, pp. 90–115. London: Hogarth Press.
Galanter M (1982) Charismatic religious sects and psychiatry: an overview. *American Journal of Psychiatry 139,* 1539–48.
Gallese V (2007) Embodied simulation: from mirror neuron systems to interpersonal relations. *Novartis Foundation Symposium 278,* 3–12.
Goodwin FK and Jamison KR (1990) *Manic–Depressive Illness.* New York: Oxford University Press.
Hamelin S, Rohr P, Kahane P, Minotti L and Vercueil L (2004) Late onset hyperekplexia. *Epileptic Disorders 6,* 169–72.
Hamilton M (1989) Frequency of symptoms in melancholia (depressive illness). *British Journal of Psychiatry 154,* 201–6.
Hare E (1981) The two manias: a study of the evolution of the modern concept of mania. *British Journal of Psychiatry 138,* 89–99.
Hofter RL, Manoach DS and Barton JJ (2005) Perception of facial expression and facial identity in subjects with social developmental disorders. *Neurology 65,* 1620–5.
Howard R and Ford R (1992) From the jumping Frenchmen of Maine to posttraumatic stress disorder: the startle response in neuropsychiatry. *Psychological Medicine 22,* 695–707.
Huxley A (1952) *The Devils of Loudun.* London: Chatto & Windus.
James W (1884) What is an emotion? *Mind 9,* 188–205.
James W (1902) *The Varieties of Religious Experience: a Study in Human Nature.* New York: Longmans, Green.
Jamison KR (1993) *Touched With Fire: Manic–Depressive Illness and the Artistic Temperament.* New York: Free Press.
Jamison KR (1995) *An Unquiet Mind. A Memoir of Moods and Madness.* New York: Knopf.
Katon W, Kleinman A and Rosen G (1982) Depression and somatization: a review. Part 1. *American Journal of Medicine 72,* 127–35.
Keane J, Calder AJ, Hodges JR and Young AW (2002) Face and emotion processing in frontal variant frontotemporal dementia. *Neuropsychologia 40,* 655–65.
Kirmayer LJ and Robbins JM (1993) Cognitive and social correlates of Toronto Alexithymia Scale. *Psychosomatics 34,* 41–52.
Klein DF (1974) Endogenomorphic depression. *Archives of General Psychiatry 31,* 447–54.
Kraepelin E (1905) *Lectures on Clinical Psychiatry,* 3rd edn (transl. Johnston T, 1917). New York: W. Wood.
Lewis A (1934) Melancholia: a clinical survey of depressive states. *Journal of Mental Science 80,* 277–378.
Lewis IM (1971) *Ecstatic Religion: an Anthropological Study of Spirit Possession and Shamanism.* Harmondsworth: Penguin
Lieberman S (1978) Nineteen cases of morbid grief. *British Journal of Psychiatry 132,* 159–63.
López Ibor JJ (1966) *Neuroses as Mood Disorders.* Madrid: Editorial Gredos.
Meinck HM (2006) Startle and its disorders. *Neurophysiologie Clinique 36,* 357–64.
Mill JS (1873) *Autobiography* (ed. Robson JM, 1989). London: Penguin.
Mumford DB (1992) Detection of psychiatric disorders among Asian patients presenting with somatic symptoms. *British Journal of Hospital Medicine 47,* 202–4.
Murphy HBM, Wittkower ED and Chance NA (1967) Cross-cultural inquiry into the symptomatology of depression: preliminary report. *International Journal of Social Psychiatry 13,* 6–15.
Nakao M, Barsky AJ, Kumano H and Kuboki J (2002) Relationship between somatosensory amplification and alexithymia in a Japanese psychosomatic clinic. *Psychosomatics 43,* 55–60.

Nemiah JC and Sifneos PE (1970) Affect and fantasy in patients with psychosomatic disorders. In Hill OW (ed.) *Modern Trends in Psychosomatic Medicine 2*, pp. 26–34. London: Butterworth.

Parkes CM (1971) Psycho-social transitions: a field for study. *Social Science and Medicine 5*, 101–15.

Parkes CM (1976) The psychological reaction to loss of a limb: the first year after amputation. In Howells JG (ed.) *Modern Perception in the Psychiatric Aspects of Surgery*, pp. 515–33. London: Macmillan.

Parkes CM and Napier MM (1975) Psychiatric sequelae of amputation. In Silverstone T and Barraclough B (eds) *Contemporary Psychiatry*, pp. 440–6. Ashford: Headley Brothers.

Parkes CM, Benjamin B and Fitzgerald RG (1969) Broken heart: a statistical study of increased mortality among widows. *British Medical Journal i*, 740–3.

Paykel ES (1992) *Handbook of Affective Disorders*, 2nd edn. Edinburgh: Churchill Livingstone.

Pell MD (1996) On the receptive prosodic loss in Parkinson's disease. *Cortex 32*, 693–704.

Powell M and Hemsley DR (1984) Depression: a breakdown of perceptual defence? *British Journal of Psychiatry 145*, 358–62.

Rack P (1982) *Race, Culture and Mental Disorder*. London: Tavistock.

Ribot T (1896) *La Psychologie des Sentiments*. Paris: Félix Alcan.

Rizzolatti G and Craighero L (2004) The mirror-neuron system. *Annual Review of Neuroscience 27*, 169–92.

Rizzolatti G and Fadiga L (1998) Grasping objects and grasping action meanings: the dual role of monkey rostroventral premotor cortex (area 5). *Novartis Foundation Symposium 218*, 81–95.

Schachter S and Singer J (1962) Cognitive, social and physiological determinants of emotional state. *Psychological Review 69*, 379–99.

Schneider K (1920) The stratification of emotional life and the structure of the depressive states. *Zeitschrift fuer Gesundheitswesen Neurologie und Psychiatrie 59*, 281.

Shepherd M (1993) Historical epidemiology and the functional psychoses. *Psychological Medicine 23*, 301–4.

Shulman K and Post F (1980) Bipolar affective disorder in old age. *British Journal of Psychiatry 136*, 26–32.

Sifneos PE (1972) *Short-term Psychotherapy and Emotional Crisis*. Cambridge: Harvard University Press.

Simpson CJ (1984) The stigmata: pathology or miracle? *British Medical Journal 289*, 1746–8.

Sims A (1994) 'Psyche' – spirit as well as mind? *British Journal of Psychiatry 165*, 441–6.

Sirois F (1982) Epidemic hysteria. In Roy A (ed.) *Hysteria*, pp. 101–16. Chichester: John Wiley.

Snaith RP (1993) Anhedonia: a neglected symptom of psychopathology. *Psychological Medicine 23*, 957–66.

Styron W (1990) *Darkness Visible: a Memoir of Madness*. London: Cape.

Taylor G (1984) Alexithymia: concept, measurement and implications for treatment. *American Journal of Psychiatry 141*, 725–32.

Trethowan WH (1979) Affective disorders. In Trethowan WH (ed.) *Psychiatry*, 4th edn. London: Baillière Tindall.

Ungerleider JT and Wellisch DK (1979) Coercive persuasion (brainwashing), religious cults, and deprogramming. *American Journal of Psychiatry 136*, 279–82.

Van Heeringen K, Hawton K and Williams JMG (2000) Pathways to suicide: an integrative approach. In Hawton K and Van Heeringen K (eds) *The International Handbook of Suicide and Attempted Suicide*. Chichester: John Wiley.

Vere J (1778) *A Physical and Moral Enquiry into the Causes of That Internal Restlessness and Disorder in Man, Which Has Been the Complaint of All Ages*. London: White & Sewell.

Vuillemier P, Ghika-Schmid F, Bogousslavsky J, Assal G and Regli F (1998) Persistent recurrence of hypomania and prosoaffective agnosia in a patient with right thalamic infarct. *Neuropsychiatry, Neuropsychology and Behavioural Neurology 11*, 40–4.

Weniger G and Irle E (2002) Impaired facial affect recognition and emotional change in subjects with transmodal cortical lesions. *Cerebral Cortex 12*, 258–68.

Wernicke C (1906) *Fundamentals of Psychiatry*. Leipzig: Thieme.

Whybrow PC (1997) *A Mood Apart: Depression, Mania and Other Afflictions of the Self*. New York: Basic Books.

World Health Organization (1992) *The ICD-10 Classification of Mental and Behavioural Disorders: Clinical Description and Diagnostic Guidelines*. Geneva: World Health Organization.

Zilboorg G and Henry GW (1941) *A History of Medical Psychology*. New York: Norton.

Anxiety, Panic, Irritability, Phobia and Obsession

19

> "Montanus speaks of one that durst not walk alone from home for fear that he should swoon or die. A second fears every man he meets will rob him, quarrel with him or kill him. A third dares not venture to walk alone, for fear he should meet the devil, a thief, be sick; fears all old women as witches; and every black dog or cat he sees he suspecteth to be a devil; every person comes near him is malificiated; every creature, all intend to hurt him, seek his ruine; another dares not go over a bridge, come near a pool, rock, steep hill, lye in a chamber where cross beams are for fear he be tempted to hang, drown or precipitate himself. If he be in a silent auditory, as at a sermon, he is afraid he shall speak aloud, at unawares, something undecent, unfit to be said. If he be locked in a close room, he is afraid of being stifled for want of air, and still carries bisket, aquavitae, or some strong waters about him for fear of deliquiums, or being sick; or if he be in a throng, middle of a church, multitude, where he may not well get out, though he sit at ease he is certase affected. He will freely promise, undertake any business beforehand; but when it comes to be performed he dares not adventure, but fears an infinite number of dangers, disasters, etc. . . . They are afraid of some loss, danger, that they shall surely lose their lives, goods, and all they have; but why they know not. *Robert Burton (1621)*

The five abnormal phenomena of this chapter are frequent among those with neurotic disorders. What makes them abnormal is their severity, their prolonged duration, their occurrence in reaction to what could be considered an inadequate situational stress and the deleterious effect they have on social functioning. Each of them has a normal, even necessary, aspect: it is appropriate to be anxious at the beginning of a speech in public; it is normal for a parent to express irritability when an 8-year-old son breaks a window – it is a necessary learning experience for him; fear is necessary for coping when an individual suddenly discovers him- or herself to be surrounded by poisonous snakes; meticulous checking and checking again is an important part of learning to be a competent airline pilot; even panic is normal, in a statistical sense, in some situations of extreme mass disaster.

Anxiety, irritability, phobia and obsession may all occur together, especially in response to increased situational stress. They may also occur in pairs. Anxiety and irritability are phenomenologically related; in irritability, aggressiveness is added to the subjective experience of tension. Panic is, in fact, *episodic paroxysmal anxiety* (ICD-10; World Health Organization, 1992: 139). Anxiety and phobia are related, in that phobia is anxiety occurring in a specific situation. Phobia and obsession are related in that those experiencing either of them suffer a loss of freedom of action and, in both, a self-examining attitude is maintained (Scharfetter, 1980). Panic and phobia occur more frequently together than separately. These five states are all more likely to occur with personality disorders of any type and with other neurotic disorders. They often occur with depressive illness and may be associated with depersonalization or hypochondriasis.

In any modern consideration of anxiety disorders, anxiety, panic and phobia would be included both as states of emotion and as distinct syndromes (Noyes and Hoehn-Saric, 1998). Irritability is a distinct and important mood state that occurs in several different conditions, and obsession is both an individual symptom and an essential feature of obsessive–compulsive disorder. Obsession, unlike phobia, is not a type of anxiety, but it could be construed as a means to regulate anxiety. Obsessive–compulsive disorder is not an anxiety disorder, unlike phobic disorder, and although anxiety may occur with the condition it is not an essential feature and is not always present in this condition.

Patients may have insight and present themselves as suffering from 'phobia', 'obsession' or 'anxiety state'. However, the lay meaning of each of these terms is significantly different from psychiatric use, and it will be more usual for the clinician to diagnose the state from a description of the mood or thought process.

Mood in neurotic disorders is an exaggeration or distortion of the normal mood that might occur in similar circumstances. It is characteristic of the mood in neurosis that it is ineffective in producing action to deal appropriately or effectively with the problems that provoked it. It is therefore maladjusted as a response to the factors that caused it and in the effects that it facilitates.

ANXIETY

Anxiety is a universal emotion that, at times, it would be maladaptive not to experience; it is a necessary part of the response of the organism to stress. Lader and Marks (1971) have discussed the features of anxiety in terms of the emotion being normal or pathological. In rather concrete terms, a man who discovers that he is sharing a field with a bull feels acutely anxious and runs at top speed for the gate; if, 6 weeks later, when back in the city, he has a panic attack and has to lie down because someone mentions a part of the city called the Bullring, his response is clearly maladaptive and his anxiety pathological.

Anxiety may also, arbitrarily, be polarized between *state* and *trait* (Sims and Snaith, 1988). Anxiety state is the quality of being anxious now, at this particular time, probably as a reaction to provoking circumstances. Anxiety trait is the tendency over a long time, perhaps throughout life, to meet all the vicissitudes of life with a habitual excessive degree of anxiety; it is often associated with anxious personality disorder (Chapter 21). Anxiety as a description of the experience of normal emotion is not different in quality, only quantitatively, from anxiety state (Hamilton, 1959). Characteristic of the mood of anxiety are feelings of *constriction*. The word is etymologically associated with the idea of narrowness, stricture, 'straits', and in early usage was located in the praecordium and prominently associated with angina (Sims, 1985). The patient with anxiety state may feel restless, uncertain, vulnerable, trapped, breathless, choked. As well as feeling frightened and worried, hypochondriacal ideas and even feelings of guilt are often prominent. Symptoms of anxiety occur pathologically in *anxiety states* without obvious external cause. The anxiety is not attached to any specific provoking object, and so it is termed *free-floating anxiety*.

There is also a contrast between the experience of anxiety as a subjective emotion and the objective occurrence of physiological somatic changes normally associated with that affect; some of the commoner symptoms are shown in Box 19.1 (Tyrer, 1982). Tyrer considers irritability to be a symptom *of* anxiety state, but Snaith and Taylor (1985) made the case for irritability being an independent mood state that may be associated with anxiety – or any other mood disorder. Although it is usual to find the psychological and physical aspects of anxiety associated and related in intensity, this may not necessarily be so. The patient may complain of feeling extremely anxious but show minimal somatic expression; in dissociation, marked physical changes have been described when the patient does not complain at all of feeling anxious. These three dichotomous aspects of anxiety are represented in Figure 19.1.

Both major classifications make a distinction between three anxiety syndromes: generalized anxiety disorder, social and specific phobias and panic disorder. Those who suffer from generalized anxiety disorder experience persistent anxiety and worry that is out of proportion to actual events or circumstances (Spiegel and Barlow, 2000). The worry is typically focused on

Box 19.1 Symptoms of anxiety

Somatic and autonomic
- Palpitations
- Difficulty in breathing
- Dry mouth
- Nausea
- Frequency of micturition
- Dizziness
- Muscular tension
- Sweating
- Abdominal churning
- Tremor
- Cold skin

Psychic (psychological)
- Feelings of dread and threat
- Irritability
- Panic
- Anxious anticipation
- Inner (psychic) terror
- Worrying over trivia
- Difficulty in concentrating
- Initial insomnia
- Inability to relax

(From Tyrer, 1982, with permission.)

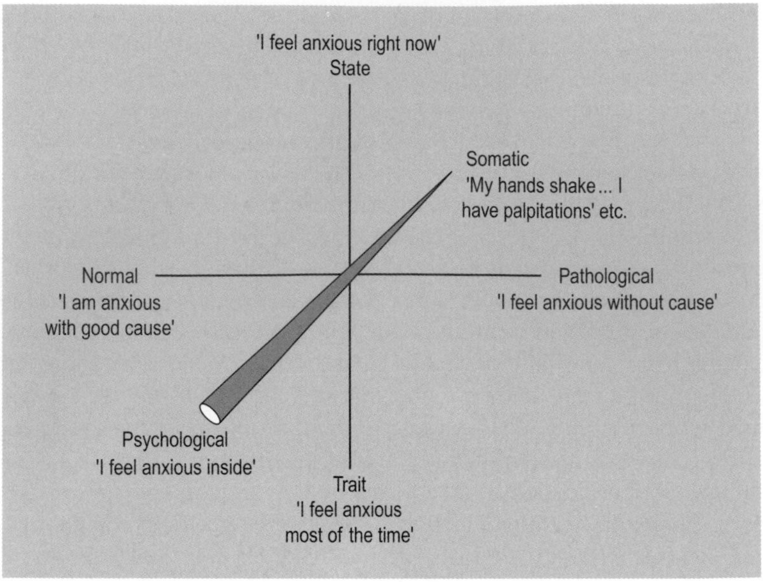

Figure 19.1 Three-dimensional model of anxiety symptoms.

everyday matters, and over time it shifts from item to item; the subject is almost never free from anxiety.

Patients with anxiety disorder describe characteristic ideational components, concentrating on themes of personal danger and especially physical harm (Hibbert, 1984). The 'most important' thought of patients included 'I may panic in front of others', 'I may die of a heart attack while asleep' and 'I am going to have a heart attack'. Fear of physical, psychological or social disaster also occurred during panic attacks. Stressful life experiences in the preceding 12 months, and some physiological disturbance other than anxiety immediately before the symptoms, were commonly described.

Other psychological functions are affected by acute anxiety. The capacity for reflection is decreased and the field of conscious awareness narrowed; this obviously has survival value for instant physical action but is a disadvantage when planning, reviewing and taking a variety of different factors into consideration are important. The variations of activity with anxiety are seen, for instance, after the experience of disaster: some victims will be numb and inert; others tense, restless and constructively overactive; and others still terrified, almost literally 'petrified', and incapable of sustained activity.

In the Present State Examination (Wing *et al.*, 1974), *general anxiety* is contrasted with *situational anxiety*, that is, the tendency to become anxious in certain defined situations. This latter is discussed later with phobic states. Under *general anxiety* are included free-floating autonomic anxiety; panic attacks (despite the current fashion for categorizing them separately); and the observation during interview that the patient appears to be anxious, tense, worried or apprehensive. Free-floating anxiety comprises such autonomic components as blushing, 'butterflies in the stomach', choking, difficulty in getting the breath, dizziness, dry mouth, giddiness, palpitations, sweating and trembling, dilated pupils, raised blood pressure; parasympathetic aspects include nausea, vomiting, frequency of micturition and diarrhoea.

The psychological quality of *feeling anxious* or *tense* is more difficult to quantify than its physiological correlates. Words are idiosyncratic in their meaning, and so there is a tendency to judge the veracity of the patient's statement that he is 'terribly anxious' according to the severity of the autonomic symptoms occurring concurrently. However, it is possible by using serial rating scales to compare the patient's subjective experience at different times; one much used example of this is the Hospital Anxiety and Depression Scale (Zigmond and Snaith, 1983). Serial recordings of a patient who showed both anxiety and depressive symptoms that responded to treatment at different times are shown in Figure 19.2. Self-description of anxiety includes worry, brooding, sleeplessness through preoccupation with contents of the thoughts and so on.

Panic attacks and disorder

Panic attacks occur as discrete episodes of somatic or autonomic anxiety associated with marked psychic anxiety as an extreme sense of fear. The attack ends either with a complete interruption to the patient's current stream of behaviour so that he lies on the floor, rushes into the open air, runs back into the house or 'collapses', or he terminates his current behaviour voluntarily so that the attack remits more gradually. In either case, there is something about his mode of activities before the attack that was precipitating panic. The patient makes this association for himself, and he goes to elaborate lengths to avoid provoking a panic attack. This may be the antecedent condition for development of a phobic state. The duration of the attack varies from less than a minute to several hours but is normally about 10 to 20 minutes. These attacks may occur many times per day, although usually less frequently.

Panic disorder has been established as a separate diagnostic category in ICD-10 (World Health Organization, 1992) and DSM-IV (American Psychiatric Association, 1994). Panic disorder is also called episodic paroxysmal anxiety; recurrent severe attacks of anxiety occur, often unpredictably. Onset is sudden, with many anxiety symptoms such as palpitations, chest pain or discomfort, choking or smothering feelings, dizziness, feelings of unreality, dyspnoea, paraesthesiae, hot flushes, sweating, faintness, trembling or fear of dying or going mad.

There are distinctions and similarities between panic disorder and generalized anxiety disorder. Forty-one generalized anxiety disorder subjects,

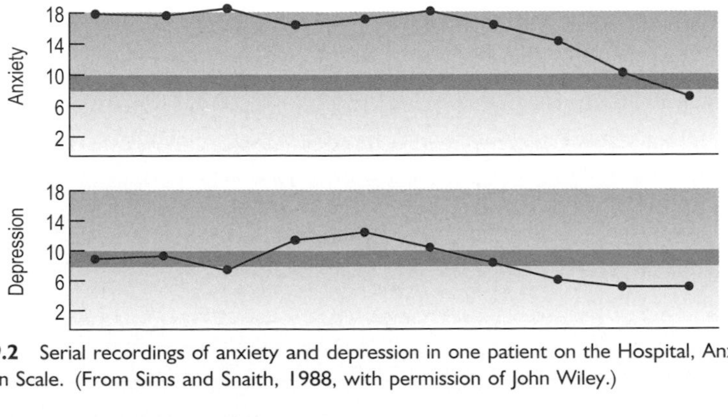

Figure 19.2 Serial recordings of anxiety and depression in one patient on the Hospital, Anxiety and Depression Scale. (From Sims and Snaith, 1988, with permission of John Wiley.)

who had never had panic attacks, were compared with 71 subjects with panic disorder (Noyes *et al.*, 1992). The generalized anxiety disorder subjects had an earlier, more gradual onset of symptoms and more often suffered from simple phobias, while the panic disorder subjects tended to report depersonalization and agoraphobia. In general, those with panic disorder had a more severe degree of illness and were more likely to give a history of major depression.

Phobic states

Phobias, or unreasonable fears, have been described for many centuries. For example, Benjamin Rush (1798) defines phobia as 'a fear of an imaginary evil, or an undue fear of a real one' and then produces a list of 18 phobias, partly humorously intended; this is reproduced in Box 19.2. *Agoraphobia* was originally described by Westphal (1871); this condition, literally 'fear of the market-place', causes very severe disability. Animal phobias have been contrasted by Marks (1970):

> " If ever we are tempted to think that all phobic states are a unity which reflects the same disorder and aetiology, we can quickly dispel this illusion simply by looking at the startling contrast between animal phobias and agoraphobias. These two conditions differ radically in onset, course, symptomatology, response to treatment and psychological measures.

Solyom *et al.* (1986) divided the symptomatology of 199 patients into three categories: agoraphobia (80 patients), social phobia (47 patients) and simple phobia (72 patients). Agoraphobia included 'fear of leaving home, of being alone at home or on the street, in crowds, of travelling by car, bus or train'. Social phobia

Box 19.2 Species of phobia according to Rush (1798)

- The cat phobia
- The rat phobia
- The insect phobia
- The odour phobia
- The dirt phobia
- The rum phobia
- The water phobia
- The solo phobia
- The power phobia
- The faction phobia
- The want phobia
- The doctor phobia
- The blood phobia
- The thunder phobia
- The home phobia
- The church phobia
- The ghost phobia
- The death phobia

involved 'fear of performing – speaking, writing, eating, urinating in public or in the presence of others'. Simple phobia described a single but life-disrupting fear, such as of animals, heights, disease, aeroplanes, insects and so on.

A more comprehensive subdivision of phobic states is contained in Box 19.3 from Marks (1969). As agoraphobia literally means 'fear of the marketplace', this is frequently appropriate nowadays, as often the most phobic situation for such people is in the supermarket. Agoraphobia is, in fact, a heterogeneous collection of disorders and not an entity; the patient does not only fear a throng of people but has multiple avoidance responses to many different stimuli (Snaith, 1991). It includes both those who have a fear of being under public scrutiny, and therefore who avoid public places, and those with illness fears in either a public place where they become noticeable or an exposed place where they will not be able to receive help.

Social phobias are common conditions that have been relatively neglected over recent years (Swinson, 1992). They are particularly likely to occur in association with other disorders of mood or other types of anxiety. There are a variety of different manifestations, but social phobia can be considered to be an extreme variant of shyness. However, avoidance is more typical of the established disorder.

Illness phobia is different from hypochondriacal preoccupation in that, with the former, avoidance occurs. Thus the criteria for phobia, according to Marks (1969), are:

- fear is out of proportion to the demands of the situation
- it cannot be explained or reasoned away
- it is not under voluntary control
- the fear leads to an *avoidance* of the feared situation.

A 28-year-old married woman said,

> “ My fear problems are worst... I am afraid of catching cancer. I am afraid of catching it from the hospital [radiotherapy hospital 1 mile away]... I bought a scarf from a shop and the assistant frightened me ... the look of her, she hardly had any hair and looked very old... I thought I had caught it from her and so I had to wash the house. I cleaned the whole house and it made me poorly. I had to move house because of the hospital and I cannot go back to that shop ever again.

Box 19.3 Subdivisions of phobic neurosis

Phobias of external stimuli
- Agoraphobia
- Social phobias
- Animal phobias

Phobias of internal stimuli
- Illness phobias
- Obsessive phobias
- Miscellaneous specific phobias

(After Marks, 1969, with permission.)

Phobias are unreasonable and inappropriate fears. Subjectively, they take the form of *situational anxiety*; anxiety is associated with specific circumstances or objects and results in *avoidance*. Situational autonomic anxiety, unlike free-floating anxiety, arises only with specific causes. Such fear-provoking situations include being in a crowded place (agoraphobia), or a confined space (claustrophobia), or perhaps on one's own or looking down from a high place; phobias may follow a stimulus that is idiosyncratic to this particular person. Provoking causes are quite frequently animals or parts of animals, for example cat, mouse, spider, snake, feathers or bird. This specific type of anxiety may then generalize, so that the person starts by being phobic for cats but becomes so frightened that she might meet a cat that all the time she spends outside her home she lives in a state of dread; eventually, this fear and avoidance bears only a tenuous relationship with the original cause.

There is also some relationship between phobias, especially agoraphobia, and depression (Schapira *et al.*, 1970). Persistent fear and foreboding, often of a situational nature, may occur with other depressive symptoms. Phobic states, as also panic disorder, may respond to antidepressant therapy.

Roth (1959) described the *phobic–anxiety–depersonalization syndrome* as a separate nosological entity, but saw it as a form of anxiety neurosis on which the additional symptoms are superimposed in some individuals; phobic symptoms are usually social and agoraphobic. This occurs most often in younger married women. Typically, such a patient shows agoraphobia so that she cannot travel on a bus or go shopping in a supermarket for fear of being conspicuous in public – either fainting or being taken suddenly ill in one of these places. She is likely to describe panic attacks on some of the occasions when she has attempted these things in the past. She develops a relationship of complete dependency on her husband, whom she may describe as 'a golden husband'. His work and other interests outside the home are severely curtailed because of her importunate demands. Fear of leaving the house unaccompanied may result in the husband staying off work to cope with her fears and household duties. The children are often involved in her symptoms also: they may be constrained to stay home from school so that she does not have to be on her own. This sets the scene for the development of separation anxiety and school phobia in the children. The phobic patient herself is chronically anxious and may experience depersonalization, either as episodes that come and go unaccountably or as a continuously unpleasant state.

Phobias are overpowering and compelling in their nature, dominating the whole of life. Like obsessions, they are repetitive, resisted unsuccessfully, regarded by the subject as senseless and irrational but at the same time as coming from inside of him- or herself. Some authors therefore describe them as *obsessional fears*. Often compulsive behaviour, such as hand washing, arises out of a phobia, for instance fear of dirt and contamination. Prominent in the subject's description of his phobia is that he is controlled by it, that the fear is something from inside himself (in no way controlled from outside).

Anxiety in other disorders

Obviously, most consideration of anxiety and its different forms and manifestations has been given in the context of the *anxiety disorders*. However, anxiety is a common symptom and is frequently a part of other illnesses, both psychiatric and physical. Among psychiatric conditions, the most frequent comorbidity is with depressive illness; most patients with depression have some anxiety symptoms, most of those with more severe anxiety disorders also have some feelings of depression. Anxiety is a frequent symptom in the prodromal stages of schizophrenia and is also associated with relapse (Tarrier and Turpin, 1992). Anxiety often occurs with organic psychosyndromes, both exacerbating the restlessness of acute organic psychosyndromes or delirium and manifesting as an additional cause of subjective distress in chronic organic states or dementia. Anxiety occurs in those with learning disability but requires experience to diagnose and evaluate (Chapter 11).

Anxiety is an understandable reaction to physical illness and its consequent distress, pain, physical and social disability and threat to life (Sims and Snaith, 1988). In the following conditions, it may also be a direct expression of the morbid process: hypoglycaemia, hyperthyroidism, phaeochromocytoma, carcinoid syndrome, some cardiac and ictal disorders and states of withdrawal from psychoactive substances. These conditions therefore need to be considered in the differential diagnosis of anxiety, and the component of anxiety in their symptomatology must be dealt with in their treatment.

IRRITABILITY

Irritability of the patient may be observed by others or experienced subjectively directed towards others (outward) or towards the self (inward). Irritability, outwardly expressed, is considered to be a disorder of mood in its own right and independent of anxiety, depression or other mood state (Snaith and Taylor, 1985): 'Outwardly expressed irritability is an independent mood disorder and not merely one which is symptomatic of states of depression or anxiety'. Outwardly expressed irritability is particularly commonly associated with puerperal mood disorder, while inwardly directed irritability was described in those with obsessive–compulsive disorder. In the Irritability, Depression and Anxiety Scale, two subscales were developed for irritability (Snaith *et al.*, 1978): outwardly directed irritability and inwardly directed irritability. Snaith and Taylor (1985) have defined irritability for use in the context of psychopathology as:

> “Irritability is a feeling state characterized by reduced control over temper – which usually results in irascible verbal or behavioural outbursts, although the mood may be present without observed manifestation. It may be experienced as brief episodes, in particular circumstances, or it may be prolonged and generalized. The experience of irritability is always unpleasant for the individual and overt manifestation lacks the cathartic effect of justified outbursts of anger.

It is a prominent symptom in post-traumatic stress disorder, in which it is listed as one of the symptoms of increased arousal. Relatives described an individual survivor of disaster: 'He has completely changed his character. He has become nasty tempered and swears at us all the time'.

The severity of irritability probably has an inverse correlation with age; it occurs in both men and women. It is useful to make a distinction between the subjective mood of irritability and the observation of violent behaviour, although these may overlap. Severe irritability may cause considerable distress to patients, relatives and healthcare professionals; there may be no other psychiatric symptomatology present. The factors that predispose to irritability are not clearly known. 'The state of irritability is primarily a mood which may be translated into behaviour' (Snaith, 1991).

OBSESSIONS AND COMPULSIONS

There is no necessary association between obsessions, or obsessive–compulsive disorder, and anxiety or any type of anxiety disorder; certainly, it is not an anxiety disorder. Isolated obsessions or obsessive–compulsive disorder may occur with or without anxiety; with or without depression; and with or without personality disorder, anankastic or otherwise. It is a distinct and separate phenomenon.

The patient may be troubled by thoughts that he knows to be his own but that he finds repetitive and strange; he finds he is unable to prevent their repetition. These obsessional thoughts have, according to Lewis (1936), three essential features: a feeling of subjective compulsion, a resistance to it and the preservation of insight. These features distinguish obsession from voluntary repetitive acts and social ceremonies. The word *obsession* is usually reserved for the thought and *compulsion* for the act. The sufferer knows that it is his own thought (or act), that it arises from within himself and that it is subject to his own will whether he continues to think (or perform) it; he can decide not to think it on this particular occasion (but it does and will recur). He is tormented by the fear of what may happen if he disturbs the routine. There is no disturbance of consciousness or of the awareness of the possession of his own thought. The person usually functions satisfactorily in other areas of his life uncontaminated by the obsessional thought, but as the obsessions become more severe there is increasing social incapacity and misery that can grossly disrupt his whole lifestyle.

John Bunyan, in his poignant autobiography *Grace Abounding to the Chief of Sinners* (1666), describes gross, obsessional thoughts and ruminations that are connected with, but can be clearly separated from, his underlying religious beliefs. For example:

> “ 33. Now you must know, that before this I had taken much delight in ringing, but my Conscience beginning to be tender, I thought that such a practice was but vain, and therefore forced myself to leave it, yet my mind hankered, wherefore I should go to the Steeple house, and look on: though I durst not ring.
> But I thought this did not become Religion neither, yet I forced my self and would look on still; but quickly after, I began to think, How, if one of the bells should fall: then I chose to stand under a main Beam that lay over thwart the Steeple from side to side thinking there I might stand sure; But then I should think again, Should the Bell fall with a swing, it might first hit the Wall, and then rebounding upon me, might kill me for all this Beam; this made me stand in the Steeple door, and now thought I, I am safe enough for if a Bell should fall, I can slip out behind these thick walls, and so be preserved not with-standing.

> "34. So after this, I would yet go to see them ring, but would not go further than the Steeple door; but then it came into my head, how if the Steeple it self should fall, and this thought, (it may fall for ought I know) would when I stood and looked on, continually so shake my mind, that I durst not stand at the Steeple door any longer, but was forced to fly, for fear it should fall upon my head. *(p. 13)*

The *obsessional symptom* and the *religious belief* expressed in this passage are not the same phenomenologically, although they are interconnected. The nature of the obsessional thought is demonstrated in the way that Bunyan felt compelled to think through this elaborate chain of arguments; he resisted his ideas, but unsuccessfully. There is no lack of insight into its being his own behaviour. The behaviour was compulsive in that it was the acting out of ambivalent, obsessional notions. There is more than a hint of underlying obsessional personality, for instance in the numbering of the paragraphs.

A midwife, aged 32, kept thinking after she had finished her spell of duty at hospital that she might have pushed an airway down the throat of a baby that she had delivered. She would telephone the ward repeatedly to check that the infant was well. She frequently made sure that her dog's collar was secure when she was out walking in case he escaped and was killed by traffic. When a little boy and his mother visited her home, she gave him a glass of 'pop'. However, she had to drink what she had just poured out for him herself, although she disliked it, to make sure it really was pop and not something harmful. The accumulation of more and more symptoms eventually prevented her from working or carrying out any reasonable social life. She knew that these were her own notions, that they were stupid, but she could not stop herself thinking and performing them.

The compulsive behaviour often provokes further anxiety in the patient, the need both to perform the action and to preserve social acceptability. Although wide areas of life are often implicated in compulsive rituals, it is often striking how the obsessional person omits other areas from his obsessionality. The patient who excoriates his hands by excessive washing and devotes a substantial portion of each day to the pursuit of cleanliness may drive to work in a dirty and ill-serviced car and work in an untidy office! The dilemma of obsessional symptoms remains that they are both reckoned as part of the patient's own behaviour and resisted unsuccessfully, that is, they are under voluntary control but not altogether experienced as voluntary. The patient has an awareness that this particular act or thought is voluntary and can be resisted, with difficulty, but the overall pattern of thinking or behaving is experienced subjectively as inevitable – it is ultimately futile to struggle. The action sometimes 'appears to be against the will of the patient, and often seems to have the quality of disgust or repulsion; this urge to do something yet to be repelled by it, is said to be a singular characteristic of the obsessional state' (Beech, 1974).

Obsession may occur as thoughts, images, impulses, ruminations or fears; compulsions as acts, rituals, behaviours. Schneider's definition (1959) emphasizes that there is no loss of contact with reality: 'An obsession occurs when someone cannot get rid of a content of consciousness, although when it occurs he realizes that it is senseless or at least that it is dominating and persisting without cause'. Thus, hallucinations, delusions and mood disturbances cannot be obsessional in form; they are not experienced as senseless, nor is there an attempt to get rid of them. The craving of an alcoholic for his beverage or the abnormal drive of sexual deviation is not compulsive in a strict sense. They do not contravene the person's will, although he may dislike himself intensely for having such wishes.

Obsessional *ideas* may be simple or complicated. A tune or a few notes may become repetitive and be resisted, or a sequence of words, for example 'the British Socialist Party', be reiterated irritatingly inside his head. The obsessions or compulsions may be more complex and ritualistic, for example a patient who tried to shut the car door after getting out found this very difficult because he was afraid that the act of shutting would produce unpleasant, obscene, repetitive thoughts. For this reason, he had to go to elaborate lengths to put the car in a certain place, check all the doors before getting out, check them all again after getting out and turn the key while looking in a particular direction.

The *images* of obsessional thinking may be vivid but are always known by the patient to be his own thoughts. These images have been considered by De Silva (1986) to be one of four types.

1. The *obsessional image* depicts repetitively the unwanted intrusive cognition – images of blood flowing, injuries and so on.
2. The *compulsive image* depicts compulsive behaviour by rectifying either an obsessional image – the woman who saw corpses in coffins and had to imagine the same people standing – or an independent compulsive image.
3. The *disaster image* affects compulsive checkers who may not only fear that disaster will occur unless they check but also 'see' the disaster happening in fantasy – the house burning down if the gas taps are not turned off.
4. The *disruptive image* may intrude while compulsive rituals are being carried out and necessitate the ritual being recommenced.

Ruminations are often pseudophilosophical, irritatingly unnecessary, repetitive and achieve no conclusion. A priest has an inner impulse to utter swear words in church, or a mother an impulse to harm her child – both quite frequent complaints of obsessional patients. Reassurance that he will not harm himself or others or act on the impulses can be given to the obsessional, provided it is truly obsessional in form, that he is not concurrently depressed and that there is not coexisting dissocial personality disorder.

Obsessions occur in the context of obsessive–compulsive disorder as the major symptom of the condition. However, they also occasionally occur in other circumstances. The depressed patient with obsessional (anankastic) personality may show obsessions and compulsions that clear when his illness is treated. Obsessional states are more common when obsessional personality is present, but this personality type is not a prerequisite. Obsessional symptoms may occur in schizophrenia, when they usually have a bizarre character. Apparent obsessional symptoms may arise *de novo* in an older person, associated with an organic psychosyndrome. However, the element of resistance characteristic of obsessionality is usually not present. It seems that the person carries out repetitive behaviour in order to cope with the uncertainties of his life caused by his failing memory and performance. Repetition and stereotyped behaviour in those with mental retardation has sometimes been labelled compulsive;

however, this is psychopathologically incorrect, as there is no resistance or conflict of urge and repulsion. Similarly, repetitiveness and stickiness of thinking occur with epilepsy, following head injury and with other organic states, but again, this is not truly obsessional in nature.

There is a striking similarity between the clinical presentation of obsessive–compulsive disorder in children and adolescents and in adults (Swedo *et al.*, 1989). In 70 consecutive juvenile patients, washing and grooming, repeating, checking and touching rituals were the most frequent compulsions, and obsessions were contamination fears, concerns about disasters happening to the patient or those close to him, symmetry and scrupulousness. Although the condition was frequently familial, the actual presenting symptoms were not shared by relatives, even by monozygotic twins.

Obsessionality and anankastic personality

The discussion above has been concerned with obsessive–compulsive disorder. The following description is more concerned with *trait* obsessionality, the features of the person with obsessional or *anankastic personality*. The general features of this personality type are discussed in Chapter 21. However, because there is so much confusion between obsessive–compulsive symptoms and obsessionality as a way of life, it is appropriate to digress and give some attention to the latter at this point.

In their thinking, anankasts tolerate ambiguity less readily than normals. They like to have decisions made but will delay making a decision until they have reached a greater degree of certainty than is required by other people. As they grow older, they become increasingly rigid in their thinking. They constrict their thinking to deal more comfortably with daily events, and this requires them to make sweeping generalizations of a narrow-minded and prejudiced sort. Reed (1969) has considered the thinking of the obsessional to be *under-inclusive*, that is, in a test for over-inclusiveness he will put too few members into a category. This is a further example of the anankast's indecision and doubt in performing new tasks and his craving for certainty. He has to be completely sure of getting it right.

Janet regarded as the central experience of patients suffering from obsessional neurosis *sentiment d'incomplétude, incompleteness* (Cooper and Kelleher, 1973). This was demonstrated as a personality trait present in a proportion of normal subjects when a principal components analysis was carried out on the Leyton Obsessional Inventory, completed by 302 supposedly normal men and women. The three distinct components of this personality trait demonstrated were *clean and tidy, incompleteness* and *checking*.

Two other features of the anankastic personality connected with intolerance of uncertainty and feelings of incompleteness are *insecurity* and *sensitivity*. Even when every possible check and precaution has been introduced, the anankast still feels insecure about his activities. Fundamentally, this is associated with the way he sees himself in relation to others: he is uncertain about the way they regard him and extremely sensitive concerning the slightest suggestion of criticism.

It is very important to make the distinction between the *form* of obsessions or compulsions and anankastic thinking. Often they overlap: a person with anankastic personality may have discrete episodes of obsessive–compulsive disorder. However, in terms of understanding the patient's symptoms, in diagnosis, in prognosis and for treatment these two phenomena should be considered separately.

REFERENCES

American Psychiatric Association (1994) *Diagnostic and Statistical Manual of Mental Disorders*, 4th edn, revised. Washington: American Psychiatric Association.

Beech HR (1974) *Obsessional States*. London: Methuen.

Bunyan J (1666) *Grace Abounding to the Chief of Sinners: or, a Brief and Faithful Relation of the Exceeding Mercy of God in Christ, to his Poor Servant John Bunyan* (ed. Sharrock R, 1962), p. 13. Oxford: Oxford University Press.

Burton R (1621) *The Anatomy of Melancholy, What It Is. With All the Kinds, Causes, Symptomes, Prognostickes, and Several Cures of it by Democritus Junior*. Oxford: Cripps.

Cooper J and Kelleher M (1973) The Leyton Obsessional Inventory: a principal components analysis on normal subjects. *Psychological Medicine 3*, 204–8.

De Silva P (1986) Obsessional–compulsive imagery. *Behaviour Research and Therapy 24*, 333–50.

Hamilton M (1959) The assessment of anxiety states by rating. *British Journal of Medical Psychology 32*, 50–5.

Hibbert GA (1984) Ideational components of anxiety: their origin and content. *British Journal of Psychiatry 144*, 613–24.

Lader MH and Marks IM (1971) *Clinical Anxiety*. London: Heinemann.

Lewis AJ (1936) Problems of obsessional illness. *Proceedings of the Royal Society of Medicine 29*, 325–36.

Marks IM (1969) *Fears and Phobias*. London: Heinemann.

Marks IM (1970) The classification of phobic disorders. *British Journal of Psychiatry 116*, 377–86.

Noyes R and Hoehn-Saric R (1998) *The Anxiety Disorders*. Cambridge: Cambridge University Press

Noyes R, Woodman C, Garvey MJ, et al (1992) Generalized anxiety disorder versus panic disorder. Distinguishing characteristics and patterns of comorbidity. *Journal of Nervous and Mental Disease 180*, 369–79.

Reed GF (1969) 'Under-inclusion': a characteristic of obsessional personality disorder I and II. *British Journal of Psychiatry 115*, 781–90.

Roth M (1959) The phobic anxiety–depersonalization syndrome. *Proceedings of the Royal Society of Medicine 52*, 587–95.

Rush B (1798) On the different species of phobia. *The Weekly Magazine of Original Essays, Fugitive Pieces, and Interesting Intelligence, Philadelphia*. In Hunter R and McAlpine I (1963) *Three Hundred Years of Psychiatry* 1535–1860, pp. 669–70. London: Oxford University Press.

Schapira K, Kerr TA and Roth M (1970) Phobias and affective illness. *British Journal of Psychiatry 117*, 25–32.

Scharfetter C (1980) *General Psychopathology: an Introduction*. Cambridge: Cambridge University Press.

Schneider K (1959) *Clinical Psychopathology*, 5th edn (transl. Hamilton MW). New York: Grune & Stratton.

Sims ACP (1985) Anxiety in historical perspective. *British Journal of Clinical Practice Supplement 38*, 4–9.

Sims ACP and Snaith P (1988) *Anxiety in Clinical Practice*. Chichester: John Wiley.

Snaith P (1991) *Clinical Neurosis*, 2nd edn. Oxford: Oxford University Press.

Snaith RP and Taylor CM (1985) Irritability: definition, assessment and associated factors. *British Journal of Psychiatry 147*, 127–36.

Snaith RP, Constantopoulos AA, Jardine MY and McGuffin P (1978) A clinical scale for the self assessment of irritability, anxiety and depression. *British Journal of Psychiatry 132*, 164–71.

Solyom L, Ledwige B and Solyom C (1986) Delineating social phobia. *British Journal of Psychiatry 149*, 464–70.

Spiegel DA and Barlow DH (2000) Anxiety disorders. In Gelder M, Lépez-Ibor JJ and Andreasen NC (eds) *New Oxford Textbook of Psychiatry*. Oxford: Oxford University Press.

Swedo SE, Rapoport JL, Leonard H, Lenane M and Cheslow D (1989) Obsessive–compulsive disorder in children and adolescents. *Archives of General Psychiatry 46*, 335–41.

Swinson RP (1992) Phobic disorders. *Current Opinion in Psychiatry 5*, 238–44.
Tarrier N and Turpin G (1992) Psychosocial factors, arousal and schizophrenic relapse. The psychophysiological data. *British Journal of Psychiatry 161*, 3–11.
Tyrer P (1982) Anxiety. *British Journal of Hospital Medicine 27*, 109–16.
Westphal C (1871) Die Agoraphobie: eine neuropathische Erscheinung. *Archiv fuer Psychiatrie und Nerven Krankheiten 3*, 138–61.
Wing JK, Cooper JE and Sartorius N (1974) *The Measurement and Classification of Psychiatric Symptoms*. Cambridge: Cambridge University Press.
World Health Organization (1992) *The ICD-10 Classification of Mental and Behavioural Disorders: Clinical Description and Diagnostic Guidelines*. Geneva: World Health Organization.
Zigmond AS and Snaith RP (1983) The Hospital Anxiety and Depression Scale. *Acta Psychiatrica Scandinavica 67*, 361–70.

Disorders of Volition and Execution

20

“ For I know that in me (that is, in my flesh,) dwelleth
no good thing; for to will is present with me; but how to
perform that which is good I find not.
For the good that I would I do not: but the evil which
I would not, that I do.
Now if I do that I would not, it is no more I that
do it, but sin that dwelleth in me.
I find then a law, that, when I would do good,
evil is present with me...
But I see another law in my members, warring against
the law of my mind, and bringing me into captivity to
the law of sin which is in my members. *The Epistle of Paul the Apostle to the Romans*

“ Dying
Is an art, like everything else.
I do it exceptionally well.
I do it so it feels like hell.
I do it so it feels real
I guess you could say I've a call. *Sylvia Plath (1962)*

This is the most unsatisfactory subject area in clinical psychopathology. The dissatisfaction derives from the loss of interest in the subject since the end of the nineteenth century and the lack of conceptual clarity that has resulted from the impoverished literature. As Berrios (1996) put it, 'The "will" no longer plays a role in psychiatry and psychology. A hundred years ago, however, it was an important descriptive and explanatory concept, naming the human "power, potency or faculty" to initiate action'. The distinctions between related but distinct concepts such as instinct, urge, impetus, impulse, drive, motivation, will, involuntary and voluntary movements and responsibility have until very recently ceased to be regarded as proper subjects of inquiry. A distinction can correctly but theoretically be drawn between the instinct and thus desire to carry out an action in order to satisfy a particular need, the drive and motivation to effect the action and the will to execute the action. All these are different from the end product, the observable action or behaviour itself (Figure 20.1).

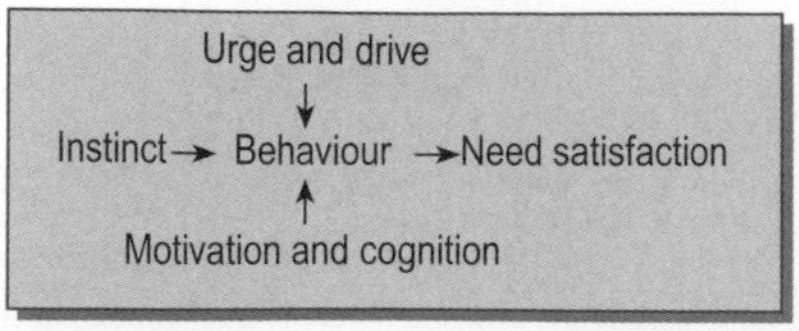

Figure 20.1 Relationship between instinct, need and behaviour.

URGE, DRIVE AND WILL, AND THEIR DISTURBANCE

Jaspers (1959) distinguishes between the different experiences of primary, contentless non-directional *urge*; natural *instinctual* drive directed towards some target; and the *volitional act* with a consciously conceived goal and an awareness of how to achieve it and its consequences. Thus, for Jaspers, there is a distinction, subjectively, between impulsive acts, awareness of inhibition of will and awareness of loss of will or availability of will-power.

Definitions proposed by Scharfetter (1980) are as follows.

- *Need* (a phenomenological concept): a striving towards a particular object, state or action that is experienced as a desire.
- *Drive*: (a) as a construct, an inclination to satisfy certain primary, that is, innate, needs; (b) as activity, the individual's basic mode of expression.
- *Instinct* (a construct): an innate pattern of behaviour that leads to drive satisfaction.
- *Motivation*: (a) as a phenomenological concept, a more or less clearly experienced mood or affect that is governed by needs and that moves us to actions that satisfy these needs; (b) as a construct, a hypothetical activating factor.
- *Will* (a phenomenological concept): a goal-directed striving or intention based on cognitively planned motivation.

Scharfetter then describes those primary needs that are innate and not learned as *hunger, thirst, breathing, urination* and *defecation, sleep* and *self-preservation*. Other needs are not essential for survival; their demands can be postponed and they are more affected by acquired patterns of behaviour, such as sexual need and prosocial need. Secondary needs are acquired and vary with the individual, for example smoking. Human beings are so complex that, although primary needs require rapid satisfaction, they account for only a small proportion of the individual's subjective experience and psychological activity. While I write this, I allow myself to become aware of the primary need for breathing, but I shall not be giving it a thought 10 minutes from now. The acquired primary needs and secondary needs have a greater influence on the individual mental state than innate primary needs.

Drive can be conceived as a state of tension that initiates directed behaviour. In this view, it can either activate or determine selectivity or strength of actions. Hull (1943) introduced the concept of need as a preliminary to introducing the more mechanical concept of drive. For Hull, 'When a condition arises for which action on the part of the organism is a prerequisite to optimum probability of survival of either the individual or the species, a state of need is said to exist' and 'Animals may almost be regarded as aggregations of need. The function of the effector apparatus is to mediate the satiation of these needs. The drive apparatus is synonymous with effector apparatus'. In this scheme, drive has the role of initiating behaviour that satisfies needs.

Instinct may be defined as 'an inherited or innate psycho-physical disposition which determines its possessor to perceive, and to pay attention to, objects of a certain class, to experience an emotional excitement of a particular quality, and to act in regard to it in a particular manner, or at least, to experience an impulse to act' (McDougall, 1908). For Freud, instinct 'appears as a borderline concept, being both the mental representative of the stimuli emanating from within and penetrating to the mind, and at the same time a measure of the demand made upon the energy of the latter in consequence of its connection with the body' (Freud, 1915).

Motivation, as a phenomenological concept, is readily understood by the layman but is ultimately tautologous: 'I do it because I am motivated', 'I am motivated to do it'. However, it is a concept that in psychiatry and psychology we cannot do without. It has both an emotional aspect as well as a cognitive aspect. In other words, it includes the pleasurable rewards that govern and regulate behaviour as well as the reasons proffered for behaviour. There are intrinsic as well as extrinsic motivating factors. Intrinsic factors are those that are internal to the person, and extrinsic factors are those, such as supermarket reward cards, that are external incentives to behave in particular ways. Thus, the term motivation refers not only to the goal towards which behaviour is directed but also to emotional states that set it off as well as those that act to reward the behaviour. And it also refers to the reasons, justifications or explanations of an action.

Similarly, *will* is a necessary concept but we have great difficulty in comprehending it. Thomas Reid (1710–1796), founder of the Scottish School of Common Sense, regarded the will as the power to put to effect our voluntary actions. For Reid, 'all our power is directed by our will, we can form no conception of power, properly so called, that is not under the direction of will. And therefore our exertions, our deliberations, our purposes, our promises, are only in things that depend upon our will. Our advices, exhortations, and commands, are only in things that depend upon the will of those to whom they are addressed. We impute no guilt to ourselves, nor to others, in things where the will is not concerned'. Other authorities make similar points but emphasize different aspects of will: 'Will has a consciously conceived goal and is accompanied with an awareness of the necessary means and consequences. It implies decision making ability, intention and responsibility' (Jaspers, 1959).

The range of definitions and understandings of the various terms underlines the intrinsic complexity of the subject area and the current absence of a unifying theory or model for making sense of the subject.

CLASSIFICATION OF ABNORMALITIES OF NEED, INSTINCT, MOTIVATION AND WILL

In terms of the self-description of the subject, any of the following phenomenological abnormalities resulting in observed disturbance of volition may occur. There may be a disturbance of *need*, which may involve hunger, thirst, exploratory behaviour or sleep. An absence of hunger can result in anorexia occurring in chronic physical illness, an increase in hunger causing hyperphagia in Kleine–Levin syndrome and a perversion in pica. Abnormality of thirst can take the form of increased thirst in lithium-induced polydipsia (diabetes insipidus) or of compulsive water drinking in psychosis, which can result in hyponatraemia. Abnormality of exploratory behaviour can take the form of diminution, which is manifest as lack of curiosity and exploration of the environment. This can be found in schizophrenia and depression. Exploratory behaviour can be increased in mania. Abnormalities of sleep are common and varied. There are different patterns of insomnia, including initial insomnia, which is more often associated with anxiety-based disorders, and early morning wakening, which is characteristic of depression. Hypersomnia can occur in narcolepsy, Kleine–Levin syndrome and Pickwickian syndrome.

Abnormality of drive can involve diminution, increase or perversion. Diminution of drive towards primary needs occurs in schizophrenia and depression and is probably indistinguishable from abnormalities of need. It is manifest as absence of the activating tension that initiates behaviour and is observable as apathy. Exacerbation of drive to satisfy sexual need is most prominent in mania but can occur as part of Kleine–Levin syndrome or indeed following acquired brain injury or in L-dopa-induced hypersexuality in Parkinson's disease. If drive determines strength and selectivity of goal of behaviour, then perversion of drive will include such conditions as fetishism.

Abnormality of *motivation* may involve diminution or exacerbation. In schizophrenia and depression, the pleasurable intrinsic motivation that acts as incentive for behaviour may be lost. This is most accurately described as anhedonia, the absence of pleasure in relation to usually pleasurable activities. In mania, it may be increased so that mundane activities become unduly fascinating and rewarding. Disorder of motivation can also be understood as involving the abnormalities of reasoning, justification and explanation, as described in the psychoanalytic literature. This is outside the scope of this book.

Disturbance of *will* can be manifest as loss of volition. This can be in the form of the will to act in schizophrenia and severe depression. It is difficult to distinguish between absence of need, drive, motivation or will. The observable end result is lack of action in the absence of any motor abnormality impairing action. Other abnormalities of will include indecisiveness in depression, ambivalence or ambitendency in schizophrenia. These abnormalities have, at their core, contrasting conceived goals with oscillating decision making that is observable as indecision or alternating and contrasted motor behaviours. Passivity experiences are by definition abnormalities of volition (Box 20.1).

Organic causes

Biological drives such as appetite, sleep and thirst are located anatomically in and around the midbrain. Localized disease in this area, of either a structural or biochemical nature, is therefore likely to result in disturbance of drive and hence volition. Hormonal, metabolic and neurophysiological mechanisms affect volition. Thus, the need for food, expressed in hunger and resulting in seeking food, is affected by the state of fullness of the gastrointestinal tract, by the

Box 20.1 Classification of abnormalities of need, drive, motivation and will

ABNORMALITIES OF NEED

Appetite

- Absence in anorexia
- Increase, as hyperphagia in Kleine–Levin syndrome
- Perversion in pica

Thirst

- Increase in diabetes insipidus, resulting in polydipsia and, in compulsive water drinking, resulting in hyponatraemia

Exploratory behaviour

- Decrease in schizophrenia and depression
- Increase in mania

Sleep

- Decrease in anxiety and depressive disorders
- Increase in hypersomnia in Kleine–Levin syndrome and Pickwickian syndrome

Abnormalities of drive

- Decrease in schizophrenia and depression
- Increase in mania
- Perversion in fetishism

Abnormalities of motivation

- Diminution, resulting in anhedonia in depression and schizophrenia
- Increase in mania

Abnormalities of will

- Absence or loss, resulting in apathy in schizophrenia and depression
- Oscillating will, resulting in indecisiveness, ambivalence or ambitendency
- Anomalous will in passivity experiences and made actions

secretion of insulin from the pancreas and by sensory innervation of the gut wall, as well as by regulation in a putative 'appetite centre'. Physical illnesses have both a specific and a generalized effect on volition.

Excessive appetite (bulimia) may occur with conditions such as tumour affecting the hypothalamus and result in gross obesity, obesity may be associated with hypoventilation and excessive sleeping (hypersomnia) in the Pickwickian syndrome (Burwell *et al.*, 1956), periodic somnolence and intense hunger with voracious over-eating occur in the Kleine–Levin syndrome (Critchley, 1962). Excessive thirst and fluid intake (polydipsia) occur with disease of the posterior pituitary or the kidney (nephrogenic diabetes insipidus, for example, with lithium treatment). Loss of appetite (anorexia) may occur with localized disease of the midbrain, resulting in severe cachexia; however, weight loss is much more common as a general feature of any severe debilitating physical illness.

Schizophrenic disturbance of volition

In schizophrenia, the disturbance of volition is much more at the level of *motivation* or *will* than of *need*. There may be abnormality of appetite with polyphagia and consequent obesity, as occurs in some chronic schizophrenic patients; however, this is not usual. Patients with schizophrenia who believe that their food is being poisoned may refrain from eating as a consequence; that is, of course, a deliberate act of will. The more conspicuous disturbance, however, is *loss of volition* that results in withdrawal from normal social interaction, for instance lack of motivation to obtain and continue in employment or diminished sexual drive resulting in decreased fecundity, especially in male schizophrenic patients.

This symptom was described by Bleuler (1911) as *disturbance of initiative*, according to Lehmann (1967). It is also recognized among the so-called negative symptoms of what Crow (1980) has designated type 2 schizophrenia. The *negative traits* – emotional apathy, slowness of thought and movement, underactivity, lack of drive, poverty of speech and social withdrawal – are a major barrier to effective rehabilitation in chronic schizophrenic patients (Wing, 1978). Although positive symptoms, such as delusions, hallucinations and thought disorder, are more conspicuous, especially in the earlier stages of a schizophrenic illness, the prognosis is probably affected to a greater extent by the loss of volition.

Andreasen has developed an instrument for measuring the negative symptoms of schizophrenia, the Scale for the Assessment of Negative Systems (Andreasen 1982, 1989). It is very obvious that the patient's quality of life and also that of his carer is impaired by the consequences of these negative symptoms, especially flatness of affect and loss of volition. What is not so clear is whether he has a subjective awareness of these symptoms or whether he suffers as a result of them. Selten *et al.* (1993) have developed a self-rating scale, the Subjective Experience of Negative Symptoms, to measure the subjective experience of affective flattening, alogia, avolition and apathy, anhedonia and asociality and impaired attention; the scale looks at awareness, causal attribution, disruption and distress.

Affective disturbance of volition

Abnormalities of volition in affective illnesses are associated with abnormality of activity, retardation being prominent in depression and overactivity in mania. In depression, motivation is impaired rather than will. A severely depressed managing director continued to worry about his plans for his company, but he found himself unable to make himself do anything about it. Loss of motivation occurs alongside loss of other affect. *Anhedonia* (see Chapter 18) or loss of ability to experience enjoyment is a prominent symptom in depressive illness (Snaith, 1993) that also occurs in schizophrenia. Depressed patients normally describe loss of interest in their previous hobbies and enjoyments in life. This anhedonia can be construed as part of the loss of motivation to carry out these activities. Such patients also describe lack of appetite and loss of all interest in food; this may result in marked loss of weight.

A 45-year-old male patient, previously highly successful as a salesman, developed severe and persistent depressive symptoms (Sims, 1994). As a result,

2 years prior to admission he had left his job, his home, his wife and his two children and drifted around the country, being admitted for short periods of time to several psychiatric hospitals. He described his subjective state: 'I feel very anxious, uncomfortable and depressed. It is like having the same person in the same body as me. It is like two different people inside one body. One person is holding back – that's like me. The other person is trying to let go – the other is different, quite strong'. *'Me'* was described as 'frightened, depressed, unsure', and the *'other person'* as 'confident, affable, a great salesman'. 'Self' and his 'other self' are compared in Figure 20.2. When he was healthy, he was energetic, extrovert and able to function well in a pressured situation. When he became depressed, he was miserable, unsure of what to do, frightened and lacking in all energy for any sort of activity. When depressed, he saw 'self' as being his real identity and 'other self' as 'like a fantasy'.

In mania, commonly there is increased activity, a subjective feeling of greater energy, effectiveness and self-confidence; such a person may initiate all sorts of new projects. Manic patients are prone to drink too much alcohol, but they do not usually over-eat, perhaps because they are readily distracted and tend to interrupt their meals with other new enterprises. Such people describe it as being very easy to make decisions, and their flight of ideas results in starting many tasks that they do not carry through to completion.

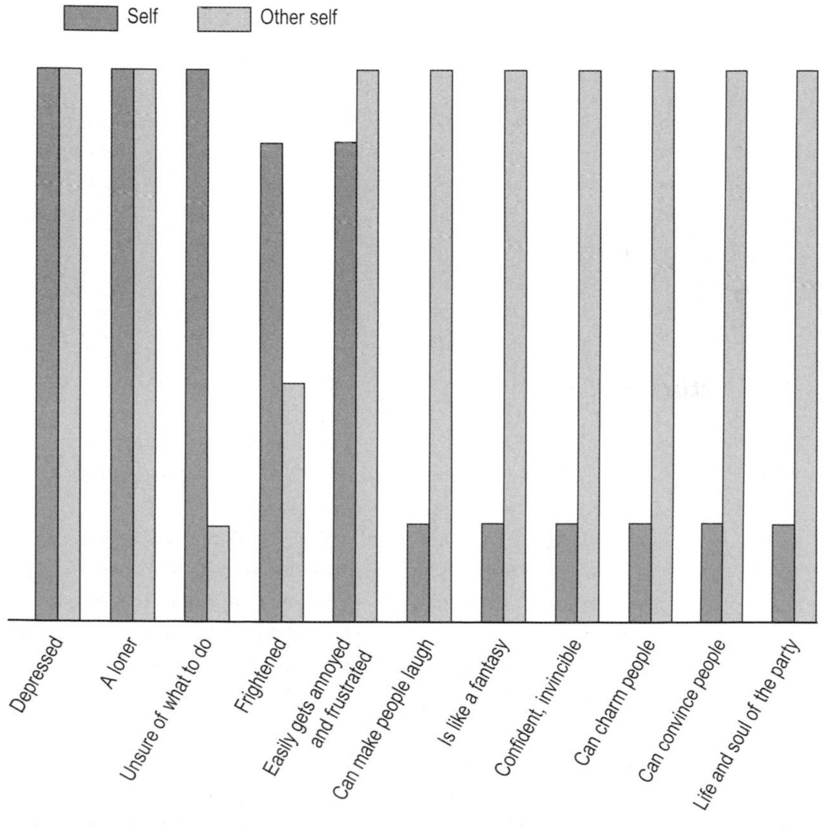

Figure 20.2 'Myself and my other self.'

An elderly man lived with his wife in a late-nineteenth-century semi-detached house in an industrial town. The first intimation of his manic illness was a desperate cry for help from his wife to their family doctor that he was destroying the house. At interview at home, one could see his many uncompleted building projects in the house. He said that he had thought it improper that every time his wife went to the toilet she should have to go through the backyard, where she could be seen by the neighbours. He had therefore knocked a hole in the wall between the kitchen and toilet to give internal access. Before he could get round to tidying the brickwork and putting in a new door, he had realized that the electric wiring was very old and so he had removed all the cables from the ground floor of the house. He was thinking next of renewing the wiring, but then decided that his wife would like a brand new bathroom. It was at this point that his wife realized that he was ill and consulted their doctor.

Disturbance with neurotic and personality disorders

Neurotic and personality disorders overlap to a considerable extent: 60 per cent of a population previously treated for neurotic disorder were found to show abnormality of personality at follow-up, while only 25 per cent of an apparently normal group showed abnormality to the same extent (Sims and Gooding, 1975). Neurotic reaction is more prone to occur in those whose abnormal personality predisposes them. Personality disorder is present when the abnormality of personality is of such degree as to cause the patient himself or other people to suffer (Schneider, 1950). The disturbance of volition with antisocial personality disorders is discussed by Dolan and Coid (1993) and in Chapter 21.

In neurotic disturbance, there is no loss of *need*; in fact, the needs are felt more keenly. Motivation and will are present but, because of neurotic attitudes and patterns of thinking, they fail to achieve the desired goals. Chronic low self-esteem and anxious over-involvement with self result in a paralysis of willing. There is no loss of will or of motivation, but there is a conflict of direction of motivation; or, as in the quotation from Shakespeare, 'I am at war 'twixt will and will not'. The patient has low self-esteem and devalues himself; he assumes he will not be able to cope with the demands made on him and feels incapable of effective action. He considers himself to be a victim of circumstances, 'the tyranny of inevitability' (Sims, 1983), in that he cannot materially alter his environment. He does not know what he can hope to achieve and therefore attempts either nothing or the unattainable (see Chapter 22).

Dissociative disorder, with automatism affecting volition, is phenomenologically quite different from passivity of volition – a delusion of control occurring as a schizophrenic symptom. In both, the subjective experience of activity is that it is not under personal control. In made volitional acts or passivity, the action is carried out in conditions in which there is awareness of self (Jaspers, 1959); the person shows normal consciousness at the time and has full memory for the action afterwards. However, in dissociative states there is dissociation from the self or ego: the patient is not aware of the act and of the self at the same time. During dissociation, there is diminished experience of self at the time of the automatic act, and in retrospect there is limited recollection for the time during which automatism occurred.

IMPULSIVE AND AGGRESSIVE ACTS

The term *impulsivity* is usually reserved for maladaptive behaviour. The behaviour universe thought to reflect impulsivity encompasses actions that appear poorly conceived, prematurely expressed, unduly risky or inappropriate to the situation and that often result in undesirable consequences. When such actions have positive outcomes, they tend not to be seen as signs of impulsivity but as indicators of boldness, quickness, spontaneity, courageousness or unconventionality (Daruna and Barnes, 1993). Eysenck (1993) distinguishes between impulsivity and venturesomeness as follows: 'Our concept of impulsiveness and venturesomeness can best be described by analogy to a driver who steers his car around a blind bend on the wrong side of the road. A driver who scores high on *Imp* never considers the danger he might be exposing himself to and is genuinely surprised when an accident occurs. The driver who scores high on *Vent*, on the other hand, considers the position carefully and decides consciously to take the risk'.

Impulsive acts are 'executed forcefully with no deliberation or reflection, under the influence of a compelling pressure that restricts the subject's freedom of will. Since reflective control or consideration is lacking, the consequences of such acts are not thought out or taken into consideration' (Scharfetter, 1980). It will be seen that this is not an all-or-nothing phenomenon. Voluntary inhibitions will be present to a varying extent from completely preventing the act, modifying it or delaying it to not existing at all, when the act takes place unrestrained.

In the past decade, there has been increasing interest in impulsivity as a concept as well as in defining a number of impulse control disorders. Impulsivity is seen as a predisposition towards rapid, unplanned reactions to internal or external stimuli and without due regard to the negative consequences of these actions for the impulsive individual or for others (Moeller *et al.*, 2001). The essential elements are predisposition, rapid unplanned action and without regard to consequences. This suggests that the term is now being used to identify a trait rather than isolated behaviour that is associated with an episode of illness. The current psychological literature, in turn, focuses on behaviourist concepts that are derived from experimental animal models. These schemes identify the features of impulsivity as (a) perseverance of behaviours despite punishment, (b) preference for a small but immediate reward over a delayed larger reward and (c) making premature responses or inability to prevent a response in a response disinhibition attentional paradigm. Once again, these conceptualizations of impulsivity suggest that impulsivity is a trait.

On the other hand, the older psychiatric literature focused on impulsive behaviour as part of episodes of illness: 'of all the morbid desires, the violent *impulse* [my emphasis] to muscular activity, to bodily movement, is particularly to be noticed, as it is seen, especially in states of mania, as a constant necessity to restless motion hither and thither, beating about, screaming, etc., a state which frequently involves the injury and destruction of what is within reach of the patient, without his having any definite purpose in doing so' and 'the involuntary nature of these acts; the patient often complains that he cannot resist the desire; and further these acts have something instinctive in the manner in which they show themselves; they come on in fits with lucid intervals, they are frequently accompanied by other symptoms of derangement' (Griesinger, 1882). Bleuler (1911) distinguishes between impulsive acts and compulsive acts: 'The action appears to him as something beyond his voluntary control. ... The patient does something he does not want to do; however he does not offer any resistance'. Thus, in this view, it is resistance to the impulse to act that defines compulsion.

Disorders of impulse control include impairment of control resulting in disinhibition and can be manifest in acquired brain injury, schizophrenia, mania, episodic dyscontrol syndrome and antisocial and emotionally unstable personality disorders. Excessive control of impulses can result in inhibited behaviour and lack of spontaneity, present in anxiety-related disorders including avoidant personality disorder.

Aggression is defined as 'a verbal or physical attack on other living creatures or things' (Scharfetter, 1980), and *aggressiveness* as a readiness to be aggressive. In general ethological terms, this is required by animals for survival and by humans to cope with individual conflicts and problems in their society. However, in a more restricted psychopathological sense, aggression involves deliberate or reckless damage and destruction and is accompanied by negative emotions such as anger, fear, despair, spite or rage.

The two concepts of aggression that Scharfetter contrasts are an *innate drive* and an *acquired response*. The former theory is followed both by ethologists such as Lorenz (1963) and in classical psychoanalysis in the writings of Freud and of Adler (1929); if aggression is an innate drive, it must find some form of expression. Learning theory would suppose that aggression is an acquired reaction in response to external stimuli, especially the expression of others' aggressive behaviour, and it is reinforced by the success it achieves.

Examples of impulsive acts follow.

> “We had a party. On the way home I was seized by an idea out of the blue – swim across the river in your clothes. It was not so much a compulsion to be reckoned with but simply one, colossal, powerful impulse. I did not think for a minute but jumped straight in ... only when I felt the water did I realise it was most extraordinary conduct and I climbed out again. The whole incident gave me a lot to think about. For the first time something inexplicable, something quite sporadic and alien, had happened to me. *(Jaspers, 1923)*

> “A 19-year-old was hospitalised for mutism. She sat motionless for prolonged periods, disinterested in her surroundings, although she appeared alert... She ate and moved slowly but was not stiff. On the second day, suddenly and without warning, she leapt from the chair and grabbed the throat of a passing therapist, severely damaging the therapist's thyroid. *(Fink and Taylor, 2003)*

> “He complained of headaches, was irritable, and occasionally exploded in a rage with minimal or trivial precipitants. Destruction of property occurred, including holes punched in walls and furniture broken plus poorly coordinated assaults on family members and some neighbours. *(Benson and Blumer, 1982)*

Although impulsivity is often demonstrated by aggression, this is not invariably the case. Gambling, misuse of substances, sexual acts associated with disinhibition and stealing are but some of the behaviours that can occur impulsively.

Responsibility

The legal term *diminished responsibility* has relevance, as a defence, only in murder cases in England and Wales (Wasik, 1990). The Homicide Act, 1957, states: 'where a person kills or is party to a killing of another, he shall not be convicted of murder if he was suffering from such abnormality of mind (whether arising from a condition of arrested or retarded development of mind or any inherent causes or induced by disease or injury) as substantially impaired his mental responsibility for his acts and omissions in doing or being party to the killing'. However, the concept of individual responsibility has much greater significance for forensic psychiatry than homicide alone, and for all types of management and treatment of mental illness it is relevant.

'To be judged mentally ill is judged, to a greater or lesser extent, not responsible' (Kennedy, 1981). Distinction is often made between *psychosis* and *neurosis* (see Chapter 23). The concept of psychosis, because of defect of insight and reality judgement, implies a different understanding of personal responsibility from neurosis, in which morbid subjective experiences are not confused with external reality. Whether a person is decreed responsible, in both a layperson's and a legal sense, depends ultimately on whether he is considered to be ill; but, as Kennedy has pointed out, *illness* itself is a judgemental term that depends on the perspective of the observer. Clearly, there are important legal, philosophical, moral and theological issues involved, but they are not the concern of a work on psychopathology. More detailed consideration of this complex subject from both the psychiatric and the forensic standpoint is found in Whitlock (1963, 1990).

Automatism occurring in the context of epilepsy is important, both clinically and legally. An accused person must have acted voluntarily to be guilty of the act; in this context, automatism is defined in law as the state of a person who, although capable of action, is not conscious of what he is doing. *Insane automatism* implies disease of the mind, especially psychomotor epilepsy, and is equivalent to a plea of insanity. It is important to demonstrate that epilepsy and automatic behaviour were present before the homicidal act. *Non-insane automatism* occurs when the dysfunction of the mind is transitory, such as following consumption of alcohol or drugs, following anaesthesia or associated with sleep abnormality such as sleepwalking.

Psychopathology of impulsive and aggressive behaviour

> “ Criminal acts may arise from delusions of one kind and another, from hallucinations of the various senses, from loss of control, which may act in various different ways; the most difficult point of all to decide upon is the so-called impulsive insanity, in which a patient loses self-control, and commits an act, the details of which he remembers, but which he truthfully

> says he was unable to prevent. Such insane impulses undoubtedly do occur, and I have been consulted by patients who have told me that loss of control of this kind would come upon them like a storm, and that they would seek shelter anywhere to avoid the danger which might arise to themselves or others. It is simple enough when these impulses occur in persons who have suffered from mental unsoundness, but it is much more difficult when the only evidence of insanity is the existence of these impulses; for it may be said that they are but the result of uncontrolled pleasure of power, which is common to all. I should hesitate before accepting impulses, unless I had evidences of insanity in other members of the family, or neuroses such as neuralgia or epilepsy in the patient himself. *(Savage, 1886)*

There is nothing that is likely to result in referral to psychiatric services more quickly than the public exhibition of inexplicable impulsive and aggressive acts. Also, there is nothing more likely to be labelled as madness by the lay public. In practice, such public behaviour is quite commonly associated with mental illness. In a study of mentally disturbed people coming to the attention of the police, there was a tendency for such people to create their disturbance near the city centre rather than at the periphery. Of the situations resulting in the involvement of the police, assault and damage were frequent, but it was the bizarreness of the behaviour that marked the person as being mentally ill, for example a man who proffered a windscreen wiper as fare for travelling on a bus, or a woman who presented herself mute at a hostel. On subsequent admission to hospital, diagnosis was predominantly of psychotic illness (57 per cent), schizophrenia accounting for 40 per cent (Sims and Symonds, 1975).

Excessive aggression, and especially unprovoked inappropriate or misdirected aggression, is much more often presented for psychiatric evaluation than a pathological lack of aggressive behaviour. However, the latter may also be a manifestation of illness. Excessive aggression may be considered both in terms of the underlying psychiatric illness and according to the specific nature of the behaviour.

Psychiatric illness and aggressive behaviour

Aggressive behaviour may be shown with almost any psychiatric condition. It is, of course, not necessarily associated with the illness but may be an expression of the individual's underlying personality and constitution and of the specific frustrations in his current social context. The McNaughton Rules, as applied to homicide, were an attempt by the judiciary, albeit not a wholly successful one, to apportion how much blame should be ascribed to the consequences of the mental illness in terms of delusions consequent on it, and how much to the moral turpitude of the individual (West and Walk, 1977). This distinction between mental illness and criminality as cause of homicidal behaviour was based, therefore, on phenomenology, on the patient's own subjective assessment of the meaning of his behaviour. The abnormal mental phenomena occurring and accounting for violence will depend for its form on the nature of the psychiatric illness.

Personality disorder

Impulsive and aggressive behaviour are particularly characteristic of what ICD-10 describes as *emotionally unstable personality disorder – impulsive type*:

> "there is a marked tendency to act impulsively without consideration of the consequences, together with affective instability. The ability to plan ahead may be minimal, and outbursts of intense anger may often lead to violence or 'behavioural explosions'; these are easily precipitated when impulsive acts are criticized or thwarted by others. Outbursts of violence or threatening behaviour are common, particularly in response to criticism by others. *(World Health Organization, 1992)*

A person whose usual mood may be equable shows what is regarded as a grossly excessive expression of emotion in response to relatively minor stimuli; the emotion may be of anger, fear, misery, anxiety or rage and often results in violent behaviour. So the violence here results from the phenomenon of a sudden, excessive and uncontrolled explosion of emotion.

Impulsive and aggressive acts may also be associated with the *dissocial, asocial* or *psychopathic personality*. Such people are heedless of the consequences of their actions; they especially do not empathize with the emotions experienced by others consequent on their own destructive behaviour. A sociopathic curate experienced sorrow when he was discovered by his vicar scrounging sums of money from an elderly female parishioner, but he had no feeling of remorse or understanding for how the vicar felt in having misplaced his confidence in him. Henderson (1939) described *creative, inadequate* and *aggressive* psychopathy. Those with dissocial personality will show different kinds of impulsive behaviour depending on which of these three qualities predominate.

Neurosis, depression and mania

Aggressiveness is not, generally, a characteristic of neurotic illness, although impulsively inappropriate behaviour may occur. Irritability is a regular feature and may on occasion find expression in impulsive aggression, for example non-accidental injury of a child by its neurotic, socially deprived and frustrated parent (Smith *et al.*, 1973). In both neurosis and depressive illness, impulsive action may result from disturbance in attitudes and emotion.

There is a very great risk of suicide with depressive illness (Lönnqvist, 2000). More than half of those who are clinically depressed have suicidal thoughts, suicidal ideation is significantly related to severity of depression and there is a 20-fold increased risk of suicide with major depression. Suicidal ideas may be consistent, experienced over a considerable time and resisted because of feelings of duty towards family or glimmerings of hope for a successful outcome to treatment, or they may be a sudden impulse to 'end it all' superimposed on consistently lowered mood. In this latter instance, close relatives sometimes describe an amelioration of mood in the few hours or days before successfully completed suicide, as if having finally made the decision brings some relief. Retardation and apathy, which are frequently present in depressive illness, may render suicide less likely. However, the earlier stages of effective treatment, for instance with electroconvulsive therapy, may result in initial lessening of retardation without concurrent improvement in mood, and so the risk of suicide may be temporarily increased. Other self-destructive behaviour may occur with depression, and homicide followed by attempted suicide also occurs occasionally. A case is described in Chapter 18 of a depressed man who intended to drown his greatly loved young son and himself but only succeeded in the former. With depressive illness, motor retardation may render any concerted activity less likely. However, if retardation does not completely inhibit action, the mood of hopelessness may make suicidal behaviour more likely.

In mania, the mood disturbance may result in aggressive behaviour. There may be frenzied violence of an ineffective kind or the patient may be consistently more irritable, resulting in aggression on relatively slight provocation. However, most of the assaults carried out by those with this diagnosis are not serious; it is rarely associated with homicide (Higgins, 1990). Not only aggressive but other impulsive behaviour of florid kind may occur in mania: one manic patient, a doctor, 'cured' a pilot with a phobia for flying by suggestion and then immediately persuaded him to hire an aeroplane to fly himself and two other in-patients from their hospital in the north of England so that they could all visit their unsuspecting psychiatrist, who was on holiday in Italy (Ropschitz, 1957).

Schizophrenia

The mental illness most consistently associated with increased risk of violent behaviour is schizophrenia (Mullen, 2000). Apparently meaningless, aggressive or self-destructive acts may take place as a result of the abnormal mental state. However, it can usually be shown that these actions take place in direct response to abnormal phenomena such as auditory hallucinations, delusions or passivity experiences. A man cycling along a canal towpath was assaulted by another man walking in the opposite direction and carrying a long length of rubber tubing. The police apprehended the assailant and after questioning requested a psychiatric opinion. The man, who proved to be suffering from schizophrenia, said, 'As I walked along I had a pain in my stomach. Then I heard a voice which said, "If you hit him the pain will go". So I hit him with the rubber pipe'. The aggressive act was a direct response to an auditory hallucination and, in fact, it is this psychopathological form, and also delusion, that most frequently accounts for violence in schizophrenia. The homicidal attack on 20 January 1843 by Daniel McNaughton on Edward Drummond, the Prime Minister's Private Secretary, was a direct response to his persecutory delusion. McNaughton believed 'The Tories in my native city have compelled me to do this. They follow and persecute me wherever I go, and have entirely destroyed my peace of mind ... in fact, they wish to murder me. It can be proved by evidence' (West and Walk, 1977). It was shown that, in London, about 15 per cent of homicide offenders were suffering from schizophrenia (Taylor and Gunn, 1984).

It has been postulated that the very rare phenomenon of *clinical vampirism*, drinking the blood of a victim, is usually associated with a schizophrenic disorder (Prins, 1984). This condition, which overlaps to some extent with necrophilia, needs to be seen in its symbolic and anthropological context.

Investigating the contribution made to acts of extreme violence by schizophrenic psychopathology, Taylor (1985) concluded that in 82 per cent of those who were schizophrenic and had committed a violent act the offence was attributable to the illness. Two hundred and three male prisoners who had committed a violent offence and were remanded for psychiatric examination were interviewed; 121 of these were psychotic, with active symptoms in all but 9 cases. Twenty per cent of actively ill men were directly driven to offend by their psychotic symptoms and a further 20 per cent probably so. Passivity delusions were especially frequent in precipitating violent acts in this series.

Undirected, frenzied violent behaviour may occur with acute catatonic schizophrenia. However, this is now extremely rare. Other impulsive actions, which are not at all aggressive in nature, may occur in schizophrenic patients in response to hallucinations, delusions or associated with loss of volition or blunting of social behaviour. This could include hoarding or unhygienic and antisocial behaviour. This was more common in those who were institutionalized and showed chronic defect states.

Impulsive and aggressive acts are not uncommon in schizophrenia; such patients tend to be over-represented in the statistics for crimes of violence, and the crimes are often bizarre, reflecting schizophrenic psychopathology (Tidmarsh, 1990). They may occur in response to auditory hallucinations – voices that command or invite the patient to carry out certain actions. Alternatively, the violence may be directed against what the patient believes to be the source of the voices in order to get rid of them. Delusions of persecution may result in action to eradicate the presumed perpetrator. With passivity experiences or delusions of control, violence may be directed at an external influence that is believed to be controlling the person in some way.

Organic states

Inexplicable impulsive acts of aggression, episodes of irritable mood, bad temper of sudden onset and without adequate provocation and petty behaviour of unexpected spitefulness and malevolence may occur with various organic psychosyndromes, often as an early sign of illness, in people who previously did not show such traits of character. These symptoms may herald a dementing process with increasing irritability and loss of control; such behaviour is characteristic of postencephalitic parkinsonism, following head injury or in epileptic automatism during convulsive discharge. The old-established dogma, maintained by such luminaries as Maudsley, Gowers, Hack and Tuke, that epilepsy and violence are particularly associated has not, however, been supported by recent epidemiological research (Toone, 1990).

A recent deterioration in behaviour without adequate social causation and with the occurrence of inexplicable aggression should always raise the suspicion of a developing organic lesion, and detailed examination neurologically and of the mental state should be carried out.

Aggressive outbursts may occur, often associated with alteration of consciousness and hallucinosis, in acute, toxic confusional states. Irritability and aggression are commonly seen with hypoglycaemia after excess dosage of insulin in diabetes and with hypoxia in incipient respiratory failure. It may occur with other metabolic illness. Of particular importance are the acute organic psychosyndromes due to intoxication with alcohol or other drugs. The relationship between alcohol abuse and crime is complex: 'the variations on the alcohol–crime connection are legion' (Edwards, 1982); repeated episodes of acute alcohol intoxication combined with uncontrollable violence are a particular problem.

Modes of behaviour

Psychiatric associations have been sought for different types of impulsive or aggressive behaviour. There is a temptation for the layperson to make the illogical leap 'because that act was so appalling and so incomprehensible *to me*, the person who committed it must have been mad'. Thus, some have thought that all murderers must be mentally ill. Careful investigation of the psychopathology will correct this misunderstanding. Violent sexual behaviour has already been discussed in Chapter 16; in most instances of rape, gaining satisfaction from violence is more prominent in the psychopathology than sexual gratification. The following terms are considered only very briefly; more detailed description will be found in textbooks of forensic psychiatry (Bluglass and Bowden, 1990; Gunn and Taylor, 1993).

Fire setting (arson)

Although fire setting is considered here with impulse control disorders, this behaviour may be preplanned, deliberate and apparently convey a non-verbal message. Thus Geller (1984) described

> “ arson by consumers of public sector mental health services who want to communicate a wish and/or a need for a change in location of those services. Fires may be set to return to a state hospital, to preclude placement from the hospital to a 'less restrictive' setting, or to express dissatisfaction with one's current locus of services.

Of 14 such patients, 8 were diagnosed as psychotic (6 schizophrenic) and 3 as showing mental retardation. In another series of 17 cases, 7 showed mental retardation, 8 had neurotic reactions and 2 were classified under personality disorder (Zeegers, 1984).

Scott (1977), in reviewing *malicious fire raising*, considered that incendiarists could be divided into those with clear-cut motives and those whose motives are either blurred or absent. An example of the former is the person who plans to profit by insuring a building and then arranging for it to be burnt down. Fire has also been used to conceal murder and is of course regularly used in vengeance or retribution or by political extremists. Apparently motiveless arson may occur among those with overt psychiatric disorder or organic brain disease, for example half-accidentally in a demented person or in response to hallucinatory voices in schizophrenia. It may also occur without overt psychiatric illness following adverse circumstances but out of proportion to them, for example a student failing his examination sets light to the college library. There is also a group of people, the 'firebugs' (Lewis and Yarnell, 1951), with psychopathic personality, who repeatedly set fires to satisfy such inner desires as wishing to help firemen, to be a hero or to enjoy destruction; some of these may gain sexual satisfaction only through this act and masturbate while watching their conflagration – fire fetishists. Fire setting is quite commonly associated with a degree of mental retardation. It is usually a male activity (6:1, males: females) and most commonly occurs between the ages of 16 and 25 years.

Of the various motives given for fire setting, revenge is the most common, although only occurring in one-third of a series of 153 adult arsonists (Rix, 1994). Most of these were young men; one-half had disorder of personality and one-tenth mental retardation, and a quarter had clear evidence of educational disadvantage. Many of the perpetrators were intoxicated at the time of the crime. Rehousing was a motive for some, more often for women than for men. A classification for arson has been proposed by Gunn and Taylor (1993), and this is represented in Box 20.2.

Acute binge drinking

The history of Western Europe and the lands populated by its emigrants is steeped in alcohol: the ceremonies of all life epochs and rites of passage are solemnized with alcohol, and contracts and relationships are symbolically sealed by drinking together. Alcohol is used for important events in the family, and the greatest effects of its abuse are also on the family: a person with an alcohol problem usually affects the lives of others around him (Orford and Harwin, 1982). In medical practice, alcohol abuse is also important. The most conservative estimate is that at least 15 per cent of patients admitted to general hospitals (in New Zealand) had an alcohol-related illness or disability, and in a further 10 to 20 per cent it is a significant contributing factor to admission; in about 50 per cent of fatal traffic accidents, alcohol is involved (Bieder *et al.*, 1982).

Box 20.2 A psychiatric classification of arson (fire setting)

- Profitable arson: fraudulent insurance claim, avoiding detection of crime, etc.
- Political arson: fire setting and bombing for political ends
- Accidental fire setting: for example setting light to rubbish by an intoxicated person
- Revenge fire setting: against society in general, against employers, jealous revenge
- Fire setting for pleasure and excitement:
  hero fire setters
  firebugs
  erotic fire setters
- Psychotic and organic fire setters: for example in the context of schizophrenia or Alzheimer's disease
- Suicide by fire: may have a political motivation
- Child fire setters: often in association with other behavioural disturbance

(From Gunn and Taylor, 1993, with permission.)

Acute binge drinking, with a pattern of repeated loss of control, is one of the many patterns of the *alcohol dependence* syndrome (Royal College of Psychiatrists, 1979). The elements of this syndrome are:

- subjective awareness of a compulsion to drink
- narrowing of the drinking repertoire (drinking in order to relieve or avoid withdrawal symptoms, and therefore a similar amount each day)
- primacy of drinking over other activities
- altered tolerance to alcohol (initially increased tolerance but eventually decreased in the late stages of alcohol dependence)
- repeated withdrawal symptoms (from shakiness, tremor, sweating, nausea, agitation and tenseness to convulsions and delirium tremens)
- relief or avoidance of withdrawal symptoms by further drinking
- reinstatement after abstinence.

Glue sniffing (solvent abuse)

Impulsive and self-destructive behaviour follows fashions and is in part determined by learning and by availability. This is exemplified by the phenomenology of intoxication with toluene-based adhesives and butane (Evans and Raistrick, 1986). Prevalence varies in different communities, for instance it is very frequent among adolescents in community homes and assessment centres (Parrott, 1990). Solvent intoxication is similar to alcohol in that initial stimulation of central nervous function is followed by depression. Both toluene and butane abusers described elevation of mood and hallucinations; nearly one-quarter of subjects experienced the dangerous delusion of being able to fly or swim. Among the group of toluene abusers, thoughts were more likely to be slowed, time appeared to pass more quickly and tactile hallucinations were more commonly reported than in the butane group. The toluene subjects were more likely to sniff only in a group setting and were more definite in their sanction against taking other drugs.

Shoplifting (kleptomania)

Stealing from shops is a major economic problem, estimated to cost the honest shopper about 2 per cent of the cost of what he or she buys (Segal, 1977). Unlike much other crime, shoplifting is predominantly a female activity (83 per cent), with 50 per cent of offenders being aged under 18 years and about 4.5 per cent of shoppers stealing at each shop, irrespective of city or country studied (Fisher, 1984). In one study, one in ten shoplifters were found to be recidivists, and these frequently also had convictions for prostitution and drug-related offences. More recently, the female predominance of shoplifting has been questioned; with high unemployment, young males are now more frequently involved.

Shoplifting becomes pathological stealing when there is a repeated failure to resist impulses to steal objects that are not acquired for personal use or monetary gain (ICD-10; World Health Organization, 1992). Those referred for clinical evaluation described irresistible impulses or urges to steal, relief of tension during or shortly after theft and, often, pleasurable feelings during the act (McElroy *et al.*, 2000).

In different series, about 2 per cent of shoplifters were referred for psychiatric assessment by the courts, but when all women accused were assessed nearly 20 per cent were found to have identifiable psychiatric disorder. Summing different studies, diagnostically 33 per cent of psychiatrically disturbed shoplifters were suffering from neuroses, psychosomatic disorders or compulsive behaviour; 17 per cent from personality disorders; 15 per cent from psychotic disorders; 11 per cent from mental handicap; 5 per cent from organic disorders such as dementia; and 3 per cent from alcohol and/or drug abuse. Gibbens *et al.* (1971) have particularly commented on the association between depression and shoplifting. Significant recent or current physical illness was also an important factor. Discussion of those shoplifters who show psychiatric disturbance, with illustrative case examples, is to be found in the account by Bluglass (1990).

The word *kleptomania* implies a 'thieving disease' and is used in DSM-IV (American Psychiatric Association, 1994). Fisher has classified stealing from shops into five categories, in some of which adverse psychological and social factors make a contribution:

- 'professional' shoplifters
- shoplifters with a severe functional or organic psychiatric disorder at the time of the offence
- reactive shoplifters (transient reaction to emotional stress)
- young shoplifters (may reflect underlying social, emotional or family problems)
- shoplifting as an abnormal learned behaviour.

Violence and homicide

Psychiatrists are usually requested to report when offenders plead guilty or are found guilty of charges of *homicide*, a term that covers murder, manslaughter and infanticide (Bluglass, 1979). There is, therefore, considerable knowledge of the mental state some time after homicide, but it is often difficult to extrapolate to the perpetrator's subjective state at the time he committed the act. Murder is classified as *normal* or *abnormal* depending on the legal outcome, and at least one-third of murders are classified as abnormal. Although most of the perpetrators of homicide are male, this ratio is less extreme for abnormal homicide. Homicide by females most often takes place in the context of depressive illness, and the victims are usually young children, frequently the child of the perpetrator. Male homicides are quite often suffering from schizophrenia and may have a history of previous physical violence. When the person who commits homicide suffers from depression, suicide or a suicide attempt often follows the killing. Delusions may be the precipitant of a murderous attack. Bluglass reported a patient who, because he believed that a piece of cotton in his car indicated that his girlfriend had been having sexual relations with his father, strangled her and drove the body to a police station. More rarely, homicide may be associated with mental subnormality, epilepsy or cerebral tumour.

Homicide may frequently follow the ingestion of alcohol (in Scotland, alcohol was implicated in 58 per cent of male and 30 per cent of female perpetrators of homicide; Gillies 1976). Other drugs are less common, but cannabis, lysergic acid diethylamide, amphetamines and barbiturates have been implicated. Hypnotic trance has been incriminated on rare occasions. Murder with the motivation of obtaining drugs also occurs not infrequently.

Dissocial personality disorder may be found to be present in a convicted murderer and is sometimes cited (as the Mental Health Act term *psychopathic disorder*) in a plea of diminished responsibility.

An individual claiming *amnesia* at the time of the act is difficult to evaluate. This is rarely associated with organic or psychotic disorder, more often with low intelligence, dissociation, alcohol intoxication, sexual excitement or rage. Malingering, dissociative amnesia and other psychogenic explanations for amnesia are virtually impossible to distinguish and may be a matter of degree (Gibbens and Hall-Williams, 1977).

Deliberate self-harm

With regard to attempted suicide and deliberate self-harm, the place of descriptive psychopathology is chiefly in the study of motivation for such actions. There has been much attention to risk factors for both suicide and deliberate self-harm (Black, 1992). Kessel (1965) introduced the term *self-poisoning* as a behavioural description of people who take an overdose of drugs. Over the 20 years from 1960 to 1980, admission to hospital for this behaviour became about six times more frequent in the United Kingdom. The term *deliberate self-harm* has been used by Morgan *et al.* (1975) 'as a non-fatal act, whether physical injury, drug overdosage or poisoning, carried out in the knowledge that it was potentially harmful and, in the case of drug overdosage, that the amount taken was excessive'.

The reasons people gave for taking overdoses were studied by Bancroft *et al.* (1976). These authors interviewed 128 subjects in Oxford immediately after the subjects recovered from taking an overdose. Forty-four per cent of subjects expressed a 'wish to die'; it was considered that in some cases this was used as a socially acceptable motive and did not always express suicidal intent. Thirty-three per cent were 'seeking help', 42 per cent 'escaping from the situation', 52 per cent 'obtaining relief from a terrible state of mind' and 19 per cent 'trying to influence someone'. The mood state of these patients at the time of the attempt was, in order of frequency, 'lonely', 'failed', 'worried', 'angry' and 'sorry'; in 92 per cent, at least one of these affects was described. Williams and Pollock (2000) consider that contemporary research supports a 'cry of pain' model for suicidal behaviour. The individual attempts to escape from a feeling of entrapment but believes there is no escape from an external situation or an inner turmoil and no prospect of rescue. Attempted suicide takes place out of the consequent sense of hopelessness.

Trying to investigate the self-experience at the time of suicide can, of course, only be conjectural. Barraclough *et al.* (1974) have found evidence of mental illness in 93 per cent, and of depressive illness in 70 per cent, of completed suicides. The symptoms of these depressives appeared to have been similar in type but more severe than in an unselected sample of depressed patients. There is a difference in mental state between those using violent methods such as jumping, drowning, hanging and shooting and those using less violent methods such as coal gas poisoning in past decades and self-poisoning nowadays.

Self-mutilation using physical acts, for example wrist slashing, probably demonstrates a different psychopathology from self-poisoning (Morgan, 1979).

Soranus, in the first century AD, recognized the danger of mentally ill people destroying themselves by jumping from a height, and he recommended looking after them on the ground floor (Zilboorg and Henry, 1941). In a study of people jumping out of buildings in a psychiatric hospital population, nearly 75 per cent were suffering from schizophrenia and related conditions (Sims and O'Brien, 1979). Self-poisoning represented 95 per cent of episodes of self-harm (Morgan *et al.*, 1975); of those who received a psychiatric diagnosis, it was usually associated with neurotic or depressive illness.

Diminished aggression

Decreased aggressiveness may accompany reduced drive; it is seen sometimes in organic, psychotic and psychogenic disturbance. It is frequently associated with apathy in acute organic disorders such as encephalitis, or in progressive dementia, although irritability and fractiousness may also occur. Generalized debilitating physical illness is normally accompanied by listlessness and apathy.

In schizophrenia, aggression is usually markedly reduced, with lack of volition and failure to initiate any directed activity; however, unprovoked violence may also occasionally occur. In depressive psychosis also, reduced aggression is much the most common presentation; however, homicide, quite often associated with suicide, is certainly described among severely depressed individuals with depressive delusions.

A consistently low level of aggressiveness may occur as a personality characteristic, for example with dependent disorder of personality. It may be seen as part of a neurotic reaction or during adverse life situations, for instance with the grief of bereavement or the unhappiness of feeling lonely. A certain degree of aggression is necessary for many of the social activities of normal life, and its absence impairs functioning. Pathological lack of aggression is closely associated with disorder of volition.

DISTURBANCE OF MOVEMENT AND BEHAVIOUR

Behavioural and movement disturbances may have crucial diagnostic significance, especially when there is difficulty with verbal explanation. However, as the emphasis of this book is on subjective description of abnormality, these disorders are discussed only briefly. The distinction between movement and behaviour is arbitrary, as will be shown, especially when schizophrenia is considered.

Disturbance of movement

Movement may be increased or speeded up, reduced or slowed down, or it may show various qualitative abnormalities. Some of these disorders of movement are involuntary and are appropriately regarded as neurological, some are voluntary but carried out unconsciously and some are deliberate actions (of the will). The words used mostly describe the objective characteristics of the action to an outside observer, not the subjective experience of the actor.

These disorders of movement are now considered briefly, starting with abnormalities of increased movement – *agitation* and *hyperactivity*, and decreased movement – *retardation*. The movement disorders of some psychiatric conditions are then described. There are psychiatric sequelae of primary movement disorders including parkinsonism, and often there is disorder of movement associated with conditions that are primarily psychiatric.

Agitation

Agitation implies mental disturbance causing physical restlessness and increased arousal; it is phenomenologically a description of a subjective mood state associated with and resulting in physical expression. The patient may describe his affect as 'feeling agitated', and both he and the external observer see motor restlessness as being logically connected with this. It is demonstrated in many different mental states; pathologically, it may occur with affective psychoses, with schizophrenia, with organic psychosyndromes such as senile dementia or with neurotic and personality disorders, especially states of anxiety. Agitation is quite often a symptom with physical illness, for example hyperthyroidism or hypoparathyroidism. It is an important component of some states of severe depressive illness. Although retardation is more commonly seen with 'endogenous depression' or melancholia, agitation may occur, either without retardation in alternating phase with retardation or concurrently with retardation in a *mixed affective state*. *Agitated depression* is an old term for one variant of a severe depressive episode with or without psychotic component (ICD-10; World Health Organization, 1992). It is alternatively known as *melancholia*. Practical clinical importance of this mood state ensues from the fact that, whereas suicidal impulses may be prevented from expression by retardation, agitation with restlessness may render such behaviour more likely. An early response to treatment following electroconvulsive treatment or effective antidepressant medication may result in the patient becoming less retarded and therefore at greater suicidal risk.

Hyperactivity

This describes the state in which there is increased motor activity, possibly with aggressiveness, over-talkativeness or uncoordinated physical activity. The term is descriptive of behaviour rather than of a subjective psychological state. Restlessness is poorly defined in the psychiatric literature and has diverse and multitudinous causes (Sachdev and Kruk, 1996). Restless hyperactivity or *hyperkinesis* may occur with a variety of different physical assaults on the brain but is especially prominent as a sequel to head injury in children, in whom it may be associated with impulsive disobedience and explosive outbursts of anger and irritability (Black *et al.*, 1969); it is also associated with childhood epilepsy when there is brain damage.

Over recent years, the condition of attention deficit/hyperactivity disorder (ADHD, in DSM-IV; American Psychiatric Association, 1994), previously described as occurring only in children, has been diagnosed in adults; the childhood disorder does sometimes persist into adult life, and the prevalence of the disorder in adulthood is low compared with that in childhood (Sachdev, 1999).

There is a pattern of persistent inattention in all areas of life, overactivity with fidgeting and restlessness and impulsivity with impatience and difficulty in delaying responses. These psychological characteristics result in disturbed behaviour in all areas of life. In adult life, there are persistent difficulties in relationships, usually a poor work record, and sometimes also a criminal record. The individual is particularly distractible and prone to be disruptive in a group setting.

Considerable comorbidity in children occurs with conduct disorder, oppositional deficit disorder, mood and anxiety disorders and mental retardation (Biederman *et al.*, 1991). Between 30 per cent and 70 per cent of children who are diagnosed as having ADHD will continue to show symptoms of the condition as adults (Bellak and Black, 1992). In a study of adults with ADHD, both genders had the manifestations of the condition but females, who unlike the situation in childhood were in the majority, had higher rates of depression, anxiety disorders and conduct disorder than normal control subjects (Biederman *et al.*, 1994). This is clearly a condition to which those practising in general adult psychiatry will have to pay more attention in future, and it is worthy of more detailed psychopathological study.

Retardation

Retardation has two quite different meanings in psychiatry. *Motor retardation*, the sense in which it is used here, implies slowness of the initiation, execution and completion of physical activity; it is frequently associated with retardation of thought, for example in severe depressive illness. The patient subjectively describes himself as having difficulty with thinking – 'my thoughts are slowed up' – and also with initiating and carrying out spontaneous activity. *Mental retardation* is a synonym for mental handicap, mental subnormality or learning disability. It is an unfortunate term as, although there is intellectual deficit, there may be no physical slowness; in fact, there may be overactivity, especially if there is coexisting brain damage. Also, the sufferer is unlikely to complain, subjectively, of slowness in the thinking process.

Retardation is so prominent a symptom of the severe endogenous type of depression that in the past it was used to name the condition, *retarded depression*. There is restricted movement, a static posture of dejection and decrease of muscular tone. Gesticulation is reduced, as is the emotional component of facial expression.

Retardation with slowness of motor activity is also seen with other causes of mental slowness, as in various organic psychosyndromes and with physical illnesses. The extreme of retardation – no voluntary movement at all – is known as *akinesis* and occurs with muteness in *stupor.*

Disorder of movement in schizophrenia

For the sake of convenience, three types of abnormality may be recognized in schizophrenia: isolated abnormalities of movement and posture, which are now discussed; more complex patterns of disordered behaviour, described later in the chapter; and the presumed effects on movement of the neuroleptic drugs, which are often used in large dosage and for a long time in schizophrenia.

Extrapyramidal side effects are described later in this chapter, but brief mention should be made of the *neuroleptic malignant syndrome*, with rapid onset of severe generalized muscular hypertonicity with hyperpyrexia and akinetic mutism and autonomic disturbance; death occurs in about 15 per cent of sufferers (Kellam, 1987). Some of the odd motor disorders that occur are described first, and then the disturbances of chronic schizophrenia are mentioned.

MOTOR DISORDERS

Catatonia means a state of increased tone in muscles at rest, abolished by voluntary activities and thereby distinguished from extrapyramidal rigidity. The syndrome *catatonic schizophrenia* was originally described by Kahlbaum (1873) and is characterized by the presence of the motor disorders described below. In reviewing Kahlbaum's concept, Johnson (1993) considers catatonia, the 'tension insanity', to be a neuropsychiatric syndrome caused by a large variety of organic disease processes manifesting catalepsy with an abnormal mental state. It is very difficult to classify the precise nature of the odd and abnormal posture in catatonic schizophrenia. *Waxy flexibility* (flexibilitas cerea) and *psychological pillow* occur but are both rare conditions. In waxy flexibility, when the limbs of the patient are put into any posture by the interviewer they will be retained in that position for a sustained period (a minute or more). Psychological pillow, when the patient's head is maintained a few inches above the bed, may continue for hours. In *stereotypy*, a bizarre uncomfortable-looking posture also may be retained for some hours.

The very varied symptoms of catatonia always involve motor activity and posture. There may be hyper- or hypoactivity, mutism, stereotypical posturing and movement, waxy flexibility, stupor and uncontrollable excitement (Fink, 1993). Some variants of catatonia are *lethal (pernicious) catatonia*, with high fever, rigidity and extreme hyperactivity and/or stupor; *neuroleptic malignant syndrome*, with rigidity, fever, autonomic instability and stupor, associated with the use of neuroleptic drugs; *periodic catatonia*, characterized by periods of excitement followed by catatonic stupor; *manic excitement*, with confusion; and *stupor* in the context of delirium.

There are two types of abnormal movement in schizophrenia: *idiosyncratic voluntary movements* or *mannerisms* and *spontaneous involuntary movements*. Mannerisms are shown in odd, stilted, voluntary movements and patterns of behaviour. The patient may claim to be unaware of these acts or explain them in terms of his delusions.

It is sometimes difficult to distinguish mannerisms from the purposeless movements or postures that are not goal-directed but are carried out in an unvarying way in any individual patient. It is important to attempt to distinguish either of these types of movement from the abnormal movements of *parkinsonian syndromes*, which occur quite frequently in schizophrenic patients treated with phenothiazine and butyrophenone drugs. *Grimacing* is a common feature in schizophrenia; *Schnauzkrampf* (literally 'snout spasm') is a characteristic facial expression in which the nose and lips are drawn together in a pout.

Abnormality of the *execution of movement* may result from the internal experiences of the schizophrenic patient. At times, he resists stimuli, for example the interviewer's request to raise his right arm, and shows *negativism*. At other times, he demonstrates excessive compliance amounting to *automatic obedience*: not only does he raise his right arm but he raises the other arm and then stands up with both arms raised in dramatic response to the request. This alternation of cooperation and opposition produces the diffident, unpredictable behaviour of *ambitendency*.

Obstruction is the equivalent in the flow of action to thought blocking in the flow of speech. While carrying out a motor act, the patient stops still in his tracks. After a pause, he continues with the act or he may proceed to do something else. Usually, he cannot account for his obstruction but may do so in terms of passivity: 'my action was stopped'.

Abnormal movements manifested in the interaction with the interviewer may reveal excessive cooperation or opposition. *Mitgehen, echopraxia, automatic obedience* and *advertence* are symptoms of excessive cooperation. In Mitgehen (literally, German, 'to go with'), the interviewer can move the patient's limbs or body by directing him with fingertip pressure, 'as if one was moving an anglepoise lamp' according to Hamilton (1984). When the patient imitates the interviewer's every action, the symptom is called *echopraxia*; this occurs despite the doctor asking him not to. *Automatic obedience* denotes a condition in which the patient carries out every command in a literal, concrete fashion, like an automaton. To demonstrate these symptoms of excessive cooperation, the patient should be asked to resist the interviewer. Mitgehen and echopraxia still occur. This inability to accede to instructions to resist occurs with *forced grasping*. The interviewer presents his hand to be shaken but at the same time asks the patient not to shake it; every time the patient does shake hands, the interviewer has great difficulty in getting his hand away again. In *advertence*, the patient turns towards the examiner when he addresses him; again, it has a bizarre, exaggerated and inflexible quality.

Opposition occurs as a negative response to all the approaches of the examiner. The patient resists the examiner when the latter attempts to move his limbs. When addressed, the patient turns away – *aversion*. *Negativism* is not just a refusal of the patient to do what he is asked: it is an active process of resisting all attempts to make contact with him. Opposition may sometimes manifest itself in muteness.

The abnormal movements of schizophrenia are strongly suggestive of neurological abnormality. In the opinion of Cutting (1985), the movement disorders of schizophrenia including catatonia, perseveration, involuntary movements and disturbed voluntary movements may, in some cases, represent a disorder of conation resulting from hemispheric imbalance.

DISORDER IN CHRONIC SCHIZOPHRENIA

Motor disorder in the mentally ill may be ascribed to the abnormal mental state, to treatment or to independent undiagnosed neurological disease (Rogers, 1985). Rogers studied motor disorders in 100 extremely chronic psychiatric in-patients, 59 women and 41 men, with a mean length of current admission of 42.8 years. Ninety-two of these patients had had a diagnosis of schizophrenia at some time, and all of them showed some current motor disorder.

Motor disorders were listed under the 10 categories of Table 20.1. These abnormalities were as follows.

Table 20.1 Percentage of patients with current motor disorder ($n = 100$)

Motor disorder	Percentage of whole group
Purposive movement	97
Speech production	95
Posture	86
Tone	85
Facial movements or postures	74
Head, trunk or limb movements	67
Activity	64
Stride or gait	48
Eye movements	48
Blinking	38

(From Rogers, 1985, with permission.)

- Difficulty with the initiation, efficient execution of or persistence with *purposive motor activity*, resulting in restriction of the motor repertoire available.
- *Speech production*, with 22 patients usually mute; 25 never initiating spontaneous conversation; 53 showing 'outbursts' of shouting, singing or talking; and 51 inarticulate or barely audible at interview.
- *Posture* and
- *tone*, with a tendency to flexion associated with varying degrees of rigidity and typically affecting the head or neck.
- *Abnormal movement* or *postures* of *orofacial muscles*, with rapid or slow contractions of different muscle groups.
- Abnormal movements of the *head, trunk* or *limbs*, which might be brief, jerky and semipurposive in quality.
- *Abnormal activity* might occur in outbursts or continuously with behaviour, such as hitting out at others, stamping, touching or following other people.
- *Stride* or *gait* might show shuffling, slowness, not swinging the arms, or turning with head and neck 'in one piece'.
- Conjugate deviation of the *eyes*, often up and laterally with deviation of the head in the same direction.
- Blinking markedly increased or decreased in rate, sometimes in 'bursts'.

Ninety-eight of these 100 patients had had motor disorder recorded prior to 1955, before there was any treatment with neuroleptic drugs. There was considerable variability between the type of motor disorder recorded before 1955 and observed currently. Disorder of eye movements, tone, gait and blinking were recorded less commonly in the past. Movement disorder in this group of patients was compared between those currently receiving neuroleptic drugs; those not treated for 1 month, 1 year or 5 years; and those never having received medication. With the possible exception of facial movements, which were more frequent in those having received treatment in the past year, there was no difference in the frequency of abnormal movements.

Motor disorder in parkinsonism

The disturbance of basal ganglia resulting in parkinsonian symptoms has two main causes of relevance to psychiatry: Parkinson's disease and symptoms secondary to the exhibition of psychotropic drugs. Some of the motor symptoms are similar in these two conditions, but the overall clinical picture differs.

PARKINSON'S DISEASE

In Parkinson's disease, as well as motor symptoms there are often sensory, autonomic and psychiatric abnormalities. Parkinson's original description in 1817 implied an absence of perceptual (as opposed to sensory) abnormality and does not comment on 'psychiatric status', which would then have been an unknown concept.

Primary or secondary sensory abnormalities may occur, and there may be autonomic under- or overactivity. However, the most conspicuous symptoms are in motor function: slowing of emotional and voluntary movement (Walton, 1985); muscular rigidity; akinesia; tremor; and disorders of gait, speech and posture. There is not necessarily any mental change; however, depression is very common (Mindham, 1970), intellectual deterioration may occur and personality disorder is sometimes associated. Psychotic episodes have also been described. A graphic description of the symptoms and subjective experience of parkinsonism was Sacks' account, *Awakenings* (1973).

EXTRAPYRAMIDAL SIDE EFFECTS OF NEUROLEPTIC DRUGS

The extrapyramidal movement disorders produced by antipsychotic drugs are described in detail by Marsden *et al.* (1986). These include drug-induced parkinsonism with the classical parkinsonian triad of muscle rigidity, tremor and akinesia, and also such symptoms as abnormalities of gait, speech, and posture; excessive salivation; difficulty with swallowing; the characteristic *facies*; and greasy skin. *Akinesia* varies from being mild in degree (dyskinesia), with an immobile, blank, expressionless face; limited movements with loss of such associated motor activity as the arms swinging when walking; and lack of spontaneity; to more severe and generalized absence of movement – this may start soon after beginning neuroleptic medication. Cogwheel rigidity and 'pill rolling' of the fingers, tremor of the hands or periorbital tremor may occur but are less common than akinesia. Extrapyramidal side effects of antipsychotic drugs are listed in Box 20.3 (from Gervin and Barnes, 2000).

Akathisia, motor restlessness, occurs frequently. There is a subjective experience of motor unease, with a feeling of being unable to sit still, a need to get up and move about and to stretch the legs, tap the feet, rock the body (Box 20.4). Akathisia may occur at the same time as the akinesia of drug-induced parkinsonism and presents the contrasting state of a subjective urge to move and physical impairment of movement. In order to distinguish akathisia from other causes of inner restlessness, restlessness of the legs should be found to be especially prominent.

Acute dystonic reactions include a variety of intermittent or sustained muscular spasms and abnormal postures. Dystonia has been defined as 'a syndrome

Box 20.3 Extrapyramidal side effects of antipsychotic drugs

Acute movement disorders
- Parkinsonism
- Acute akathisia
- Acute dystonia

Chronic movement disorders
- Tardive dystonia
- Chronic akathisia
- Tardive dyskinesia

(From Gervin and Barnes, 2000, with permission.)

Box 20.4 Subjective components of akathisia

Commonly experienced
- Sense of inner restlessness
- Mental unease
- Unrest or dysphoria
- Feeling unable to keep still
- An irresistible urge to move the legs
- Mounting inner tension when required to stand still

Less commonly experienced
- Tension and discomfort in the limbs
- Paraesthesiae and unpleasant pulling or drawing sensations in the muscles of the legs

(From Gervin and Barnes, 2000, with permission.)

dominated by sustained muscle contractions, frequently causing twisting and repetitive movements, or abnormal postures' (Fahn *et al.*, 1987). There may be protrusion of the tongue, grimacing, oculogyric crises, blepharospasm, torticollis, opisthotonus and other hyperkinetic exaggerated actions of the face, head, trunk or limbs. Owens (1990) has considered the major clinical types of dystonia to be acute dystonias, oculogyric spasms, focal dystonias including torticollis, blepharospasm, writer's cramp and other occupational dystonias, and laryngopharyngeal dystonia, segmental dystonias, generalized dystonia, drug-related (symptomatic) dystonias and psychogenic dystonia.

The frequency of association of so-called tardive dyskinesia, in which repetitive, purposeless movements of the facial muscles, mouth and tongue occur (sometimes with choreoathetotic limb movement and respiratory grunting) with the exhibition of psychotropic drugs is disputed. There is no doubt that faciobuccolinguomasticatory dyskinesia occurs in many chronic, especially elderly, psychotic patients on neuroleptic medication, but is it causally connected with drugs? The word *tardive* is used as the syndrome was considered to be a late consequence of drug treatment; however, there are cases described in patients who have never received neuroleptic drugs, and the precise relationship remains to be elucidated – it may be simply a late stage of the illness. In practice, the extrapyramidal symptoms secondary to medication are difficult to evaluate and measure in terms of severity – problematic in accounting for aetiologically but important in the satisfactory treatment of the patient. At a 3-year follow-up of psychiatric patients receiving antipsychotic medication, orofacial dyskinesia increased from 39 per cent to 47 per cent of the sample, with a few individuals developing the disorder anew and a few remitting (Barnes *et al.*, 1983). There was an association between dyskinesia and age over 50 years and the presence of akathisia, but none with the use of antipsychotic drugs; in fact, those on high dosage were unlikely to have the condition. These dyskinesic symptoms also occur in Huntington's chorea and in senile chorea.

Huntington's chorea

This is a hereditary condition, inherited as a Mendelian dominant, which manifests usually in early middle life and is characterized by choreiform movements and dementia. Jerky, rapid, involuntary movements start in the face and upper limbs. Dysarthria and disorders of gait also usually occur before intellectual impairment develops. The progressive dementia, with inertia and apathy, may be accompanied by irritability and occasional outbursts of excited behaviour. Occasionally, the dementia occurs as the first sign of the illness.

Various psychological abnormalities have been described in the prodromal stage before manifestation of chorea and dementia. These may be anxiety, reactive depression and the features of personality disorder, especially antisocial behaviour. It is not known if this is truly an early symptom of the illness or part of the psychosocial reaction to this appalling and doom-laden condition.

Other dementing illnesses

Non-specific deterioration of motor behaviour occurs with other dementing illnesses, especially increasing clumsiness and incoordination, and eventually inertia and akinesia. In Alzheimer's disease, which is much commoner in females than in males, the course is usually steadily and smoothly progressive. Death generally occurs within 5 years of the onset of the condition, from intercurrent infection or progressive inanition. In vascular dementia, males and females are approximately equally affected; the course is fluctuating and stepwise in progression and usually slower in achieving its eventually fatal outcome than dementia in Alzheimer's disease.

Tics and Gilles de la Tourette's syndrome

Tics are rapid, repetitive, coordinated and stereotyped movements, most of which can be mimicked, and are usually reproduced faithfully by the individual (Macleod, 1987). In Gilles de la Tourette's syndrome, multiple tics are accompanied by forced vocalizations that often take the form of obscene words or phrases – *coprolalia* (Lishman, 1997). The condition starts in childhood, under the age of 16; there are multiple motor tics and unprovoked loud utterances that may amount to shouted obscenities.

The condition is more common in boys than in girls and usually starts between the ages of 5 and 8 with simple tics. The vocalizations usually begin as unrecognizable sounds but may progress to 'four-letter' swear words. Both tics and utterances are likely to occur with emotional stress. The subject often tries desperately hard not to vocalize the word, and this may be accompanied by considerable anxiety. An interesting study compared adult sufferers with depressed adults and normal controls on measures of obsessionality, depression and anxiety (Robertson *et al.*, 1993). Gilles de la Tourette's syndrome sufferers scored as high as depressives on measures of obsessionality but were intermediate between them and normal subjects for both depression and anxiety.

Disturbance of behaviour

There is no clear demarcation between disturbance of movement and of behaviour, and the distinction made here is arbitrary. Thus with parkinsonism, and to an even greater extent catatonic schizophrenia, an individual abnormal movement may be elaborated into an abnormal pattern of behaviour.

Behavioural disorders of schizophrenia

Disorder of movement is characteristic of *catatonia,* in which the patient may become immobilized in one attitude because of increased muscle tone at rest; it is usually seen in schizophrenia but has been described with frontal lobe tumour and some other organic conditions. There are abnormalities of posture and of movement, frequently shown in the actions made in relation to another person – the interviewer. Thus, in *waxy flexibility* the posture of the limbs is so described because it is maintained indefinitely after being manipulated into that attitude by the observer. Behaviour, the composite of movements, may also be abnormal, and this is characteristic of *catatonic schizophrenia,* with more than just one isolated abnormality of posture. It has often been commented that the incidence of catatonic schizophrenia has markedly declined. However, Mahendra (1981) has queried the existence of catatonic schizophrenia as a condition with classical Kraepelinian schizophrenic features *and* catatonia in the same patient. He believes many of the patients with catatonia suffered from neurological disease, perhaps postencephalitis, following epidemic and endemic viral infections. If this were so, the presumed association between schizophrenia and catatonia was accidental.

One could make a vast catalogue of the bizarre, and sometimes unpleasant, behaviour demonstrated by chronic schizophrenic patients, but this would never be exhaustive. Certain types of behaviour pattern are described here with examples. Schizophrenic *stupor* occurs, although rarely. The patient is mute and akinetic, although from the alertness of the eyes and the occasional excursion into abrupt activity or speech he is clearly conscious. It can be distinguished from depressive or manic stupor by the obvious abnormalities of mood in the stupor of the affective psychoses. A schizophrenic patient sat mute and motionless with her arms held in stereotyped, twisted posture for hours at a time. This symptom is almost never seen nowadays with adequate treatment of schizophrenic symptoms.

Negativism, as described above under motor disorders, may influence the behaviour of the patient substantially. A schizophrenic patient was interviewed in prison. He was brought to the door of the doctor's examination room. When the doctor invited him to enter, he took two steps backwards. To get him to enter, the doctor had to ask him to go away. When the doctor put his hand out to shake hands, the patient put his hand behind his back and reversed behind the desk. He would not sit down until he was politely asked to remain standing.

Excitement may occur associated with catatonia but can also be seen without this state; sometimes, a patient is mute and motionless for a time and then unpredictably becomes overactive and aimlessly destructive. A chronic schizophrenic patient, normally calm, would suddenly and unaccountably rush headlong across the ward and charge head first into the wall. On occasion this behaviour was directed at a window, and he had cut himself severely on the glass in the past.

Impulsive behaviour may not always be manifested as excitement; it may be carried out in contradistinction to the patient's habitual behaviour. A normally respectable and tranquil elderly female patient would suddenly and unpredictably make sexual assaults on unsuspecting male visitors to the hospital.

Hoarding is a common feature in chronic schizophrenics and is not confined to those in institutions. A patient used to put in a small tin insects and pieces of rubbish found around the hospital, such as cigarette ends and small pieces of string. She did not appear to use her assortment but was constantly collecting more items.

Water intoxication due to grossly excessive water drinking has been described in schizophrenia, although it may occur, but much less commonly, in almost any psychiatric disorder (Ferrier, 1985). The symptom is potentially dangerous (Singh *et al.*, 1995) and can even result in death from hyponatraemia, often associated with convulsions. The water drinking may be explained by the patient in terms of delusions, or there may be a failure of the normal thirst–fluid intake homeostatic mechanism, or both.

There may be *mannerisms* and idiosyncrasies of behaviour as well as of single movements. One totally mute male chronic patient used to retire to the top of a remote staircase above a ward, where he ingeniously and delicately cut keys that would open any door in the hospital. He would exchange these for cigarettes with other patients, despite remaining utterly silent.

Gross self-neglect has been described, especially among elderly reclusives who have sometimes been well educated, intelligent and wealthy. This syndrome has, rather unfortunately, been called the Diogenes syndrome after the Greek philosopher who rejected social norms and worldly luxuries (Clark *et al.*, 1975). An early case was described by Daniel Hack Tuke (1874) of a rich old man, 'mad Lucas', who died in a filthy state, half-naked and alone in his decaying mansion. He remained as a hermit for 25 years, continually terrified that his younger brother would seize his house and kill him. He and similar recluses usually suffer from a paranoid schizophrenic illness, although the term Diogenes syndrome itself is purely descriptive (Aquilina, 1992).

Multitudinous other forms of abnormal behaviour are manifested in schizophrenia. Flagrant stealing occurs, sometimes with a manneristic flavour, such as the hospital in-patient who 'stole' bedsprings, much to the discomfort of the occupants. Unprovoked aggression and 'nastiness' sometimes occur. Patients may exhibit childish naughtiness or grotesque dirtiness, and self-immolation and suicide have occasionally occurred. This may take place in obedience to auditory hallucinations or as part of a delusion. One patient regularly heard a voice that instructed him to jump out of the window; he was prevented on many occasions but finally took the reinforced window frames with him in leaping to his death.

Behavioural signs of emotional disturbance

Psychiatrists have learned that they must *listen* to their patients; it is also important to *observe* them and form useful, testable hypotheses from these observations. Internal medicine has, traditionally, made great diagnostic use of physical signs, and psychiatry also would do well to use behavioural signs as possible indicators, not positive proof, of psychological disturbance. Trethowan (1977) has noted, in addition to the evidence for catatonia and parkinsonism, the following *behavioural*, as opposed to neurological, signs, which may be of value diagnostically in psychiatry.

- *The handshake* may be limp and lifeless, as in the asthenic adolescent or sufferer from simple schizophrenia, or vice-like in mania. The hand of the schizophrenic patient with negativism may be withdrawn when the interviewer offers his, or the manic or personality disordered patient may insist on shaking hands, contrary to the doctor's intention.
- *Other forms of hand behaviour* that may be significant include bitten or picked nails, clenched hands with blanched knuckles and restless fidgeting with the fingers; all these may indicate acute or chronic anxiety. Heavily cigarette-stained fingers obviously reflect the large number of cigarettes smoked and the extent to which each cigarette is consumed; this may demonstrate a degree of tension. Tremor may reveal alcoholism with alcohol withdrawal. In 'Trethowan's wedding ring sign', a woman during history taking unconsciously reveals her marital difficulties by constantly sliding her wedding ring on and off her finger.
- *The feet* may be used for restless pacing in agitated depression. Akathisia, as described on p. 385, with an inability to keep the feet still, may indicate excessive medication with phenothiazine drugs.
- *Depressive facies* and *posture* sometimes lead to diagnosis before the patient speaks. The patient may be slumped in the chair with a fixed expression of unmitigated grief on his face and a prominent 'crow's foot' between the eyebrows. Trethowan (1977) has commented on the greatly reduced blink rate with severely retarded depressives.
- *Clothing* in mania may be distinctive and suggestive of both the diagnosis and the hypereroticism that sometimes accompanies it. Hair, make-up and dress may be unequivocal demonstrations of manic mood: 'Thus Stella, normally a fairly modest girl, appeared one day in my consulting room wearing an all black outfit consisting of net stockings, a mini-skirt which extended barely to vulva level, and a top with so deep a cleavage as almost to expose her umbilicus. As if this were not enough she had stuffed her red, white and blue jubilee panties into the top of her open handbag, for all to see' (Trethowan, 1977).

- *Stroking the cheek* may be an indicator of emotional distress, as described by Gillett (1986): 'During the initial history-taking and assessment, there was one over-ridingly important emotive issue, as evident from observation of her body language signs. When she spoke of her son dying at the age of three, her body stiffened, the muscle tension in her face increased, as if trying to stifle expression, lacrimation increased (though only just perceptibly), and her voice rose in pitch and wavered. She then lightly stroked her right cheek with the tip of her fore-finger, as if wiping away an imaginary tear – a common sign which usually indicates a desire to cry at the same time as a wish not to show it'.

This list is far from exhaustive. The point is that clinicians should use their eyes and their previous clinical experience to form hypotheses in observation that they can subsequently test in the history or examination of mental state.

Behaviour of dissociative (conversion) disorders: hysteria

In the *International Classification of Diseases*, 9th edition (World Health Organization, 1977), disturbances in hysteria were described: 'There may be dramatic but essentially superficial changes of personality sometimes taking the form of a fugue (wandering state). Behaviour may mimic psychosis, or, rather, the patient's idea of psychosis'. Patients still complain of similar symptoms and manifest the same behaviour, although the terminology of ICD-10 (World Health Organization, 1992) now describes hysteria as dissociative (conversion) disorder. Conversion symptoms include such motor disturbances as dissociative paralyses, astasia–abasia and other disorders of gait and tremor, and also sensory disturbances.

The word *conversion* implies the conversion of an unpleasant and unacceptable emotion into a physical symptom. This is, of course, a theoretical interpretation of the dynamics of aetiology of the symptom. A characteristic example of conversion was a girl, aged 20, who had spent a lot of time during her childhood in hospital. Four years previously, she had been unable to walk and was pushed into the neurological ward in a wheelchair. No organic pathology was found. She was then transferred to a psychiatric ward and without further specific treatment her function gradually returned to normal. Two years later, she complained of backache and, after 6 months importuning, she persuaded an orthopaedic surgeon to operate on an intervertebral disc. Following the operation, she walked with a stick, dragging one leg and saying the backache was unchanged. On physical examination, there was no voluntary movement of flexion or extension at the knee or ankle on the right side. However, there was no wasting or fasciculation of muscles. Tone was normal, knee and ankle jerks were brisk and equal and both plantar responses were flexor. There was stocking anaesthesia of the right leg. She smiled as she described the way her disability limited her lifestyle and how limited was the effectiveness of the medical profession. When offered admission to hospital with the prognosis of complete relief of symptoms, she refused, saying that she could not afford the time off work.

Behaviour in chronic fatigue syndrome

This condition is characterized by severe and prolonged fatigue, affecting both physical and mental functioning, exacerbated by relatively minor exertion

(Fukuda *et al.*, 1994). Thus, the core symptom of chronic fatigue syndrome (CFS) is fatigue, but this also occurs in many other physical and mental conditions. Discussion concerning CFS has been bedevilled by the Cartesian dilemma: psychiatric explanations being regarded as 'purely mental' and neurological as 'real disease'. Lawrie *et al.* (1997) have proposed the hypothesis that CFS is a primary disturbance of the *sense of effort*. This would place the condition firmly within psychopathological disorders of volition and execution. They observe the patients' reports of fatigue and muscle weakness alongside neurophysiological investigations that demonstrate normal muscular strength but an increased perception of effort on both isometric contraction and isotonic exercise.

Fatigue has been measured physiologically, isometrically and isotonically for muscular fatigue (Kent-Braun *et al.*, 1993; Sisto *et al.*, 1996). Physical assessment in clinical practice may be more satisfactory when carried out functionally, for example how many steps can be climbed. Measurement is hindered by the problem of motivation. Measurement of fatigability and comparison with other conditions, such as myasthenia gravis, may have benefits in demonstrating to the patient progress towards recovery.

Behaviour in anorexia and bulimia nervosa

The name *anorexia nervosa* is a misnomer: although some patients may claim to have no appetite, others admit to a voracious appetite that, with almost superhuman effort, they successfully control. The behavioural abnormality is a feeding disturbance or eating disorder; carbohydrate deprivation with carbohydrate starvation is characteristic.

The patient may resist the encouragement of her parents and the hospital staff to eat, often using deception such as hiding food in her clothes, holding it in her mouth and depositing it in a WC or throwing it out of the window. She may make herself vomit or take purgatives to expel food and hence calories. Anorexia may alternate with episodes of bulimia, when she eats excessively. This over-eating is often bizarre in nature, for example a 16-year-old girl persuaded her parents to lock the pantry door to prevent her stealing food and each parent had then to keep a key on their person. One evening, when they were both out, she broke the pantry window, climbed in and consumed everything she could. On the day she came to hospital, she got up at 5.30 a.m. and ate 1 lb of raw sausages and a whole loaf of bread. Patients often feel very guilty about eating and obtain a feeling of satisfaction from starving themselves and reducing their weight to cachexia. They, and their families, tend to use food as currency; that is, food is used as a reward and positive feelings are expressed in terms of food. Food and eating behaviour also take on moral overtones: there is 'good' and 'bad' food, to eat 'bad' food makes one feel guilty and to refrain from eating gives the patient a feeling of smug satisfaction (Sims, 1994).

Ritualistic behaviour may be shown in the preparation and eating of food. Very frequently, cooking or dietetics is their hobby, with an array of exotic cooking books on the kitchen shelf. They are very interested in what other people eat: a married anorexic cooked her husband into obesity, 'like a Michelin man' she admitted, while she starved herself. Another patient recounted that if she were reading a novel and came to a description of food or eating, she would go back and read that passage several times with gloating excitement before continuing the book.

Abnormalities in sexuality, gender role and attitudes towards maternity of anorexic patients have been described (Bruch, 1973). Worries about oral impregnation, fatness resulting in childbirth and so on appear to be much rarer in the better informed adolescents of today. However, there is often an expressed wish not to become an adult, a mother or a woman. An anorexic patient occupied the same room as a young woman admitted to hospital with her baby son. The anorexic girl intensely disliked and refused to look at the baby boy. She resented the attention that he received, which was therefore no longer directed at her, previously having been the youngest person on the ward. She disliked him because he was male and would become a man. She hated the reminder that she was becoming a woman and would be capable of having a baby. It is quite common for the patient to be pleased that she is amenorrhoeic and to try to limit weight gain so that periods do not recur. She may take the returning attention of boys, as she begins to put on weight and become attractive, as a signal that she needs to lose weight again. Sometimes, her denial of food is seen as a self-imposed penalty for sexual thoughts or misdemeanours that occurred when she was at normal weight.

Laterality

It is increasingly being realized that many aspects of psychiatric assessment and treatment are influenced by issues of laterality and hemispheric dominance. Humankind has been described as the lopsided animal (Coren, 1992), as about 90 per cent are right-handed, and this has a major influence on all human activities. Laterality and hemispheric dominance has been considered important in the pathogenesis of schizophrenia. Developmental difficulties resulting in emotional disturbance may occur in those who are left-handed, especially if forced to use their right hands. Increased premature mortality has also been shown among left-handed people, although it is not known why.

REFERENCES

Adler A (1929) *Problems of Neuroses*. London: Kegan Paul, Trench, Trubner.

American Psychiatric Association (1994) *Diagnostic and Statistical Manual of Mental Disorder*, 4th edn. Washington: American Psychiatric Association.

Andreasen NC (1982) Negative symptoms in schizophrenia. Definition and reliability. *Archives of General Psychiatry 39*, 784–8.

Andreasen NC (1989) Scale for the Assessment of Negative Systems (SANS). *British Journal of Psychiatry 155* (suppl. 7), 53–8.

Aquilina C (1992) Diogenes syndrome. *Psychiatric Bulletin 16*, 573.

Bancroft JHJ, Skrimshire AM and Simkin S (1976) The reasons people give for taking overdoses. *British Journal of Psychiatry 128*, 538–48.

Barnes TRE, Kidger T and Gore SM (1983) Tardive dyskinesia: a 3 year follow-up study. *Psychological Medicine 13*, 71–81.

Barraclough GM, Bunch J, Nelson B and Sainsbury P (1974) A hundred cases of suicide: clinical aspects. *British Journal of Psychiatry 125*, 355–73.

Bellak L and Black RB (1992) Attention-deficit hyperactivity disorder in adults. *Clinical Therapeutics 14*, 138–47.

Benson DF and Blumer D (1982) *Psychiatric Aspect of Neurologic Disease*, vol. 2. New York: Grune & Stratton.

Berrios GE (1996) *The History of Mental Symptoms*. Cambridge: Cambridge University Press.

Bieder L, O'Hagan J, Whiteside E and Paton A (1982) *Handbook on Alcoholism for Health Professionals*. London: Heinemann.

Biederman J, Newcorn J and Sprich S (1991) Comorbidity of attention deficit hyperactivity disorder with conduct, depressive, anxiety, and other disorders. *American Journal of Psychiatry 148*, 564–77.

Biederman J, Faraone SV, Spencer T, Wilens T, Mick E and Lapey KA (1994) Gender differences in a sample of adults with attention deficit hyperactivity disorder. *Psychiatry Research 53*, 13–29.

Black DW (1992) Suicide and suicidal behaviour. *Current Opinion in Psychiatry 5*, 201–6.

Black P, Jeffries JJ, Blumer D, Wellner A and Walker AE (1969) The post-traumatic syndrome in children. In Walker AE, Caveness WF and Critchley M (eds) *The Late Effects of Head Injury*. Springfield: Thomas.

Bleuler E (1911) *Dementia Praecox or the Group of Schizophrenias* (transl. Zinkin J, 1950). New York: International Universities Press.

Bluglass R (1979) The psychiatric assessment of homicide. *British Journal of Hospital Medicine 22*, 366–77.

Bluglass R (1990) Shoplifting. In Bluglass R and Bowden P (eds) *Principles and Practice of Forensic Psychiatry*. Edinburgh: Churchill Livingstone.

Bluglass R and Bowden P (1990) *Principles and Practice of Forensic Psychiatry*. Edinburgh: Churchill Livingstone.

Bruch H (1973) *Eating Disorders: Obesity, Anorexia Nervosa and the Person Within*. London: Routledge & Kegan Paul.

Burwell CS, Robin ED, Whaley RD and Bickelmann AG (1956) Extreme obesity associated with alveolar hypoventilation – a Pickwickian syndrome. *American Journal of Medicine 21*, 811–8.

Clark ANG, Manikar GD and Gray I (1975) Diogenes syndrome: a clinical study of gross neglect in old age. *Lancet i*, 366–73.

Coren S (1992) *Left Hander: Everything You Need to Know About Left Handedness*. London: John Murray.

Critchley M (1962) Periodic hypersomnia and megaphagia in adolescent males. *Brain 85*, 627–56.

Crow TJ (1980) Molecular pathology of schizophrenia: more than one disease process? *British Medical Journal 280*, 66–8.

Cutting J (1985) *The Psychology of Schizophrenia*. Edinburgh: Churchill Livingstone.

Daruna JH and Barnes PA (1993) A neurodevelopmental view of impulsivity. In McCown WG, Johnson JL and Shure MB (eds) *The Impulsive Client: Theory, Research and Treatment*. Washington: American Psychological Association.

Dolan B and Coid J (1993) *Psychopathic and Antisocial Personality Disorders*. London: Gaskell.

Edwards G (1982) *The Treatment of Drinking Problems: a Guide for the Helping Professions*. London: Grant McIntyre.

Epistle of Paul the Apostle to the Romans (1662), Chapter 7, 18–23, Authorized Version.

Evans AC and Raistrick D (1986) *Phenomenology of intoxication with toluene based adhesives and butane gas*. Unpublished text.

Eysenck SGB (1993) The 17: development of a measure of impulsivity and its relationship to the superfactors of personality. In McCown WG, Johnson JL and Shure MB (eds) *The Impulsive Client: Theory, Research and Treatment*. Washington: American Psychological Association.

Fahn S, Marsden CD and Calne B (1987) Classification and investigation of dystonia. In Marsden CD and Fahn RS (eds) *Movement Disorders 2*. London: Butterworth.

Ferrier IN (1985) Water intoxication. *British Medical Journal 291*, 1594–6.

Fink M (1993) Catatonia: a treatable disorder, occasionally recognized. *Directions in Psychiatry 13*, 1–8.

Fink M and Taylor MA (2003) *Catatonia: a Clinician's Guide to Diagnosis and Treatment*. Cambridge: Cambridge University Press.

Fisher C (1984) Psychiatric aspects of shoplifting. *British Journal of Hospital Medicine 31*, 209–12.

Freud S (1915) Instincts and their vicissitudes. In *Collected Papers*, vol. 4. London: Hogarth Press.

Fukuda K, Straus SE, Hickie I, Sharpe MC, Dobbins JG and Komaroff A (1994) The chronic fatigue syndrome: approach to its definition and study. *Annals of Internal Medicine 121*, 953–9.

Geller J (1984) Arson: an unforeseen sequela of deinstitutionalization. *American Journal of Psychiatry 141*, 504–8.

Gervin M and Barnes TRE (2000) Assessment of drug-related movement disorders in schizophrenia. *Advances in Psychiatric Treatment 6*, 332–41.

Gibbens TCN and Hall-Williams JE (1977) In Whitty CWM and Zangwill OL (eds) *Amnesia*. London: Butterworth.

Gibbens TCN, Palmer C and Prince J (1971) Mental health aspects of shoplifting. *British Medical Journal 3*, 612–5.

Gillett R (1986) Short term intensive psychotherapy – a case history. *British Journal of Psychiatry 148*, 98–100.

Gillies H (1976) Homicide in the west of Scotland. *British Journal of Psychiatry 111*, 1087–94.

Griesinger W (1845) *Mental Pathology and Therapeutics* (transl. Robertson CL and Rutherford J, 1882). New York: William Wood & Co.

Gunn J and Taylor PJ (1993) *Forensic Psychiatry: Clinical, Legal and Ethical Issues*. Oxford: Butterworth-Heinemann.

Hamilton M (1984) *Fish's Schizophrenia*, 3rd edn. Bristol: Wright.

Henderson DK (1939) *Psychopathic States*. New York: Norton.

Higgins J (1990) Affective psychoses. In Bluglass R and Bowden P (eds) *Principles and Practice of Forensic Psychiatry*. Edinburgh: Churchill Livingstone.

Hull CL (1943) *Principles of Behaviour*. New York: Appleton-Century-Crofts.

Jaspers K (1923) *General Psychopathology* (transl. Hoenig J and Hamilton MW, 1963) Manchester: Manchester University Press.

Jaspers K (1959) *General Psychopathology*, 7th edn. (transl. Hoenig J and Hamilton MW, 1963). Manchester: Manchester University Press.

Johnson J (1993) Catatonia: the tension insanity. *British Journal of Psychiatry 162*, 733–8.

Kahlbaum KL (1873) Die Katatonie, oder das Spannungs Irresein. In *Catatonia* (transl. Levi Y and Pridan T, 1973). Baltimore: John Hopkins University Press.

Kellam AMP (1987) The neuroleptic malignant syndrome, so called: a survey of the world literature. *British Journal of Psychiatry 150*, 752–9.

Kennedy I (1981) *The Unmasking of Medicine*. London: George Allen & Unwin.

Kent-Braun JA, Sharma KR, Weiner MW, Massie B and Miller RG (1993) Central basis of muscle fatigue in chronic fatigue syndrome. *Neurology 43*, 125–31.

Kessel WIN (1965) Self poisoning. *British Medical Journal ii*, 1265–70, 1336–40.

Lawrie SM, MacHale SM, Power MJ and Goodwin GM (1997) Is the chronic fatigue syndrome best understood as a primary disturbance of the sense of effort? [editorial] *Psychological Medicine 27*, 995–9.

Lehmann HE (1967) Schizophrenia. In Freedman AM and Kaplan HI (eds) *Comprehensive Textbook of Psychiatry*. Baltimore: Williams & Wilkins.

Lewis NDC and Yarnell H (1951) Pathological firesetting. In *Nervous and Mental Disease Monographs*, no. 82.

Lishman WA (1997) *Organic Psychiatry*, 3rd edn. Oxford: Blackwell Scientific.

Lönnqvist JK (2000) Psychiatric aspects of suicidal behaviour: depression. In Hawton K and Van Heeringen K (eds) *The International Handbook of Suicide and Attempted Suicide*. Chichester: John Wiley.

Lorenz K (1963) *On Aggression* (transl. Latzke M, 1966). London: Methuen.

McDougall W (1908) *An Introduction to Social Psychology*. London: Methuen.

McElroy SL, Arnold LM and Beckman DA (2000) Impulse control disorders. In Gelder M, López-Ibor JJ and Andreasen NC (eds) *New Oxford Textbook of Psychiatry*. Oxford: Oxford University Press.

Macleod J (1987) *Davidson's Principles and Practice of Medicine*, 13th edn. Edinburgh: Churchill Livingstone.

Mahendra B (1981) Where have all the catatonics gone? *Psychological Medicine 11*, 669–71.

Marsden CD, Mindham RHS and MacKay AVP (1986) Extrapyramidal movement disorders produced by antipsychotic drugs. In Bradley PB and Hirsch SR (eds) *The Psychopharmacology and Treatment of Schizophrenia*. Oxford: Oxford University Press.

Mindham RHS (1970) Psychiatric symptoms in Parkinsonism. *Journal of Neurology, Neurosurgery and Psychiatry 33*, 188–91.

Moeller FG, Barratt ES, Dougherty DM, Schmitz JM and Swann AC (2001) Psychiatric aspects of impulsivity. *American Journal of Psychiatry 158*, 1783–93.

Morgan HG (1979) *Death Wishes? The Understanding and Management of Deliberate Self-Harm*. Chichester: Wiley.

Morgan HG, Burns-Cox CJ, Pocock H and Pottle S (1975) Deliberate self-harm: clinical and socio-economic characteristics of 368 patients. *British Journal of Psychiatry 127*, 564–74.

Mullen PE (2000) Dangerousness, risk and the prediction of probability. In Gelder M, López-Ibor JJ and Andreasen NC (eds) *New Oxford Textbook of Psychiatry*. Oxford: Oxford University Press.

Orford J and Harwin J (1982) *Alcohol and the Family*. London: Croom Helm.

Owens DGC (1990) Dystonia – a potential psychiatric pitfall. *British Journal of Psychiatry 156*, 620–34.

Parrott J (1990) Solvent abuse. In Bluglass R and Bowden P (eds) *Principles and Practice of Forensic Psychiatry*. Edinburgh: Churchill Livingstone.

Plath S (1962) Lady Lazarus. In Ted Hughes (ed.) (1981) *Sylvia Plath: Collected Poems*. London: Faber & Faber.

Prins H (1984) Vampirism – legendary or clinical phenomenon. *Medicine, Science and the Law 24*, 283.

Reid T (1863) In *The Works of Thomas Reid* (ed. Hamilton W). Edinburgh: Maclachlan & Stewart.

Rix KJB (1994) A psychiatric study of adult arsonists. *Medicine, Science and the Law 34*, 21–34.

Robertson MM, Channon S, Baker J and Flynn D (1993) The psychopathology of Gilles de la Tourette's syndrome: a controlled study. *British Journal of Psychiatry 162*, 114–7.

Rogers D (1985) The motor disorders of severe psychiatric illness: a conflict of paradigms. *British Journal of Psychiatry 147*, 221–32.

Ropschitz DH (1957) Folie à deux: a case of folie imposée à quatre and à trois. *Journal of Mental Science 103*, 589–96.

Royal College of Psychiatrists (1979) *Alcohol and Alcoholism*. London: Tavistock.

Sachdev P (1999) Attention deficit hyperactivity disorder in adults [editorial]. *Psychological Medicine 29*, 507–14.

Sachdev P and Kruk J (1996) Restlessness: the anatomy of a neuropsychiatric symptom. *Australian and New Zealand Journal of Psychiatry 30*, 38–53.

Sacks OW (1973) *Awakenings*. London: Duckworth.

Savage G (1886) *Insanity and Allied Neuroses: Practice and Clinical*. London: Cassell.

Scharfetter C (1980) *General Psychopathology: an Introduction*. Cambridge: Cambridge University Press.

Schneider K (1950) *Psychopathic Personalities* (transl. Hamilton MW, 1958). London: Cassell.

Scott D (1977) Malicious fire-raising. *Practitioner 218*, 812–7.

Segal M (1977) Psychiatry and the shoplifter. *Practitioner 218*, 823–7.

Selten J-PCJ, Sijben NES, van den Bosch RJ, Omloo-Visser J and Warmerdam H (1993) The Subjective Experience of Negative Symptoms: a self-rating scale. *Comprehensive Psychiatry 34*, 192–7.

Sims A (1983) *Neurosis in Society*. London: Macmillan.

Sims A (1994) Myself and my other self: the 'double phenomenon' in neurotic disorders. In Sensky T, Katona C and Montgomery S (eds) *Psychiatry in Europe: Directions and Developments*. London: Gaskell.

Sims ACP and Gooding KM (1975) The psychiatric outcome of 'normal' people at follow-up. *Journal of Psychiatric Research 12*, 167–75.

Sims ACP and O'Brien K (1979) Autokabalesis: an account of mentally ill people who jump from buildings. *Medicine, Science and the Law 19*, 195–8.

Sims ACP and Symonds RL (1975) Psychiatric referrals from the police. *British Journal of Psychiatry 127*, 171–8.

Singh S, Padi MH, Bullard H and Freeman H (1985) Water intoxication in psychiatric patients. *British Journal of Psychiatry 146*, 127–31.

Sisto SA, LaManca J, Cordero DL, et al (1996) Metabolic and cardiovascular effects of progressive exercise tests in patients with chronic fatigue syndrome. *American Journal of Medicine 100*, 634–40.

Smith SM, Hanson R and Noble S (1973) Parents of battered babies: a controlled study. *British Medical Journal iv*, 388–91.

Snaith RP (1993) Anhedonia: a neglected symptom of psychopathology. *Psychological Medicine 23*, 957–66.

Taylor PJ (1985) Motives for offending among violent and psychotic men. *British Journal of Psychiatry 147*, 491–8.

Taylor PJ and Gunn J (1984) Violence and psychosis. I. Risk of violence among psychotic men. *British Medical Journal 288*, 1945–9.

Tidmarsh P (1990) Schizophrenia. In Bluglass R and Bowden P (eds) *Principles and Practice of Forensic Psychiatry*. Edinburgh: Churchill Livingstone.

Toone B (1990) Organically determined mental illness. In Bluglass R and Bowden P (eds) *Principles and Practice of Forensic*

Psychiatry. Edinburgh: Churchill Livingstone.
Trethowan WH (1977) Psychiatry's physical signs. *World Medicine November 16*, 19–21.
Tuke DH (1874) The hermit of Red Coats' Green. *Journal of Mental Science 20*, 361–72.
Walton J (1985) *Brain's Diseases of the Nervous System*, 9th edn. Oxford: Oxford University Press.
Wasik M (1990) Insanity, diminished responsibility and infanticide: legal aspects. In Bluglass R and Bowden P (eds) *Principles and Practice of Forensic Psychiatry*. Edinburgh: Churchill Livingstone.
West DJ and Walk A (1977) *Daniel McNaughton: His Trial and the Aftermath*. Ashford: Headley Brothers.
Whitlock FA (1963) *Criminal Responsibility and Mental Illness*. London: Butterworth.
Whitlock FA (1990) Criminal responsibility. In Bluglass R and Bowden P (eds) *Principles and Practice of Forensic Psychiatry*. Edinburgh: Churchill Livingstone.
Williams IMG and Pollock LR (2000) The psychology of suicidal behaviour. In Hawton K and Van Heeringen K (eds) *The International Handbook of Suicide and Attempted Suicide*. Chichester: John Wiley.
Wing JK (1978) *Reasoning About Madness*. Oxford: Oxford University Press.
World Health Organization (1977) *International Classification of Diseases*, 9th revision. Geneva: World Health Organization.
World Health Organization (1992) *The ICD-10 Classification of Mental and Behavioural Disorders: Clinical Description and Diagnostic Guidelines*. Geneva: World Health Organization.
Zeegers M (1984) Criminal fire-setting: a review and some case studies. *Medicine and Law 3*, 171–6.
Zilboorg G and Henry GW (1941) *A History of Medical Psychology*. New York: Norton.

Section Six

VARIATIONS OF HUMAN NATURE

The Expression of Disordered Personality

21

> "But the impressions and actions of human beings are not solely the result of their present circumstances, but the joint result of those circumstances and of the characters of the individuals: and the agencies which determine human character are so numerous, (nothing which has happened to the person throughout life being without its portion of influence), that in the aggregate they are never in any two cases exactly similar. Hence, even if our science of human nature were theoretically perfect, that is, if we could calculate any character as we can calculate the orbit of any planet, from given data; still, as the data are never all given, nor even precisely alike in different cases, we could neither make positive predictions, nor lay down universal propositions. *John Stuart Mill (1811)*

Mill states succinctly the difficulty of forming a theory of personality that is useful in clinical practice in *predicting* behaviour.

The term *personality disorder* is an abstraction built on several tenuous theories. It is an untidy concept, but it carries clinical usefulness. The way in which the term has been developed and its relationship with *neurosis* are dealt with elsewhere (Sims, 1983). The intention here is to discuss only the effects different types of personality have on actions and behaviour. The clinician builds on a profile for personality disorder starting with the meaning of the term *personality*, which Schneider (1958) has defined as 'the unique quality of the individual, his feelings and personal goals'. This leads to a characteristic pattern of behaviour that allows us, to some extent, to predict his future actions and that makes this individual different. The clinical designation of personality is purely descriptive and carries no theoretical implications, otherwise there is a logical flaw in describing personality type in terms of consistent behaviour and at the same time claiming the *type* accounts for definite patterns of behaviour. Acute and detailed observation of the characteristics of personality and its evaluation is a useful psychiatric skill that has, regrettably, been much neglected for many years.

These characteristics of behaviour, including the capacity for and nature of relationships with other people, are brought together to describe *traits* or *personality types*; obviously, to be clinically relevant these traits must have implications for the functioning of the individual. The distinction between *trait*, the predisposition associated with personality, and *state*, the current mental condition, is very important. These classifications of personality disorder based on such lists of traits were categorized by Schneider (1923) and more recently in ICD-10 (World Health Organization, 1992) and in DSM-IV (American Psychiatric Association, 1994). Certain characteristics have clinical significance, such as the degree to which the person is aware of the feelings, and sensitive to the judgements, of other people. Abnormal personality is found when a personality trait considered to be clinically significant is present to either too small or too great an extent to conform statistically with the mass of mankind. The concepts of personality and personality disorder were discussed by Tantam (1988), and more recently personality disorder has been reviewed by Tyrer and Stein (1993).

Although Schneider's typology has been largely superseded by ICD-10 in general clinical use, it did show considerable reliability (Standage, 1979). When psychiatrists rated according to Schneider's criteria, satisfactory reliability was found for *asthenic, explosive, depressive* and *affectionless* types; *insecure* and *attention-seeking* types were overused; and low reliability was found for the *fanatic, labile* and *hyperthymic* types.

Abnormality of personality has been described in terms of trait. What then is *personality disorder*? Here Schneider's definition will suffice. Personality disorder is present when that abnormality of personality causes either the patient himself or other people to suffer (Schneider, 1958).

- A highly conscientious and meticulous Post Office sorter was promoted to foreman sorter after many years' reliable service. The appropriate response might have been to be pleased at the increased pay and to spend the first week's increment before receiving it. However, this man was fearful about the promotion. He worried that he might not be able to cope with the job, that he might not be able to persuade the men in his charge to sort letters to his own high standards, that he would not be able to mix socially with his superiors and equals, that he would make a fool of himself and that other people would laugh at him. He became miserable, anxious and lacking confidence, and he had to stop work. Because of his abnormal, obsessional (anankastic) personality, he responded to the stress of promotion by becoming acutely distressed and developing neurotic depressive symptoms.
- A bland and plausible confidence trickster extracted without compunction the means of subsistence from an elderly widow. His psychopathic blunting of appreciation for the way others would experience his behaviour and their consequent feelings resulted in his causing suffering to others.

Personality abnormality is a part of the individual's constitution. Whether or not it manifests as personality disorder depends to a considerable extent on social circumstances. A highly abnormal personality that in one situation may be considered criminal psychopathy and be possessed by a convicted prisoner, in another situation will be the driving force in a highly successful and relatively creative political revolutionary. Personality in an individual cannot be divorced from its social and cultural setting.

Having ascertained whether personality disorder is present, its type should be categorized using an accepted system. However, a caution is needed here. It is often extremely difficult to fit people into arbitrary categories of personality, and the whole topic of classification is still highly unsatisfactory. It may be much better to use a few descriptive sentences for the personality, and probably it is best to combine description with categorization. The systems used in ICD-10 and DSM-IV can be recommended; the typological classification of personality disorder introduced by Tyrer and Alexander (1979) was also satisfactory but has not been widely used. Table 21.1 is a composite of these classifications. They all start from the same bases: the definition of personality, the evaluation of abnormality and the observation of certain influential and regularly occurring traits. Tyrer and Alexander's five discrete categories of abnormal personality followed from a cluster analysis of personality data and is therefore a simplification of ICD-9 (World Health Organization, 1977), which itself was based originally on Schneider. DSM-IV has certain different terms that have proved important in American psychiatry, although they are not necessarily found helpful elsewhere. These include *narcissistic* personality disorder, which is discussed later in this chapter; *avoidant*, which is similar to *anxious* personality disorder in ICD-10; and *schizotypal* personality disorder, which ICD-10 classifies with *schizophrenia, schizotypical* and *delusional disorders* (F2).

The following descriptions are based on the categorization found in ICD-10. It is important to realize that these categories are not mutually exclusive: mixed personality types are more frequent than a single personality type in pure form. Readers in the United Kingdom or in countries influenced by British psychiatry should be aware of an ongoing source of confusion perpetuated by recent discussion of the legal and administrative aspects concerning 'dangerous people with severe personality disorder' (Haddock *et al.*, 2001; Mullen, 1999). In terms of descriptive psychopathology, this debate is almost entirely concerned with dissocial personality disorder, but those taking part in the discussion tend to ignore other personality types, thus causing confusion for the assessment and classification of those with other personality disorders such as anankastic or anxious avoidant personality disorder. This can result in inappropriate treatment or lack of treatment administered by mental health professionals and unjustifiable stigmatization experienced by the sufferers.

Table 21.1 Comparison of personality types

Tyrer and Alexander (1979)[a]	ICD-10[b]	DSM-IV[c]
	F60.0 Paranoid	Paranoid
Schizoid	F60.1 Schizoid	Schizoid
Sociopathic		Schizotypal
	F60.2 Dissocial	Antisocial
	F60.3 Emotionally unstable	
	.30 Impulsive	
	.31 Borderline	Borderline
	F60.4 Histrionic	Histrionic
Anankastic	F60.5 Anankastic	Obsessive–compulsive
Dysthymic	F60.6 Anxious	Avoidant
Passive dependent	F60.7 Dependent	Dependent
	F60.8 'Other'	Narcissistic

[a]Tyrer and Alexander (1979).
[b]World Health Organization (1992).
[c]American Psychiatric Association (1994).

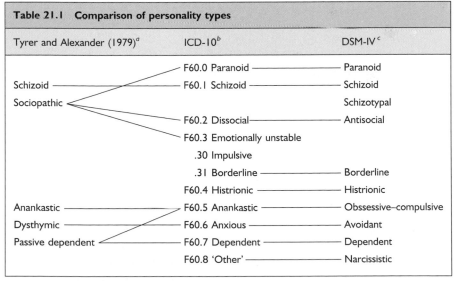

PARANOID PERSONALITY DISORDER

The essential feature of this type of personality disorder is self-reference, the proper psychiatric sense of the word *paranoid*; such people misinterpret the words and actions of others as having special significance for, and being directed against, themselves. Theoretically, self-referent ideas could imply that others are always noticing them in an admiring and benevolent way; in practice, such people would not consult a psychiatrist and those presenting in psychiatry have ideas of persecution. They mistrust other people and are very sensitive and suspicious, believing that others are against them and that what they say about them is derogatory. There are active and passive types of paranoid personality disorder; both types feel that others are 'getting at them' but their response differs.

The active paranoid personality manifests suspiciousness and is hostile and untrusting. Such a person is quarrelsome, litigious, quick to take offence, intensely suspicious and sometimes violent; he will go to enormous lengths to defend his rights or to address real or imagined injustices. He is extremely vigilant and tenacious in taking precautions against any perceived threat. This is the sort of person who will march fearlessly across a field of young corn because he sees there is a public right of way on his map and the farmer has no right to violate this. They repudiate blame and may be regarded by others as devious, scheming and secretive. Such a person is intensely jealous of what he regards as his own belongings, which may be people as well as objects, and he spends a lot of time planning to 'get his own back'. He may be self-important and fanatical. Morbid jealousy may be shown, and such a person may be involved in acts of violence because of imagined injustice. Such a personality may find creative expression in social and political life but is likely to be very destructive within the family. A patient commented on this ruefully, 'I have scarcely talked to my wife for the last 10 years', because of his succession of court cases against those with whom he came into contact.

A person with passive paranoid personality faces the world from a position of submission and humiliation. He assumes that whatever happens to him will be damaging. Like the active type, he is suspicious, sensitive and self-referent and misconstrues circumstances and other people. He believes that other people will dislike him and that they will ultimately let him down. However, he accepts 'the slings and arrows of outrageous fortune' passively, bowing to the inevitable; he is vulnerable and frequently feels humiliated and unable to initiate any assertive activity. Other people tend to take advantage of him, thus fulfilling his pessimistic expectations.

A frequent manifestation of psychopathology within the context of paranoid personality is the presence of an overvalued idea (Chapter 8). This, alternatively described as a fixed idea (idée fixe), is a belief that might seem reasonable both to the patient and to other people. However, it comes to dominate completely the person's thinking and life, and instead of testing its validity he tends to consider that every circumstance of life substantiates it; it becomes the basis for action that is sometimes aggressive or self-destructive. It is quite distinct phenomenologically from both *delusion* and *obsessional idea*.

SCHIZOID PERSONALITY DISORDER

This personality disorder is characterized by a lack of need for, and defect in, the capacity to form social relationships. Such people show withdrawal from social involvement; emotional coolness and detachment; and indifference to the praise, criticism and feelings of other people.

These individuals are 'loners' with a disinclination to mix, and they appear somewhat aloof. They lack tender feelings, have little interest in sexual experience and are not interested in the company of others. They are not depressed in mood, nor are they shy or sensitive towards other people, but they are solitary and prefer not to be involved in social occupations. Their interests and hobbies usually tend to increase their isolation from other people, as they are more interested in things, objects and machines.

Close relatives may complain of the subject's emotional detachment, an inability to inspire strong feelings in others, a lack of any real sense of pleasure, oddness and eccentricity and callous indifference to others' suffering. In a follow-up of former schizoid subjects, they were found to use psychological constructs less than a control group, and this pointed to the schizoid individual's lack of empathy (Chick *et al.*, 1979).

Those with schizoid personality and poor social adjustment have been considered more likely to develop schizophrenia. In a large study based on the previous personality assessment of 50 054 male recruits to the Swedish army, aspects of personality were found to be risk factors for the subsequent development of schizophrenia (Malmberg *et al.*, 1998).

DISSOCIAL PERSONALITY DISORDER

The essential, phenomenological abnormality of dissocial (asocial, antisocial or psychopathic) personality disorder is primarily one of empathy. There is a defect in the capacity to appreciate other people's feelings, especially to comprehend how other people feel about the consequences of this person's own actions. This personality type, or abnormality, includes those people considered to suffer from psychopathic personality within the meaning of the Mental Health Act, 1983 (Bluglass, 1983). A normal person is prevented most of the time, by shame or by his capacity for empathy, from carrying out unpleasant actions towards other people. He does not want to be disliked and feels very keenly how it would be passively to be the recipient of such behaviour. It is this inability to feel for himself the discomfort that others experience as a result of his antisocial activities that appears to be absent in the psychopath. Despite such comprehensive descriptions as that of Cleckley (1941), in *The Mask of Sanity*, and others, there are still considerable doubts as to whether this personality type forms a distinct category or not, and if it does, whether it should be considered within or outside psychiatry. This is succinctly expressed by Wooton (1959): psychopaths are 'extremely selfish persons and no one knows what makes them so'.

The confusion of terminology is explained partly by the varied nature of presentation; partly by the conflicting desires of professionals not to stigmatize and also not to cast blame on those who cannot control their actions; and partly by the requirements of classification for different professional groups and settings – lawyers, criminologists, psychiatrists, psychologists and so on. A comprehensive account of diagnostic issues, developmental history and methods of treatment is to be found in Dolan and Coid (1993).

The concept of *moral derangement* was introduced by Benjamin Rush (1812), and of *moral insanity* by Prichard (1835), who considered this to occur among criminals who showed loss of feeling, of control, and of ethical sense, equivalent to mental disease but at a different level. It is important to stress that not all psychopaths are criminal, nor are all criminals psychopathic. Henderson (1939) described *creative, inadequate* and *aggressive psychopathy*, citing Lawrence of Arabia as an example of a creative psychopath. Dissocial personality disorder, with conspicuous lack of conscience and human sympathy, is found more often in males than in females.

This personality disorder should not be diagnosed unless the subject is aged over 18 years. However, in childhood or adolescence many of the following may have been demonstrated by the person subsequently diagnosed as dissocial: truancy, expulsion or suspension from school for misbehaviour, delinquency, running away from home, persistent lying, repeated casual sexual intercourse, repeated drunkenness, substance abuse, theft, vandalism, school performance below expectation, repeated violation of rules at home and school and fighting. Of course, such behaviour may occur in normal children, especially with social deprivation, but it is their persistence and the presence of so many of these signs of disturbed behaviour that may predict subsequent psychopathy. There is also debate concerning the manifestation of attention deficit disorder in childhood and subsequent antisocial behaviour in young adult life (Hinshaw, 1994).

Such a person may be meaninglessly cruel, callous and aggressive, and emotionally cold, rejecting social norms and showing irresponsibility in his relationships. He is often unable to maintain consistency at work, with frequent unemployment, changes of occupation, absenteeism and poor relationships. Similarly, there are unsatisfactory relationships with sexual partners, with a history of several separations or divorces, promiscuity with heterosexual or homosexual preferences, desertion and repeated marital arguments. Poor parenting results in conspicuous physical and psychological problems among his children, and the individual's aggressiveness may result in child abuse with non-accidental injury. As he ages, he is less likely to be in conflict with the law and less likely to be violent, but his affectionless inability to see the consequences of his actions, and the way other people suffer because of them, remains destructive within the family and in other institutions. There is a failure to accept society's norms as regards social behaviour, drugs and alcohol and personal property. A lengthy criminal record is frequently seen, as he fails to learn from his experiences (Craft, 1966). Such a person may feel miserable and even suicidal when discovered in an unacceptable act, but this does not amount to the normal sense of feeling guilt. There is a failure to identify with the victim.

The definition of psychopathy proposed by Whiteley (1975) is as follows: the psychopath is an individual (a) who persistently behaves in a way that is not in accord with the accepted social norms of the culture or times in which he lives, (b) who appears to be unaware that his behaviour is seriously at fault and (c) whose abnormality cannot be readily explained as resulting from the 'madness' we commonly recognize nor from 'badness' alone.

Failure to plan ahead and failure to honour obligations, for example matrimonial or financial commitments, are repeated. There is a disregard for truth and also for safety, both for the individual himself and for others.

EMOTIONALLY UNSTABLE PERSONALITY DISORDER

Impulsive type

This personality disorder is not often encountered. The essential feature is liability to intemperate and uncontrolled outbursts of mood, most frequently violent anger but occasionally inconsolable grief, extreme anxiety or uproarious hilarity. It is usually aggressiveness that brings individuals with this disorder to the attention of the psychiatrist; with very slight provocation, they may have become irritable and on occasions violent. They are treated with extreme circumspection by other people, and their ill humour therefore becomes reinforced as it enables them to get their own way. They may exploit other people's fears of them to achieve their objectives, for example the arbitrarily violent husband whose wife is completely dominated by him through fear. Such personalities are disruptive and unpopular.

Those with this personality structure behave normally for most of the time and only occasionally explode in impulsive irritability, which is more common in younger people and may appear in either sex (Snaith and Taylor, 1985). In the system of classification advocated by Tyrer and Alexander, this personality type is not retained as distinct but combined with paranoid and asocial personality to form a category of *sociopathic personality disorder*.

Borderline type

This very confused diagnostic term has been used variously to describe a group of apparently neurotically disturbed patients who became psychotic while undergoing psychoanalysis; an enduring, unstable and vulnerable personality structure; and a group of patients who 'almost' had schizophrenia (Anonymous, 1986). It is considered that at least five of the following should be present for the diagnosis to be made (DSM-IV; American Psychiatric Association, 1994):

- frantic efforts to avoid real or imagined abandonment
- a pattern of unstable and intense interpersonal relationships
- identity disturbance in areas such as self-image, gender identity or long-term goals
- impulsivity or unpredictability in areas that are potentially self-damaging
- recurrent suicidal behaviour, gestures or threats or self-mutilating behaviour
- affective instability due to a marked reactivity of mood
- chronic feelings of emptiness
- inappropriate intense anger or difficulty in controlling anger
- transient, stress-related paranoid ideation or severe dissociative symptoms.

Although psychodynamically inclined psychiatrists have used this category extensively, there appears to be no phenomenological thread linking the very different criteria that are required for its diagnosis. Carrasco and Lecic-Tosevski (2000) have described it as the most controversial of all personality disorders and 'best understood as a heterogeneous syndrome manifested by egosyntonic affective instability and impulsivity (behavioural dys-control) and propensity to cognitive–perceptual distortions in the context of chronically unstable interpersonal relationships'.

HISTRIONIC PERSONALITY DISORDER

The word *histrionic* is derived from 'playing on the stage'; it is a better term than *hysterical* for this disorder, which is characterized by theatrical behaviour, craving for attention and excitement, excessive reaction to minor events and outbursts of mood, especially temper tantrums. In summarizing the descriptions of 22 different authors, De Alarcon (1973) found the greatest agreement for hysterical personality disorder in the following features: histrionic behaviour, egocentricity, emotional lability, excitability, dependency, suggestibility and seductiveness.

Characteristic of the disturbance of histrionic personality is the nature of relationships, with limited ability to experience profound affect and communicate such feelings. There is a shallowness and lability of emotion, and this is seen by others as lacking in genuineness, even though they are superficially charming – 'the life and soul of the party'. They form excellent and rapid acquaintanceships with new people, but they have great difficulty sustaining a close long-term, mutually rewarding, exclusive relationship.

Mood is fluctuating and inconsistent, and they display towards other people a craving for attention, affection and appreciation. They are seen as egocentric, self-indulgent and inconsiderate of others. There is often extreme but superficial involvement with many different people in a short space of time, and such a person is seen as being manipulative, vain and demanding; the manipulativeness is often ineffectual and self-destructive. They are often superficially found very attractive and achieve their short-term goals while being unable to sustain long-term relationships, for instance marriage frequently ends in divorce. They may be dependent and helpless, constantly seeking reassurance and the approval of others. Gestures of deliberate self-harm, hysterical conversion symptoms and abuse of alcohol and other drugs are common. Reactive depression is also frequently encountered, especially when a breakdown of relationships occurs. In a hospital study of those with hysterical personality disorder, Thompson (1980) found 83 per cent of subjects to be female; there was a clear association with neurotic depression, overdosage, self-mutilation, abuse of alcohol and a history of criminality and sometimes violence. Tyrer and Alexander do not regard this as a distinct personality disorder but combine it with dependent personality disorder in a category of *passive dependence*.

ANANKASTIC PERSONALITY DISORDER

Anankastic personality traits in moderate amount are valuable in society and for the success of the individual; they are frequently observed in professionals such as lawyers or doctors. However, when these are developed to an abnormal extent and interfere with the person's functioning, personality disorder is present and is characterized by perfectionism, rigidity, sensitivity, indecisiveness, a lack of capacity to express strongly felt emotion and excessive conscientiousness. The anankast's pervading sense of insecurity is associated with extreme self-doubt and feelings of sensitivity concerning how other people view him.

Perfectionism and excessive attention to detail interfere with the overall grasp of subjects or situations. There is gross preoccupation with rules, efficiency, trivial details, procedures and protocol. One patient was making lists of the lists she had previously set herself. She could not throw away a list until everything on it had been completed and, as some of the items on the lists were things that she wished to remind herself to do regularly, she was accumulating such an ever-increasing number of lists as to be unmanageable. Efficiency and perfection are aimed at, but the excessively detailed manner in which the attempt to achieve them is made undermines the possibility of success. Often, extreme orderliness in one area of life results in chaos in another, for example the medical practitioner who kept the top of his desk in immaculate tidiness but tipped all his case notes and other papers into the back of his car.

Rigidity in patterns of behaviour is characteristic. The individual values accuracy and thoroughness highly and respects other obsessional people for these qualities. He tends to keep fixed times and live to a regular programme, altered only with the greatest misgivings. These constraints are extended to other people in that he insists that they submit to his way of doing things. There is often a lack of awareness of the feelings in others evoked by his behaviour. This anankastic control of other people is typified by Mrs Ogmore-Pritchard in Dylan Thomas' *Under Milk Wood* (1954), who imposes on her dead husband the dictum 'I must put my pyjamas in the drawer marked pyjamas... I must take my cold bath which is good for me'.

The anankast is extremely sensitive to the criticism, real or suspected, of other people; the slightest censure is 'taken very much to heart'. This awareness of other people's opinion makes him a conformist, not prepared to step out of line, always wishing 'to keep up with the Joneses'. He is rigid, formal and self-controlled, not only in his public business but also at home and with his more intimate relationships. Insecurity about his abilities and his relationships makes the anankast indecisive. He doubts his own capacity and only too easily finds himself agreeing in secret with those who criticize him. He vacillates and has great difficulty in making choices, constantly looking at situations from different points of view, 'weighing up the pros and cons'. He often finds himself in a position of ambivalence and may overcompensate for this indecisiveness by making arbitrary decisions that then become immutable on insufficient evidence, or he may compensate for his legalistic rigidity by flaunting the law ostentatiously. Even in this, his basic obsessionality and perfectionism are still manifest. The anankast finds the initiation or completion of any activity very difficult, but hard work is highly prized, and he is therefore prepared to carry on the middle part of the task indefinitely.

The obsessional's need for formality, and his feelings of sensitivity about how other people view him, results in restricted ability to express tender emotion. He is unduly conventional, serious and formal. Stinginess may be shown both with money and with the expression of feelings. Such a person actually experiences very strong affect but is quite unable to express this appropriately towards other people.

The different facets of the anankastic personality disorder are, of course, interlocked. As traits of personality, they are seen very frequently, not least among members of the medical profession. However, developed as a personality disorder, this way of life may be incapacitating, especially the indecisiveness and inability to express strong emotion. Depression, obsessive–compulsive neurosis and hypochondriasis are not uncommonly associated with this abnormality of personality.

ANXIOUS (AVOIDANT) PERSONALITY DISORDER

This is a disorder of *trait*, while anxiety disorder is a disorder of *state* (see Chapter 19). There is often free-floating anxiety that is exacerbated by any overt predisposing cause. Such people often find the public side of life, for example at work, very much more stressful than the private side, within the family. *Trait* anxiety is present when the development of the individual's personality results in some level of abnormal anxiety being a persistent background part of their constitution (Sims and Snaith, 1988); this could alternatively be described as anxious temperament or anxiety-prone personality. Such people describe themselves as 'born worriers'.

This personality disorder is characterized by persistent and pervasive feelings of terror and apprehension; a belief that one is socially inept, unattractive or inferior; excessive preoccupation with criticism and rejection by others; hesitancy in new social relationships; restriction of lifestyle because of the need for security; and avoidance of those social situations that might provoke disapproval (ICD-10; World Health Organization, 1992).

DEPENDENT PERSONALITY DISORDER

The dependent personality is characterized by feelings of inadequacy concerning self and dependence on other people. There is gross lack of self-confidence, initiative and drive. Such a person is unable to react to the changing demands of life and allows other people, sometimes one other person, to assume responsibility for major areas of life. He may function reasonably well and appear inconspicuous when carried along through life by a dominant close relationship. However, when external stress occurs he lacks confidence and is unable to cope and craves long-term support and encouragement from relatives, a close friend, his family doctor, his social worker, his minister, his employer or his surrounding social organizations. He may, for example, flourish in the armed forces but be unable to adjust to civilian life.

Such people tend to go through life with one dominant dependent relationship; for a man, this may be initially his mother and subsequently his wife, who takes over his mother's role. Crises resulting in psychiatric referral may occur when a parent dies or becomes incapable, his marriage breaks down, he loses his job, after detection in crime or following physical illness. It is usually only after such situations that a person with this type of personality disorder comes to the attention of the caring professions. Dependence amounts to passive compliance with the aims and demands of the more dominant partner. There is a lack of vigour in maintaining aims and goals and in attempting to achieve these. They may describe themselves as depressed, but it is more a feeling of inertia and an inability to cope with their problems than the symptoms of affective disorder.

PERSISTENT MOOD DISORDERS

In ICD-9 (World Health Organization, 1977), these conditions were classified as disorder of personality. However, in ICD-10 they have been listed as a subcategory of affective disorders because they are genetically related to mood disorders and sometimes respond to the same methods of treatment. They are retained in this chapter because they conform with the psychopathology of personality disorders. Akiskal (1993) has made a convincing case for depressive personality to be returned to the generic category of personality disorders rather than being classified with *axis 1 mood (affective) disorders*. There is a persistent lifelong abnormality of mood, not amounting to illness, as opposed to those reactive or endogenous disturbances of affect that are of shorter duration and are regarded as illness. The most frequent types of affective personality disorder show excessive lability of mood or persistent depressive stance towards life. Other abnormalities of personality may occur, such as persistent hypomania, but these rarely present to the psychiatrist.

Those with *cyclothymia* show marked fluctuations of mood, for instance for a day or a week they may be optimistic, energetic, creative and garrulous, then for a period they may become gloomy, morose, taciturn and unable to turn themselves to any useful activity. These cycles may be linked to other biological rhythms such as the menstrual cycle; they may, however, appear out of the blue, apparently unprovoked. A premorbid cyclothymic personality is thought to predispose to manic–depressive psychosis. Certainly, Goodwin and Jamison (1990), in a study of manic–depressive illness and creativity, found that among poets especially there was an excess of cyclothymic personality, depressive illness and suicide.

Dysthymia is manifested by all-pervasive and permanent gloom and apprehension. It leads to the diagnostic quandary 'Is this depressive state or depressive trait?' Such people are usually gentle and sensitive; they take themselves and their activities seriously; they are often safety-conscious and hypochondriacal. An acquaintance with this personality structure coined aphorisms that revealed his mental state, such as 'there is no situation in life so bad as to be incapable of further deterioration' or 'every silver lining has its cloud'.

OTHER PERSONALITY DISORDERS

DSM-IV (American Psychiatric Association, 1994) includes two other personality disorders. They are described below, in brief, for completeness.

Narcissistic personality disorder

This is categorized by a grandiose sense of self-importance or uniqueness; preoccupation with fantasies of unlimited success, power, brilliance, beauty or ideal love; an exhibitionistic need for constant attention and admiration; indifference, anger or humiliation in response to criticism or indifference from others; and characteristic disturbances in interpersonal relationships, such as feelings of entitlement to special favours, taking advantage of other people, relationships with others that alternate between the extremes of over-idealization and devaluation, and lack of empathy.

Avoidant personality disorder

This personality disorder is, in fact, very close to the anxious personality disorder of ICD-10; it is characterized by excessive sensitivity to rejection, humiliation or shame. There is unwillingness to enter into a relationship unless the person receives strong guarantees of uncritical acceptance. There is social withdrawal, despite a need for affection and acceptance, and the person has very low self-esteem, devaluing his own achievements, and is very aware of his personal shortcomings. Such people are exquisitely sensitive to the way they believe others will react to them.

In DSM-IV, the helpful notion of three *clusters* of personality types is based on descriptive similarities. Cluster A includes *paranoid, schizoid and schizotypal personality disorders*. In cluster B are *antisocial, borderline, histrionic and narcissistic personality disorders*. Cluster C contains *avoidant, dependent and obsessive–compulsive personality disorders*. In practice, of course, patients may show features from different clusters, and the validity of this subclassification is still being questioned.

Why is a text on psychopathology concerned with personality classification and disorder? The accurate observation and delineation of personality characteristics is valuable in clinical practice for diagnosis, prognosis and the rational planning of treatment. The skills of a trained psychopathologist are ideally suited to the observation of consistent personality traits and forming an opinion unprejudiced by preconceived theoretical considerations.

REFERENCES

[Anonymous] (1986) Management of borderline personality disorders [leading article]. *Lancet ii*, 846–7.

Akiskal HS (1993) Proposal for a depressive personality (temperament). In Tyrer P and Stein G (eds) *Personality Disorder Reviewed*. London: Gaskell.

American Psychiatric Association (1994) *Diagnostic and Statistical Manual of Mental Disorders*, 4th edn. Washington: American Psychiatric Association.

Bluglass RS (1983) *A Guide to the Mental Health Act, 1983*. Edinburgh: Churchill Livingstone.

Carrasco JL and Lecic-Tosevski D (2000) Specific types of personality disorder. In Gelder M, López-Ibor JJ and Andreasen NC (eds) *New Oxford Textbook of Psychiatry*. Oxford: Oxford University Press.

Chick J, Waterhouse L and Wolff S (1979) Psychological construing in schizoid children grown up. *British Journal of Psychiatry 135*, 425–30.

Cleckley HM (1941) *The Mask of Sanity*. London: Kingston.

Craft M (1966) *Psychopathic Disorders*. Oxford: Pergamon Press.

De Alarcon RD (1973) Hysteria and hysterical personality disorder. *Psychiatric Quarterly 47*, 258–75.

Dolan B and Coid J (1993) *Psychopathic and Antisocial Personality Disorders: Treatment and Research Issues*. London: Gaskell.

Goodwin FK and Jamison KR (1990) *Manic–depressive Illness*. New York: Oxford University Press.

Haddock A, Snowden P, Dolan M, Parker J and Rees H (2001) Managing dangerous people with severe personality disorder: a survey of forensic psychiatrists' opinions. *Psychiatric Bulletin 25*, 293–6.

Henderson DK (1939) *Psychopathic States.* New York: Norton.
Hinshaw SP (1994) *Attention Deficits and Hyperactivity in Children.* Thousand Oaks: Sage Publications.
Malmberg A, Lewis G, David A and Allebeck P (1998) Premorbid adjustment and personality in people with schizophrenia. *British Journal of Psychiatry 172,* 308–13.
Mill JS (1811) *A System of Logic Volume II,* 3rd edn. London: John W. Parker.
Mullen PE (1999) Dangerous people with severe personality disorder. *British Medical Journal 319,* 1146–7.
Prichard JC (1835) *A Treatise on Insanity and Other Disorders Affecting the Mind.* London: Sherwood, Gilbert & Piper.
Rush B (1812) *Medical Inquiries and Observations Upon the Diseases of the Mind.* Philadelphia: Kimber & Richardson.
Schneider K (1923) *Psychopathic Personalities* (transl. Hamilton MW, 1958). London: Cassell.
Schneider K (1958) *Clinical Psychopathology,* 5th edn (transl. Hamilton MW, 1959). New York: Grune & Stratton.
Sims ACP (1983) *Neurosis in Society.* Basingstoke: Macmillan.
Sims A and Snaith R (1988) *Anxiety in Clinical Practice.* Chichester: John Wiley.
Snaith RP and Taylor CM (1985) Irritability: definition, assessment and associated factors. *British Journal of Psychiatry 147,* 127–36.
Standage KF (1979) The use of Schneider's typology for the diagnosis of personality disorder – an examination of reliability. *British Journal of Psychiatry 135,* 238–42.
Tantam D (1988) Personality disorders. In Granville-Grossman K (ed.) *Recent Advances in Clinical Psychiatry,* no. 6. Edinburgh: Churchill Livingstone.
Thomas D (1954) *Under Milk Wood.* London: Dent.
Thompson DJ (1980) *A comprehensive study of hysterical personality disorder.* MSc Thesis, University of Manchester.
Tyrer P and Alexander J (1979) Classification of personality disorder. *British Journal of Psychiatry 135,* 163–7.
Tyrer P and Stein G (1993) *Personality Disorder Reviewed.* London: Gaskell.
Whiteley JS (1975) The psychopath and his treatment. In Silverstone T and Barraclough B (eds) *Contemporary Psychiatry.* Ashford: Headley Brothers.
Wooton BF (1959) *Social Science and Social Pathology.* London: Allen & Unwin.
World Health Organization (1977) *International Statistical Classification of Diseases, Injuries and Causes of Death,* 9th revision. Geneva: World Health Organization.
World Health Organization (1992) *The ICD-10 Classification of Mental and Behavioural Disorders: Clinical Description and Diagnostic Guidelines.* Geneva: World Health Organization.

Psychopathology of Neurotic Disorders

22

> “The poor girl lived beneath a stethoscope, and bore all their pokings and tappings with exquisite patience. She herself believed that she was dying, and so she repeatedly told her mother. Mrs Woodward could only say that all was in God's hands, but that the physicians still encouraged them to hope the best. *Anthony Trollope (1858),* The Three Clerks

Throughout this book, there have been allusions to different 'neurotic' or non-psychotic symptoms and syndromes. It seemed useful at this stage to draw some of the various threads together, as there does appear to be, psychopathologically, a common core to neurotic thinking and behaviour. *Neurotic disorders*, using the term generically, are enormously diverse, and one cannot hope in a short space to do more than point out some of the broad outlines of their descriptive psychopathology. They are the most common of the conditions presenting to the psychiatrist and far and away the most common psychiatric presentation to general practitioners or hospital specialists other than psychiatrists. Neurosis is an important factor in influencing social relationships at all levels, although it may not be obvious to the doctor that that is an underlying problem; it affects communication in families, offices, factories, schools, hospitals and all other institutions and segments of society.

THE TERM *NEUROSIS*

The term *neuroses* was introduced into the English language by Cullen (1784) 'to describe all those preternatural affections of sense and motion ... which do not depend upon a topical affection of the organs, but upon a more general affection of the nervous system, and of those powers of the system upon which sense and motion more especially depend'. Neurosis can be defined as 'a psychological reaction to acute or continuous perceived stress, expressed in emotion or behaviour ultimately inappropriate in dealing with that stress' (Sims, 1983). Of course, the individual suffering the neurotic disorder may not perceive the stress in the same way or even as having the same nature as an outside observer, but he undoubtedly experiences stress, uncomfortable pressure or conflict. One young man described his situation as intolerable at work: 'it's not surprising I'm anxious, everyone is getting at me all the time, they are always chivvying and harassing me'. In fact, his employer described his chronic indecisiveness as having a major deleterious effect on his performance and said that he required a great deal of encouragement to get anything done at all. Other related terms, such as *hysteria* (Jordern, 1603), *hypochondriasis* (Sydenham, 1682) and *neurasthenia* (Beard, 1880), have a long history.

Objectively, then, neurotic behaviour is carried out as a response to the stimulus of a problem or source of conflict that requires resolving; however, the particular behaviour manifested is inappropriate in solving that problem. Subjectively, the neurotic subject describes himself as being either unable to cope or coping only with supreme effort and considerable distress. All of us occasionally show neurotic behaviour and suffer neurotic thoughts. In the neurotic *state*, however, these inappropriate thoughts and behaviours have become habitual, the response is out of proportion to the stimulus and all actions become tinged with this neurotic failure; the person with a neurotic disorder comes to see all his problems through neurotic eyes and so all difficulties become insurmountable – 'the tyranny of the inevitable'.

Neurosis is chameleon-like in its presentation: it takes on the predominant colouring of the culture or organization in which it occurs. Only rarely do we see nowadays the grosser manifestations of hysteria that seemed to be so common in Charcot's day, although such cases are more common in developing countries. The 'housebound' housewife or agoraphobic presentation of phobic neurosis appeared almost to reach epidemic proportions in the 1960s and 1970s (Buglass *et al.*, 1977), while disordered eating behaviour, especially bulimia nervosa, became extremely common in the 1980s and 1990s. Chronic fatigue syndrome, which was so common under the rubric *neurasthenia* in the past, is seen frequently once again in the present (Lawrie and Pelosi, 1994). The type of behaviour manifested tends to be appropriate to the source of help the sufferer wishes to enlist: somatic symptoms are usually presented to the general practitioner; problems in coping with financial matters and interpersonal conflicts to the social worker; and feelings of guilt, personal inadequacy and doubts to the minister of religion. However, the constellation of problems in the way the neurotic subject evaluates himself, relates to other people and copes with his environment may be similar in all three different presentations.

THE DEBATE ON TERMINOLOGY AND CLASSIFICATION

Even now, the term *neurosis* holds widely different meanings for different psychiatrists. As a broad generalization, in Europe it has been contrasted with *psychosis* so that psychosis is present in those disorders in which reality judgement is significantly disturbed, whereas in the majority of cases in which it is not, neurosis is present. In North America the word neurosis was understood to have psychodynamic connotations with the implicit presence of unconscious conflict, and the term was therefore abandoned in the third edition of the *Diagnostic and Statistical Manual*, DSM-III (American Psychiatric Association, 1980). In the ninth edition of the *International Classification of Diseases*, ICD-9 (World Health Organization, 1977), neurosis was used as a generic term to include anxiety states, hysteria, phobic state, obsessive–compulsive disorders, neurotic depression, neurasthenia, depersonalization syndrome, hypochondriasis and 'other neurotic disorders'. 'Neurotic disorders' were part of a larger, generic category that also included 'personality disorders, sexual deviations and disorders, alcohol dependence syndrome, drug dependence, non-dependent abuse of drugs, physiological malfunctioning arising from mental factors, special symptoms or syndromes not elsewhere classified, acute reaction to stress and adjustment reaction'. The generic nature of neurosis became somewhat attenuated in ICD-10 (World Health Organization, 1992); in particular, what was previously called *neurotic depression* has become separated from other neurotic disorders and submerged within 'mood (affective) disorders'. One can safely predict that many of what are now classified as affective disorders will ultimately be returned to this generic grouping, although probably under different names.

There is still a need for a generic term to cover the various features that neurotic disorders hold in common and that are different from other psychiatric conditions. The individual neurotic disorders are not fundamentally distinct from each other, and many cases cross over from one neurotic diagnosis to another over time (Tyrer, 1985). The methods of treatment and provision of services are held in common for many neurotic disorders but are quite different from other conditions, both psychotic and physical (Sims, 1985). There are intermediate and mixed cases, which belie the spuriously clear definitions between individual neurotic diagnoses (Gelder, 1986). As well as these practical and administrative distinctions between neurosis and other psychiatric disorders, there do appear also to be psychopathological and phenomenological distinctions, which are described later.

One of the unfortunate consequences of eliminating the concept of neurosis as a distinct generic term has been the need to introduce the alternative term *comorbidity*. Increasingly in recent research on the conditions that used to be subsumed within neurosis, authors repeatedly refer to the fact that the condition (generalized anxiety disorder, panic disorder, dysthymia, etc.) is frequently complicated and hence exacerbated by comorbidity with other neurotic conditions (Sims, 1992). The finding, regularly reciprocated in these papers, is that neurotic disorders show protean manifestations, with sometimes different neurotic syndromes occurring in the same patient at different times and sometimes concurring in the same patient at the same time.

Depression and neurosis

Different schools of psychiatric thought have either emphasized the unitary nature of depressive illness or the dichotomy between endogenous, psychotic, biological types of depression and reactive, neurotic, psychosocial conditions. There are undoubtedly many cases in which no distinction is possible, either because they are between the two extremes or because they have many positive features of both types of depression. Equally, there is a very clear qualitative difference between typical examples at the two extremes of the dichotomy. It is not the function of this account to enter into the merits of these two approaches.

It is important to note that coexisting depressive symptomatology may be present with any of those disorders that are designated 'neurotic, stress-related and somatoform disorders' in ICD-10 (World Health Organization 1992: 132). Thus *anxiety disorder*, be it phobic, generalized, or panic disorder, *obsessive–compulsive* disorder, *reactions to severe stress*, *dissociative* and *somatoform disorders*, *neurasthenia* and *depersonalization* may all occur with mild, moderate or severe degrees of depression; they may also occur in virtually any combination with each other. Depression is particularly likely when the neurotic disorder is chronic, severe or both; depression may result from the loss of self-esteem due to experiencing the symptoms, from the disturbance in relationships that comes from neurotic disability or from the underlying conflicts that are responsible for the neurotic disturbance. When depressive symptomatology of any degree of severity is found to occur with other neurotic symptoms, then, in using ICD-10 as a diagnostic classification, both diagnoses should be made.

Neurosis and personality disorder

Whereas a single episode of neurotic behaviour occurs when an act in response to a stressor is carried out in a way that is inappropriate to deal with that stress or its consequences, *neurotic disorder* could be said to occur when there is a pattern of behaviour or thinking that is maladaptive in resolving conflicts in response to a continuing stress, a repeated similar stress or several different types of stress. An example of a single episode of neurotic behaviour could be the husband who breaks down his own front door with his fists because his wife locks him out. Neurotic illness might be shown in a spouse responding inappropriately but consistently to the long-term stress of an unsatisfactory marriage, for instance in several acts of self-poisoning. Alternatively, repeated stresses of a similar nature, such as sitting examinations, may provoke anxiety state, or dissimilar but stressful stimuli accumulate, leading to neurotic reaction. Contrasted with these *reactions* or *states* as an episodic condition interfering with a normal pattern of life is neurotic personality, neuroticism, abnormality of personality or personality disorder as a lifelong characteristic. In these latter conditions, similarly inappropriate behaviour occurs in the context of a lifelong pattern, so the anxious, sensitive schoolboy who shows school refusal and anxiety when threatened with separation from his mother may develop into the anxious avoidant employee who responds to threats and challenges at work by repeated absences with minor ailments.

Thus the self-experience of neurotic thinking and behaviour is similar to that of personality abnormality and disorder; the difference is more in the duration, severity and appropriateness. Clearly, a person who has experienced low self-esteem and sensitive feelings and ideas concerning the criticism of other people for the whole of his adult life is likely to be more intractable to treatment and to have more severe symptoms than a person who has manifested such thought and behaviour for only a few months.

DESCRIPTIVE PSYCHOPATHOLOGY OF NEUROSES

In neurotic disorder, there is no fundamental disturbance in reality judgement and yet the individual persists in behaviour and in patterns of thought that are counterproductive in achieving that individual's own goals, aspirations and sources of enjoyment and comfort. Although the reasons for this are outside the scope of this book, the way in which this neurotic thinking and behaviour cause disturbance in the whole person and in the functioning of each part is relevant. If one briefly reviews the functions of descriptive psychopathology, as amplified in the chapters of this book, it can be shown how neurotic disorder is global, affecting all these functions.

Consciousness

Normal consciousness was contrasted with three quite different meanings of unconsciousness in Chapter 3: coma, deep sleep and the unconscious mind. Coma and its lesser stages of clouding, drowsiness and sopor occur with organic impairment of the brain; a neurotic disorder may coexist but cannot be the cause of this type of alteration in consciousness.

It was recounted in the *Times* (1994) that every time a woman from Cincinnati, who was suffering from hysterical conversion disorder, heard the word 'sex', even if spelt out with the individual letters, she fell down in a faint. It was claimed that a man, knowing of this response, had whispered the word sex and raped her while she was immobile; at the ensuing court case, proceedings were repeatedly interrupted by her lapses into unconsciousness whenever sex was mentioned, necessarily quite often. This exemplifies how neurotic disorder of dissociative type may result in temporary unconsciousness that may be indistinguishable from that with organic aetiology.

Impairment of attention and concentration also occurs very frequently with various neurotic disorders. Active, voluntary attention may be impaired by severe background anxiety or by persistent depressive affect. Concentration may be disturbed by feelings of self-reference, sensitivity and low self-esteem; it may also be interfered with by persistent unproductive daydreaming. It is, for example, one of the symptoms listed under 'increased arousal' in post-traumatic stress disorder.

As discussed in Chapter 4, sleep is a function that is almost universally disturbed in the course of neurotic disorder. Complaints of disturbed sleep, restlessness at night, inability to get to sleep and poor quality of sleep when it is at last achieved are frequently made by patients with anxiety disorders, reactive depression and other neurotic disorders. Unpleasant dreams and nightmares are also a frequent complaint. Sleep disorder is often associated with unpleasant feelings of sleepiness, impaired concentration and diminished alertness during the day.

Memory and time

Affective and psychogenic disturbance of memory is described in Chapter 5. Both organic and psychological factors may result in impairment of memory. Selective forgetting and falsification of memory are the result of the strong influence of the affective state on the processes of memory, especially recall for previously registered and retained information. In dissociative fugue in the Ganser state, and in multiple personality disorder (dissociative identity disorder, DSM-IV; American Psychiatric Association, 1994), there is amnesia subsequently for the time during which the individual was acting and thinking abnormally. There may be lesser degrees of dissociation in which the amnesia is not total but the state of consciousness appears to be altered.

There may also be affective and neurotic disturbances of time and time sense. The underlying emotional state and the satisfaction and enjoyment with which an activity is associated will affect the judgement made on its duration, hence the expression 'doesn't time fly when you're having fun?' Alongside so many other situational causes of anxiety, anxious patients also complain about pressures of time and their being anxious in that sphere. Depressed patients may complain of wasted time, loss of time, encroaching doom and other symptoms that demonstrate both disturbance concerned with time and the underlying affective change. Depersonalization is also associated with altered time sense, for example time 'standing still' and feeling oneself to be 'outside time'.

Perception

Sensory distortions and false perceptions may both occur with neurotic disorder and especially with disturbances of affect such as anxiety, fear, irritability or depression. There may be changes in the intensity of perception, for example objects appearing to be dull or lustreless with depression. There are often changes in the feelings associated with perception, especially with depersonalization: 'I can see everybody else quite clearly but they seem to be a million miles away from me'. Affective illusion is frequently associated with states of increased anxiety including persistent free-floating anxiety in generalized anxiety disorders. 'True' hallucinations do not occur with neurotic disorder alone but, as is made clear in Chapter 7, the distinction between hallucination and pseudohallucination and vivid imagery may on occasions be difficult to determine.

Ideation, thinking and speech

Although true, or primary, delusions do not occur when neurotic disorder is the sole diagnosis, various other types of pathological ideation are experienced. Overvalued idea is quite often associated with hypochondriasis and also with other disorders in which neurotic thinking is prominent, such as dysmorphophobia, anorexia nervosa, transsexualism and personality disorder, especially of paranoid type. Similarly paranoid, self-referent ideas are frequently associated with the low self-esteem and sensitivity occurring frequently with both neurotic and personality disorders.

The thinking process may be disturbed among those suffering from neurotic symptoms in that undirected fantasy thinking may dominate consciousness, resulting in subjective feelings of fear, inadequacy and dissatisfaction and objectively in a lack of appropriate behaviour to solve current problems. Persistent daydreams may, rarely, be confused with reality and acted on. This abnormality is intimately connected with the disturbances of self-concept, and especially loss of self-esteem, which is so prominent among those who are neurotically disordered. Cognitive factors concerning both the nature of self and the traumatic experience are of great significance in post-traumatic stress disorder (Dunmore *et al.*, 1999).

Abnormality of speech may occur in those suffering from neuroses, although the aphasias of disturbed brain function and the grosser forms of schizophrenic language disorder are not seen. Mutism is a not uncommon dissociative symptom, and speech usually returns when the immediate conflicts have been resolved. Neurotic disturbance affecting attention, concentration and motivation may produce temporary disturbance in intellectual performance so that individuals who are affected may perform at work or in study well below their intellectual capacity.

Volition and behaviour

All the functions of urge, drive, will, impulse and behaviour may be affected by neurotic thinking and the resultant disturbance in self-evaluation and relationships. Problems in this realm particularly result from conflicts in which the subject feels constrained to act in different directions from his own wishes, resulting in either frustrated inactivity or inappropriate actions that fail to solve the underlying problems.

Chronic fatigue syndrome is an area of concern and debate that has become more prominent in recent years (Natelson, 2001). One area of conflict is whether chronic fatigue syndrome (sometimes known previously as myalgic encephalomyelitis) is a physical or mental illness. Lawrie and Pelosi (1994) find this dilemma incomprehensible semantically, because the distinction between physical and psychological is unhelpful, unnecessary and ultimately counterproductive. The usual outcome of the syndrome is quite long-term disturbance of function; with a mean follow-up of 3.2 years, only 6 of 139 subjects had no symptoms. Psychological factors such as illness attitudes and coping styles were more important predictors of long-term outcome than immunological or demographic variables (Wilson *et al.*, 1994).

PHENOMENOLOGY OF NEUROTIC DISORDER

Psychopathological functions of neurotic disorder resulting from neurotic thinking occur in the areas of:

- self-experience
- disturbance of mood
- bodily symptoms
- experience of relationships.

These abnormalities give rise to the characteristic phenomenology of neurotic disorder (Sims, 1991).

Phenomenology attempts to delineate the inner world, the subjective experience of the neurotic patient. Whereas psychotic thinking is, in the terminology of Jaspers (1959), ultimately ununderstandable, neurotic thinking and behaviour, however inappropriate and socially unacceptable, are understandable when the doctor talks with his patient in detail, exploring subjective space, so that the doctor might say, 'if I had been in that situation with that past experience, I can understand how I could have done (felt) that'. It should be possible to make the distinction between what is regarded as neurotic experience and behaviour and what is not on phenomenological grounds. That is, we should be able to obtain from the patient himself an account of how the motivation for the action or the manner in which it was carried out was inappropriate in achieving his own immediate or long-term life goals. This will not necessarily be presented by the patient with a logical, methodical or objective explanation but in his attribution of how things have gone wrong because of circumstances outside his control. This may be approached from the perspective of *attributional theory* (Antaki and Brewin, 1981), or the way the individual structures his world, past experiences, *attitudes* and *cognitions* and the effect this has on present mood state (Beck, 1967), or in terms of *locus of control*, in which the subject showing neurotic thinking believes that control is external to himself (Rotter, 1966). In all these ways, the person with continuing neurotic thinking believes that there is no way in which he can change his circumstances – the *tyranny of inevitability*. This vitally affects the manner in which the neurotic subject considers himself to be responsible for his thoughts and actions. At the same time he is responsible for his behaviour, in that his reality judgement is not disturbed nor are there psychotic symptoms, but his belief is that his own freedom of action is severely limited.

Self-experience

The disturbance of self-experience in neurotic disorder varies very considerably both in severity and in form. Different neurotic disorders, however, tend to have in common consistent and chronic low self-esteem with impaired judgement of the sufferer's own personal capabilities. This results either in chronic indecision and an inability to initiate appropriate corrective activity, or in hasty unconsidered activity undertaken with the expectation that it will be unsuccessful. There is anxious deprecatory over-involvement with self; pessimistic self-absorption that proceeds to fear of failure, resulting in inability to control adverse emotions and attitudes causing guilt, shame and resentment; and consequent loss of confidence in self, with further pessimistic self-absorption. This cycle of *demoralization* (Figure 22.1) has been described by Frank (1974). Self-devaluation causes further demoralization. The

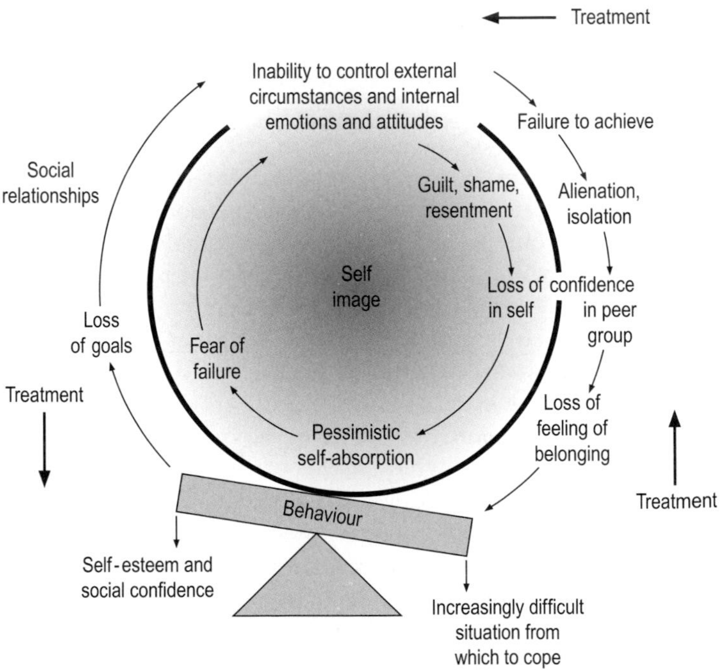

Figure 22.1 Cycle of demoralization.

disturbance of self-image is often associated with distortion of body image in which the person perceives himself as unattractive; this further contributes to low self-esteem.

The dimensions of self-awareness, described by Jaspers and Scharfetter, have been discussed in Chapter 13: being, activity, unity, identity and the boundaries of self. Each of these may be disordered neurotically, and this differs markedly from the nature of disorder seen in schizophrenic illness, in which passivity is often the dominant feature.

Awareness of one's essential being is disturbed in the symptom of depersonalization. Typically, there is a loss of feelings about oneself that are normally taken for granted: 'I feel unreal ... feel *as if* I don't exist ... I feel like a cardboard cut-out, an automaton'.

Awareness of activity may be disordered in the neurotic individual: 'my actions are my own but I have no freedom of action. I am constrained by external circumstances, by things outside myself'. This is exemplified by the individual who accumulates debts and is quite unable to initiate any appropriate action to deal with this and even may attempt, and complete, suicide rather than sort out the underlying circumstances, which may, in fact, have been amenable to remedial action.

Awareness of unity may be disturbed in neurosis either with *dissociative identity disorder* (*multiple personality disorder*) or with the *double phenomenon*. The individual may describe himself as having more than one personality, experiencing different aspects of himself, which, although both are acknowledged as self, seem to be in conflict with each other; or he (or more often she) may be apparently unaware of quite different 'personalities' resident within his or her body.

Awareness of identity may reveal itself in neurotic disorder in a person who describes himself thus: 'I am irretrievably flawed because throughout my life everything has conspired against me and is outside my control'. He feels a sense of discontinuity with his past and has no feeling of confidence about his role and his performance in the future.

Awareness of the boundaries of self may be disturbed in neurosis: the individual retains the sense of definition of self, but there is a feeling of loss of capacity to influence the outside world and a corresponding feeling of the outside world impinging on him whether he wishes it or not.

Disturbance of mood

In their description of *subclinical neurosis syndrome*, Taylor and Chave (1964) listed the fundamental symptoms as 'nerves, depression, undue irritability and sleeplessness'. Thus, emotional disorder has always been seen as a prominent part of neurosis, especially anxiety, depression and irritability. Depersonalization is also an important symptom that has an affective component. With feelings of *self-reference*, the individual *feels* himself to be the object of adverse attention, and this results in sensitivity regarding other people's attitudes towards his self-presentation and behaviour.

The depression that occurs with neurotic disorder has been described in more detail in Chapter 18; depression is the emotion of the experience of loss.

Four different psychopathological variants of *anxiety* may be listed:

- generalized diffused anxiety, as described a century ago by Freud (1895)
- situational anxiety or phobia, with either external stimuli, as in agoraphobia, or internal stimuli with illness phobia
- panic disorder or episodic anxiety
- the anxiety that invariably occurs with post-traumatic stress disorder and related conditions.

Anxiety is described in more detail in Chapter 19. Snaith and Taylor (1985) have described irritability, which is also dealt with in Chapter 19.

The relationship of the mood of depression to neurotic disorders has been much disputed. Tyrer (1989) has grappled with the difficult distinction of anxiety from depression in psychiatric classification. He has introduced the term *general neurotic syndrome* to cover 'the demonstration of primary anxiety and depressive symptoms that show changes in primacy at different times, are manifest in the absence of major life events and which commonly occur against a background of personality disturbance in which dependent and/or inhibited qualities are prominent'.

Bodily symptoms

An account has been given in Chapter 15 of how bodily symptoms may occur without physical illness. Among neurotic conditions, physical symptoms may play a prominent part in dissociative disorders, especially in the manifestation of motor disorders, convulsions, anaesthesia and other sensory loss; in somatoform disorders with somatization, hypochondriasis and persistent somatoform pain disorder; and also in dysmorphophobia. Such conditions have to be distinguished from what ICD-10 calls *elaboration of physical symptoms for psychological reasons and intentional production or feigning of symptoms or disabilities, either physical or psychological* (factitious disorder) (World Health Organization, 1992: 222). These disorders of body awareness and physical symptoms have been described in earlier chapters and will not be discussed further.

Disturbance of the experience of relationships

Fundamental to the neurotic condition is a disturbance in relationships and the manner in which the individual sufferer experiences this. All areas of life may be affected, including work, sexual, marital and family relationships and external circumstances such as social status, financial situation, criminal activity and establishing and maintaining friendships. The characteristic disturbance in relationships of neurotic disorder has been given the term *anophelia* by Henderson *et al.* (1981): 'a state of real or perceived deficiency in relationships ... a state of not receiving care, concern, comfort, interest or support from others'. This characteristic has been quantified in terms of (a) fewer people available for attachment, (b) those who are available are perceived as having lower adequacy for attachment, (c) there is less availability of congenial people for social interaction and (d) a lower perceived adequacy in this area. With severely neurotically disordered individuals, there is lack of availability and low perceived adequacy in all social relationships. This disturbance in the ability for congenial relationship is illustrated by C. Day Lewis in the poem with which Chapter 14 started.

The manner in which satisfactory relationships reinforce the sense of well-being of the individual is well exemplified by Francis Bacon, who wrote,

> "But one thing is most admirable, which is that this community of a man's self to his friends works two contrary effects; for it redoubleth joys and cuts griefs in half. For there is no man that imparteth his joys to his friends, but that he joyeth the more; and no man that imparteth his grief to his friend but he grieveth the less.

Clearly, when relationships fail there is failure in all other areas of adaptation.

The social and relationship consequences of neurotic thinking tend to be acted out in decisions affecting life course, especially in early adulthood. These decisions, which have been made neurotically, vitally affect all subsequent activity for the rest of life. A number of adverse factors, such as precipitation of the condition by marital, sexual, family or occupational problems, long duration of illness or development of illness in those aged under 20 and coexisting personality disorder or abnormality in such people tend to come together at this age and then become self-perpetuating (Sims, 1975). The tyranny of inevitability, the lack of feeling of capacity to control outside circumstances, low self-esteem and failure of relationships all concur to produce a reinforcing vicious circle that is likely to perpetuate itself. For instance, both in the work record and in the marital and social relationships of the individual, adverse factors combine to produce a downward spiral of impaired social functioning (Figure 22.2).

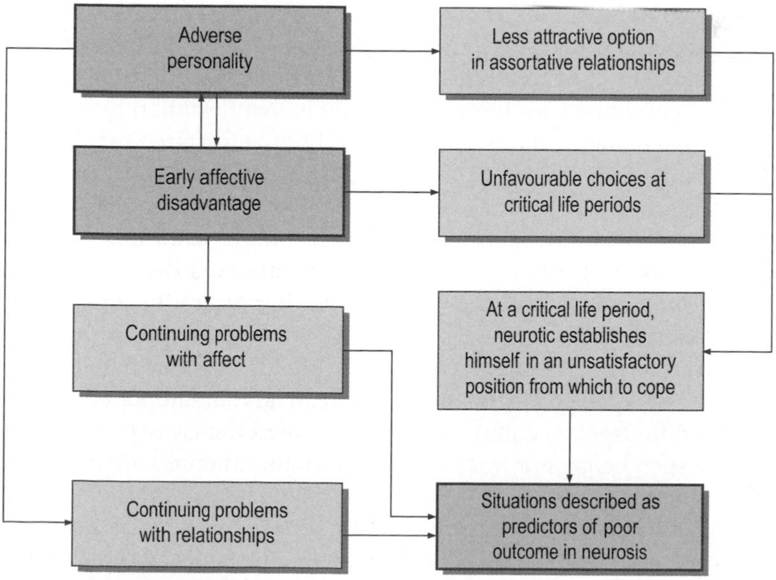

Figure 22.2 Neurotic paradigm.

As far as work is concerned, the paradigm would indicate that an individual, because of his personality problems, is seen as a less desirable person to employ and therefore obtains a post that is inferior to what could be expected from his qualifications. At the same time, because of an unsatisfactory childhood, he escapes his family background as early as possible, for example perhaps by joining the armed services even though he is not suited to this. Because of this unsatisfactory job that does not match his abilities, he becomes established in a work situation that consistently produces further problems. Personality problems persist into adult life with continuing relationship difficulties, an unhappy childhood progresses to misery in early adult life, and these together compound the existing work problems to cause further difficulties and subjective experience of dissatisfaction at work. The paradigm can be worked through in a similar way for marital relationships and partnerships.

This subjective feeling of problems with relationships is experienced in the different categories of neurotic disorder. For example, a schoolteacher in her thirties with anxiety disorder, depersonalization, post-traumatic stress disorder and depression described her feelings about other people since the onset of her condition thus: 'I am not really connecting with people and events and it is as if one is going through the motions ... kind of numbness ... being with people and looking at things from the outside rather than being part of it'. There is considerable variation in the precise description, but the common thread is difficulty in personal relationships at a greater level and of a different nature compared with before the illness.

CULTURAL VARIATION

All psychiatric conditions are modified in their manifestation by the wider culture and peer group pressures on the individual, but none more so than neurotic disorders. This has been demonstrated with epidemiological precision in the classical paper by Rawnsley and Loudon (1964) on the evaluation of islanders from Tristan da Cunha following an earthquake. Some conditions have been described that are found only within certain cultures, for example among the anxiety disorders *koro* (Kiev, 1972) or *brain fag syndrome* (Guinness, 1992). Other conditions are influenced in their manifestation by local cultural changes and the demands met on the individual sufferer by those around him: the 'housebound housewife' presentation of phobic disorder became especially common when young mothers from close-knit families were moved to new housing estates distant from their own mother and family of origin.

One has to be extremely careful not to assume patterns of behaviour and expression to be evidence of mental illness and collect recurring themes into syndromes simply because the observer does not understand the cultural background. Bartholomew (1994) has commented that 'examples of this bias include the mislabelling of dancing manias, tarantism and demonopathy in Europe since the Middle Ages as culture-specific variants of mass psychogenic illness'. Episodes of such behaviour 'may involve normal, rational people who possess unfamiliar conduct codes, world views and political agendas'.

Although the *content* of specific cultural conditions may be geographically localized and may differ markedly from the content of conditions appearing elsewhere, the *form* of these neurotic disorders is remarkably uniform. Thus the ascription given by patients in different cultures for the cause of their symptoms will vary according to the environment (demons, the bosses, increased maintenance for second family), but the symptoms of anxiety, for example both physical and psychological, are broadly similar. When the stresses on people in different cultures are examined epidemiologically, it has often been found that although the nature of the stress in precise terms, the content, varies very greatly, the total emotional impact of stress is surprisingly similar between different cultures. It was found, for example, in Taiwan that a higher risk of minor psychiatric morbidity was present among women with chronic stressors than others in a large community sample; acute life events predicted the presence of such morbidity (Cheng, 1989a). It appeared that chronic psychosocial stressors had a stronger effect in female subjects, and this accounted for higher prevalence of minor psychiatric morbidity in women. This morbidity tended to have a longer mean duration in women, so that the ratio of incidence between the sexes was closer to unity (Cheng, 1989b).

NEUROTIC SYNDROMES

Table 22.1 shows the conditions in which neurotic thinking predominates listed against their ICD-10 designation (World Health Organization, 1992). The term neurosis has been used to encompass a smaller group of conditions in ICD-10 than the generic term 'neurotic disorders, personality disorders and other non-psychotic mental disorders' used in ICD-9 (World Health Organization, 1977). Obviously, the more comprehensive category used in ICD-9 was untidy and imprecise, but it was useful to have a generic term to include neuroses, personality disorders and other related conditions. For comparative purposes, this generic category is listed in Table 22.2.

In considering the descriptive psychopathology of neurotic disorders, one cannot exclude the reactive, psychosocial end of the continuum of affective disorders, because so much of the phenomenology is held in common between

Table 22.1 Disorders manifesting neurotic psychopathology, with their designation in ICD-10

Designation	Disorder
F34.1	Dysthymia
F40	Phobic anxiety disorders
F41	Other anxiety disorders
F42	Obsessive–compulsive disorder
F43	Reaction to severe stress, and adjustment disorders
F44	Dissociative (conversion) disorders
F45	Somatoform disorders
F48	Other neurotic disorders
F48.0	Neurasthenia
F48.1	Depersonalization–derealization syndrome

(From World Health Organization, 1992, with permission.)

Table 22.2 Generic category of neurotic disorders, personality disorders and other non-psychotic mental disorders (300 to 316) in ICD-9

Code	Disorder
300	Neurotic disorders
300.0	Anxiety states
300.1	Hysteria
300.2	Phobic state
300.3	Obsessive–compulsive disorders
300.4	Neurotic depression
300.5	Neurasthenia
300.6	Depersonalization syndrome
300.7	Hypochondriasis
300.8	Other neurotic disorders
301	Personality disorders
302	Sexual deviations and disorders
303	Alcohol dependence syndrome
304	Drug dependence
305	Non-dependent abuse of drugs
306	Physiological malfunctioning arising from mental factors
307	Special symptoms or syndromes not elsewhere classified
308	Acute reaction to stress
309	Adjustment reaction
310	Specific non-psychiatric mental disorders following organic brain damage
311	Depressive disorder, not elsewhere classified
312	Disturbance of conduct, not elsewhere classified
316	Psychic factors associated with diseases classified elsewhere

(From World Health Organization, 1977, with permission.)

those with the neurotic type of depression and those with other neurotic disorders. As has been stated above, comorbidity between depression and other neurotic conditions is actually more frequent with severer degrees of neurotic disorder than a single neurotic syndrome occurring on its own. In one series of patients with severe neurotic disorder, although other neurotic syndromes were also described, neurotic depression invariably occurred (Sims *et al.*, 1993). Even when another neurotic diagnosis is not made, there are often features from other neurotic syndromes found among those suffering from depressive illness arising as a reaction to a stressor.

There are many similarities in the modes of thinking and the motives for carrying out behaviour between neurotic disorders and those conditions listed in ICD-10 as 'behavioural syndromes associated with physiological disturbances and physical factors' (World Health Organization, 1992: 174). These latter include:

- eating disorders such as anorexia nervosa, bulimia nervosa and over-eating and vomiting associated with psychological disturbances

- non-organic sleep disorders such as insomnia, hypersomnia, sleepwalking, sleep terrors and nightmares
- sexual dysfunction not caused by organic disorder or disease, including lack or loss of sexual desire and enjoyment, failure of genital response, orgasmic dysfunction, premature ejaculation, vaginismus, dyspareunia and excessive sexual drive
- mental and behavioural disorders associated with the puerperium, not elsewhere classified
- psychological and behavioural factors associated with disorders or diseases that are classified elsewhere
- abuse of non-dependence-producing substances such as antidepressants, laxatives, analgesics, antacids, vitamins, steroids, hormones or herbal remedies.

A neurotic mechanism in their genesis and in maintenance of symptoms is usual.

Neurotic disorder need not be diagnosed by exclusion alone from other psychiatric conditions. It has a distinctive psychopathology common to different neurotic disorders and not only the specific symptoms described within individual neurotic syndromes. The term *neurosis* is therefore a useful generic category in psychiatric nosology. The distinct neurotic syndromes are not necessarily consistent over time: they may change from one syndrome to another or they may exhibit comorbidity at different times. Mixed and intermediate states between syndromes also occur. There has been much confusion engendered in the classification of these conditions; concentrating wholly on the separate syndromes exacerbates this, while accepting a generic and unitary category with elements of psychopathology held in common is helpful for further understanding.

REFERENCES

American Psychiatric Association (1980) *Diagnostic and Statistical Manual of Mental Disorders,* 3rd edn. Washington: American Psychiatric Association.

Antaki C and Brewin C (1981) *Attributions and Psychological Change.* London: Academic Press.

Bacon F (1597) Of friendship. In *The Essays* (1985). London: Penguin.

Bartholomew RE (1994) Tarantism, dancing mania and demonopathy: the anthro-political aspects of 'mass psychogenic illness'. *Psychological Medicine 24,* 281–306.

Beard GM (1880) *A Practical Treatise on Nervous Exhaustion (Neurasthenia). Its Causes, Symptoms and Sequences.* New York: Wood.

Beck AT (1967) *Depression: Clinical, Experimental and Theoretical Aspects.* New York: Hoeber.

Buglass D, Clarke J, Henderson AS, Kreitman N and Pressley AS (1977) A study of agoraphobic housewives. *Psychological Medicine 7,* 73–86.

Cheng TA (1989a) Psychological stress and minor psychiatric morbidity: a community study in Taiwan. *Journal of Affective Disorders 17,* 137–52.

Cheng TA (1989b) Sex difference in prevalence of minor psychiatric morbidity: a social epidemiological study in Taiwan. *Acta Psychiatrica Scandinavica 80,* 395–407.

Cullen W (1784) *First Lines in the Practice of Physic,* vols I and II. Edinburgh: C. Elliot & T. Cadell.

Day Lewis C (1948) *Poems 1943–1947.* London: Cape.

Dunmore E, Clark DM and Ehlers A (1999) Cognitive factors involved in the onset and maintenance of posttraumatic stress disorder (PTSD) after physical or sexual assault. *Behaviour Research and Therapy 37*, 809–29.

Frank JD (1974) The restoration of morale. *American Journal of Psychiatry 131*, 271–4.

Freud S (1895) On the grounds for detaching a particular syndrome from neurasthenia under the description 'anxiety neurosis'. In *Standard Edition of the Complete Psychological Works of Sigmund Freud*, vol. III, pp. 90–115. London: Hogarth Press.

Gelder MG (1986) Neurosis: another tough old word. *British Medical Journal 292*, 972–3.

Guinness EA (1992) Profile and prevalence of the brain fag syndrome: psychiatric morbidity in school populations in Africa. *British Journal of Psychiatry 160* (suppl. 16), 42–52.

Henderson S, Byrne DG and Duncan-Jones P (1981) *Neurosis and the Social Environment*. Sydney: Academic Press.

Jaspers K (1959) *General Psychopathology*, 7th edn. (transl. Hoenig J and Hamilton MW, 1963). Manchester: Manchester University Press.

Jordern E (1603) *A Briefe Discourse of a Disease Called the Suffocation of the Mother*. London: John Windet.

Kiev A (1972) *Transcultural Psychiatry*. Harmondsworth: Penguin.

Lawrie SM and Pelosi AJ (1994) Chronic fatigue syndrome: prevalence and outcome. *British Medical Journal 308*, 732–3.

Natelson BH (2001) Chronic fatigue syndrome. *Journal of the American Medical Association 285*, 2557–9.

Rawnsley K and Loudon JB (1964) Epidemiology of mental disorder in a closed community. *British Journal of Psychiatry 110*, 830–9.

Rotter JB (1966) Generalized expectations for internal versus external control of reinforcements. *Psychological Monographs 80*, no. 1.

Sims ACP (1975) Factors predictive of outcome in neurosis. *British Journal of Psychiatry 127*, 54–62.

Sims ACP (1983) *Neurosis in Society*. Basingstoke: MacMillan.

Sims ACP (1985) Neurotic illness: conserving a threatened concept. *British Journal of Clinical Pharmacology 19*, 95–155.

Sims ACP (1991) The phenomenology of neurotic disorders. *Psychiatriki 2*: 23–33.

Sims ACP (1992) Neuroses and personality disorders: editorial overview. *Current Opinion in Psychiatry 5*, 187–9.

Sims ACP, Heard DH, Rowe CE, Gill MMP and Maddock V (1993) 'Neurosis' and the personal social environment. The effects of a time-limited course of intensive day care. *British Journal of Psychiatry 162*, 369–74.

Snaith RP and Taylor CM (1985) Irritability: definition, assessment and associated factors. *British Journal of Psychiatry 147*, 127–36.

Sydenham T (1682) Dissertatio epistolaris ad Gulielmum Cole, MD de affectione hysterica. In *The Entire Works of Dr Thomas Sydenham, Newly Made English from the Originals* (transl. Swan J, 1742). London: Cave.

Taylor SJLT and Chave S (1964) *Mental Health and Environment*. London: Longmans.

Times (1994) Plaintiff swoons at mention of S-word. *Times* Friday March 11, p. 15.

Trollope A (1858) *The Three Clerks*. London: Penguin.

Tyrer P (1985) Neurosis divisible? *Lancet i*, 685–8.

Tyrer P (1989) *Classification of Neurosis*. Chichester: John Wiley.

Wilson A, Hickie I, Lloyd A, *et al*. (1994) Longitudinal study of outcome of chronic fatigue syndrome. *British Medical Journal 308*, 756–9.

World Health Organization (1977) *International Statistical Classification of Diseases, Injuries and Causes of Death*, 9th revision. Geneva: World Health Organization.

World Health Organization (1992) *The ICD-10 Classification of Mental and Behavioural Disorders: Clinical Description and Diagnostic Guidelines*. Geneva: World Health Organization.

Section Seven

DIAGNOSIS

Psychopathology and Diagnosis

23

> 'There's glory for you!' 'I don't know what you mean by "glory",' Alice said. 'I meant, there's a nice knock-down argument for you!' 'But "glory" doesn't mean "a nice knock-down argument",' Alice objected. 'When I use a word,' Humpty Dumpty said in a rather scornful tone, 'it means just what I choose it to mean, – neither more nor less.' *Lewis Carroll (1872),* Through the Looking Glass

Diagnosis is much more than a word plucked out of the air and pinned on to a hapless 'patient'. It conveys meaning about the antecedents of the present state, about other conditions that are similar and, most important of all, about what is likely to happen in the future and, therefore, what should be done about it. Diagnosis is a means of communication between doctors; it should encompass a full formulation (see Chapter 2) rather than just a single word used in an idiosyncratic manner.

The importance of making a diagnosis, and the range of diagnoses, is as great in psychiatry as in the rest of medicine; the conceptual differences between different diagnostic categories are actually greater, as *mental disorders* include situational, social, emotional and psychological disturbance as well as physical illness. Understandably, most of the medical illnesses that have been described were based on signs or symptoms; this is true also for psychiatry. There is, therefore, a very close association between the observation and classification of 'symptoms in the mind' (Burton, 1621) and psychiatric diagnosis.

The importance with which diagnosis is regarded in psychiatry has developed alongside the introduction of effective remedies for many conditions. There has been a substantial change in the attitude of psychiatrists since Stengel wrote in 1959 that there was 'almost general dissatisfaction with the state of psychiatric classification, national and international'. Much of the progress made has arisen directly from the more careful application of descriptive psychopathology, for instance Kendell (1975). Schwartz and Wiggins (1987) have shown that in order to make a diagnosis an experienced clinician uses a mechanism of *typification*: 'This more fundamental capacity to recognize various mental disorders arises, not through mastering conceptual definitions, but rather through directly encountering individual patients who manifest these disorders. Through such direct encounters we learn the typical forms of the various mental disorders. We learn what is distinctive to each condition and how to distinguish these conditions from one another'. Thus the detailed examination of psychopathological functions that forms the substance of this text is a prerequisite to this, the first step for clinical diagnosis in psychiatry.

In general medicine, diagnosis is based on the complete clinical process: detailed history taking, examination of the patient and carrying out appropriate special investigations. This is true also for psychiatry. However, because of the limitations of its subject, this book does not deal with physical examination nor with physical (radiological, laboratory) or psychological (psychometric) investigations.

CONCEPTS OF HEALTH AND PSYCHOPATHOLOGY

The late Peter Sedgwick (1981) made the important discovery that 'disease is a human invention ... there are no illnesses or diseases in nature', hence the quotation at the beginning of this chapter. He rightly pointed out that humans describe potato blight as a disease solely because they want to grow potatoes: 'if man wished to cultivate parasites (rather than potatoes) there would be no "blight" but simply the necessary foddering of the parasite crop'. Sedgwick claimed that it was the human social meaning attached to the fracture of a septuagenarian femur that constituted illness or disease.

> " Out of his anthropocentric self-interest, man has chosen to consider as 'illness' or 'diseases' those natural circumstances which precipitate the death (or the failure to function according to certain rules) of a limited number of biological species; man himself, his pets and other cherished livestock, and the plant-varieties he cultivates for gain or pleasure.

Such arguments point us to the fact that medicine is not 'objective, scientific' applied biology but necessarily value-laden. This is true of the disruption of the internal state that 'patients' bring as 'complaints' to the doctor, and true also of those complaints that the doctor regards as 'symptoms'. A less extreme view of the effect of social values on the presentation of illness is the notion of the *sick role* as developed by Talcott Parsons (1951). Whatever the underlying causes of conditions, the role that the subject himself, the patient, chooses to play and the role that is forced on him by those around him because of his illness are highly significant in the way his symptoms manifest.

People differ in the way they perceive, evaluate and act on, or fail to act on, the symptoms they experience. Mechanic (1986) has called this *illness behaviour*. Somatic or psychological symptoms do, of course, frequently occur without any evidence of organic disease. When attempting to describe and classify such symptoms, it is helpful to establish a phenomenological basis; conditions are recognized because of the particular characteristics of the patient's complaints, not because of some presumed theoretical notion of cause. The bizarre lengths that result from the application of a preformed theory of disease aetiology to symptoms, rather than developing from *symptoms* to *theory*, is admirably illustrated in Engelhardt's (1981) essay 'The disease of masturbation'. In the nineteenth century, masturbation was widely believed to produce many signs and symptoms including dyspepsia, constriction of the urethra, epilepsy, blindness, vertigo, loss of hearing, headache, impotence, loss of memory, insanity, cardiac arrhythmia, rickets, leucorrhoea in women, conjunctivitis and generalized weakness, and it was held to be a dangerous disease entity.

Lewis (1953) pointed out that mental illness could be characterized in terms of psychopathology: 'disturbance of part functions as well as general efficiency'.

Part functions refer to the different aspects of psychological experience and behaviour described in previous chapters: memory, perception, forming beliefs and so on. Thus Lewis saw a disturbance in perception, for example hallucination, as a reason for establishing a *case* of mental illness – on psychopathological grounds.

USE OF SYMPTOMS TO FORM DIAGNOSTIC CATEGORIES

The relationship between signs and symptoms in psychiatry was discussed in Chapter 1. Traditionally, symptoms have been divided into those causing suffering and pain (distress) and those causing loss of function (disability). When the only disharmony is between the individual and his society, the disturbance is not regarded as mental illness. For the great majority of mental disorders, diagnostic classification is made according to the profile of symptoms presented. Exceptions to this are (a) when the aetiology is known, for example dementia in human immunodeficiency virus disease; (b) when the structural pathology is known, for example Huntington's disease; and (c) when cause is hypothesized to result from a process without conclusive evidence, for example dissociative fugue. Descriptive psychopathology is almost atheoretical in nature and thus allows the development of a generally descriptive diagnostic terminology.

Symptoms are collected into constellations that commonly occur together to form the *syndromes* of mental illness. It is usual to make a distinction between *illness*, with a definite onset after normal health, and the *lifelong* characteristics of learning disability or personality disorder.

Another fundamental distinction often made by psychiatrists and based ultimately on psychopathology is that between *psychoses* and *neuroses*. Psychoses 'are major mental illness. They are exceedingly hard to define although they are usually said to be characterized by severe symptoms, such as delusions and hallucinations, and by lack of insight' (Gelder *et al.*, 1983); there is loss of contact with reality. It is probable that the everyday use of the concept of psychosis by clinicians is based on the notion of 'unitary psychosis'; the development of this concept has been discussed by Berrios and Beer (1994). Neurosis 'is a psychological reaction to acute or continuous perceived stress, expressed in emotion or behaviour ultimately inappropriate in dealing with that stress' (Sims, 1983: 3); phenomenological characteristics held in common by neurotic patients include disturbances of self-image, of the experience of relationships and, often, bodily symptoms without organic cause (Sims, 1983).

Psychiatric diagnosis is often hierarchical, organic syndromes taking precedence over functional psychoses, these over neuroses and neuroses over situational or adjustment reactions. A patient with schizophrenia and superadded anxiety will usually receive only the diagnosis of schizophrenia. This can be a considerable disadvantage in practice for planning treatment programmes as, for instance, the prognosis of chronic schizophrenia may be determined more by the presence of neurotic symptoms than by the response of schizophrenic symptoms to treatment (Cheadle *et al.*, 1978). Foulds (1976) used this hierarchical approach to establish a system of classification of *personal illness*, with *delusions of disintegration* at the apex, taking priority over intervening levels down to *dysthymic states* as the lowest level.

An example of *categorical* classification is shown in Box 23.1. Various non-categorical methods of classification have also been used. In the *dimensional* approach as advocated by Eysenck (1970), the variations of presentation of mental illness are accounted for on just three dimensions: psychoticism, neuroticism and extroversion/introversion. *Multiaxial* classification codes different sets of information separately.

The present state examination

An example of psychiatric phenomenology applied in nosological research is the development of the Present State Examination (PSE; Wing *et al.*, 1974): 'The Present State Examination (PSE) schedule is a guide to structuring a clinical interview, with the object of assessing the present mental state of adult

Box 23.1 Classification of mental disorders

Psychoses

- Organic disorders:
  acute organic syndrome
  chronic organic syndrome (dementia)
  dysamnestic syndrome
- Schizophrenia:
  schizoaffective disorders
  paranoid states
- Affective disorders:
  mania
  depressive disorder

Neuroses and related disorders

- Neuroses:
  depressive neurosis
  anxiety neurosis
  phobic neurosis
  obsessional neurosis
  hysteria
  depersonalization syndrome
  non-specific and mixed
- Personality disorders
- Adjustment disorder
- Other disorders:
  sexual dysfunction and sexual deviations
  alcohol and drug dependence
  miscellaneous syndromes
  psychological factors associated with medical conditions
- Mental retardation
- Disorders specific to childhood

(After Gelder *et al.*, 1983, with permission of Oxford University Press.)

patients suffering from one of the neuroses or functional psychoses'. It aims to enquire about the patient's condition and subjective state and record this information in terms of symptoms. When there is conflict between clinical and statistical judgements, clinical judgement is allowed to prevail. Symptoms are aggregated into a list of syndromes. The classification of symptoms is carried out on a programme known as 'Catego', which reduces the 500 PSE items to a maximum of six descriptive categories and thence into one descriptive group for the individual patient.

An aim of the PSE has been to determine whether there are clinically recognizable symptoms on which all psychiatrists can agree and label in the same way. Wing *et al.* (1974) pose two questions:

> First, whether certain psychological and behavioural phenomena which have generally been thought by psychiatrists to be symptoms of mental illnesses can be reliably recognized and described, irrespective of the language and culture of the doctor or patient; secondly, whether rules of classification can be specified with such precision that an individual with a given pattern of symptoms will also be allocated to the same clinical grouping.

Thus the PSE starts from a psychopathological standpoint. The interviewer is trained to note the presence or absence of listed symptoms in the glossary. Groups of symptoms are collected together into syndromes by use of computerized Catego class. The end product of the PSE is diagnosis as a research tool based on phenomenology and available for study by other workers in other cultures. An example of the relationship between syndromes and symptoms in the PSE is shown in Figure 23.1.

This example of an excerpt from the PSE involves the terms used for the symptoms of schizophrenia. The *nuclear syndrome* of Wing *et al.* (1974) is composed of Schneider's (1958) first-rank symptoms. The symptoms they listed as comprising this syndrome in the ninth edition of the PSE are *thought intrusion, thought insertion, thought broadcast, thought commentary, thought withdrawal, voices about the patient, delusions of control, delusions of alien penetration* and *primary delusions*. They make the useful point that *thought insertion* is likely to be rated with a false positive if the examiner does not have the symptom in mind but some general approximation to it. *Voices about the patient* implies non-affective verbal hallucinations heard by the subject talking about him in the third person. *Delusions of control* refers, of course, to passivity experiences. *Delusions of alien forces penetrating or controlling* the mind or body is a special form of symptom already listed as belonging to the nuclear syndrome. By *primary delusions*, Wing *et al.* imply *delusional perception* and give the example of a patient undergoing liver biopsy who came to believe, as the needle was inserted, that he had been chosen by God. The emphasis placed here on the PSE is intended because it is such a direct application of descriptive psychopathology to psychiatric diagnosis (see Table 23.1).

French classification

French psychiatric classification in the nineteenth century was firmly based on the observation and coding of symptoms according to Pichot (1984). Pinel stated that 'One must be on one's guard against mixing metaphysical

Syndrome no.	Syndrome name	Symptoms (list II)	
(*a*)	(*b*)	(*c*)	
1 (NS)	*Nuclear syndrome*	55 Thought intrusion	62 Voices about patient
		56 Thought broadcast	71 Delusions of control
		57 Thought commentary	81 Delusions of alien penetration
		58 Thought withdrawal	82 Primary delusions
		0	No symptoms
		1	NS? = partial delusions only
		2	NS+ = 1 symptom
		3	NS+ = 2+ symptoms

Figure 23.1 Excerpt from the Present State Examination. (From Wing *et al.*, 1974, with permission.)

Table 23.1 First-rank symptoms of schizophrenia[a] and symptoms from the present state examination[b]

First-rank symptom	Equivalent symptom from present state examination
Delusional	
Delusional percept	Primary delusion
Auditory hallucinations	
Audible thoughts	Thought echo or commentary
Voices arguing or discussing	Voices about the patient
Voices commenting on the patient's action	Voices about the patient
Thought disorder: passivity of thought	
Thought withdrawal	Thought block or withdrawal
Thought insertion	Thought insertion
Thought broadcasting (diffusion of thought)	Thought broadcast or thought sharing
Passivity experiences: delusion of control	
Passivity of affect ('made' feelings)	Delusions of control
Passivity of impulse ('made' drives)	Delusions of control
Passivity of volition ('made' volitional acts)	Delusions of control
Somatic passivity (influence playing on the body)	Delusions of alien penetration

[a]Schneider (1958).
[b]Wing *et al.* (1974).

discussions, or certain disquisitions of the ideologists, with a science which consists of carefully observed facts' (Pichot 1984), while his pupil, Esquirol, produced a nosology 'based predominantly on the symptoms displayed by the patient at one particular time' (Pichot, 1984). However, later in that century a biological basis for illness became accepted, even in those conditions in which no organic pathology could be demonstrated. This led to an emphasis on the pattern of development to delineate specific diseases.

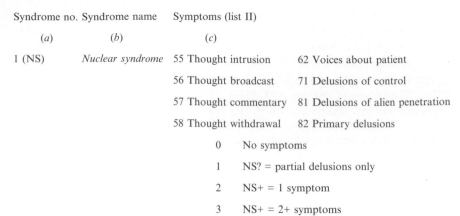

The theory of *degeneration*, a process that could be inherited over several generations, was introduced by Morel; it has been discussed in its historical context by Huertas (1992, 1993). This theory later became the basis for the system of classification devised by Magnan. The subsequent work of Kraepelin, which has so greatly influenced British as well as German psychiatry, and of Bleuler (which although starting in Switzerland was particularly influential in the United States of America) had different effects in France, especially within the classification of what in Britain would be regarded as schizophrenia. Three terms have been used in France: *schizophrenia*, which incorporated that part of Kraepelin's concept of dementia praecox that excluded the other two; *bouffées délirantes*, more or less equivalent to acute delusional states; and *chronic hallucinatory psychosis*, with chronic systematized delusions.

The ICD-10 classification

The ICD-10 Classification of Mental and Behavioural Disorders (World Health Organization, 1992) is now used internationally. There is evidence of its predecessor, ICD-9 (*International Statistical Classification of Diseases Injuries and Causes of Death*, 9th revision; World Health Organization, 1977), in ICD-10, but at the same time many confusing terms have been explained or excluded and the number of codes available in ICD-10 is much larger. ICD-10 can also be used in multiaxial form. The only other psychiatric classification widely used currently is DSM-IV (*Diagnostic and Statistical Manual of Mental Disorders*, 4th edition; American Psychiatric Association, 1994). ICD-10 has been designed for administrative, clinical and research work including large-scale epidemiological studies. One version of ICD-10, *Diagnostic Criteria for Research* (World Health Organization, 1993), has been prepared specifically for this purpose.

The distinction between *neurosis* and *psychosis* has not been made in ICD-10, as the intention in the latter has been to categorize according to major common themes. Most of the neurotic disorders of ICD-9 are still retained in the generic category in ICD-10 'neurotic, stress-related and somatoform disorders' (F40 to F48). The next two generic categories, 'behavioural syndromes associated with physiological disturbances and physical factors' (F50 to F59) and 'disorders of adult personality and behaviour' (F60 to F69), are clearly related, and there is no difficulty in using these three categories together if one wishes to see the common themes and self-experience of neurotic psychopathology. The only major difficulty in this area of neurotic psychopathology is the classification of *depression*.

'Mood (affective) disorders' (F30 to F39) in ICD-10 does not include all disturbances of mood, such as anxiety, irritability and so on, but specifically relates to depression and elation and is therefore close to older concepts of manic–depressive illness. However, the generic category also includes milder types of depression, 'recurrent depressive disorders' and 'persistent mood (affective) disorders'. Some of the conditions previously diagnosed '*neurotic* depression' will be found in one or other of these categories.

ICD-10 recommends that as many diagnoses as necessary should be recorded to give a complete clinical picture (comorbidity), and this will be particularly important for more severe neurotic disorders so that both the relevant neurotic syndrome and the appropriate mood disorder are recorded; for example, in the majority of more severe cases of post-traumatic stress disorder, comorbid depressive episode is also present (Lally and Sims, 1999). ICD-10 has been found to be somewhat cumbersome for mood disorders and does present some difficulties in practice.

As far as delusional syndromes are concerned, ICD-10 has advantages over its predecessors (Sims, 1991). It is somewhat surprising that the term *delusion* is frequently used but never defined. Delusion is referred to in the major categories F0, organic; F1, substance misuse; F2, schizophrenia; and F3, affective disorders. It is a term of exclusion from F4, neurotic syndromes, and it does not play a part in diagnosis in F5 to F9. Accurate classification relies on the diagnostician knowing what is and what is not delusion: because an individual holds a false belief does not necessarily mean he is deluded. The phenomenology of the monodelusional disorders (persistent delusional disorder in ICD-10) requires particular care for diagnosis (Munro, 1991, 1997).

'Disorders with onset specific to childhood' in ICD-10 has proved to be an improvement. However, the classification of mental retardation (F70 to F79) still remains rudimentary; the term *mental retardation* has been used in this book, as it is the usage of ICD-10 (F70 to F79). Currently, in the United Kingdom, the term *learning disability* is favoured, but this term does not make adequate discrimination from other causes of difficulty with learning. The terms *mental subnormality* and *mental handicap* are now obsolete, as are the descriptive words used in earlier editions of the *International Classification*: feeble-minded, moron, imbecile, idiot, oligophrenia. The fashion has been to change the designation every few years in a laudable but not necessarily successful attempt to lessen stigma.

DSM-IV

The *Diagnostic and Statistical Manual of Mental Disorders* (third edition, revised) was replaced by DSM-IV in 1994. DSM-IV and ICD-10 have converged to some extent, and there no longer exist the difficulties in classification and hence clinical understanding that occurred previously. DSM-IV is designed for research use as well as clinical classification and gives diagnostic criteria for each condition listed; these may demand that a certain number of items must be present out of a longer list of items, and there may also be exclusion items. A problem for administrative and epidemiological use is how to classify those cases that just fail to meet diagnostic criteria. It would be of value to world psychiatry if the convergence of these two systems could continue in subsequent revisions so that eventually they merge. It has been shown (Wilson, 1993) that the failure of the biopsychosocial model of American psychiatry in the 1970s to demarcate between the mentally ill and mentally well led to a crisis of confidence in the specialty. At the expense of limiting the scope of psychiatry, the introduction of the successive versions of DSM has legitimized practice on a basis of descriptive psychiatry.

Multiaxial classification

The concept of multiaxial diagnosis is enlisted in DSM-IV and is recommended for parts of ICD-10. This enables different types of clinical information to be evaluated for planning treatment and predicting outcome in each individual. Axis 1 of DSM-IV includes all 'clinical disorders' excluding axis 2, which includes personality disorders and mental retardation. Axis 3 is used for general medical conditions. Axis 4 is for psychosocial and environmental problems, and axis 5 for a global assessment of functioning. Axes 1, 2 and 3 are used in normal clinical practice for evaluating treatment and predicting outcome; axes 4 and 5 are mostly for research use. Child psychiatry now also makes wide use of a five-axis system originally proposed by a World Health Organization working party (Rutter *et al.*, 1975). The axes recommended are as follows.

- Axis 1: clinical psychiatric syndrome.
- Axis 2: specific delays in development.
- Axis 3: intellectual level.
- Axis 4: medical conditions.
- Axis 5: abnormal psychosocial situations.

Clinicians have found this system relatively easy to use, and it allows the systematic recording of the broader range of information required for adequate evaluation in child psychiatry. The obvious disadvantage of multiaxial classifications is, of course, their rather complicated nature, resulting in inaccurate usage when applied to general administrative diagnostic recording.

DIAGNOSTIC CRITERIA FOR SCHIZOPHRENIA

At the present time, diagnosis in psychiatry is increasingly being made on the presence of *diagnostic criteria*, which are often psychopathological entities. This is a considerable improvement on previous ways of making a diagnosis, which often had a closer resemblance to intuition than to the rigorous examination of evidence. One problem with the use of diagnostic criteria is that different authors may use different features as a yardstick. This is well exemplified by the diagnosis of schizophrenia, for which Geddes (1993) has listed seven separate sets of diagnostic criteria. The original descriptions do, of course, give much more explanatory detail, which is necessary for research and clinical use, but they are briefly summarized here purely for the purpose of comparison. The final set of criteria, DSM-IV, is not cited by Geddes.

St Louis criteria (Feighner et al., *1972)*

For a diagnosis of schizophrenia, A to C are required.

A Both of the following are necessary.
- A chronic illness with at least 6 months of symptoms prior to the index evaluation without return to the premorbid level of psychosocial adjustment.
- Absence of a period of depressive or manic symptoms.

B The patient must have at least one of the following.
- Delusions or hallucinations, without perplexity or disorientation.

- Verbal production that makes communication difficult because of a lack of logical or understandable organization.

C At least three of the following manifestations must be present for a diagnosis of 'definite' schizophrenia, and two for a diagnosis of 'probable' schizophrenia:
- single
- poor premorbid social adjustment or work history
- family history of schizophrenia
- absence of alcoholism or drug abuse within 1 year of onset of psychosis
- onset of illness prior to age 40.

Taylor and Abrams (1978)

- At least one of a to c:
  a formal thought disorder
  b at least one first-rank symptom
  c emotional blunting.
- Clear consciousness.
- No diagnosable affective disorder.
- No diagnosable coarse brain disease, no past drug abuse and no medical condition known to cause schizophrenic symptoms.

Research diagnostic criteria (Spitzer et al., 1975)

A to C are required for the episode of illness being considered.

A At least two of the following are required for definite schizophrenia.
- Thought broadcasting, insertion or withdrawal.
- Delusions of control.
- Delusions other than persecutory or jealousy, lasting at least a week.
- Delusions of any type if accompanied by hallucinations of any type for at least a week.
- Auditory hallucinations in which either a voice keeps up a running commentary on the subject's behaviours or thoughts as they occur, or two or more voices converse with each other.
- Non-affective verbal hallucinations spoken to the subject.
- Hallucinations of any type throughout the day for several days or intermittently for at least 1 month.
- Formal thought disorder.
- Catatonic behaviour.

B Illness lasting at least 2 weeks.

C At no time during the active period of illness being considered did the subject meet the criteria for manic or depressive syndrome.

Carpenter's flexible system (Carpenter et al., 1973)

Five or six of the following twelve signs and symptoms were used depending on the threshold:

- audible, broadcast or transmitted thoughts
- nihilistic delusions
- bizarre delusions
- widespread delusions
- unreliable information
- restricted affect
- poor insight
- poor rapport
- incoherent speech
- absence of elation
- depressed facies
- wakening early.

DSM-III (American Psychiatric Association, 1980)

A At least one of the following during a phase of the illness.
- Bizarre delusions.
- Somatic, grandiose, religious, nihilistic or other delusions without persecutory or jealous content.
- Delusions with persecutory or jealous content if accompanied by hallucinations of any type.
- Auditory hallucinations in which either a voice keeps up a running commentary on the individual's behaviour or thoughts, or two or more voices converse with each other.
- Auditory hallucinations.
- Incoherence, marked loosening of association, markedly illogical thinking or marked poverty of content of speech if associated with at least one of the following:
  a blunted, flat or inappropriate affect
  b delusions or hallucinations
  c catatonic or other grossly disorganized behaviour.

B Deterioration from a previous level of functioning in such areas as work, social relations and self-care.

C Duration: continuous signs of the illness for at least 6 months.

D The full depressive or manic syndrome (criteria A and B of major depressive or manic episode), if present, developed after any psychotic symptoms or was brief in duration relative to the duration of the psychotic symptoms in A.

E Onset of prodromal or active phase of the illness before age 45.

F Not due to any organic mental disorder or mental retardation.

DSM-IIIR (American Psychiatric Association, 1987)

A Presence of characteristic psychotic symptoms in the active phase: either 1, 2 or 3 for at least 1 week.
- Two of the following:
  a delusions
  b prominent hallucinations

c incoherence or marked loosening of association
d catatonic behaviour
e flat or grossly inappropriate affect.
- Bizarre delusions.
- Prominent hallucinations of a voice with content having no apparent relation to depression or elation, or a voice keeping up a running commentary on the person's behaviour or thoughts, or two or more voices conversing with each other.

B Functioning in such areas as work, social relations and self-care is markedly below the highest level achieved before onset of the disturbance.
C Schizoaffective disorder and mood disorder with psychotic features have been ruled out.
D Continuous signs of the disturbance for at least 6 months.
E It cannot be established that an organic factor initiated and maintained the disturbance.
F If there is a history of autistic disorder, the additional diagnosis of schizophrenia is made only if prominent delusions or hallucinations are also present.

ICD-10 (World Health Organization, 1992)

The following groups of symptoms have diagnostic importance.

A Thought echo, thought insertion or withdrawal and thought broadcasting.
B Delusions of control, influence or passivity, delusional perception.
C Hallucinatory voices giving a running commentary on the patient's behaviour or discussing the patient among themselves, or other types of hallucinatory voices coming from some part of the body.
D Persistent delusions of other kinds.
E Persistent hallucinations in any modality.
F Breaks or interpolations in the train of thought, resulting in incoherence or irrelevant speech, or neologisms.
G Catatonic behaviour.
H 'Negative' symptoms.
I A significant and consistent change in the overall quality of some aspects of personal behaviour.

DSM-IV (American Psychiatric Association, 1994)

Diagnostic criteria are as follows.

A *Characteristic symptoms*: two (or more) of the following.
- Delusions.
- Hallucinations.
- Disorganized speech (e.g. frequent derailment or incoherence).
- Grossly disorganized or catatonic behaviour.
- Negative symptoms, i.e. affective flattening, alogia or avolition.

B *Social/occupational dysfunction*: for a significant portion of the time since the onset of the disturbance, one or more major areas of functioning such as work, interpersonal relations or self-care are markedly below the level achieved prior to the onset.

C *Duration*: continuous signs of the disturbance persist for at least 6 months.

D *Schizoaffective and mood disorder* excludes schizophrenia.

E *Substance use, general medical condition exclusion*: the disturbance is not due to the direct physiological effects of a substance (e.g. a drug of abuse, a medication) or a general medical condition.

F *Relationship to a pervasive developmental disorder*: if there is a history of autistic disorder or another pervasive developmental disorder, the additional diagnosis of schizophrenia is made only if prominent delusions or hallucinations are also present for at least a month (or less if successfully treated).

Rather than accepting any of these generally similar but, in detail, surprisingly different approaches to the diagnosis of schizophrenia as being absolute or ultimate, it is probably better to combine two or three sets of criteria for satisfactory diagnosis (Kendell, 1982). In an investigation intended to detect whether the incidence of schizophrenia was changing in Edinburgh between 1971 and 1989, Kendell *et al.* (1993) were unable to show a change in the incidence but they did consider that there were changes over that time in the way the condition was diagnosed. McGuffin *et al.* (1991) have designed an operational checklist with a computer program for psychotic illnesses called the OPCRIT system, and this has achieved high inter-rater reliability. There is clearly considerable usefulness in the practical application of diagnostic criteria in psychiatry, but it is important that categories are not so exclusive that a substantial number of patients actually seen in the clinic cannot be classified. In current clinical practice, ICD-10 and DSM-IV are almost universally used, with well-educated clinicians knowing also how to incorporate Schneider's first-rank symptoms.

POSTSCRIPT

Fundamental to psychiatry is the need to understand what the patient is experiencing. Eisenberg (1986) has succinctly summarized the aspirations of the biological school of psychiatry: 'for every twisted thought there is a twisted molecule'. Ironically, if this association were to be achieved it would make the need for expert phenomenological skills more, rather than less, important, as it is likely to remain, from the patient's point of view, more comfortable to have his thoughts than his molecules explored. At the opposite pole of psychiatry, psychodynamics, there is also great value in descriptive psychopathology, unembellished by interpretation, as a starting point for further understanding.

Uses of psychopathology

It has been said of William of Ockham, who so courageously navigated the murky and dangerous waters of medieval philosophy and science, that he was 'an empiricist refusing to stretch knowledge beyond the bounds of ascertainable experience' (Leff, 1958). This is the position of descriptive psychopathology: aiming not to draw conclusions beyond the subjective experience of the patient and its judicious exploration by the interviewer. Every psychiatrist uses phenomenology to some extent, but it is a much more valuable tool if used rigorously.

The four practical applications of descriptive psychopathology, then, are as follows.

- *Communication*. It enables clinicians to speak and write to each other about the problems of their patients in a mutually comprehensible way. This is clearly of value both in clinical practice and for research.
- *Diagnosis*. Psychiatric diagnosis to a considerable extent is based on psychopathology, and this is wholly appropriate, especially until there is more evidence for aetiology and underlying pathology for the different conditions.
- *Therapy*. The method of empathy, that is using phenomenology to explore the patient's subjective experience, is a rational way of establishing a therapeutic relationship. It enables the therapist to understand the subjective experience of his patient and will give the patient confidence in further entrusting the secrets of his internal environment to the therapist.
- *The law*. Descriptive psychopathology is the only reasonable way of determining what is mental illness and what are the differences between mental illnesses, from a forensic point of view. Mutual enlightenment in the area between the law and psychiatry, when there is at present so much misunderstanding, will result from a clearer acknowledgement of the value of psychopathology by lawyers and doctors.

The patient's symptoms, his sufferings, are a logical starting point for the doctor's sympathy, curiosity and therapeutic endeavour. To start elsewhere turns medicine on its head and, ultimately, one arrives in a topsy-turvy world like Samuel Butler's *Erewhon* (1872), where 'illness of any sort is considered ... to be highly criminal and immoral; and that I was liable, for catching cold, to be had up before the Magistrates and imprisoned for a considerable period...' and 'if a man forges a cheque, or sets his home on fire or robs with violence from a person, or does any such things that are criminal in our own country, he is either taken to a hospital and is carefully tended at the public expense, or if he was in good circumstances, he lets it be known to all his friends that he is suffering from a severe fit of immorality ... and they come and visit him with great solicitude...' You may think this is too far-fetched; however, the less pleasant aspects of this certainly appear to have been the situation for some of the dissidents in psychiatric custody in the previous USSR (Bloch and Reddaway, 1977).

The ultimate aim of psychiatry is not, of course, knowledge but to help people to function and feel better; phenomenology is a valuable therapeutic tool. Ideally, it gives the patient, in his doctor, a person who understands what he is feeling but does not try to explain causes in terms of theory, which the patient may find unconvincing. The patient often has a great sense of relief when the doctor, however falteringly, describes back to him the symptoms, or the internal experience, that he, the patient, has found so difficult to describe.

Need for research

Psychopathology was introduced into psychiatry before the current emphasis on quantification, population surveys and experimental method. It is now imperative both for the further development of descriptive psychopathology and, more importantly, for continued progress in psychiatric research that more rigorous research methods be applied. Phenomenology has a place in psychiatric research that has not yet been fully exploited. It forms a logical bridge between research findings emanating from clinical and applied psychology and the increasing knowledge of disordered neuroanatomy – physiology and chemistry – that is resulting from more sophisticated methods of neuroimaging and assay. This is the direction that research in descriptive psychopathology should go.

Investigation of the experience of the individual has to be linked to an understanding of his biology, and it is also important to assess how normal phenomena are distributed within the population. The scientific bases of psychiatry include, as well as biological and behavioural sciences, epidemiology and phenomenology. Recognition of homogeneity includes both the symptoms within an individual patient and the features of an affected population. The PSE has been discussed earlier as a method of quantifying psychopathological information. In previous chapters, mention has also been made of repertory grids as an experimental method for investigating semantic space.

To introduce experimental methods into research in descriptive psychopathology will sometimes involve single-case studies in which variables that have been evaluated phenomenologically are altered. For example, Green and Preston (1981) amplified the quiet whispering of a chronic schizophrenic patient during the time he was auditorily hallucinated. He whispered at the same time as he heard voices, and the content of his vocalization corresponded to what the voices were reported to have said, thus demonstrating the disturbance of boundaries of self found in schizophrenia. This type of investigation has been extended further, and there are several examples in this book, for example in Chapters 10 and 13. There has been a danger in that some other psychological studies, not quoted here, have used phenomenology imprecisely and hence vitiated the significance of their findings.

An interesting development in research based on descriptive psychopathology is the application of particular psychological techniques to specific phenomenological entities. Examples of this are the use of cognitive–behaviour therapy in the treatment of persistent auditory hallucinations (Bentall *et al.*, 1994) and more general application of psychological interventions in schizophrenia (Haddock and Lewis, 1996).

It is important for progress in the treatment of patients and in research that advances in biological aspects of psychiatry are assisted by accurate psychiatric diagnosis based on phenomenology that is both reliable (that is, capable of reproduction by the same interviewer at a different time, or by different interviewers) and quantifiable. Never were the skills of the clinical phenomenologist more necessary or more likely to yield beneficial results both in understanding and in therapy. The introduction of improved neuropsychiatric methods of investigation increases the need for reliable findings from descriptive psychopathology rather than rendering it obsolete. Jaspers (1959) commented, 'phenomenology, though one of the foundation stones of psychopathology, is still very crude'. This is still true, but it is now high time that descriptive psychopathology became more sophisticated.

Phenomenology takes the doctor's art and discipline of observation inside his patient's mind. David Hume (1804) described the absence of physical examination in medicine in his essay 'Of Polygamy and Divorces'. He tells of the physician brought into the Grand Signior's seraglio in Constantinople.

> "He was not a little surprised, in looking along a gallery, to see a great number of naked arms standing out from the sides of the room. He could not imagine what this could mean; till he was told that those arms belonged to bodies, which he must cure, without knowing any more about them than what he could learn from the arms. He was not allowed to ask a question of the patient, or even of her attendants, lest he might find it necessary to enquire concerning circumstances which the delicacy of the seraglio allows not to be revealed. Hence physicians in the east pretend to know all diseases from the pulse, as our quacks in Europe undertake to cure a person merely from seeing his water.

Psychiatry must now come out of the seraglio and use all available information in the service of its patients, including phenomenology, for diagnosis, for understanding and for treatment.

REFERENCES

American Psychiatric Association (1980) *Diagnostic and Statistical Manual of Mental Disorders*, 3rd edn. Washington: American Psychiatric Association.

American Psychiatric Association (1987) *Diagnostic and Statistical Manual of Mental Disorders*, 3rd edn, revised. Washington: American Psychiatric Association.

American Psychiatric Association (1994) *Diagnostic and Statistical Manual of Mental Disorders*, 4th edn. Washington: American Psychiatric Association.

Bentall RP, Haddock G and Slade PD (1994) Cognitive–behaviour therapy for persistent auditory hallucinations: from theory to therapy. *Behaviour Psychotherapy 25*: 51–6.

Berrios GE and Beer D (1994) The notion of unitary psychosis: a conceptual history. *History of Psychiatry V*, 13–36.

Bloch S and Reddaway P (1977) *Russia's Political Hospital*. London: Gollancz.

Burton R (1621) *The Anatomy of Melancholy, What it is. With all the Kinds, Causes, Symptoms, Prognostickes, and Severall Cures of it by Democritus Junior*. Oxford: Cripps.

Butler S (1872) *Erewhon*. London: Cape.

Carpenter WT, Strauss JS and Bartko JJ (1973) Flexible system for the diagnosis of schizophrenia. *Science 182*, 1275–8.

Carroll L (1872) *Through the Looking Glass, and What Alice Found There*. London: Macmillan.

Cheadle AJ, Freeman HL and Korer J (1978) Chronic schizophrenic patients in the community. *British Journal of Psychiatry 132*, 221–7.

Eisenberg (1986) Mindlessness and brainlessness in psychiatry. *British Journal of Psychiatry 148*, 497–508.

Engelhardt HT (1981) The disease of masturbation: values and the concept of disease. In Caplan AL, Engelhardt DT and McCartney JJ (eds) *Concepts of Health and Disease*. Reading: Addison-Wesley.

Eysenck HJ (1970) A dimensional system of psychodiagnosis. In Mahrer AR (ed.) *New Approaches to Personality Classification*, pp. 169–207. New York: Columbia University Press.

Feighner JP, Robins E, Guze SB, Woodruff RA, Winokur G and Munoz R (1972) Diagnostic criteria for use in psychiatric research. *Archives of General Psychiatry 26*, 57–63.

Foulds GA (1976) *The Hierarchical Nature of Personal Illness*. London: Academic Press.

Geddes JR (1993) *A study of the clinical characteristics and outcome of schizophrenic patients with no history of admission to psychiatric hospital*. MD thesis, University of Leeds.

Gelder M, Gath D and Mayou R (1983) *Oxford Textbook of Psychiatry*. Oxford: Oxford University Press.
Green P and Preston M (1981) Reinforcement of vocal correlates of auditory hallucinations using auditory feedback: a case study. *British Journal of Psychiatry 139*, 204–8.
Haddock G and Lewis SW (1996) New psychological treatments in schizophrenia. *Advances in Psychiatric Treatment 2*, 110–6.
Huertas R (1992, 1993) Madness and degeneration. *History of Psychiatry 3*, 391–412; *4*, 1–22, 141–58, 301–20.
Hume D (1804) *Essays and Treaties on Several Subjects*, vol. 1. Edinburgh: Bell & Bradfute.
Jaspers K (1959) *General Psychopathology*, 7th edn (transl. Hoenig J and Hamilton MW, 1963). Manchester: Manchester University Press.
Kendell RE (1975) *The Role of Diagnosis in Psychiatry*. Oxford: Blackwell.
Kendell RE (1982) The choice of diagnostic criteria for biological research. *Archives of General Psychiatry 39*, 1334–9.
Kendell RE, Malcolm DE and Adams W (1993) The problem of detecting changes in the incidence of schizophrenia. *British Journal of Psychiatry 162*, 212–8.
Lally S and Sims A (1999) The treatment of post-traumatic stress disorder: a UK perspective. *Primary Care Psychiatry 5*, 89–100.
Leff G (1958) *Medieval Thoughts*. Harmondsworth: Penguin.
Lewis AJ (1953) Health as a social concept. *British Journal of Sociology 4*, 109–24.
McGuffin P, Farmer A and Harvey I (1991) A polydiagnostic application of operational criteria in studies of psychotic illness. *Archives of General Psychiatry 48*, 764–70.
Mechanic D (1986) The concept of illness behaviour: culture, situation and personal predisposition. *Psychological Medicine 16*, 1–7.
Munro A (1991) Phenomenological aspects of mono-delusional disorders. *British Journal of Psychiatry 159* (suppl. 14), 62–4.
Munro A (1997) Paranoia or delusional disorder. In Bhugra D and Munro A (eds) *Troublesome Disguises: Underdiagnosed Psychiatric Syndromes*. Oxford: Blackwell.
Parsons T (1951) Illness and the role of the physician: a sociological perspective. *American Journal of Orthopsychiatry 21*, 452–60.
Pichot PJ (1984) The French approach to psychiatric classification. *British Journal of Psychiatry 144*, 113–8.
Rutter BM, Shaffer D and Shepherd M (1975) *A Multiaxial Classification of Child Psychiatric Disorders*. Geneva: World Health Organization.
Schneider K (1958) *Clinical Psychopathology*, 5th edn (transl. Hamilton MW, 1959). New York: Grune & Stratton.
Schwartz MA and Wiggins OP (1987) Typifications: the first step for clinical diagnosis in psychiatry. *Journal of Nervous and Mental Disease 175*, 65–77.
Sedgwick P (1981) Illness – mental and otherwise. In Caplan AL, Engelhardt HT and McCartney JJ (eds) *Concepts of Health and Disease: Interdisciplinary Perspectives*, pp. 119–30. Reading: Addison-Wesley.
Sims ACP (1983) *Neurosis in Society*. London: Macmillan.
Sims ACP (1991) Delusional syndromes in ICD-10. *British Journal of Psychiatry 159* (suppl. 14), 46–51.
Spitzer RL, Endicott J and Robins E (1975) *Research Diagnostic Criteria for a Selected Group of Functional Disorders*. New York: Biometrics Research Division, New York State Psychiatric Institute.
Stengel E (1959) Classification of mental disorders. *Bulletin of the World Health Organization 21*, 601–3.
Taylor MA and Abrams R (1978) The prevalence of schizophrenia: a reasssessment using modern criteria. *American Journal of Psychiatry 135*, 945–8.
Wilson M (1993) DSM-III and the transformation of American psychiatry: a history. *American Journal of Psychiatry 150*, 399–410.
Wing JK, Cooper JE and Sartorius N (1974) *The Measurement and Classification of Psychiatric Symptoms: an Instruction Manual for the PSE and Category Program*. Cambridge: Cambridge University Press.
World Health Organization (1977) *International Statistical Classification of Diseases Injuries and Causes of Death*, 9th revision. Geneva: World Health Organization.
World Health Organization (1992) *The ICD-10 Classification of Mental and Behavioural Disorders: Clinical Description and Diagnostic Guidelines*. Geneva: World Health Organization.
World Health Organization (1993) *The ICD-10 Classification of Mental and Behavioural Disorders: Diagnostic Criteria for Research*. Geneva: World Health Organization.

Subject Index

Note: Page numbers in *italics* refer to figures or tables.

A

B

C

D

SUBJECT INDEX

E

F

G

H

I

J

K

L

M

N

SUBJECT INDEX

O

P

Q

R

S

T

U

V

W

Y

Z